I0065878

Clinical Epigenetics: Mechanisms, Diagnosis and Prognosis

Clinical Epigenetics: Mechanisms, Diagnosis and Prognosis

Edited by Elias Foster

hayle
medical

New York

Hayle Medical,
750 Third Avenue, 9th Floor,
New York, NY 10017, USA

Visit us on the World Wide Web at:
www.haylemedical.com

© Hayle Medical, 2019

This book contains information obtained from authentic and highly regarded sources. Copyright for all individual chapters remain with the respective authors as indicated. All chapters are published with permission under the Creative Commons Attribution License or equivalent. A wide variety of references are listed. Permission and sources are indicated; for detailed attributions, please refer to the permissions page and list of contributors. Reasonable efforts have been made to publish reliable data and information, but the authors, editors and publisher cannot assume any responsibility for the validity of all materials or the consequences of their use.

ISBN: 978-1-63241-803-6

Trademark Notice: Registered trademark of products or corporate names are used only for explanation and identification without intent to infringe.

Cataloging-in-Publication Data

Clinical epigenetics : mechanisms, diagnosis and prognosis / edited by Elias Foster.
    p. cm.
Includes bibliographical references and index.
ISBN 978-1-63241-803-6
1. Epigenetics. 2. Epigenesis. 3. Medical genetics. 4. Genetic disorders--Diagnosis.
5. Genetic disorders--Treatment. I. Foster, Elias.
QH450 .C55 2019
616.042--dc23

Table of Contents

Permissions

List of Contributors

Index

Preface

The study of the changes in the heritable phenotypes, which do not involve any alterations in the DNA sequence, is known as epigenetics. It usually denotes the changes which affect gene activity and expression. It can also be used to describe heritable phenotypic changes. The effects on the physiological and cellular phenotypic traits often result from external or environmental factors. Epigenetics has several medical applications. It plays a major role in congenital genetic diseases such as Prader-Willi syndrome and Angelman syndrome. The study of epigenetic modifications to the DNA of cancer cells, which do not involve a change in the nucleotide sequence, is called cancer epigenetics. The ever-growing need of advanced technology is the reason that has fueled the research in the field of clinical epigenetics in recent times. The objective of this book is to give a general view of the different areas of clinical epigenetics and their applications. As this field is emerging at a rapid pace, the contents of this book will help the readers understand the modern concepts and applications of the subject.

Significant researches are present in this book. Intensive efforts have been employed by authors to make this book an outstanding discourse. This book contains the enlightening chapters which have been written on the basis of significant researches done by the experts.

Finally, I would also like to thank all the members involved in this book for being a team and meeting all the deadlines for the submission of their respective works. I would also like to thank my friends and family for being supportive in my efforts.

Editor

Urine cell-based DNA methylation classifier for monitoring bladder cancer

Antoine G. van der Heijden[1†], Lourdes Mengual[2,6*†] (iD), Mercedes Ingelmo-Torres[2], Juan J. Lozano[3],
Cindy C. M. van Rijt-van de Westerlo[1], Montserrat Baixauli[2], Bogdan Geavlete[4], Cristian Moldoveanud[4],
Cosmin Ene[4], Colin P. Dinney[5], Bogdan Czerniak[5], Jack A. Schalken[1], Lambertus A. L. M. Kiemeney[1], Maria J. Ribal[2],
J. Alfred Witjes[1] and Antonio Alcaraz[2]

Abstract

Background: Current standard methods used to detect and monitor bladder cancer (BC) are invasive or have low sensitivity. This study aimed to develop a urine methylation biomarker classifier for BC monitoring and validate this classifier in patients in follow-up for bladder cancer (PFBC).

Methods: Voided urine samples ($N = 725$) from BC patients, controls, and PFBC were prospectively collected in four centers. Finally, 626 urine samples were available for analysis. DNA was extracted from the urinary cells and bisulfite modificated, and methylation status was analyzed using pyrosequencing. Cytology was available from a subset of patients ($N = 399$). In the discovery phase, seven selected genes from the literature (*CDH13, CFTR, NID2, SALL3, TMEFF2, TWIST1,* and *VIM2*) were studied in 111 BC and 57 control samples. This training set was used to develop a gene classifier by logistic regression and was validated in 458 PFBC samples (173 with recurrence).

Results: A three-gene methylation classifier containing *CFTR, SALL3,* and *TWIST1* was developed in the training set (AUC 0.874). The classifier achieved an AUC of 0.741 in the validation series. Cytology results were available for 308 samples from the validation set. Cytology achieved AUC 0.696 whereas the classifier in this subset of patients reached an AUC 0.768. Combining the methylation classifier with cytology results achieved an AUC 0.86 in the validation set, with a sensitivity of 96%, a specificity of 40%, and a positive and negative predictive value of 56 and 92%, respectively.

Conclusions: The combination of the three-gene methylation classifier and cytology results has high sensitivity and high negative predictive value in a real clinical scenario (PFBC). The proposed classifier is a useful test for predicting BC recurrence and decrease the number of cystoscopies in the follow-up of BC patients. If only patients with a positive combined classifier result would be cystoscopied, 36% of all cystoscopies can be prevented.

Keywords: Cytology, Biomarkers, Bladder cancer, DNA methylation, Non-invasive diagnosis, Urine

Background

Seventy to 80% of patients with bladder cancer (BC) present with non-muscle-invasive tumors, either confined to the mucosa [stage Ta and carcinoma in situ (CIS)] or submucosa (stage T1). Based on clinical and pathological characteristics, non-muscle-invasive bladder cancer (NMIBC) patients can be classified into three different prognostic groups [1]. A minority of patients (20–30%) have low-risk tumors with a recurrence rate of 20–30%, without progression. The second and also the largest group, the intermediate-risk group, consists of patients who frequently develop a non-muscle-invasive recurrence (40–60%) but seldom progress to muscle-invasive disease. Finally, a small group of patients has a relatively aggressive NMIBC at presentation. The 5-year recurrence rate in this group is as high as 68% despite maximum intravesical treatment.

---

* Correspondence: LMENGUAL@clinic.cat
†Antoine G. van der Heijden and Lourdes Mengual contributed equally to this work.
[2]Laboratory and Department of Urology, Hospital Clinic of Barcelona, IDIBAPS, University of Barcelona, Barcelona, Spain
[6]Hospital Clínic de Barcelona, Centre de Recerca Biomèdica CELLEX, office B22, C/Casanova, 143, 08036 Barcelona, Spain
Full list of author information is available at the end of the article

Furthermore, up to 34% of these high-risk patients will develop muscle-invasive bladder cancer (MIBC) [2]. For this reason, an intensive follow-up schedule is mandatory in patients with intermediate- or high-risk NMIBC.

The follow-up schedule consists of urethrocystoscopy and urine cytology. Depending on the patient's risk profile, the European Association of Urology guidelines recommend up to 15 urethrocystoscopies during the first 5 years of follow-up [3].

Urethrocystoscopy is considered the gold standard, but is invasive, expensive, and moreover misses up to 15% of the papillary and up to 30% of the flat recurrences [4, 5]. Urine cytology, on the other hand, has a high specificity (SP) but lacks sensitivity (SN) especially in low-risk tumors [6]. Additionally, the interobserver and intraobserver reproducibility of cytology is poor [7]. Recently, several non-invasive methods, NMP-22, bladder tumor antigen, and UroVysion FISH, have shown to help increase the sensitivity of urine cytology. However, due to limited specificity or sensitivity, the markers proposed to date have not been widely adopted in daily clinical practice. Therefore, there is a clear clinical need to find reliable markers to monitor the recurrence in NMIBC [8].

DNA methylation has been recognized to be important in developmental biology and cancer etiology in general [9]. DNA methylation occurs principally at CpG dinucleotides. These CpG dinucleotides are distributed throughout the genome, and the majority is normally methylated. Some regions in the genome have a high CpG density and are called CpG islands. Hypermethylation of normally unmethylated CpG islands in the promoter regions of tumor suppressor genes represses its transcription in human tumors [9, 10]. Therefore, aberrant DNA methylation is a potential biomarker for diagnosis, prognosis, and monitoring of disease after therapy [11]. Recently, it was shown that the combination of *SOX1*, *IRAK3*, and *L1-MET* provides better resolution than cytology and cystoscopy in the detection of early recurrence [12]. The objective of the present study is to investigate whether a set of methylation markers can lead to the development of a voided urine test that predicts tumor presence and may be used to stratify BC patients according to their risk of recurrence, thus allowing the reduction of the number of cystoscopies in the follow-up of BC.

Methods
Patients and clinical samples
After Institutional Review Board approval and obtaining patients' informed consents, we prospectively collected freshly voided urine samples from BC patients, controls, and patients in follow-up for bladder cancer (PFBC) at four different centers [Hospital Clínic of Barcelona (Spain); Radboud University Medical Center in Nijmegen (The Netherlands); St. John Emergency Hospital, Bucharest (Romania); MD Anderson Cancer Center, Houston, Texas, (USA)], from October 2010 to February 2012. Participating centers were asked to collect and prepare the cell pellet by urine centrifugation and freeze them for a final processing at the Hospital Clinic of Barcelona or Radboud University Medical Center, Nijmegen. We took a two-stage approach with a discovery phase (or training set) and a validation phase (or testing set) (Additional file 1: Figure S1). In the discovery phase, the inclusion criteria for the cases were patients of both sexes, 18 years of age or older, and patients with histopathological confirmation of BC at any grade or stage. Without being mandatory, we recommended patients to have cytology at cystoscopy or during the period between cystoscopy and surgery. Patients with a prior endovesical chemotherapeutic or immunotherapeutic treatment could be included. The exclusion criteria were the absence of histological confirmation of BC and patients with other urological malignancies (prostate, kidney, urinary tract tumors). The inclusion criteria for the controls were patients of both sexes, 18 years of age or older, and with non-malignant urologic pathology (infection, lithiasis, urinary incontinence, BPH) or non-urologic pathology. The exclusion criterion for controls was a histological confirmation of any urological malignancy.

The validation phase was designed as a cross-sectional study including PFBC, i.e., the indicated population for the test in daily clinical practice. For efficiency reasons, we oversampled patients with a recurrence because we focused on sensitivity instead of specificity (see also the results in the "Reducing the number of follow-up cystoscopies by using the three-gene methylation/cytology combined classifier" section). PFBC with a prior endovesical chemotherapeutic or immunotherapeutic treatment could be included. Without being mandatory, we recommended PFBC to have cytology at cystoscopy. The exclusion criterion was a histological confirmation of any other urological malignancy.

A total number of 725 voided urine samples were prospectively collected by the four participating institutions. From the total number of urines collected, 99 (13%) were excluded from the study because of technical problems during the sample collection, storage, or analysis. Finally, 626 urines were used: 111 from BC patients and 57 from controls for the discovery phase and 458 from PFBC (of whom 173 had a recurrence) for the validation phase (Tables 1 and 2). The grade and stage of the tumors were determined according to WHO 2004 criteria and TNM 2002 classification, respectively [13, 14].

Tumors were classified according to their risk of recurrence and progression into three categories: high-risk

Table 1 Clinicopathological and demographic characteristics of the study population classified by the study phase

	Discovery phase	Validation phase
	Training set	Testing set
	N bladder cancer (%)	N R-PFBC (%)
Gender		
Male	86 (77)	135 (78)
Female	25 (23)	38 (22)
Age		
Mean	72	68
Range	39–98	26–99
Stage and grade		
Tis	7 (6)	13 (8)
Ta LG	26 (23)	61 (35)
Ta HG	11 (10)	20 12)
T1 LG	20 (18)	35 (20)
T1 HG	22 (20)	44 (25)
> T2 LG	1 (1)	–
> T2 HG	24 (22)	–
Subtotals	111	173
	N control (%)	
Gender		
Male	29 (51)	–
Female	28 (49)	–
Age		
Mean	60	–
Range	22–82	–
Urinary condition		
BPH	11 (19)	–
Urolithiasis	13 (23)	–
Incontinence	2 (4)	–
Benign bladder disease	1 (2)	–
Urinary tract infections	12 (21)	–
Non-urological diseases	18 (32)	–
Subtotals	57	–
		N NR-PFBC (%)
Gender		
Male	–	217 (76)
Female	–	68 (24)
Age		
Mean	–	69
Range	–	26–92
Stage and grade previous TURBT		
Tis	–	21 (7)
Ta LG	–	100 (35)
Ta HG	–	53 (19)

Table 1 Clinicopathological and demographic characteristics of the study population classified by the study phase *(Continued)*

	Discovery phase	Validation phase
	Training set	Testing set
T1 LG	–	22 (8)
T1 HG	–	82 (29)
T2 HG	–	3 (1)
Tx LG	–	2 (1)
Tx HG	–	2 (1)
Subtotals	–	285
Total	168	458

LG low-grade, *HG* high-grade, *TURBT* transurethral resection bladder tumor, *BPH* benign prostate hyperplasia, *CIS/Tis* carcinoma in situ, *BC* bladder cancer, *R-PFBC* recurrent patients in follow-up for bladder cancer, *NR-PFBC* non-recurrent patients in follow-up for bladder cancer

(HR) NMIBC (any of the following: T1, HG/G3 tumors, or CIS), non-high-risk (nHR) NMIBC (all the other cases of NMIBC), and muscle-invasive bladder cancer (MIBC) (T2–4). None of the included patients had an upper urinary tract tumor.

Urine sample processing

Urine samples were collected before cystoscopy, the day before the transurethral resection of the bladder tumor (TURBT), or the day before cystectomy. From all patients and controls, only one single sample was included.

For urine cytology

Urine cytology was performed according to Papanicolaou staining and evaluated by expert pathologists in each center blinded to the patient's clinical history. The results were considered as positive or negative. No central cytology review was performed.

For methylation studies

Voided urine samples (50 to 100 ml) were collected in sterile containers containing 4 ml of 0.5 M EDTA, pH 8.0. Urines were immediately stored at 4 °C and processed within the next 24 h. The samples were centrifuged at $1000 \times g$ for 10 min, at 4 °C. The cell pellets were frozen at – 80 °C.

DNA isolation, bisulfite treatment, and PCR

DNAs from the urinary cell pellets were extracted using QIAamp DNA Mini Kit (Qiagen) according to the manufacturer's instructions and quantified with a Nano-Drop1000 (NanoDrop Technologies, Wilmington, DE, USA). DNA extraction was performed in each center except for Bucharest, whose cell pellets were sent in dry ice to the Radboud University Medical Center, Nijmegen (The Netherlands) for DNA extraction.

One microgram of genomic DNA was used for the bisulfite modification using EpiTect Bisulfite kit (Qiagen,

Table 2 Clinicopathological and demographic characteristics of the study population classified by the participating center

		Hospital Clinic Barcelona	Radboud University Medical Center, Nijmegen	Saint John Emergency Clinical Hospital Bucharest	MD Anderson Cancer Center Houston	Total
Discovery phase	Bladder cancer urine samples					
	Stage					
	Tis	5	–	1	1	7
	Ta	14	5	5	13	37
	T1	19	2	21	–	42
	> T2	9	–	16	–	25
	Grade					
	LG	20	2	17	8	47
	HG	27	5	26	6	64
	Subtotal	47	7	43	14	111
	Control urine samples					
	BPH	8	3	–	–	11
	Urolithiasis	13	–	–	–	13
	Incontinence	1	1	–	–	2
	Benign bladder disease	4	5	1	–	10
	Urinary tract infection	1	8	4	–	13
	Non-urological diseases	6	–	–	2	8
	Subtotal	33	17	5	2	57
Validation phase	R-PFBC URINE SAMPLES					
	Stage					
	Tis	2	1	8	2	13
	Ta	13	15	47	6	81
	T1	4	2	55	18	79
	Grade					
	LG	14	8	74	–	96
	HG	5	10	36	26	77
	Subtotal	19	18	110	26	173
	NR-PFBC urine samples					
	Stage previous TURBT					
	Tis	5	6	6	4	21
	Ta	32	56	36	26	150
	Ta + CIS	1	–	–	2	3
	T1	36	16	25	19	96
	T1 + CIS	5	–	–	3	8
	T2	3	–	–	–	3
	Tx	4	–	–	–	4
	Grade previous TURBT					
	LG	34	35	38	19	126
	HG	52	43	29	35	159
	Subtotal	86	78	67	54	285
	TOTAL	185	120	225	96	626

LG low-grade, *HG* high-grade, *TURBT* transurethral resection bladder tumor, *BPH* benign prostate hyperplasia, *CIS/Tis* carcinoma in situ, *BC* bladder cancer, *R-PFBC* recurrent patients in follow-up for bladder cancer, *NR-PFBC* non-recurrent patients in follow-up for bladder cancer.

Inc.) following the manufacturer's instructions. The modified DNA was eluted with 20 μl Tris-HCL (1 mM, pH 8.0) and stored at − 80 °C before further processing. Bisulfite modifications were performed in Hospital Clinic of Barcelona, Spain (training set), and in Radboud University Medical Center, Nijmegen, The Netherlands (testing set).

A total of seven DNA methylation markers, i.e., *CDH13*, *CFTR*, *NID2*, *SALL3*, *TMEFF2*, *TWIST1*, and *VIM2*, were selected from four recently published BC studies [15–18]. The sequences of the primers used to amplify the regions of interest of these genes and the PCR conditions are shown in Additional file 2: Table S1. PCR primers were designed using the PyroMark Assay Design software v2.0 (Qiagen). PCR was performed in a volume of 25 μl with 2 μl of converted genomic DNA, 0.6 U Ampli Taq Gold 360 DNA polymerase (Thermofisher), 0.8 μl of a mix of Primer-F and biotinylated Primer-R at 10 μM, 2 μl MgCl$_2$ 25 mM, and 0.5 μl dNTPs 10 mM. Amplification was performed according to the following thermocycling conditions: denaturation at 95 °C for 10 min, followed by 45 cycles of 95 °C for 30 s, the optimal Tm for 30 s, and 72 °C for 1 min; and a final extension at 72 °C for 7 min. The formation of PCR products with accurate size was confirmed by resolving PCR samples (1 μl) by 2% agarose gel electrophoresis, with visualization by ethidium bromide staining.

Pyrosequencing for quantitative methylation
Biotin-labeled single-stranded amplicons were isolated from 20 μl of the PCR product according to the protocol using the Pyromark Q96 Work Station and pyrosequenced with 0.3 μM sequence primer using PSQ96MD System (Biotage AB). Additional file 2: Table S1 shows the sequences of the primer sets used for bisulfite sequencing. The percent methylation for each of the CpGs was calculated using PyroQ CpG Software (Qiagen). The differences in the percentage of methylation were calculated between BC vs. control and recurrent vs. non-recurrent PFBC (R-PFBC and NR-PFBC, respectively) samples. A high correlation in the methylation percentages of the CpG dinucleotides in the same island was observed (Additional files 3 and 4: Figures S2 and S3). For this reason, hypermethylation was analyzed in all genes at the first CpG dinucleotide present (Additional file 5: Table S2).

Data analysis
Univariable and multivariable logistic regression analyses were used to examine the associations between BC and DNA methylation status of urinary sediments. A forward stepwise logistic regression was performed to determine the best classifier between BC and control samples. The inclusion criterion was p value of < 0.1. Risk probability of presenting BC was calculated in the training set. We established cutoff point value (≥ 0.464) allowing 15% false negatives in the tumor group (SN = 85%). In the subset of samples in which cytology results were available, the cutoff point value that yielded 85% SN in the training set was 0.688, and in the combined model (methylation test + cytology results), it was 0.617. If the predicted probability value derived from each classifier in each of the samples was higher than the cutoff point value, the samples were classified for each of the classifiers as tumor sample. The performance of the models was evaluated in a testing set by means of AUROC using pROC R-package [19]. Student's t test was used to evaluate statistical differences in DNA methylation. Statistical significance was established at p value of 0.05. R-software and SPSS v23.0 were used for calculations.

Results
Training set
DNA methylation of all seven selected genes was significantly increased in urine sediments from BC patients compared to controls (Fig. 1). To determine the combination of markers capable of detecting BC in urine sediments with the highest accuracy, we built a model of multiple markers by logistic regression. The best possible biomarker combination based on AUC was provided by the combination of *CFTR*, *SALL3*, and *TWIST1*. This three-gene methylation classifier achieved an AUC = 0.874 (Fig. 2a); at a fixed overall SN of 85%, the classifier provides a SP of 68%. Moreover, the SN of the three-gene methylation classifier increases through the BC risk groups and grading (Table 3).

Testing set
To examine whether the three-gene methylation BC diagnostic classifier was able to identify recurrences in a clinical setting, the classifier was validated in an independent multicenter international series of 458 urine sediments from patients in follow-up for bladder cancer (PFBC), of whom 173 had a recurrence. Recurrent PFBC (R-PFBC; N = 173) displays higher percentages of DNA methylation compared with non-recurrent PFBC (NR-PFBC; N = 285) (Fig. 3). SN of the three-gene methylation BC classifier increased in the validation series (SN = 90%), while SP drops (SP = 31%), as evidenced by the ROC curves and AUC value (AUC = 0.741) (Table 3 and Fig. 2a). Figure 4a depicts the risk probabilities derived from the three-gene methylation classifier in R-PFBC and NR-PFBC.

Comparison of test performance with urine cytology
A total of 399 urine cytologies (91 from the training and 308 from the testing set) were performed. In both

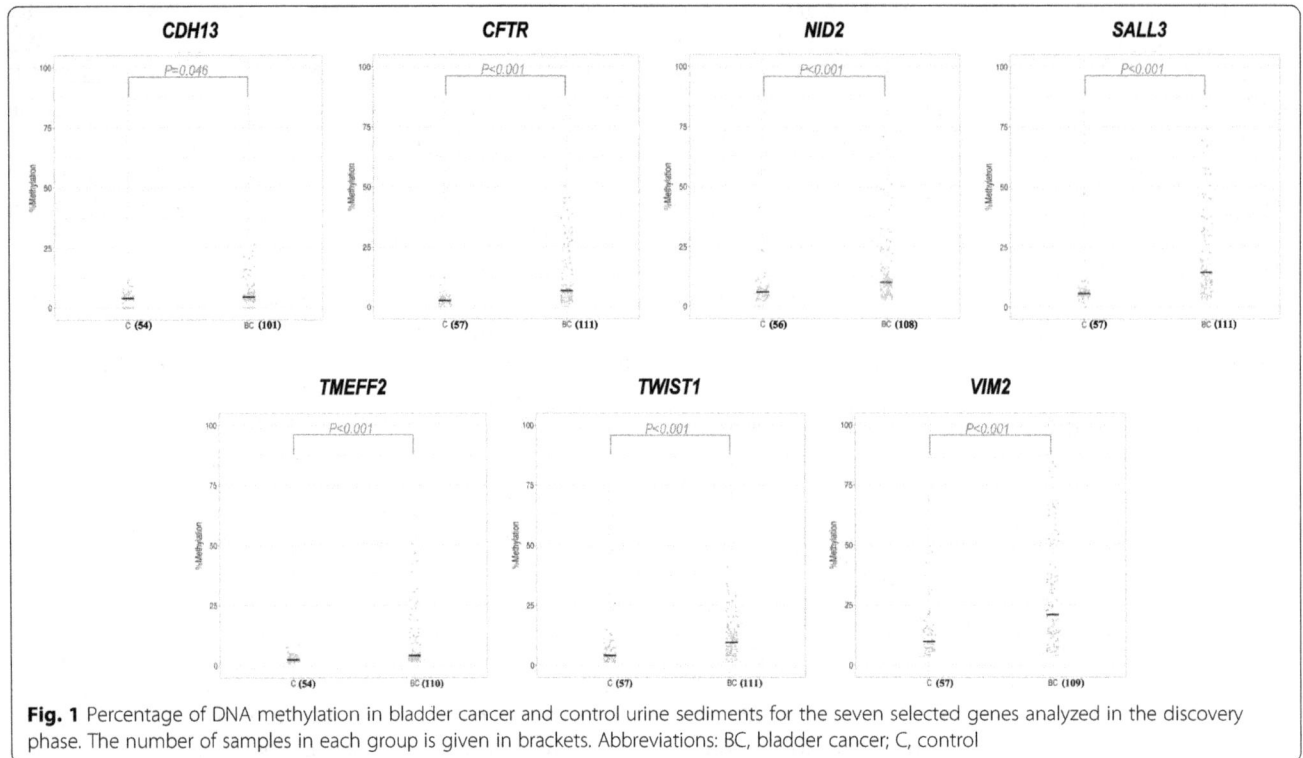

Fig. 1 Percentage of DNA methylation in bladder cancer and control urine sediments for the seven selected genes analyzed in the discovery phase. The number of samples in each group is given in brackets. Abbreviations: BC, bladder cancer; C, control

training and testing set, SN of the three-gene methylation classifier (86 and 93%, respectively) was higher than that of the urine cytology (54 and 46%, respectively) in this subset of samples (Additional files 6 and 7: Table S3 and Figure S4). In the testing set, this means that 55% of the recurrences (68 out of 124) were detected by the three-gene classifier but were missed by urine cytology. On the other hand, 12 recurrences were missed by the three-gene classifier of which half was detected by cytology (Additional file 8: Figure S5). Negative predictive value (NPV) is also higher for the three-gene methylation classifier than that of the urine cytology in training (40 and 29%, respectively) and testing set (82 and 69%, respectively). Contrary, positive predictive value (PPV) is higher for the urine cytology than for the methylation classifier in training (98 and 89%, respectively) and testing set (85 and 50%, respectively). Cytology had a SP of 93 and 94% while the three-gene methylation classifier achieved a SP, in this subset of samples, of 47 and 27%, in the training and testing set, respectively. In the testing set, 120 NR-PFBC samples were positive by the three-gene

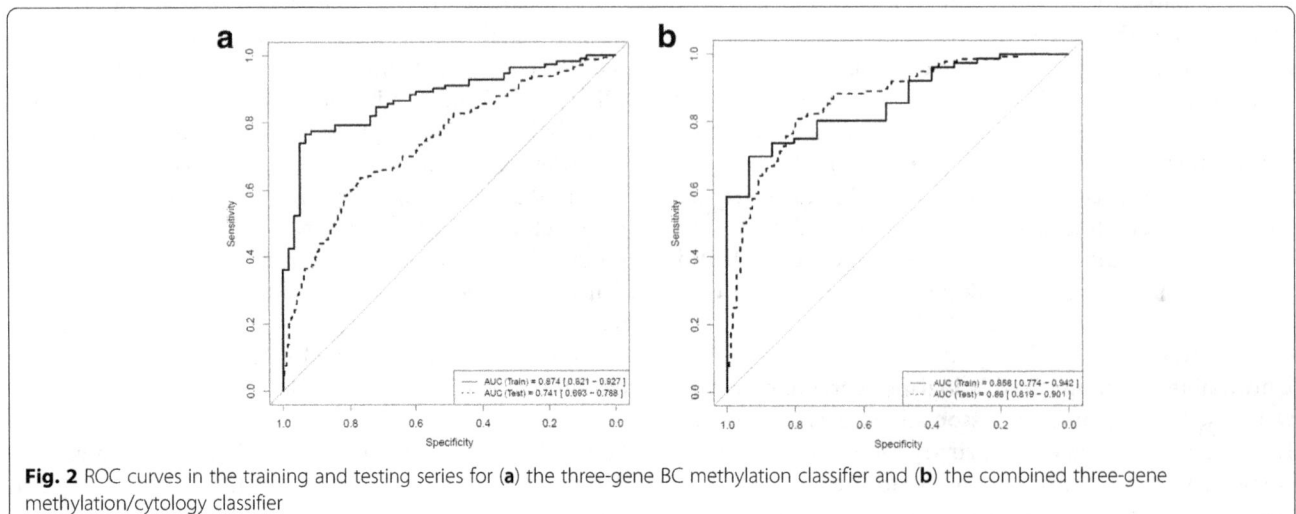

Fig. 2 ROC curves in the training and testing series for (**a**) the three-gene BC methylation classifier and (**b**) the combined three-gene methylation/cytology classifier

Table 3 Diagnostic performance of the three-gene methylation classifier in the training and testing set of samples (at fixed sensitivity of 85% in the training set)

	Training set	Testing set
Overall		
N samples	111 BC/57 C	173 R-PFBC/285 NR-PFBC
AUC	0.874	0.741
SN (%)	84.68	89.6
SP (%)	68.42	30.53
PPV (%)	83.93	43.91
NPV (%)	69.64	82.86
Non-high-risk NMIBC		
N samples	26 BC/57 C	61 R-PFBC/285 NR-PFBC
SN (%)	73.08	88.52
SP (%)	68.42	30.53
PPV (%)	51.35	21.43
NPV (%)	84.78	92.55
High-risk NMIBC		
N samples	60 BC/57 C	112 R-PFBC/285 NR-PFBC
SN (%)	86.67	90.18
SP (%)	68.42	30.53
PPV (%)	74.29	33.78
NPV (%)	82.98	88.78
MIBC		
N samples	25 BC/57C	–
SN (%)	92	–
SP (%)	68.42	–
PPV (%)	56.1	–
NPV (%)	95.12	–
Low-grade		
N samples	47 BC/57 C	96 R-PFBC/285 NR-PFBC
SN (%)	76.6	90.62
SP (%)	68.42	30.53
PPV (%)	66.67	30.53
NPV (%)	78	90.62
High grade		
N samples	64 BC/57 C	77 R-PFBC/285 NR-PFBC
SN (%)	90.62	88.31
SP (%)	68.42	30.53
PPV (%)	76.32	25.56
NPV (%)	86.67	90.62

LG low-grade, *HG* high-grade, *AUC* area under the curve, *MIBC* muscle-invasive bladder cancer, *NMIBC* non-muscle invasive bladder cancer, *NPV* negative predictive value, *PPV* positive predictive value, *SN* sensitivity, *SP* specificity, *BC* bladder cancer, *C* control, *R-PFBC* recurrent patients in follow-up for bladder cancer, *NR-PFBC* non-recurrent patients in follow-up for bladder cancer.

methylation classifier. Nine of them also had positive urine cytology (Additional file 8: Figure S5). After 1 year, two NR-PFBC with a positive test (who had a negative cytology) had a tumor recurrence.

Combination of the three-gene methylation classifier with urine cytology

Combining the three-gene methylation classifier and urine cytology results showed an improved diagnostic performance in the training (AUC 0.858) and as well as in the testing set (AUC 0.86) (Fig. 2b). A SN of 96% and a NPV of 92% are achieved in the testing set. Of note, in HG tumors, a 100% SN and NPV are achieved (Additional file 6: Table S3). The risk probabilities derived from the combined classifier in R-PFBC and NR-PFBC are shown in Fig. 4b.

Reducing the number of follow-up cystoscopies by using the three-gene methylation/cytology combined classifier

In our study, we oversampled patients with BC. We therefore cannot directly calculate predictive values from the test results. In the hospitals participating in the study, recurrence is detected in approximately 10% of all follow-up cystoscopies performed (90% of patients previously diagnosed with NMIBC are without recurrence at the time of follow-up cystoscopy). In order to calculate the predictive values that reflect values in real clinical practice, we assumed the distribution of recurrent vs. non-recurrent to be 10 vs. 90%. For this, we multiplied the NR-PFBC samples by 7. Using the SN and SP that we found in the study, the PPV and NPV in the validation phase become 15 and 99%, respectively. If patients with a negative classifier will not undergo a cystoscopy, this means that more than a third (~ 36%) of all cystoscopies can be prevented at the cost of 4% of recurrences remaining undiagnosed which all were LG tumors.

Discussion

In the present study, a set of DNA methylation markers to predict the presence of bladder cancer (BC) in urine samples has been selected. The best possible marker combination to discriminate BC from controls was the combination *CFTR*, *SALL3*, and *TWIST1*. We confirmed that these genes (and specifically CpG dinucleotides analyzed here) are hypermethylated in the bladder cancer tissue using methylation data from the TCGA Research Network [20] (Additional file 9: Figure S6). This supports their use as diagnostic markers in urine samples. In the training set, the three-gene methylation classifier achieved an AUC 0.874 while in the testing set, an AUC 0.741 was achieved to discriminate recurrent from non-recurrent patients in follow-up for bladder cancer (PFBC). These results improved significantly in

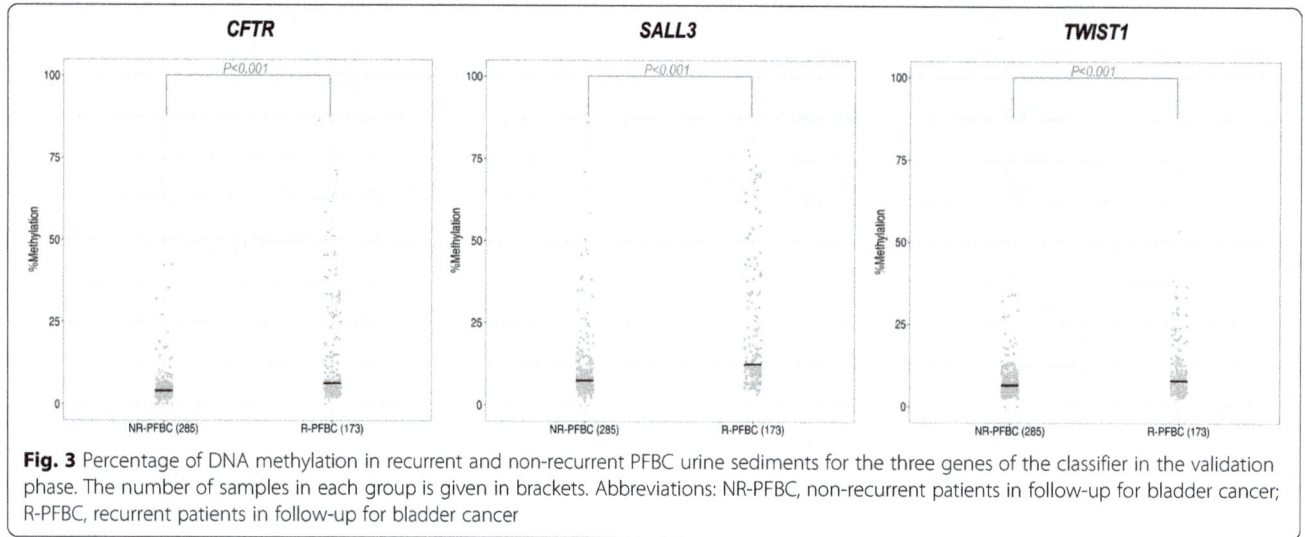

Fig. 3 Percentage of DNA methylation in recurrent and non-recurrent PFBC urine sediments for the three genes of the classifier in the validation phase. The number of samples in each group is given in brackets. Abbreviations: NR-PFBC, non-recurrent patients in follow-up for bladder cancer; R-PFBC, recurrent patients in follow-up for bladder cancer

the testing set when cytology results were included in the analysis (AUC 0.86).

TWIST1 hypermethylation in BC was first described by Renard and co-workers [16]. In a case-control study (*n* = 145 cases/321 controls), they detected *TWIST1* and *NID2* hypermethylation in urine sediments of BC patients using methylation-specific PCR. This two-gene panel achieved a SN of 90%, SP of 93%, PPV of 86%, and NPV of 95%. Nevertheless, the group of Fantony published conflicting results. They found only a SN of 67% and SP of 69% for this two-gene urine panel

[21]. However, the results were significantly better in the subgroup of active smokers. Unfortunately, we did not collect information about tobacco smoking, and therefore, we cannot perform a subset analysis for smoking behavior.

Yu and co-workers previously found in a case-control study that *CFTR* and *SALL3*, out of 59 genes that were screened, were the most frequently methylated genes to predict the presence of BC in urine [15]. However, in this study, no PFBC were included. In daily clinical practice, this group is especially of interest. It is not very

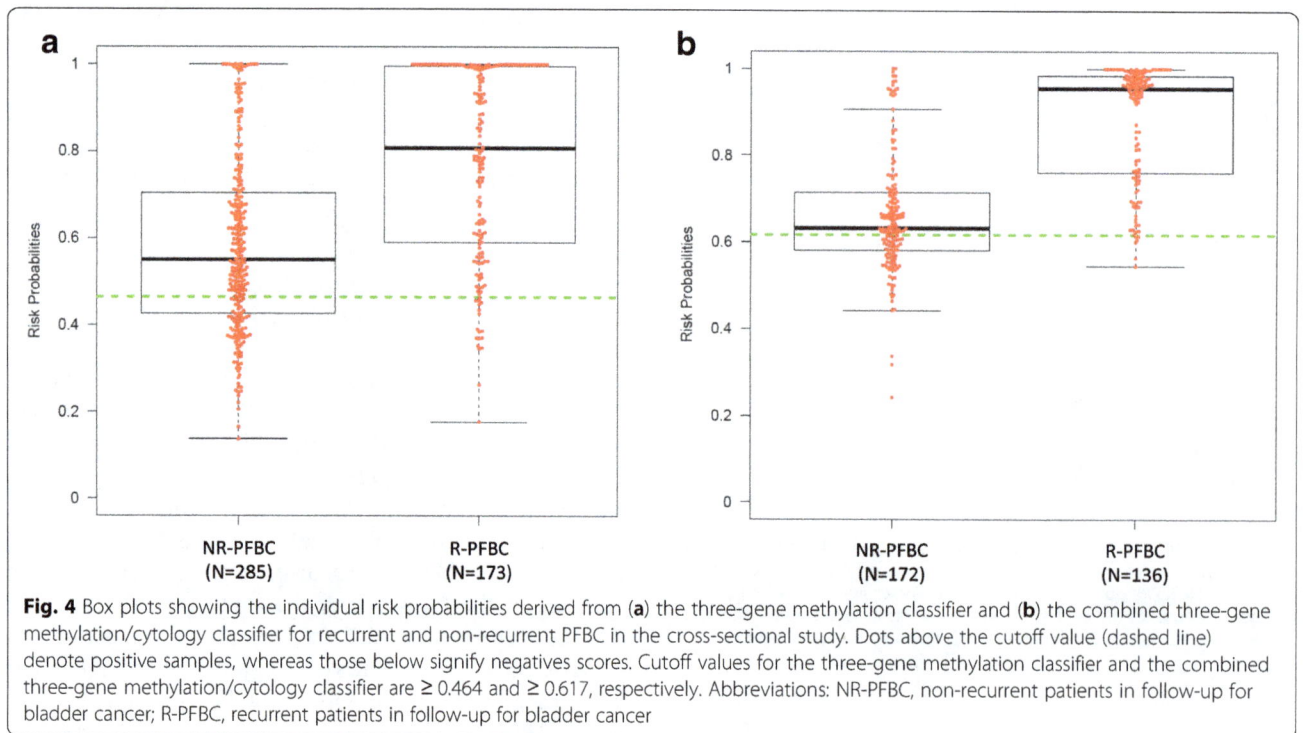

Fig. 4 Box plots showing the individual risk probabilities derived from (**a**) the three-gene methylation classifier and (**b**) the combined three-gene methylation/cytology classifier for recurrent and non-recurrent PFBC in the cross-sectional study. Dots above the cutoff value (dashed line) denote positive samples, whereas those below signify negatives scores. Cutoff values for the three-gene methylation classifier and the combined three-gene methylation/cytology classifier are ≥ 0.464 and ≥ 0.617, respectively. Abbreviations: NR-PFBC, non-recurrent patients in follow-up for bladder cancer; R-PFBC, recurrent patients in follow-up for bladder cancer

likely that biomarkers will replace ureterocystoscopy in patients with macroscopic hematuria referred to the urologist. But in PFBC, urinary biomarkers with a high SN and high NPV could make a difference, i.e., lower the number of follow-up cystoscopies. Our combined three-gene methylation/cytology classifier achieves a high SN and NPV, for both high-risk and non-high-risk NMIBC. Consequently, more than a third of all cystoscopies could be prevented.

The SP of the combined classifier in the testing set, using PFBC samples, is expected to be lower than the SP of the training set, using BC and control samples. Possible reasons for methylation observed in PFBC samples are small tumors not yet detected by cystoscopy, residual tumor cells at the resection site, or epigenetically changed urothelial cells at the resection site or else in the bladder also known as epigenetic field defect [22]. In patients with persistent hypermethylation, which does not recur within 18 months, the presence of an epigenetic field defect is most likely. Wolff and co-workers suggested that the aberrant methylation is caused by a generalized epigenetic alteration in the whole bladder urothelium, and this widespread methylated urothelium may be the cause of the high recurrence rate in NMIBC [22].

The discovery of highly sensitive methylation markers allows us to lower the number of follow-up cystoscopies in more than a third of all follow-up patients. In the clinical situation, patients supply a urine sample before cystoscopy to perform the test. If the combined test is positive, patients will undergo a cystoscopy. In our validation series, 60% of NR-PFBC had a positive combined test and should undergo a cystoscopy. This is not a major problem since in normal daily practice, follow-up patients would have undergone a cystoscopy anyway. If the combined test is negative, cystoscopy could be skipped.

However, a methylation test has also financial and logistic implications, which means that a cost-effectiveness analysis is necessary. Using our three-gene methylation/cytology classifier, 4% of PFBC are wrongly diagnosed as not having a recurrence; all of them had LG NMIBC. Of note, cystoscopy, our gold standard, misses up to 15% of the papillary and up to 30% of the flat lesions [4].

The strengths of this study lie in the fact that we have chosen for a two-stage approach using PFBC in the validation phase. Furthermore, the use of voided urine samples to analyze the DNA methylation status allows the development of a non-invasive BC diagnostic tool with an easy translation into clinical practice. However, some limitations should be mentioned. To avoid inefficiency, patients with a recurrence were oversampled by also recruiting patients who were scheduled for a TURBT of a proven bladder tumor. Consequently, the number of NR-PFBC was misrepresented in the

validation series, and we had to make an estimation to calculate the number of cystoscopies that could be skipped. Secondly, 13% of the samples had to be excluded due to technical failures. Thirdly, intravesical treatments in NMIBC patients may have influenced methylation patterns. Finally, we have evaluated only a limited number of hypermethylated genes with diagnostic value previously described in the literature.

Conclusions

In conclusion, this combined three-gene methylation/cytology classifier can reduce the number of follow-up cystoscopies in PFBC. This approach may improve the patients' quality of life. For a definitive conclusion, replication of the classifier in another series of patients and cost-effectiveness studies are needed.

Additional files

Additional file 1: Figure S1. Flowchart of the entire study. A total of seven hypermethylated genes, differentially expressed between BC patients and controls ($n = 168$), were determined in the discovery phase. With these results, a three-gene methylation classifier was developed. This three-gene classifier was tested in a cross-sectional study (validation phase; $n = 458$). Samples with available cytology results in each phase are indicated. Abbreviations: BC, bladder cancer; C, control; R-PFBC, recurrent patients in follow-up for bladder cancer; NR-PFBC, non-recurrent patients in follow-up for bladder cancer. (PPTX 75 kb)

Additional file 2: Table S1. Primer sequences used in PCR and pyrosequencing. (DOCX 13 kb)

Additional file 3: Figure S2. Pearson correlation coefficient heat map of the percentage of methylation for every CpG dinucleotide in the seven genes. Every CpG sites are correlated (via the Pearson correlation) with all others. Correlations are scaled by the color of the corresponding cell. Parameters are represented in the same order on the x- and y-axes. (PPTX 1232 kb)

Additional file 4: Figure S3. Representative pyrograms showing gene methylation patterns in DNA urine samples from a bladder cancer patient. Percentage of methylation is indicated above peaks (gray columns) corresponding to the CpG sites in this region. (PPTX 183 kb)

Additional file 5: Table S2. Percentage of methylation for each CpG dinucleotide in the seven selected genes in control and bladder cancer urine samples. Underlined in grey the CpG site used for methylation analysis. Abbreviations: SDV; Standard Deviation. (DOCX 21 kb)

Additional file 6: Table S3. Diagnostic performance of the three-gene methylation classifier, cytology, and the combined methylation/cytology classifier in the training and testing subset of samples with cytology available. Abbreviations: LG, Low Grade; HG, High Grade; AUC, area under curve; MIBC, muscle invasive bladder cancer; NMIBC, Non-Muscle Invasive Bladder Cancer; NPV, Negative Predictive Value; PPV, Positive Predictive Value; SN, Sensitivity; SP, Specificity; BC, Bladder Cancer; C, Control; R-PFBC, Recurrent Patients in Follow up for Bladder Cancer; NR-PFBC, Non Recurrent Patients in Follow up for Bladder Cancer. (DOCX 20 kb)

Additional file 7: Figure S4. Sensitivity, negative and positive predictive values of urine cytology, the three-gene methylation classifier, and the combined three-gene methylation/cytology classifier in the testing set ($N = 308$). Overall specificity was 94% for urine cytology, 27% for the three-gene methylation classifier, and 40% for the combined three-gene methylation/cytology classifier. Abbreviations: LG, low-grade; HG, high-grade; NMIBC nHR, non-muscle-invasive bladder cancer non-high risk; NMIBC HR, non--muscle-invasive bladder cancer high risk; NPV, negative predictive value; PPV, positive predictive value. (PPTX 189 kb)

Additional file 8: Figure S5. Flow diagram of participants in the cross-sectional study according a) to the three-gene methylation classifier and cytology results and b) to the combined three-gene methylation/cytology classifier. Abbreviations: R-PFBC, recurrent patients in follow-up for bladder cancer; NR-PFBC, non-recurrent patients in follow-up for bladder cancer; Cytol, cytology; NA, non-available; Test, combined three-gene methylation/cytology classifier. (PPTX 85 kb)

Additional file 9: Figure S6. DNA methylation profiles for bladder cancer and control tissue samples for the three-gene classifier. Data obtained from Wanderer Web page: http://maplab.imppc.org/wanderer/. The red arrow indicates the CpG dinucleotide analyzed in each of the three genes. (PPTX 203 kb)

Abbreviations

AUC: Area under the curve; BC: Bladder cancer; BPH: Benign prostatic hyperplasia; C: Control; CIS/Tis: Carcinoma in situ; HG: High-grade; HR: High-risk; LG: Low-grade; MIBC: Muscle-invasive bladder cancer; NA: Not available; nHR: Non-high risk; NMIBC HR: Non-muscle-invasive bladder cancer high risk; NMIBC nHR: Non-muscle-invasive bladder cancer non-high risk; NMIBC: Non-muscle-invasive bladder cancer; NPV: Negative predictive value; NR-PFBC: Non-recurrent patients in follow-up for bladder cancer; PPV: Positive predictive value; R-PFBC: Recurrent patients in follow-up for bladder cancer; SN: Sensitivity; SP: Specificity; TURBT: Transurethral resection of the bladder tumor

Acknowledgements

We thank the technical support from the staff of the Servei Veterinari de Genètica Molecular, Facultat de Veterinària, Universitat Autònoma de Barcelona. Part of the work was developed at the building Centre de Recerca Biomèdica Cellex, Barcelona. Furthermore, funding from CERCA Programme/Generalitat de Catalunya is gratefully acknowledged.

Funding

This work was supported by grants from the Dutch Cancer Society.

Authors' contributions

AGvdH, LM, LALMK, MJR, JAW, and AA contributed to the conception and design. AGvdH, LM, MI-T, CCMvR-vdW, MB, LALMK, MJR, JAW, and AA contributed to the methodology, collection, and assembly of data. All authors contributed to the data analysis and interpretation and manuscript writing and reviewing. All authors approved the final manuscript.

Competing interests

The authors declare that they have no competing interests.

Author details

[1]Department of Urology Radboud University Medical Center, Nijmegen, The Netherlands. [2]Laboratory and Department of Urology, Hospital Clinic of Barcelona, IDIBAPS, University of Barcelona, Barcelona, Spain. [3]CIBERehd, Plataforma de Bioinformática, Centro de Investigación Biomédica en red de Enfermedades Hepáticas y Digestivas, Barcelona, Spain. [4]Saint John Emergency Clinical Hospital, Bucharest, Romania. [5]MD Anderson Cancer Center, Houston, Texas, USA. [6]Hospital Clínic de Barcelona, Centre de Recerca Biomèdica CELLEX, office B22, C/Casanova, 143, 08036 Barcelona, Spain.

References

1. Oosterlinck W, Lobel B, Jakse G, et al. Guidelines on bladder cancer. Eur Urol. 2002;41:105–12.
2. Fernandez-Gomez J, Madero R, Solsona E, et al. Predicting nonmuscle invasive bladder cancer recurrence and progression in patients treated with bacillus Calmette-Guerin: the CUETO scoring model. J Urol. 2009;182:2195–203.
3. Babjuk M, Bohle A, Burger M, et al. EAU Guidelines on Non-Muscle-invasive Urothelial Carcinoma of the Bladder: update 2016. Eur Urol. 2016;71:447–61.
4. Grossman HB, Gomella L, Fradet Y, et al. A phase III, multicenter comparison of hexaminolevulinate fluorescence cystoscopy and white light cystoscopy for the detection of superficial papillary lesions in patients with bladder cancer. J Urol. 2007;178:62–7.
5. Fradet Y, Grossman HB, Gomella L, et al. A comparison of hexaminolevulinate fluorescence cystoscopy and white light cystoscopy for the detection of carcinoma in situ in patients with bladder cancer: a phase III, multicenter study. J Urol. 2007;178:68–73.
6. Brown FM. Urine cytology. It is still the gold standard for screening? Urol Clin North Am. 2000;27:25–37.
7. Sherman AB, Koss LG, Adams SE. Interobserver and intraobserver differences in the diagnosis of urothelial cells. Comparison with classification by computer. Anal Quant Cytol. 1984;6:112–20.
8. Parker J, Spiess PE. Current and emerging bladder cancer urinary biomarkers. ScientificWorldJournal. 2011;11:1103–12.
9. Esteller M. Epigenetics in cancer. N Engl J Med. 2008;358:1148–59.
10. Saxonov S, Berg P, Brutlag DL. A genome-wide analysis of CpG dinucleotides in the human genome distinguishes two distinct classes of promoters. Proc Natl Acad Sci U S A. 2006;103:1412–7.
11. Shames DS, Minna JD, Gazdar AF. DNA methylation in health, disease, and cancer. Curr Mol Med. 2007;7:85–102.
12. Su SF, Castro Abreu AL, Chihara Y, et al. A panel of three markers hyper- and hypomethylated in urine sediments accurately predicts bladder cancer recurrence. Clin Cancer Res. 2014;20:1978–89.
13. Sobin LH, Wittekind CH. TNM classification of malignant tumours. International union against cancer. 6th ed. New York: Wiley; 2002.
14. Lopez-Beltran A, Sauter G, Gasser T, et al. Tumours of the urinary system. In: Eble JN, Sauter G, Epstein JI, Sesterhenn IA, editors. Pathology and genetics of tumours of the urinary system and male genital organs. World Health Organization classification of tumours. Lyon: IARC Press; 2004. p. 89–157.
15. Yu J, Zhu T, Wang Z, et al. A novel set of DNA methylation markers in urine sediments for sensitive/specific detection of bladder cancer. Clin Cancer Res. 2007;13:7296–304.
16. Renard I, Joniau S, van Cleynenbreugel B, et al. Identification and validation of the methylated TWIST1 and NID2 genes through real-time methylation-specific polymerase chain reaction assays for the noninvasive detection of primary bladder cancer in urine samples. Eur Urol. 2010;58:96–104.
17. Brait M, Begum S, Carvalho AL, et al. Aberrant promoter methylation of multiple genes during pathogenesis of bladder cancer. Cancer Epidemiol Biomark Prev. 2008;17:2786–94.
18. Costa VL, Henrique R, Danielsen SA, et al. Three epigenetic biomarkers, GDF15, TMEFF2, and VIM, accurately predict bladder cancer from DNA-based analyses of urine samples. Clin Cancer Res. 2010;16:5842–51.
19. Robin X, Turck N, Hainard A, et al. pROC: an open-source package for R and S+ to analyze and compare ROC curves. BMC Bioinformatics. 2011;12:77.
20. Diez-Villanueva A, Mallona I, Peinado MA. Wanderer, an interactive viewer to explore DNA methylation and gene expression data in human cancer. Epigenetics Chromatin. 2015;8:22.
21. Fantony JJ, Abern MR, Gopalakrishna A, et al. Multi-institutional external validation of urinary TWIST1 and NID2 methylation as a diagnostic test for bladder cancer. Urol Oncol. 2015;33:387–6.
22. Wolff EM, Chihara Y, Pan F, et al. Unique DNA methylation patterns distinguish noninvasive and invasive urothelial cancers and establish an epigenetic field defect in premalignant tissue. Cancer Res. 2010;70:8169–78.

CDX2 in colorectal cancer is an independent prognostic factor and regulated by promoter methylation and histone deacetylation in tumors of the serrated pathway

Janina Graule[1†], Kristin Uth[1,2†], Elia Fischer[1], Irene Centeno[1], José A. Galván[1], Micha Eichmann[1], Tilman T. Rau[1], Rupert Langer[1], Heather Dawson[1], Ulrich Nitsche[3], Peter Traeger[4], Martin D. Berger[5,6], Beat Schnüriger[7], Marion Hädrich[7], Peter Studer[7], Daniel Inderbitzin[8], Alessandro Lugli[1], Mario P. Tschan[1,2†] and Inti Zlobec[1*†]

Abstract

Background: In colorectal cancer, CDX2 expression is lost in approximately 20% of cases and associated with poor outcome. Here, we aim to validate the clinical impact of CDX2 and investigate the role of promoter methylation and histone deacetylation in CDX2 repression and restoration.

Methods: CDX2 immunohistochemistry was performed on multi-punch tissue microarrays ($n = 637$ patients). Promoter methylation and protein expression investigated on 11 colorectal cancer cell lines identified two CDX2 low expressors (SW620, COLO205) for treatment with decitabine (DNA methyltransferase inhibitor), trichostatin A (TSA) (general HDAC inhibitor), and LMK-235 (specific HDAC4 and HDAC5 inhibitor). RNA and protein levels were assessed. HDAC5 recruitment to the CDX2 gene promoter region was tested by chromatin immunoprecipitation.

Results: Sixty percent of tumors showed focal CDX2 loss; 5% were negative. Reduced CDX2 was associated with lymph node metastasis ($p = 0.0167$), distant metastasis ($p = 0.0123$), and unfavorable survival (multivariate analysis: $p = 0.0008$; HR (95%CI) 0.922 (0.988–0.997)) as well as BRAF[V600E], mismatch repair deficiency, and CpG island methylator phenotype. Decitabine treatment alone induced CDX2 RNA and protein with values from 2- to 25-fold. TSA treatment ± decitabine also led to successful restoration of RNA and/or protein. Treatment with LMK-235 alone had marked effects on RNA and protein levels, mainly in COLO205 cells that responded less to decitabine. Lastly, decitabine co-treatment was more effective than LMK-235 alone at restoring CDX2.

Conclusion: CDX2 loss is an adverse prognostic factor and linked to molecular features of the serrated pathway. RNA/protein expression is restored in CDX2 low-expressing CRC cell lines by demethylation and HDAC inhibition. Importantly, our data underline HDAC4 and HDAC5 as new epigenetic CDX2 regulators that warrant further investigation.

Keywords: Colorectal cancer, CDX2, Methylation, Histone modification, Prognosis, Biomarker

* Correspondence: inti.zlobec@pathology.unibe.ch
†Janina Graule, Kristin Uth, Mario P. Tschan and Inti Zlobec contributed equally to this work.
[1]Institute of Pathology, University of Bern, Murtenstrasse 31, Room L310, 3008 Bern, Switzerland
Full list of author information is available at the end of the article

Background

CDX2 is a homeobox protein responsible for the maintenance of the intestinal phenotype [1, 2]. Over the last decade, CDX2 has been linked to colorectal cancer (CRC) progression, with reduced expression of the protein associated with more advanced tumor stage, vessel invasion, and metastasis [3–7]. Many studies, including the work by Dalerba et al., underline the unfavorable survival time in patients with a complete absence of CDX2 in the tumor [8], a feature that occurs in approximately 5% of patients [7, 8]. Furthermore, they demonstrate that CDX2-negative CRC patients may benefit from chemotherapy, particularly in a stage II setting [8].

Reduced CDX2 protein expression is related to certain molecular alterations during colorectal tumorigenesis. Previous work by our group and others shows that nearly all sporadic microsatellite unstable (MSI) cancers show some degree of loss of the protein in the tumor, whether in a small or substantial percentage of cells [3, 5, 9]. This loss is not however limited to MSI-high cancers, but is also found in microsatellite stable (MSS) tumors with BRAF mutation and high-level CpG island methylator phenotype (CIMP), in other words, in cancers deriving from the so-called serrated pathway [10]. More than 20% of CRCs show some degree (or complete loss) of CDX2 protein in the tumor, which is often reported along with a preponderance for female gender and right-sided tumor location, two features frequently associated with serrated lesions [11].

Since CDX2 mutations are extremely rare events in CRCs [12], we hypothesized that epigenetic changes, such as promoter hypermethylation or histone deacetylation could be responsible for significant downregulation or absence of CDX2, particularly in the group of tumors displaying "serrated" molecular features (BRAF mutation, MSI, and CIMP) [13]. In fact, human serrated adenomas with high-grade dysplasia have been shown to have significantly greater frequencies of CDX2 hypermethylation than other polyp types (like classical adenomas) [14].

In this study, we aim (1) to validate the clinical relevance of CDX2 in a large group of CRC patients ($n = 637$), (2) to determine whether epigenetic modifications contribute to CDX2 repression, and (3) to restore CDX2 expression in vitro by targeting methylation and histone deacetylation.

Methods

Patients

Two retrospective cohorts were investigated. Patient characteristics are found in Additional file 1: Table S1.

Cohort 1 (Germany)

The cohort initially included 341 primary resected colon cancer (no rectal cancer) patients treated at the Department of Surgery at the Technical University Munich (TUM)

hospital, Munich, Germany, between 1993 and 2005. Clinical and pathological features for this cohort included age at diagnosis, gender, tumor location, TNM stage (UICC 6th ed.), R classification, and tumor grade. After exclusion of patients with unavailable tumor material for this study, the final cohort comprised 252 patients of which 237 (94%) had information on therapy and survival. Overall 5-year survival rate was 66.6%.

Cohort 2 (Switzerland)

This cohort encompasses 385 surgically treated CRC patients. Clinical features retrieved from patient charts were age at diagnosis, tumor location, and gender. Survival information, follow-up, and therapy information were available for 286 (82.9%). Histopathology was re-reviewed according to the TNM 7th edition and is summarized in Additional file 1: Table S1. MSI status determined by PCR was available for 128 patients. Adjuvant treatment for high-risk stage II and stage III colon cancer consisted of a 5-FU or capecitabine-based chemotherapy (5-FU orcapecitabine ± oxaliplatin). Palliative first-line chemotherapy for stage IV patients comprised either the FOLFOX, XELOX, or FOLFIRI regimen with or without bevacizumab/cetuximab, while anti-EGFR treatment was applied only to KRAS wild-type patients. Overall 5-year survival was 60.7%.

Ethics, consent, and permissions

The ethics committees of the Klinikum rechts der Isar and Canton of Bern approved the use of data and patient material for this study (nos. 1926/7 and 200/2014, respectively).

Next-generation tissue microarray (ngTMA®) construction

Tissues from all 637 patients were retrieved from the corresponding archives of the Institutes of Pathology at the TUM and University of Bern. One to two H&E slides were sectioned from each block, and the slides were scanned (P250 Flash II, 3DHistech, Hungary). Digital slides were annotated using a tissue microarray tool by placing six to eight different circles onto various histological areas (Additional file 1: Figure S1) [15]. The annotated digital slide was then aligned with the tumor block and cored using a 0.6-mm-diameter TMA tool (TMA Grandmaster, 3DHistech, Hungary). In addition, the TMA tool of 1.0 mm diameter was used to punch out cores from cohort 1, which were placed into tubes for downstream molecular analysis.

Cell lines and treatment

CRC cell lines (LS174T, T84, LS180, HCT15, HT29, SW620, COLO205, HCT116, COLO320, LoVo, CaCo2) were obtained from the American Type Culture Collection (ATCC, Manassas, VA, USA) and grown in media with supplements as described in Additional file 1: Table S2 under humidified atmosphere of 5% CO2.

Treatment with DNA methyltransferase inhibitor (DNMTi): 3.5×10^4 COLO205 or SW620 cells were seeded in six-well plates and treated with 0.5% DMSO, 1.25 µM, 2.5 µM, 5 µM, and 10 µM of decitabine (Stock 50 mM in DMSO, Cat.#S1200, Selleckchem, Houston, TX, USA) for 48 h.

Treatment with histone deacetylase inhibitors (HDACi): 3.5×10^4 COLO205 or SW620 cells were seeded in six-well plates and treated with 0.01% DMSO, 50 nM trichostatin A (Stock 5 mM in DMSO, Cat.# T8552, Sigma-Aldrich, St. Louis, MO, USA) and 20 nM LMK-235 (Stock 10 mM in DMSO, Cat.# S7569, Selleckchem) alone or in combination with 2.5 µM, 5 µM, and 10 µM of decitabine for 48 h.

3.5×10^4 HT29, SW620, LS174T, and LoVo cells were seeded in six-well plates and treated with 8×10^{-3} DMSO, 5 nM, 10 nM, 20 nM, 40 nM, and 80 nM of LMK-235 for 48 h.

RNA extraction and real-time quantitative RT-PCR (qPCR)

RNA was extracted using the miRCURY RNA Isolation Kit (Prod.#300110; Exiqon, Vedbaek, Denmark) according to the manufacturer's instructions. RNA concentrations were measured using NanoDrop (Thermo Scientific) and adjusted to 500 ng/10 µL. cDNA Synthesis Reagent (5xRT Super Mix, Cat. #B24403; Biotool, Houston, TX, USA) was added to the diluted RNA, RT-PCR performed using a Veriti 96-well Thermal Cycler (Model #9902; Applied Biosystems, Rotkreuz, Switzerland), and H$_2$O added to an final concentration of 10 ng/µL cDNA. qPCR was performed using 10 ng/µL cDNA and TaqMan Fast Universal PCR Master Mix (Applied Biosystems). For quantification of *CDX2* and *HIC1* mRNA, the Taqman® Gene Expression Assay Hs01078080_m1 and Hs00359611_s1 (both Applied Biosystems), respectively, was used. *HMBS* primers and probes have been described earlier [16]. Raw Ct values were normalized to *HMBS* and to the untreated controls and are shown as *n*-fold changes ($2^{-\Delta\Delta Ct}$ analysis).

Western blot analysis

Cell lysates were prepared using a buffer containing 8 mM urea, 0.5% Triton-X, and proteinase inhibitors (25× PIC Complete, Rosch), protein concentration determined with Bradford Assay (Bio-Red Protein Assay; BioRad, Cressier, Switzerland) and 10 µg samples, mixed with loading buffer (4× Laemmli Sample Buffer, Cat: #161-0747, BioRad) and loaded on Mini-Protean TGX Stain Free Gels (12%, 15-well, Cat. #456-8095; BioRad). After UV activation, proteins were transferred to a PVDF membrane (0.2 µm PVDF, Cat. #170-4156; BioRad) using a Trans-Blot Turbo Transfer Pack (Mini format; BioRad). Membranes were blocked with 5% TBS-milk for at least 45 min. Blots were incubated with anti-CDX2 (1:500 in BSA, EPR2764Y—28.8 µg/mL, Rabbit

Monoclonal, Cell Marque; Sigma-Aldrich) over night at 4 °C followed by incubation with anti-rabbit (1:10,000 in milk; Cell Signalling Technology, Leiden, The Netherlands) for at least 2 h at RT. Detection took place using ECL (Clarity Western ECL Substrate, Cat. #170-5060; BioRad) and ChemiDoc (MP, Serial #731BR00765; BioRad). Quantification was performed with ImageJ.

Chromatin immunoprecipitation (ChIP)

HEK-293T cells have been transiently transfected using calcium phosphate [17] and 2 µg of FLAG-HDAC5 (Addgene #32213) expression plasmid in a 10-cm dish. After 48 h, cells were harvested and processed for ChIP using the ChIP-IT Express Chromatin Immunoprecipitation Kit (ChIP-IT Express, Active Motif, Carlsbad, CA, USA) according to the manufacturer's recommendations. In parallel, FLAG-HDAC5 expression was determined by Western blotting (data not shown). For immunoprecipitation, 2.5 µg anti-Flag antibody (Sigma, Cat.#F3165) was used. Antibodies against acetyl-histone H3 (Cell Signalling, Cat.#9715) and mouse IgG (PP64B, Upstate, Millipore) served as positive and negative controls, respectively. PCR was performed using JumpStart *Taq* (Sigma-Aldrich) and the following primers, specifically selected to cover a 2500-bp genomic region upstream of the transcription start site (TSS) of the *CDX2* gene: 2000–2500 bp, F: 5′-CTTTCCATGGCTGG AGCACT-3′, R: 5′-CGCTGGCTAATTGTCCCTGT-3′; 1500–2000 bp, F: 5′-CATTCCCACCCCATCAGGTC-3′, R: 5′-CCAAGGAGCTGTGCACTCAA-3′; 1000–1500 bp, F: 5′-ACAGACAAGTGCAGGTCTCC-3′, R: 5′-CCCA GCTCGGTTTCAGCA-3′; and TSS–500 bp, F: 5′-TGGA GGTTAAAGTGCACCAGGT-3′, R: 5′-GACACCAAT GGTTGGAGACG-3′. As a positive control for HDAC5 recruitment, we amplified a genomic region of the HDAC5 repressed fibroblast growth factor 2 (*FGF2*) gene using the following published primers: F: 5′-TGGAGGTTAAAGTG CACCAGGT-3′ and R: 5′-GACACCAATGGTTGGAGAC G-3′ [18].

DNA extraction and CDX2 methylation analysis

Genomic DNA was extracted from selected tumoral area of FFPE tissues using QIAamp DNA FFPE Tissue Kit (Qiagen; Hilden, Germany). Bisulfite conversion and pyrosequencing were used to analyze *CDX2* methylation in two different promoter regions. Both regions are located on chromosome 13, GRCh38.p7 Primary Assembly (NC_000013), region 1: 27970684-27970645 and region 2: 27970508-27970478. PCR conditions and details on primer sequences and region to analyze are outlined in Additional file 1: Methods.

MS-MLPA for CIMP status

Methylation-specific multiplex ligation-dependent probe amplification (MS-MLPA) was performed according to standard protocol for CIMP status evaluation and *BRAF*^{V600E}

mutation. Promoter methylation of *CACNA1G, IGF2, NEU-ROG1, RUNX3, SOCS1, CDKN2A, MLH1*, and *CRABP1* was analyzed by SALSA MLPA probemix ME042-C1 (MRC Holland, Amsterdam, Netherlands). A gene was considered methylated when one fourth (25%) or more probes were at least 30% methylated. This cutoff was set as it corresponds with the highest background methylation value in the healthy tissue control.

Immunohistochemistry and in situ hybridization

All ngTMA blocks were sectioned at 2.5 µm, and immuno-histochemistry was performed on an automated immunos-tainer (Leica Bond Rx or Ventana Benchmark Ultra) for CDX2 (clone ERP2764Y, Cell Marque, 1:400, Tris 95° 30′), *BRAF*^{V600E} protein (clone VE1, Roche, CC1 99° 72′), and MLH1 (clone ES05, Leica Novocastra, 1:200, Tris 95° 30′). CDX2 and MLH1 protein expression was evaluated by estimating the number of immunoreactive nuclei in each tumor punch, then an average positive count across all cores from the same patient lead to the final marker value for statistical analysis. Since CDX2 is normally present in all cells of the normal colonic mucosa, we quantified the percentage of immunoreactive cells in the tumor then defined a "reduced or loss of" expression when less than 100% of cells were stained and a complete loss of expression when 0% of cells where stained. VE1 was scored as positive or negative. Any doubt regarding positive staining of VE1 was confirmed by pyrosequencing. RNA expression was evaluated semi-quantitatively [19] across all tumor punches in cohort 1 using RNAscope 2.0 FFPE assay and probes for *CDX2*, the bacterial gene *dapB*, as negative control and the housekeeping gene *PPIB* as positive control (Advanced Cell Diagnostics, Inc.). Scoring was performed as previously described [17]. Briefly, score 0 = no staining, score 1 = difficult to see under 40x, score 2 = difficult to see under 20x but easy under 40x, score 3 = difficult to see under 10x but easy under 20x, and score 4 = easy to see under 10x.

Immunohistochemistry was also performed on cell lines. 1×10^6 cells of COLO205 and SW620 cell lines were seeded, treated with decitabine and/or TSA or LMK-235 and harvested using trypsin after 48 h and 72 h. Cells were washed with PBS, formalin-fixed and paraffin embedded (FFPE), and immunohistochemically stained for CDX2. Slides were scanned with a Pannoramic 250 Flash II (3DHistech Ltd., Budapest, Hungary). Cell quantification was performed with the open source image analysis software QuPath [20], using watershed cell detection on optical density sum images and subsequent random trees classification of the detected cells.

Statistics

Descriptive statistics, non-parametric Wilcoxon rank sum test or chi-square tests were used to analyze differences in CDX2 staining with categorical features.

Survival time analysis was performed using both log-rank tests and Kaplan-Meier curves and Cox propor-tional hazards regression models in multivariable analysis, adjusting for potential confounding factors. Hazard ratios and 95%CI were used to determine the effect differences. Spearman correlation coefficients were calculated to de-termine the strength of relationship between methylation and protein expression. Student's *t* test was used to compare mean methylation percentage in CDX2-positive or CDX2-negative cell lines. For statistical analysis of four biological replicates of qPCR and Western blot results, Mann-Whitney test was performed. *p* values < 0.05 were considered statistically significant. No adjustment for multiple comparisons was performed [21]. Analyses were performed using SAS V9.3 (The SAS Institute, Cary, NC) and PRISM, GraphPad Software.

Results

Distribution of CDX2 protein expression scores

CDX2 protein expression ranged from 0 to 100%. Additional file 1: Figure S2 highlights the distribution of expression from cohort 2 (A) as well as representative immunostaining (B-D). Thirty-nine patients (5.0%) showed a complete absence of CDX2 protein in the tumor. The percentage of CDX2 immunostained tumor cells was 66% on average, with a median of 78.8%. In terms of different tumor areas, there was no difference in expression between the tumor center and invasion front; however, tumor budding cells were frequently seen with an absent CDX2 staining.

Relationship between mRNA ISH scores and protein expression

One thousand four hundred sixty-one punches were evaluated for mRNA ISH with corresponding protein data. There was a strong and statistically significant correlation between the CDX2 protein expression scores in the tumors and the corresponding mRNA ISH scores ($r = 0.99$, $p < 0.0001$) indicating that RNA expression and protein expres-sion were highly associated. The mean percentage of CDX2 protein expression across all tumors was 44.2% (score 0), 52.7% (score 1), 65.8% (score 2), 76.2% (score 3), and 90.8% (score 4) ($p < 0.0001$) (Additional file 1: Figure S3).

Clinicopathological features associated with progressive CDX2 loss

In cohort 1, there was a significant correlation between reduced CDX2 expression and female gender ($p = 0.0338$); more advanced pT classification ($p = 0.0068$), lymph node metastasis ($p = 0.0167$), and distant metastasis ($p = 0.0123$); and higher tumor grade ($p = 0.0163$) (Table 1). Similar correlations could be found for cohort 2 with significant associations between reduced CDX2 and histo-logical subtype ($p = 0.009$), right-sided tumor location (p

Table 1 Association of progressive CDX2 loss with clinicopathological features in two cohorts

Clinicopathological feature	COHORT 1 ($n = 252$)		COHORT 2 ($n = 385$)	
	CDX2% (mean/median)	p value	CDX2% (mean/median)	p value
Gender				
Male	61.5/71.7	0.0338	72.6/85	0.5675
Female	52.6/56.7		67.6/83.1	
Histological subtype				
Adeno	n/a		71.9/85	0.009
Mucinous	n/a		66.6/75	
Other	n/a		41.9/51.3	
Tumor location				
Left	58.2/60.8	0.812	69.5/86.3	0.0135
Right	57.3/65.8		75.6/90	
Rectum	–		68.1/75	
pT				
pT1	62.3/75.0	0.0068	83.8/93.8	0.002
pT2	55.8/63.3		68.7/82.5	
pT3	55.9/64.5		73.7/84.4	
pT4	37.0/26.7		56.3/66.7	
pN				
pN0	61.6/71.7	0.0167	72.5/86.3	0.1891
pN1-2	52.6/58.8		69.0/82.5	
pM				
pM0 (c)	65.2/76.7	0.0123	72.5/85	0.0337
pM1-2	48.9/60		60.2/71.3	
Tumor grade				
G1-2	65.4/76.7	0.0163	74.8/85	0.0004
G3	47.0/40.0		57.2/70.4	
Lymphatic invasion				
L0	n/a	–	74.7/88.8	0.0136
L1	n/a		68.9/75.8	
Venous invasion				
V0	n/a	–	74.2/84.4	0.0706
V1	n/a		67.7/80	
Perineural invasion				
Pn0	n/a	–	70.0/80	0.7978
Pn1	n/a		69.8/85	
BRAF				
Wild-type	59.6/66.7	0.0044	76.0/87.5	< 0.0001
Mutated	43.0/38.3		26.4/4.4	
MMR status				
Deficient	48.1/47.5	0.0077	43.5/50	0.0005
Proficient	61.8/71.7		69.5/79.4	

n/a not available

= 0.0135), more advance pT stage ($p = 0.0002$), distant metastasis ($p = 0.0337$), higher tumor grade ($p = 0.0004$), lymphatic vessel invasion ($p = 0.00136$), and a trend to venous vessel invasion ($p = 0.0706$).

CDX2 is an adverse and independent prognostic factor

Survival analysis was performed on the combined set of patients; 599 patients were available for analysis. In univariate analysis, reduced CDX2 expression was significantly related to worse overall survival (Cox regression analysis using percentage of positive cells) ($p = 0.0008$; HR (95%CI) 0.992 (0.988–0.997)). The survival effect of CDX2 was also evaluated using two different cutoff values, found in the literature: 0% (versus any expression) [8] and a threshold of 75% (focal versus diffuse) [10]. Thirty-four of 599 patients had tumors with 0% expression, and 16 (47.1%) died over the course of follow-up (Fig. 1).

Five hundred and sixty-five patients had tumors with any CDX2 expression, and 139 died during follow-up. In both instances, there was a significant and marked effect of CDX2 absence/loss on survival. However, of the two cutoffs interrogated, only the 0% cutoff was found to have an independent prognostic effect on outcome, after adjusting for TNM stage and postoperative therapy (Table 2). Our analysis of CDX2-negative patients with and without chemotherapy shows no difference in the overall survival with postoperative treatment. However, due to low statistical power of the negative subgroup, we cannot adequately evaluate the survival benefit with chemotherapy here.

CDX2 loss is associated with molecular features of the serrated pathway

$BRAF^{V600E}$ mutation was found in 10.4% of patients, while mismatch repair (MMR) deficiency in 12.2% of all patients in both cohorts. Expression of CDX2 was significantly reduced in tumors with $BRAF^{V600E}$ mutations ($p = 0.0044$ cohort 1; $p < 0.001$ cohort 2) and tumors with defective MMR ($p = 0.0077$ cohort 1; $p = 0.0005$ cohort 2). Additional file 1: Figure S4 outlines the progressive loss of CDX2 protein with changes in both MMR status (proficient or deficient) and BRAF status (wild-type or mutation) across both cohorts ($n = 590$). In comparison to MMR-proficient/BRAF WT tumors (70.1% CDX2), those with MMR-deficient/$BRAF^{V600E}$-mutated cancers (29.3% CDX2) have a significantly reduced expression ($p < 0.0001$).

CDX2 promoter methylation is a mechanism of protein loss in CRC cell lines

To test whether hypermethylation of CDX2 promoter could explain mRNA and protein loss in CRCs, 11 different CRC cell lines were fixed in formalin, embedded in paraffin, and immunostained for CDX2. Diffuse, partial, or absent CDX2 expression was evaluated and correlated to the analysis of methylation status at two

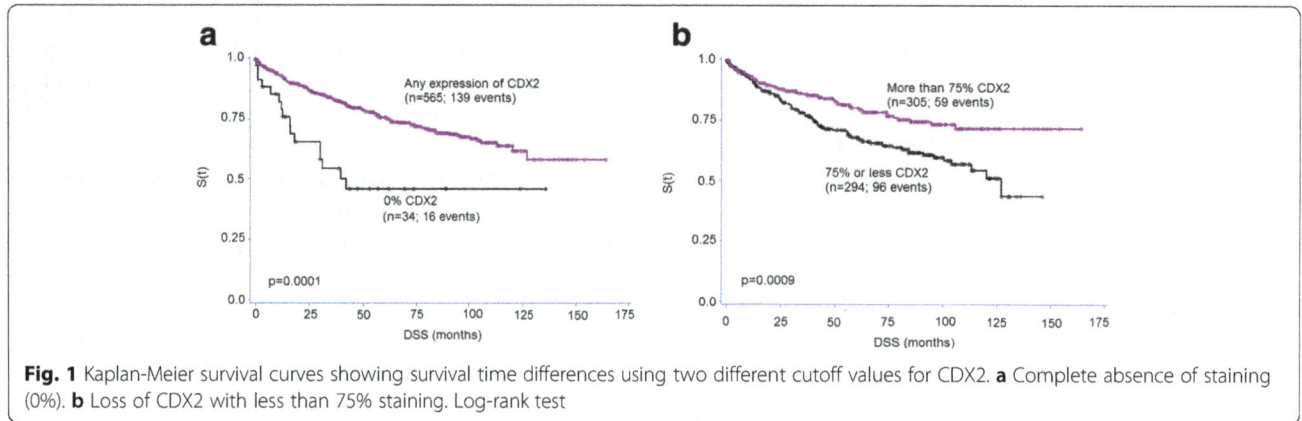

Fig. 1 Kaplan-Meier survival curves showing survival time differences using two different cutoff values for CDX2. **a** Complete absence of staining (0%). **b** Loss of CDX2 with less than 75% staining. Log-rank test

promoter regions. LS174T, T84, LS180, and HCT-15 were moderately to strongly positive and showed minimal methylation percentages at both sites. In contrast, HT29, SW620, COLO205, and HCT-116 showed a complete absence of CDX2 or only few CDX2-positive cells at the protein level and a high (> 80%) degree of methylation (Fig. 2). The association between higher percentage of methylation and absence of protein expression was significantly correlated ($p = 0.0295$). The remaining three cell lines, LoVo, CaCo2, and COLO320, showed no correlation between protein expression and methylation status.

CDX2 promoter hypermethylation and protein expression in CRCs

We selected 39 patients from cohort 1, including all tumors with BRAF mutation and MMR deficiency ($n = 9$), and performed both a CDX2 promoter methylation analysis as well as CIMP analysis. All nine cases were CIMP-high. CDX2 hypermethylation (> 20% methylation across all CpG sites) was found in 23 patients. Pyrosequencing results for these patients can be found in Additional file 1: Table S3. There was a striking inverse correlation between CDX2 protein and percentage of methylation, which was limited to the serrated tumor group ($r = -0.7$). Cancers without these serrated molecular features had no correlation between CDX2 protein expression and methylation ($r = -0.07$).

DNA methyltransferase inhibitor (DNMTi) treatment restores CDX2 expression

To test whether global demethylation can restore CDX2 expression, we treated two CRC cell lines (COLO205 and SW620) showing low/absent CDX2 expression with the DNMTi, decitabine. Upon 48 h treatment with decitabine, a significant 2- and 15-fold induction of CDX2 RNA could be observed for SW620 and COLO205, respectively, with the latter showing a dose-dependency (Fig. 3a). Importantly, SW620 cells show a 4-fold higher CDX2 basal level expression of mRNA compared to COLO205 cells.

As a control for the efficiency of the decitabine treatment, we determined the mRNA induction of hypermethylated in cancer 1 (HIC1) in SW620 and COLO205 cells, a gene with known promoter hypermethylation in cancer. We found a significant increase in HIC1 mRNA levels in both cell lines upon decitabine treatment (Additional file 1: Figure S5).

On a protein level, a major induction in CDX2 protein was observed in SW620 and to a lesser extent in COLO205 cells, as seen on both Western blot and immunohistochemistry (Figs. 3b).

Combination of DNMTi and HDACi or HDAC4/5i treatment improves restoration of CDX2 expression

Since DNA demethylation affects CDX2 restoration, we asked whether other epigenetic modifications, in particular, histone acetylation could have an additional impact on CDX2 gene regulation. In a first step, we treated COLO205 and SW620 cells with a general HDACi, trichostatin A (TSA). We observed an up to 10-fold induction of CDX2 RNA upon TSA treatment alone and an up to 23-fold induction of CDX2 RNA when combined with decitabine in COLO205 cells (Fig. 4a), as well as on protein level (Fig. 4b, c). This result indicates that the combination treatment of TSA and decitabine is more effective at restoring CDX2 expression than decitabine or TSA alone in COLO205. In comparison, TSA treatment alone or in combination did not have a comparable impact on CDX2 restoration in SW620 cells (Additional file 1: Figure S6). Since TSA is a general HDACi with varying specificity in HDAC inhibition, we asked whether inhibition of specific HDACs might be involved in CDX2 regulation.

We therefore treated cells with LMK-235, a specific inhibitor of HDAC4 and HDAC5. In COLO205, our results show an even more pronounced induction of CDX2, both upon single-treatment with LMK-235 (up to 25-fold) or in combination with decitabine (up to 35-fold) (Fig. 4a). These results are again underlined by

Table 2 Multivariable analysis of CDX2 (absence versus any positive expression) adjusting for TNM stage and postoperative therapy

	HR (95%CI)	p value
CDX2		
Negative	1.0	
Positive	0.35 (0.17–0.71)	0.0037
TNM stage		
TNM I (vs IV)	8.85 (4.05–19.2)	< 0.0001
TNM II (vs IV)	6.33 (3.65–10.9)	< 0.0001
TNM III (vs IV)	3.62 (2.18–6.02)	< 0.0001
Postoperative therapy		
None	1.0	
Treated	1.01 (0.83–1.23)	0.9172

increased protein expression assessed by Western blotting and immunohistochemistry (Fig. 4b, c). A similar effect can be observed in SW620 cells, namely a marked increase in both *CDX2* RNA and protein is seen upon LMK-235 treatment alone and in combination with DNMTi (Additional file 1: Figure S6).

Next, we asked whether CDX2 protein restoration could be induced by LMK-235 in HT29, a cell line known to be only minimally responsive to DNMTi treatment. Indeed, upon LMK-235 treatment, HT29 cells showed a significant and dose-dependent increase of CDX2 on RNA level and remarkably on protein level as well (Fig. 5). We further observed a pronounced CDX2 induction upon LMK-235 treatment, independent of CDX2 promoter methylation status of two other cell lines, LS174T and LoVo (Additional file 1: Figure S7).

To test if HDAC5 localizes to the *CDX2* promoter region and is directly involved in repression *CDX2* gene expression,

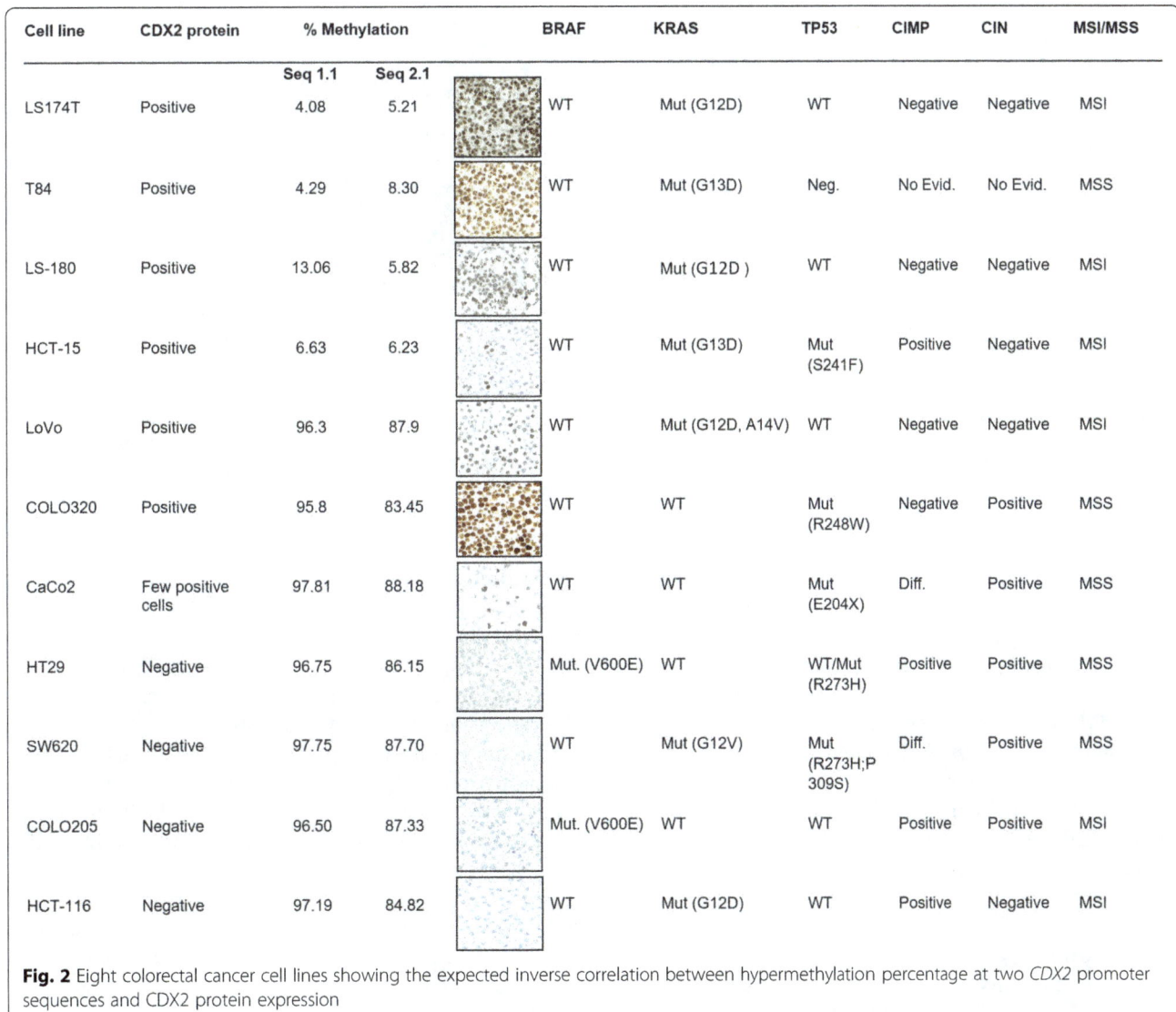

Cell line	CDX2 protein	% Methylation Seq 1.1	% Methylation Seq 2.1		BRAF	KRAS	TP53	CIMP	CIN	MSI/MSS
LS174T	Positive	4.08	5.21		WT	Mut (G12D)	WT	Negative	Negative	MSI
T84	Positive	4.29	8.30		WT	Mut (G13D)	Neg.	No Evid.	No Evid.	MSS
LS-180	Positive	13.06	5.82		WT	Mut (G12D)	WT	Negative	Negative	MSI
HCT-15	Positive	6.63	6.23		WT	Mut (G13D)	Mut (S241F)	Positive	Negative	MSI
LoVo	Positive	96.3	87.9		WT	Mut (G12D, A14V)	WT	Negative	Negative	MSI
COLO320	Positive	95.8	83.45		WT	WT	Mut (R248W)	Negative	Positive	MSS
CaCo2	Few positive cells	97.81	88.18		WT	WT	Mut (E204X)	Diff.	Positive	MSS
HT29	Negative	96.75	86.15		Mut. (V600E)	WT	WT/Mut (R273H)	Positive	Positive	MSS
SW620	Negative	97.75	87.70		WT	Mut (G12V)	Mut (R273H;P 309S)	Diff.	Positive	MSS
COLO205	Negative	96.50	87.33		Mut. (V600E)	WT	WT	Positive	Positive	MSI
HCT-116	Negative	97.19	84.82		WT	Mut (G12D)	WT	Positive	Negative	MSI

Fig. 2 Eight colorectal cancer cell lines showing the expected inverse correlation between hypermethylation percentage at two *CDX2* promoter sequences and CDX2 protein expression

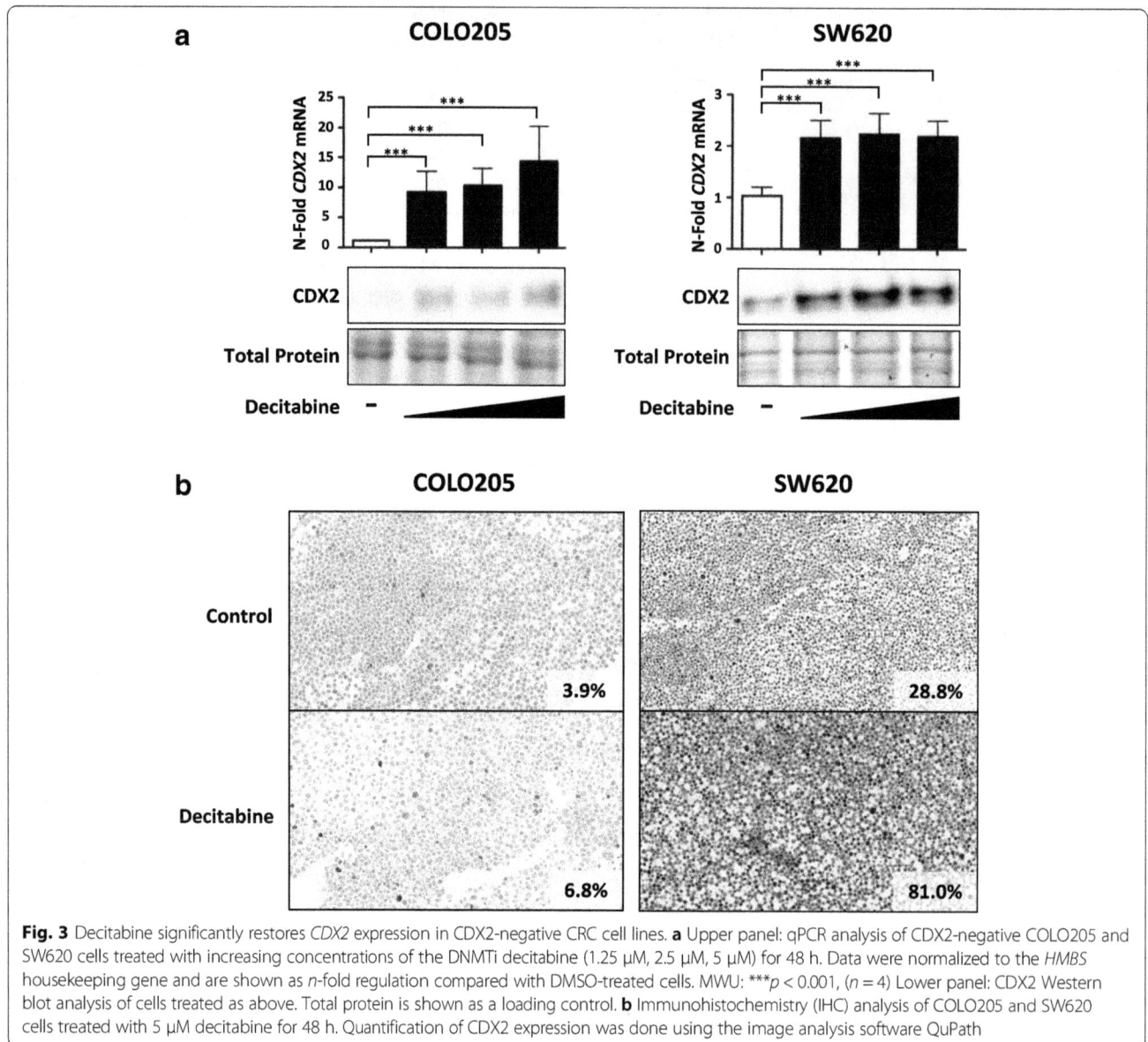

Fig. 3 Decitabine significantly restores *CDX2* expression in CDX2-negative CRC cell lines. **a** Upper panel: qPCR analysis of CDX2-negative COLO205 and SW620 cells treated with increasing concentrations of the DNMTi decitabine (1.25 μM, 2.5 μM, 5 μM) for 48 h. Data were normalized to the *HMBS* housekeeping gene and are shown as *n*-fold regulation compared with DMSO-treated cells. MWU: ***$p < 0.001$, ($n = 4$) Lower panel: CDX2 Western blot analysis of cells treated as above. Total protein is shown as a loading control. **b** Immunohistochemistry (IHC) analysis of COLO205 and SW620 cells treated with 5 μM decitabine for 48 h. Quantification of CDX2 expression was done using the image analysis software QuPath

we performed an HDAC5 chromatin immunoprecipitation (ChIP) assay. Indeed, HDAC5 is found at a genomic region upstream of the transcriptional start site indicating direct *CDX2* repression by HDAC5 (Fig. 6). As a positive control for HDAC5 repressed gene expression, we amplified a genomic region of the fibroblast growth factor 2 (FGF2) gene [18].

In summary, combining decitabine with the HDAC4/5 inhibitor LMK-235 allows for improved CDX2 expression in CRC cells, particularly in cells with a low sensitivity to DNMT inhibition, whereby HDAC5 is directly involved in *CDX2* gene expression by localizing to the *CDX2* gene promoter region.

Discussion

The novel findings of this study show that CDX2 in CRC can be regulated by either promoter methylation

and more markedly by histone acetylation. In particular, treatment of cell lines by specific HDAC4 and HDAC5 inhibitor LMK-235 (with and without DNMTi) leads to a marked upregulation and re-expression of CDX2 RNA and protein, implying that both enzymes are involved in the repression of *CDX2* transcription.

CDX2 is an important prognostic factor. Its loss has been linked to more aggressive tumor features such as TNM stage, metastasis, and vessel invasion [3–5, 8, 10, 19]. Recent reports have shown that a complete loss of protein (0% staining) provides information on overall survival and chemotherapy benefit [8]. However, our study demonstrates that any loss of CDX2 can be informative, with a reduction in protein related to poorer clinical outcome in a stage-independent manner. Nolte and colleagues published a detailed analysis of CDX2 by digital image analysis on a

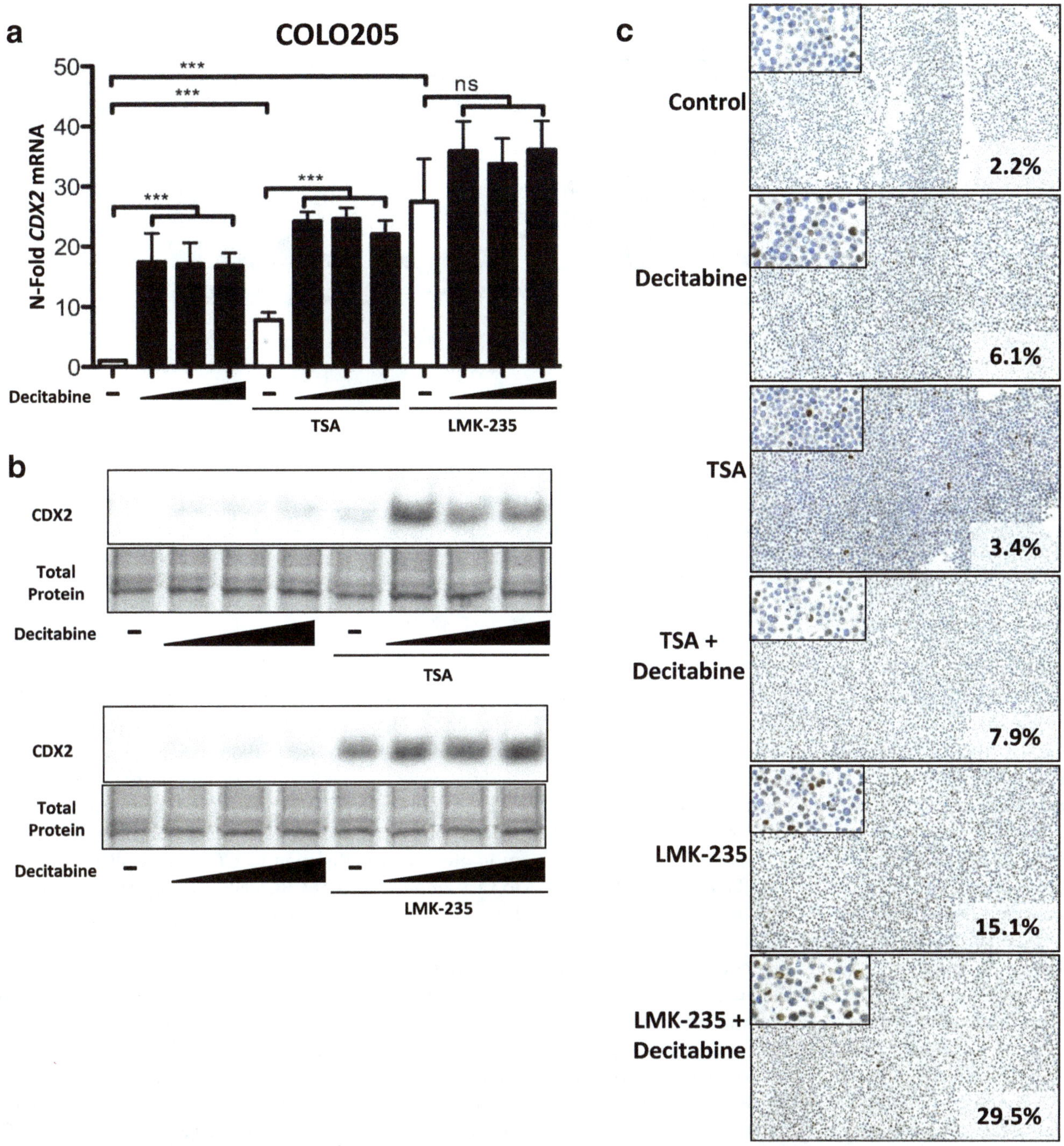

Fig. 4 Improved CDX2 restoration in COLO205 cells upon combining DNMTi and HDACi treatment. **a** qPCR analysis of COLO205 cells treated for 48 h with DNMTi decitabine (2.5 μM, 5 μM, 10 μM) alone and in combination with the general HDACi trichostatin A (TSA; 50 nM) or the specific HDAC4/5 inhibitor LMK-235 (20 nM). Analysis as in Fig. 5a. MWU: ***$p < 0.001$, ($n = 4$). **b** CDX2 Western blot analysis of COLO205 cells treated as in **a**. Total protein is shown as a loading control. **c** Immunohistochemistry (IHC) analysis of COLO205 cells treated with decitabine (5 μM), TSA (50 nM), or LMK-235 (20 nM) alone or combination treatments with decitabine and TSA or LMK-235

similar number of cases, highlighting the range of possible CDX2 values expressed by CRCs [22]. They used the full information from staining intensity and percentage of positive cells and underline that any loss of protein is related to more aggressive features. Our results are in line with this observation: here, we validate the independent prognostic effect of both progressive and complete CDX2 loss of protein expression. Regardless of the large number of patients in this study ($n = 599$ for survival analysis), we cannot confirm the predictive effect of CDX2 to chemotherapy response.

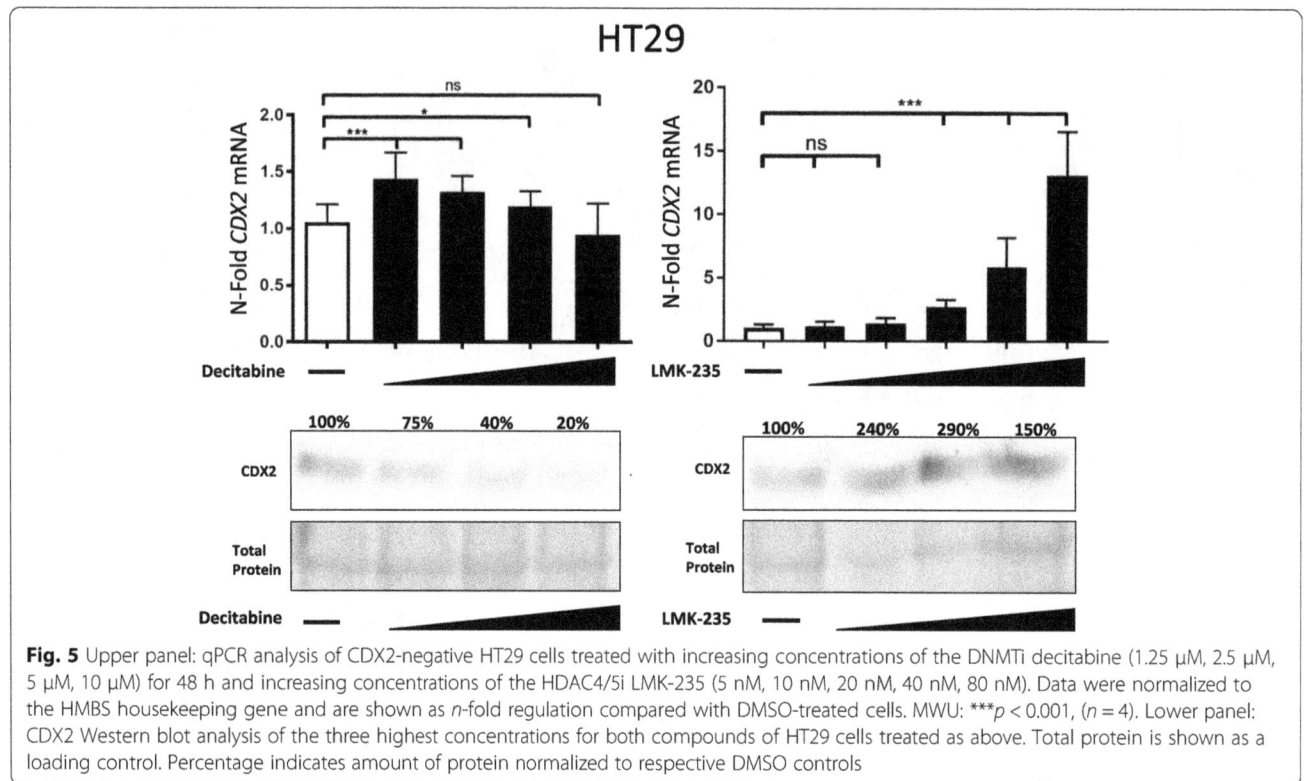

Fig. 5 Upper panel: qPCR analysis of CDX2-negative HT29 cells treated with increasing concentrations of the DNMTi decitabine (1.25 µM, 2.5 µM, 5 µM, 10 µM) for 48 h and increasing concentrations of the HDAC4/5i LMK-235 (5 nM, 10 nM, 20 nM, 40 nM, 80 nM). Data were normalized to the HMBS housekeeping gene and are shown as n-fold regulation compared with DMSO-treated cells. MWU: ***$p < 0.001$, ($n = 4$). Lower panel: CDX2 Western blot analysis of the three highest concentrations for both compounds of HT29 cells treated as above. Total protein is shown as a loading control. Percentage indicates amount of protein normalized to respective DMSO controls

Our group has previously shown that a loss of CDX2 is specific for *BRAF* mutation and for the CIMP-high phenotype and that both MSI and MSS cancers may show loss of CDX2 in this context [9, 10]. Here, we validate these findings by showing a gradual reduction in the percentage of positive cells with single (MSI or $BRAF^{V600E}$) and double (MSI + $BRAF^{V600E}$) alterations, findings that are in line with work from other groups [3, 23, 24]. Since the molecular characteristics of CDX2-negative tumors are predominantly those with *BRAF* mutation, CIMP, and MSI and frequently found in female patients with right-sided tumors, we hypothesized that CDX2 loss could play a functional role in tumors derived from the serrated pathway, a route of CRC development originating from the serrated adenoma. Dhir and colleagues report that CDX2 is lost in high-grade dysplastic areas of sessile serrated adenomas and may occur due to promoter hypermethylation, an observation that is directly in line with our hypothesis in cancers [14]. We therefore investigated hypermethylation as a possible mechanistic reason for the gradual loss of the CDX2 protein.

Of 11 CRC cell lines investigated, we initially selected two low-expressing cell lines (SW620 and COLO205) to evaluate whether mRNA and protein could be re-expressed upon demethylation with a broad DNMTi, decitabine, already used in clinics for treatment of some patients with myelodysplastic syndrome (MDS) and acute myeloid leukemia (AML). Here, we could demonstrate a strong re-expression of CDX2 at mRNA and protein level, thus providing a functional link between promoter methylation and protein. Although restoration of CDX2 has been previously shown for COLO205 [12], reports show that HT29 cells are not induced to express CDX2 at the protein level upon DNMTi treatment [25, 26]. The contribution of DNA promoter hypermethylation to *CDX2* gene silencing seems to vary among different CRC cells possibly reflecting a similar situation in CRC patients.

We next investigated whether HDAC inhibition could help to further restore CDX2 RNA and protein either alone or in combination with decitabine in CRC cells. We hypothesized that the more open state of chromatin coupled to demethylation would have a synergistic or additive effect on restoration of CDX2. We found that combining decitabine with a general HDACi TSA resulted in marked CDX2 induction. However, LMK-235, a specific HDAC4/5 inhibitor, had a considerably more potent effect on CDX2 restoration as compared to TSA, independent of response to decitabine treatment. Highlighting this further, protein expression of CDX2 could be restored in HT29 cells upon LMK-235 treatment, a result that is not seen upon treatment with DNMTi. Furthermore, we found direct recruitment of HDAC5 to the *CDX2* promoter region indicating that this HDAC directly represses *CDX2* gene transcription. Further, studies are needed to investigate if HDAC4 and other HDACs are also involved in repressing *CDX2* gene expression.

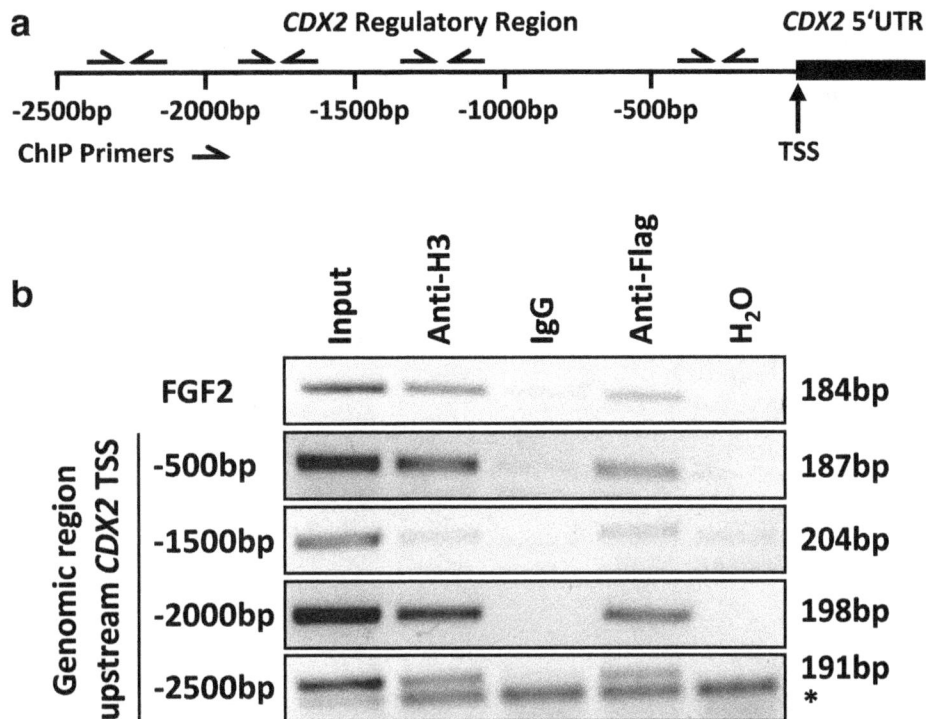

Fig. 6 HDAC5 regulates CDX2 expression by binding to the promoter region of the *CDX2* gene. **a** Schematic representation of the genomic region upstream of the transcriptional start site (TSS) of the *CDX2* gene. ChIP primer locations are indicated by arrows. **b** In vivo binding of HDAC5 to the indicated genomic regions upstream of the *CDX2* TSS was shown by ChIP in 293T cells transfected with FLAG-tagged HDAC5 using antibodies against FLAG. Antibodies against acetyl-histone H3 and mouse IgG were used as positive and negative controls, respectively. Amplification of a genomic region in the *FGF2* gene was shown as a positive control for a genomic region bound by HDAC5. *unspecific PCR band

In human disease, it appears that loss of CDX2 is an early event in the progression of cancers via the serrated pathway [14] [27]. In our study, we can show that methylation of *CDX2* in cancers with the serrated profile have different degrees of hypermethylation that correlate with CDX2 protein in a dose-dependent manner. Few studies have examined methylation of *CDX2*. Wang and colleagues determine that the rate of hypermethylation of *CDX2* is 78.5% in colorectal cancers when compared to a normal population control (43.5%). However, this normal control group was composed of patient with colorectal polyps, likely explaining the high number of hypermethylated cases [27]. CDX2 has on the one hand been described as a tumor suppressor and its loss is associated with development of adenomas in mice [28]. On the other, it is reported as an amplified lineage-survival oncogene, sometimes amplified in CRCs and required for proliferation and survival of CRC cells [29]. Although amplification of *CDX2* was not investigated in this study, future studies may focus on this mechanism as an alternative explanation for the lack of correlation between DNA methylation and protein expression outside of the serrated tumors. Since *CDX2* mRNA (detected by ISH) and protein were so tightly linked in this study, we speculate that post-transcriptional or post-translational modification of CDX2 may play only a minor role in CRC progression.

Conclusion

Our findings underline the independent and adverse prognostic effect of CDX2 and the involvement of epigenetic modifications in the silencing of *CDX2* gene expression, in particular of promoter methylation and histone deacetylation by HDAC4 and HDAC5. These results open a new epigenetic landscape into CDX2, which should be further investigated.

Acknowledgements
Deborah Shan-Krauer is gratefully acknowledged for the excellent technical support. Tissues for cohort 2 were provided by Tissue Bank Bern.

Funding
This study was supported by the Swiss National Science Foundation (31003A_166578/1 to IZ and MPT). The funding body did not play a role in the design of the study and collection, analysis, and interpretation of data and in writing the manuscript

Authors' contributions

JG, KU, EF, IC, ME, and JAG carried out and helped design the experiments. AL, HD, and RL performed the histopathological review. UN, PT, MDB, BS, MH, and DI obtained the clinical data. TR and PS gave critical inputs. MPT and IZ designed the study, oversaw the experiments, performed the statistical evaluation, and wrote and edited the manuscript. All authors approved the final version of the paper.

Author details

[1]Institute of Pathology, University of Bern, Murtenstrasse 31, Room L310, 3008 Bern, Switzerland. [2]Graduate School for Cellular and Biomedical Sciences, University of Bern, Freiestrasse 1, 3012 Bern, Switzerland. [3]Department of Surgery, Klinikum rechts der Isar, Technische Universität München, Ismaninger Strasse 22, Munich 81675, Germany. [4]Careanesth AG, Nelkenstrasse 15, Zürich 8006, Switzerland. [5]Department of Medical Oncology, University Hospital of Bern, 3010 Bern, Switzerland. [6]Division of Medical Oncology, Norris Comprehensive Cancer Center, Keck School of Medicine, University of Southern California, Los Angeles 90033, CA, USA. [7]Department of Visceral and Internal Medicine, University Hospital of Bern, 3008 Bern, Switzerland. [8]University of Bern and Bürgerspital Solothurn, Schöngrünstrasse 42, 4500 Solothurn, Switzerland.

References

1. Lorentz O, Duluc I, Arcangelis AD, Simon-Assmann P, Kedinger M, Freund JN. Key role of the Cdx2 homeobox gene in extracellular matrix-mediated intestinal cell differentiation. J Cell Biol. 1997;139(6):1553–65.
2. Suh E, Chen L, Taylor J, Traber PG. A homeodomain protein related to caudal regulates intestine-specific gene transcription. Mol Cell Biol. 1994; 14(11):7340–51.
3. Baba Y, Nosho K, Shima K, Freed E, Irahara N, Philips J, et al. Relationship of CDX2 loss with molecular features and prognosis in colorectal cancer. Clin Cancer Res. 2009;15(14):4665–73.
4. Bae JM, Lee TH, Cho NY, Kim TY, Kang GH. Loss of CDX2 expression is associated with poor prognosis in colorectal cancer patients. World J Gastroenterol. 2015;21(5):1457–67.
5. Lugli A, Tzankov A, Zlobec I, Terracciano LM. Differential diagnostic and functional role of the multi-marker phenotype CDX2/CK20/CK7 in colorectal cancer stratified by mismatch repair status. Mod Pathol. 2008;21(11):1403–12.
6. Mallo GV, Rechreche H, Frigerio JM, Rocha D, Zweibaum A, Lacasa M, et al. Molecular cloning, sequencing and expression of the mRNA encoding human Cdx1 and Cdx2 homeobox. Down-regulation of Cdx1 and Cdx2 mRNA expression during colorectal carcinogenesis. Int J Cancer. 1997;74(1):35–44.
7. Zhang BY, Jones JC, Briggler AM, Hubbard JM, Kipp BR, Sargent DJ, et al. Lack of caudal-type homeobox transcription factor 2 expression as a prognostic biomarker in metastatic colorectal cancer. Clin Colorectal Cancer. 2017;16(2):124–8.
8. Dalerba P, Sahoo D, Paik S, Guo X, Yothers G, Song N, et al. CDX2 as a prognostic biomarker in stage II and stage III colon cancer. N Engl J Med. 2016;374(3):211–22.
9. Zlobec I, Bihl M, Foerster A, Rufle A, Lugli A. Comprehensive analysis of CpG island methylator phenotype (CIMP)-high, -low, and -negative colorectal cancers based on protein marker expression and molecular features. J Pathol. 2011;225(3):336–43.
10. Dawson H, Koelzer VH, Lukesch AC, Mallaev M, Inderbitzin D, Lugli A, et al. Loss of Cdx2 expression in primary tumors and lymph node metastases is specific for mismatch repair-deficiency in colorectal cancer. Front Oncol. 2013;3:265.
11. Bettington M, Walker N, Clouston A, Brown I, Leggett B, Whitehall V. The serrated pathway to colorectal carcinoma: current concepts and challenges. Histopathology. 2013;62(3):367–86.
12. Hinoi T, Loda M, Fearon ER. Silencing of CDX2 expression in colon cancer via a dominant repression pathway. J Biol Chem. 2003;278(45):44608–16.
13. Guinney J, Dienstmann R, Wang X, de Reynies A, Schlicker A, Soneson C, et al. The consensus molecular subtypes of colorectal cancer. Nat Med. 2015; 21(11):1350–6.
14. Dhir M, Yachida S, Van Neste L, Glockner SC, Jeschke J, Pappou EP, et al. Sessile serrated adenomas and classical adenomas: an epigenetic perspective on premalignant neoplastic lesions of the gastrointestinal tract. Int J Cancer. 2011;129(8):1889–98.
15. Zlobec I, Suter G, Perren A, Lugli A. A next-generation tissue microarray (ngTMA) protocol for biomarker studies. J Vis Exp. 2014;91:51893.
16. Bonora M, Wieckowsk MR, Chinopoulos C, Kepp O, Kroemer G, Galluzzi L, et al. Molecular mechanisms of cell death: central implication of ATP synthase in mitochondrial permeability transition. Oncogene. 2015;34(12):1608.
17. Tschan MP, Fischer KM, Fung VS, Pirnia F, Borner MM, Fey MF, et al. Alternative splicing of the human cyclin D-binding Myb-like protein (hDMP1) yields a truncated protein isoform that alters macrophage differentiation patterns. J Biol Chem. 2003;278(44):42750–60.
18. Urbich C, Rossig L, Kaluza D, Potente M, Boeckel JN, Knau A, et al. HDAC5 is a repressor of angiogenesis and determines the angiogenic gene expression pattern of endothelial cells. Blood. 2009;113(22):5669–79.
19. Dawson H, Galvan JA, Helbling M, Muller DE, Karamitopoulou E, Koelzer VH, et al. Possible role of Cdx2 in the serrated pathway of colorectal cancer characterized by BRAF mutation, high-level CpG Island methylator phenotype and mismatch repair-deficiency. Int J Cancer. 2014;134(10):2342–51.
20. Bankhead P, Loughrey M, Fernandez J, Dombrowski Y, McArt D, Dunne P, et al. QuPath: open source software for digital pathology image analysis. bioRxiv. 2017. https://www.biorxiv.org/content/early/2017/01/12/099796.
21. Perneger TV. What's wrong with Bonferroni adjustments. BMJ. 1998; 316(7139):1236–8.
22. Nolte S, Zlobec I, Lugli A, Hohenberger W, Croner R, Merkel S, et al. Construction and analysis of tissue microarrays in the era of digital pathology: a pilot study targeting CDX1 and CDX2 in a colon cancer cohort of 612 patients. J Pathol Clin Res. 2017;3(1):58–70.
23. Bae JM, Kim JH, Kwak Y, Lee DW, Cha Y, Wen X, et al. Distinct clinical outcomes of two CIMP-positive colorectal cancer subtypes based on a revised CIMP classification system. Br J Cancer. 2017;116(8):1012–20.
24. Kim JH, Rhee YY, Bae JM, Cho NY, Kang GH. Loss of CDX2/CK20 expression is associated with poorly differentiated carcinoma, the CpG island methylator phenotype, and adverse prognosis in microsatellite-unstable colorectal cancer. Am J Surg Pathol. 2013;37(10):1532–41.
25. Zhang JF, Zhang JG, Kuai XL, Zhang H, Jiang W, Ding WF, et al. Reactivation of the homeotic tumor suppressor gene CDX2 by 5-aza-2'-deoxycytidine-induced demethylation inhibits cell proliferation and induces caspase-independent apoptosis in gastric cancer cells. Exp Ther Med. 2013;5(3):735–41.
26. Hatano Y, Semi K, Hashimoto K, Lee MS, Hirata A, Tomita H, et al. Reducing DNA methylation suppresses colon carcinogenesis by inducing tumor cell differentiation. Carcinogenesis. 2015;36(7):719–29.
27. Sakamoto N, Feng Y, Stolfi C, Kurosu Y, Green M, Lin J, et al. BRAFV600E cooperates with CDX2 inactivation to promote serrated colorectal tumorigenesis. elife. 2017;10:6.
28. Chawengsaksophak K, James R, Hammond VE, Kontgen F, Beck F. Homeosis and intestinal tumours in Cdx2 mutant mice. Nature. 1997;386(6620):84–7.
29. Salari K, Spulak ME, Cuff J, Forster AD, Giacomini CP, Huang S, et al. CDX2 is an amplified lineage-survival oncogene in colorectal cancer. Proc Natl Acad Sci U S A. 2012;109(46):E3196–205.

Epigenetic signature of preterm birth in adult twins

Qihua Tan[1,2]* iD, Shuxia Li[2], Morten Frost[3], Marianne Nygaard[1], Mette Soerensen[1], Martin Larsen[2,4], Kaare Christensen[1,2] and Lene Christiansen[1]

Abstract

Background: Preterm birth is a leading cause of perinatal mortality and long-term health consequences. Epigenetic mechanisms may have been at play in preterm birth survivors, and these could be persistent and detrimental to health later in life.

Methods: We performed a genome-wide DNA methylation profiling in adult twins of premature birth to identify genomic regions under differential epigenetic regulation in 144 twins with a median age of 33 years (age range 30–36).

Results: Association analysis detected three genomic regions annotated to the *SDHAP3*, *TAGLN3* and *GSTT1* genes on chromosomes 5, 3 and 22 (FWER: 0.01, 0.02 and 0.04) respectively. These genes display strong involvement in neurodevelopmental disorders, cancer susceptibility and premature delivery. The three identified significant regions were successfully replicated in an independent sample of twins of even older age (median age 66, range 56–80) with similar regulatory patterns and nominal *p* values < 5.05e−04. Biological pathway analysis detected five significantly enriched pathways all explicitly involved in immune responses.

Conclusion: We have found novel evidence associating premature delivery with epigenetic modification of important genes/pathways and revealed that preterm birth, as an early life event, could be related to differential methylation regulation patterns observable in adults and even at high ages which could potentially mediate susceptibility to age-related diseases and adult health.

Keywords: Preterm birth, Twins, Epigenetics, Epigenome-wide association study, Adults

Background

Preterm birth (PTB) or premature birth is defined as birth before 37 weeks of pregnancy. With a prevalence estimated from 5 to 18% in singleton pregnancies across 184 countries according to the World Health Organization and over 50% in twin pregnancies in the USA [1], PTB is a leading cause of perinatal mortality as well as long-term morbidity and health consequences. Survivors of PTB were subject to adaptive mechanisms that might be deleterious later in life, and are more susceptible to early on-set chronic diseases [2] including cardiovascular disease [3], metabolic disorders [4], respiratory complications [5] and mental and cognitive impairments [6]. Despite the strong epidemiological evidence, the molecular mechanisms and etiology behind these phenotypes have been poorly understood. Preterm infants are exposed to various stressful conditions in the peridelivery period, a critical stage for their organ development. Molecular mechanisms including epigenetic modification may have been involved in the adaptation to adverse environment which, in the long-run, could be detrimental to health [7–9]. It has been hypothesized that epigenetic modifications such as DNA methylation induced by PTB may lead to long-term consequences and increased susceptibility to adult-onset diseases [10–12].

Advantaged by the emerging new technology in genomic analysis of DNA methylation, epigenome-wide association studies (EWAS) have been done to look for DNA methylation markers of PTB in neonates [13–16] and have reported differentially methylated sites implicated in neural function [16], or with increased risk for adverse

* Correspondence: qtan@health.sdu.dk
[1]Epidemiology and Biostatistics, Department of Public Health, Faculty of Health Science, University of Southern Denmark, J. B. Winsløws Vej 9B, DK-5000 Odense, Denmark
[2]Unit of Human Genetics, Department of Clinical Research, University of Southern Denmark, Odense, Denmark
Full list of author information is available at the end of the article

health outcomes later in life [13]. Notably, PTB-associated methylation patterns were also investigated in adolescents by Cruickshank et al. [14] and Simpkin et al. [15] in their longitudinal samples. Although relatively large numbers of CpG sites were found significantly differentially methylated in association with PTB at birth, they are largely resolved in adolescents in both studies. Nevertheless, persistent methylation differences were identified at ten CpG sites in the study by Cruickshank et al. [14] reflecting a lasting epigenetic effect of PTB.

The fact that PTB is associated with an increased risk of chronic diseases in adults suggests that it is of high importance to focus on the epigenetic signature of PTB that mediates the long-term health consequences. Given the high prevalence of PTB in twin pregnancies, epigenetic analysis of PTB in twins is therefore especially important and valuable for the health of the twin population and for the general population as well. Using relatively large numbers of adult twin samples for discovery (144 twins) and replication (350 twins), we conducted an epigenomic profiling of the DNA methylome to look for genomic sites and regions under epigenetic regulation in association with PTB in adult subjects.

Methods
The discovery samples
The discovery samples in this study consisted of 72 pairs of identical twins (144 individuals, 78 males and 66 females) aged 30 to 36 years with a median age of 33 (Table 1). Gestational ages were collected from the Danish Medical Birth Registry (DMBR) established in 1973. The median of gestational age was 39 weeks with a minimum of 33 and a maximum of 42 weeks. A total of 26 twins had their gestational ages < 37 weeks. The samples formed a subset (those born after 1973 when gestational age was

recorded by DMBR) of 150 pairs of identical twins discordant for birthweight used in an EWAS by Tan et al. [17]. Figure 1 displays the samples by plotting individual gestational age against birthweight. There is a moderate correlation of 0.52 between gestational age (PTB indicated by empty spots) and birthweight. Although no significant association was found between birthweight and DNA methylation [17], we adjusted for individual birthweight in all our analyses.

Blood sampling and DNA extraction
Blood sampling and DNA preparation were described by Tan et al. [17]. In brief, ethylene di-amine tetra acetic acid (EDTA)-anticoagulated blood samples were collected. The blood was centrifuged at $1000g$ for 10 min, and buffy-coat was frozen in aliquots at − 80 °C. DNA was isolated from the buffy-coats using the salt precipitation method applying either a manual protocol or a semi-automated protocol based on the Autopure System (Qiagen, Hilden, Germany). Bisulphite treatment of 500 ng template genomic DNA was carried out with the EZ-96 DNA methylation kit (Zymo Research, Orange County, USA) following the manufacturer's protocol.

DNA methylation data
Genome-wide DNA methylation was analysed using the Illumina Infinium HumanMethylation450 Beadchip assay (Illumina, San Diego, CA, USA) at Leiden University Medical Center or at GenomeScan B.V., Leiden, The Netherlands. The array interrogates more than 485,000 CpG sites across and beyond gene and CpG island regions in the human genome. The laboratory experiment was conducted according to the array manufacturer's

Table 1 Descriptive statistics for the discovery and replication samples

Variables	Discovery	Replication
Age, year		
Median	33	66
Range	30–36	56–80
Gestational age, week		
Median	39	0 (weeks before term)
Range	33–42	0–8 (weeks before term)
Report method	DMBR	Midwife
Sample size		
Male	78	192
Female	66	158
Total	144	350
PTB	26	40 (more than 3 weeks before term)

DMBR Danish Medical Birth Registry

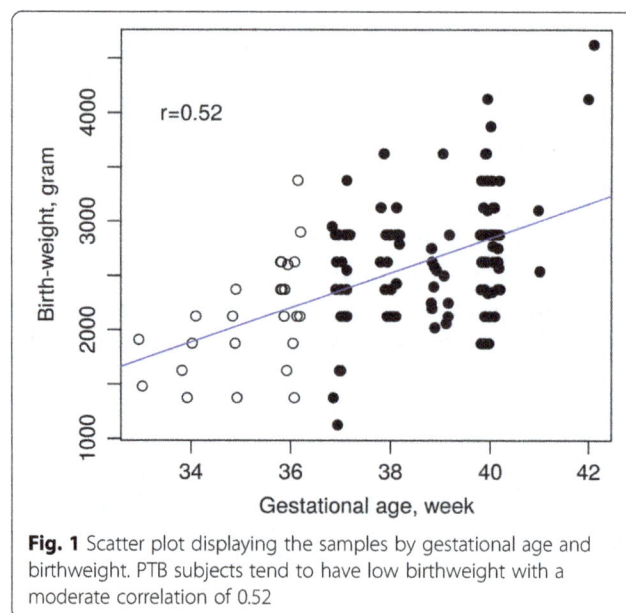

Fig. 1 Scatter plot displaying the samples by gestational age and birthweight. PTB subjects tend to have low birthweight with a moderate correlation of 0.52

instructions. Twins of each pair were processed together on the same array to minimize batch effect. The quality of DNA methylation data was controlled by calculating a detection p value defined as the proportion of samples reporting background signal levels for both methylated and unmethylated channels. The detection p was calculated using the free R package *minfi* (http://bioconductor.org/packages/release/bioc/html/minfi.html). Probes with detection $p > 0.05$ were dropped from subsequent analysis. In addition, we also removed CpG probes harbouring SNPs considering potential disruption on their methylation levels by heterozygous SNPs. As usual, we also dropped methylation data on sex chromosomes to focus on autosomal CpG sites. A total of 473,864 CpGs were available for subsequent analysis. Data normalization was done using the subset-quantile within-array normalization (SWAN) [18] implemented in *minfi*. At each CpG site, the DNA methylation level was summarized by calculating a "beta" value defined by the Illumina's formula as $\beta = M/(M + U + 100)$, where M and U are methylated (M) and unmethylated (U) signal intensities measured at the CpG site. We further removed CpGs with $\beta < 0.05$ [19] leaving 427,555 CpGs for statistical analysis. Both raw and processed DNA methylation data for the discovery samples have been deposited to the NCBI GEO database (http://www.ncbi.nlm.nih.gov/geo) under accession number GSE61496.

The replication samples

The replication sample was comprised of 175 pairs of identical twins (350 individuals, 192 males and 158 females) aged 56 to 80 years with a median age of 66 (Table 1). The estimated weeks before term birth were provided by midwives with a range from 0 to 8 weeks. Preterm birth was defined as birth at least 3 weeks before term. A total of 40 twins were found as preterm births. Blood sampling, DNA extraction and methylation analysis were performed as described for the discovery samples. The methylation data were also normalized using the Subset-quantile Within Array Normalization (SWAN) [18]. Methylation "beta" values were likewise calculated using the Illumina's formula.

Estimating and adjusting cell composition

Cell composition in whole blood can change with age. Although the age range of our discovery samples was relatively short, that of the replication samples was 24 years (Table 1). For the discovery samples, we controlled for this issue by estimating and correcting for cell composition in each individual. We estimated cell composition for six blood cell types: CD8T, CD4T, natural killer cell, B cell, monocyte and granulocyte based on our measured DNA methylation data from whole blood using an approach proposed by Houseman et al. [20], using the R package *minfi*. For the replication samples,

blood leukocyte subtypes (monocytes, lymphocytes, basophils, neutrophils and eosinophiles), counted using a Coulter LH 750 Haematology Analyser, were available. Missing blood cell counts were imputed by a modified version of the method supplied by PredictCellComposition (www.github.com/mvaniterson/predictcellcomposition). The effect of cell composition was then adjusted for by including the estimated proportion of each cell type as covariates in the regression analyses.

Data analysis

The association between DNA methylation and PTB was investigated on both single CpGs and genomic regions through fitting linear models that regressed the level of DNA methylation on PTB status adjusting for sex, birthweight and cell compositions. Before fitting the models, DNA methylation β-values were transformed into M values using logit transformation to ensure normal or approximately normal distribution.

Single-CpG-based analysis

We applied a linear regression model with a robust sandwich variance estimator to regress the methylation M values on PTB status (preterm coded as 1 and term coded as 0), sex, birthweight and estimated cell compositions. The sandwich variance estimator was introduced to take into accounts the intra-pair twin correlation on DNA methylation. By estimating and testing the regression coefficient for PTB, we were interested in identifying differentially methylated CpG probes (DMPs) of PTB. The model was fitted using the *clubSandwich* package in R (https://cran.r-project.org/web/packages/clubSandwich). P values were adjusted for multiple testing by calculating the false discovery rate [21] (FDR) with genome-wide significance defined as FDR < 0.05.

Multiple-CpG-based analysis

On top of the single-CpG-based analysis, we further extended our analysis to multiple CpGs to look for differentially methylated genomic regions (DMRs) in association with PTB. This was done using the bumphunter approach introduced by Jaffe et al. [22] implemented in the R package *minfi*. The methylation M values were first regressed on sex, birthweight and estimated cell compositions. The residuals from the regression and PTB status were then submitted to the *bumphunter()* function in *minfi*. The approach assumes that the locus-specific estimates of regression coefficients (βs) are smooth along the strand of a chromosome and applies the loess smoothing technique to smooth coefficient βs within a pre-defined chromosomal region (300 base pairs in our analysis). After smoothing, the 99th percentile of the smoothed βs can be calculated to obtain upper and lower thresholds. These thresholds are then used to define hyper- or hypo-methylated DMRs with smoothed peaks above or below the thresholds. For each DMR identified, a sum statistic is calculated by taking the sum of the absolute values of all the smoothed βs within that region. The sum statistic is then used to rank all DMRs with the top-most important DMR having the highest sum statistic value. Statistical significance of the DMRs is assessed by computer permutation (we set 1000 replications) in combination with correction for multiple testing to obtain family-wised error rate (FWER) [22].

Biological pathway analysis

Advantaged by the multiple-CpG-based analysis that outputs genomic locations of the identified DMRs, biological pathway analysis was conducted by submitting the chromosomal coordinates of the detected DMRs to the Genomic Regions Enrichment of Annotations Tool (GREAT) at http://bejerano.stanford.edu/great/public/html/ to analyse the functional significance of *cis*-regulatory regions identified by localized measurements of DNA binding events across an entire genome [23] using the Genome Reference Consortium Human Build 37 (GRCh37) as the RefSeq database. GREAT incorporates annotations from 20 ontologies and associates genomic regions with genes by defining a 'regulatory domain' for each gene such that all non-coding sequences that lie within the regulatory domain are assumed to regulate that gene. The 'two nearest genes' was assigned as the association rule from genomic regions to genes, which extends each gene's regulatory domain from its transcription start site (TSS) to the nearest upstream and downstream TSS, up to 1 MB in each direction. Both the binomial test over genomic regions and the hypergeometric test over genes were performed to provide an accurate picture of annotation enrichments [23].

Genomic plotting

Visualization and annotation of genomic segments hosting regions under differential methylation were realized by integrative plotting using R package Gviz [24]. Information on genomic annotation was taken from the UCSC hg19 assembly.

Results

Discovery EWAS

We first performed an EWAS on the 144 discovery samples using regression analysis on each of the 473,864 CpGs after filtering, measured using the Illumina Infinium HumanMethylation450 Beadchip assay (see the 'Methods' section for details). From the volcano plot (Fig. 2) and Manhattan plot (Additional file 1: Figure S1), it can be seen that no CpG reached genome-wide significance level of FDR < 0.05 for the effect of PTB (Additional file 2: Table S1). We continued our discovery

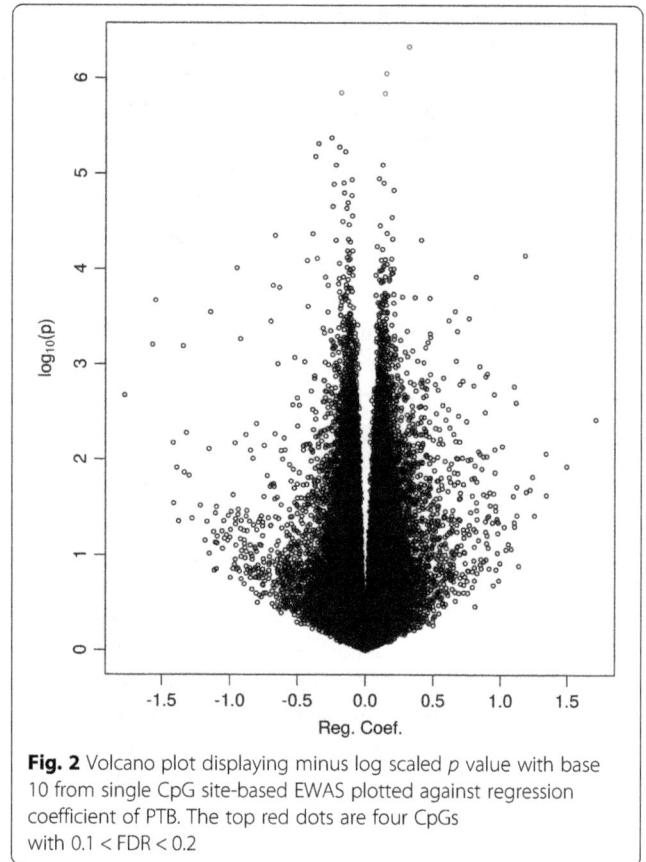

Fig. 2 Volcano plot displaying minus log scaled *p* value with base 10 from single CpG site-based EWAS plotted against regression coefficient of PTB. The top red dots are four CpGs with 0.1 < FDR < 0.2

EWAS by performing genomic region-based analysis using the *bumphunter* function in the free R package *minfi* (see the 'Methods' section for detail). By focusing on regions with a mean methylation difference of over 10% between PTB and term births, we found a list of 16,508 regions (Additional file 3: Figure S2) and among them 2651 regions with *p* value < 0.05 (Additional file 4: Table S2). Table 2 shows the top six regions with FWER < 0.1, three of them with FWER < 0.05. Among the top three DMRs, the most significant was annotated to the promotor region of *SDHAP3* gene on chromosome 5 at p15.33 exhibiting a clear pattern of hypomethylation (Figs. 3a and 4a); the second most significant DMR was hypermethylated in the gene body (second or third intron) of *TAGLN3* on chromosome 3 at q13.2 (Figs. 3b and 4b); and the third DMR was hypermethylated in the promotor region of the GSTT1 gene on chromosome 22 at q11.23 (Figs. 3c and 4c). Of the three less significant DMRs with FWER < 0.1, two were hypomethylated in the promotor region of the *DUSP22* and *NFYA/LOC221442* genes on chromosome 6 (Fig. 5a, b), and one was hypermethylated in the promotor of *mir886* on chromosome 5 (Fig. 5c). In Additional file 5: Table S3, we show the detailed information on statistical estimate and biological annotations for single CpGs in each of the DMRs in Figs. 3, 4 and 5 (Table 2). CpGs in each DMR

Table 2 Characterizations of the six identified DMRs with FWER < 0.1

DMR	Chr	Start	End	Discovery			Replication		Linked genes	Gene region	Location to CGI
				Value	p value	FWER	Value	p value			
1	5	1,594,282	1,594,863	− 0.505	4.46E−07	0.01	− 0.157	1.90E−04	SDHAP3	Body, TSS200, TSS1500	Island
2	3	111,730,545	111,730,545	1.571	7.92E−07	0.02	0.891	8.88E−05	TAGLN3	Body	NA
3	22	24,384,159	24,384,573	0.455	2.28E−06	0.04	0.184	5.03E−04	GSTT1	1stExon, 5'UTR, TSS200	Island
4	6	291,687	292,596	− 0.453	4.26E−06	0.08	0.311	2.55E−05	DUSP22	1stExon, 5'UTR, TSS200, TSS1500	Island, N-Shore
5	6	41,068,646	41,068,752	− 0.512	4.46E−06	0.08	0.382	1.70E−05	NFYA, LOC221442	3'UTR	Island
6	5	135,415,258	135,416,613	0.271	4.90E−06	0.10	0.197	8.68E−06	MIR886	Body, TSS200, TSS1500	Island, N-Shore, S-Shore

show similar direction of effect and tend to have low nominal p values that may, however, not reach statistical significance individually.

Functional analysis of significant DMRs

To study the biological functions of the 2651 regions with $p < 0.05$ (Additiona file 5: Table S2), we used the online annotation tool GREAT (see the 'Methods' section) for exploring the *cis* regulatory regions of nearby genes, making use of the Molecular Signatures Database (MSigDB) which is one of the most widely used and comprehensive databases of gene sets for performing gene set enrichment analysis. The analysis identified five MSigDB pathways, all involved in immune responses

(Table 3). Both the binomial test over genomic regions and the hypergeometric test over genes showed very high significance for the five pathways as indicated by their FDRs (FDR < 8.13e−28 for binomial test; FDR < 9.37e−03 for hypergeometric test).

Replication of top significant DMRs

Using the old twin samples, we performed independent replication analysis of the six DMRs in Table 2. For each DMR, the same set of CpGs as in the discovery stage was selected according to genomic location. Differential methylation between PTB and term birth replication samples was estimated in the same manner as for the discovery analysis (adjusting for age, sex and cell

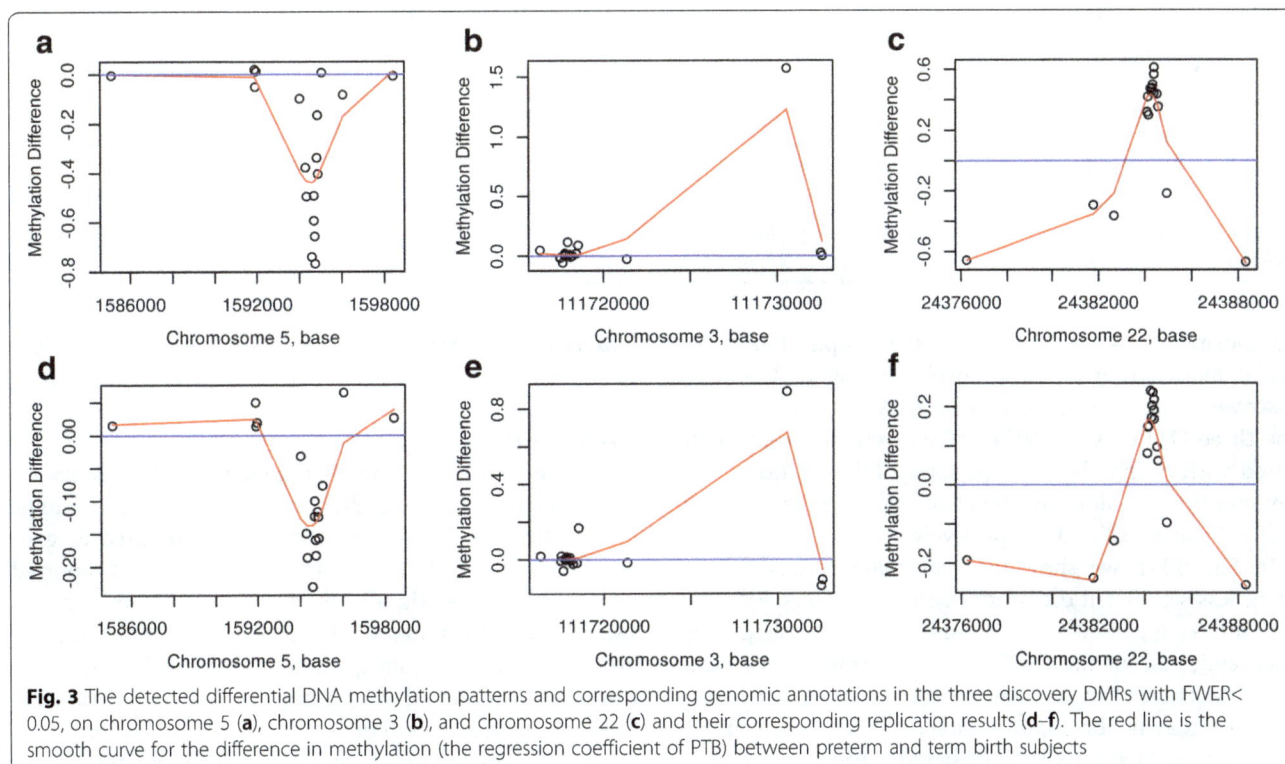

Fig. 3 The detected differential DNA methylation patterns and corresponding genomic annotations in the three discovery DMRs with FWER< 0.05, on chromosome 5 (**a**), chromosome 3 (**b**), and chromosome 22 (**c**) and their corresponding replication results (**d–f**). The red line is the smooth curve for the difference in methylation (the regression coefficient of PTB) between preterm and term birth subjects

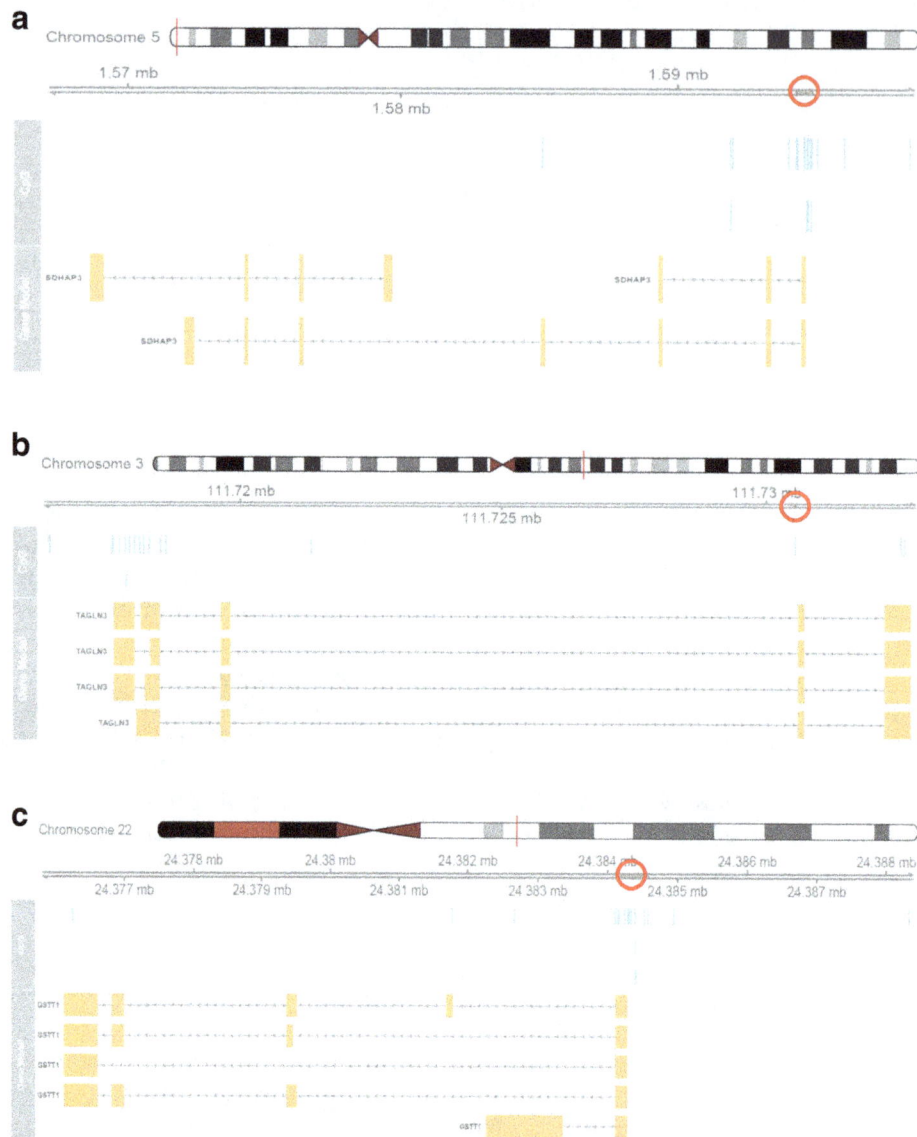

Fig. 4 Genomic regions hosting the significant discovery DMRs (indicated by the red circles) on chromosomes 5 (**a**), 3 (**b**) and 22 (**c**) plotted against the CpG sites in Fig. 3 and corresponding gene annotations

composition). Figure 3d–f displays the replicated differential methylation patterns corresponding to the three discovery-stage DMRs in Fig. 3a–c. As shown in Fig. 3, the three DMRs with FWER < 0.05 were all nicely replicated with nearly the same patterns. Table 2 shows very low nominal p values for the replication DMRs: 1.9e–04, 8.88e–05 and 5.03e–04 respectively.

In Fig. 5d–f, we show the replication results for the three less significant discovery DMRs with 0.05 < FWER < 0.1. Interestingly, although a similar methylation pattern was replicated for the DMR on chromosome 5, the other two DMRs on chromosome 6 were replicated with again similar patterns but opposite directions. The corresponding patterns in the replication samples were not random

patterns considering their very low nominal p values (2.55e–05, 1.7e–05 and 8.68e–06 respectively) (Table 2).

Discussion

We have performed the first genome-wide association study on the epigenetic effect of preterm birth in adults. Cruickshank et al. [14] investigated PTB-related epigenetic changes at birth and at 18 years of age and reported no genome-wide significant finding in their samples from 18-year-olds. Likewise, our analysis did not identify any CpG sites reaching genome-wide significance in the discovery samples of young adults. The highly valuable findings in this study come from genomic region-based association analysis that jointly tested the association of

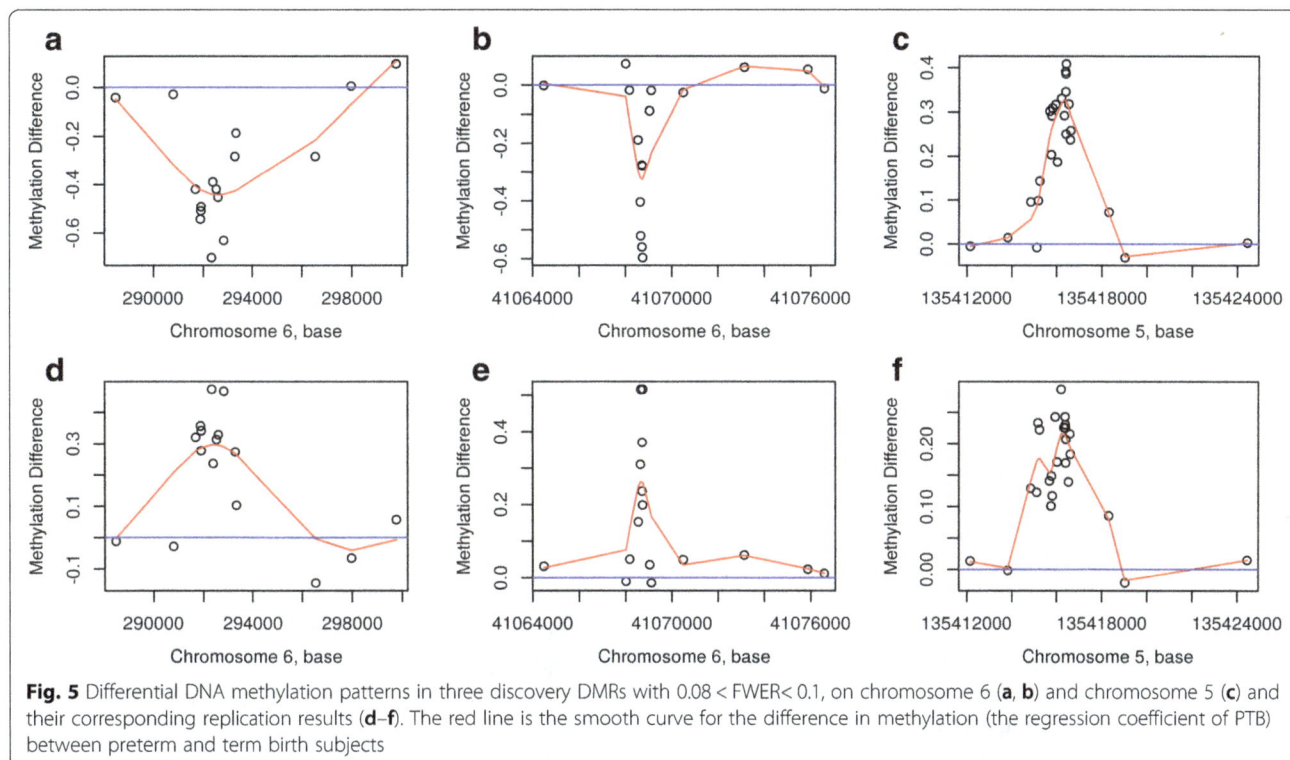

Fig. 5 Differential DNA methylation patterns in three discovery DMRs with 0.08 < FWER< 0.1, on chromosome 6 (**a**, **b**) and chromosome 5 (**c**) and their corresponding replication results (**d–f**). The red line is the smooth curve for the difference in methylation (the regression coefficient of PTB) between preterm and term birth subjects

groups of adjacent CpGs that form DMRs. As shown in Table 2, multiple genomic regions were found as differentially methylated in association with PTB. The results indicate that, as an early life event, PTB could impose differential epigenetic patterns that can be detected in the DNA methylome of adult subjects in their thirties as in the discovery samples and even at old ages as in the replication samples.

Among the genes linked to the most significant DMRs in Table 2, *SDHAP3* has very recently been implicated in smoking, as significantly decreased methylation at the CpG island within the promoter region of *SDHAP3* on chromosome 5 was reported in smoking-exposed foetuses [25]. The PTB associated methylation pattern as shown in Figs. 3a and 4a points to the same direction and genomic location although maternal smoking information is not available in our study. A differential DNA

methylation pattern was also found in *SDHAP3* when comparing autistic brains and control [26]. The second most significant DMR is in the gene body of *TAGLN3* (Fig. 4b). This gene (also known as NP22, encoding a novel cytoskeleton-associated protein) is differentially expressed in human alcoholic brain [27] and in the anterior cingulate cortex of schizophrenia [28].

Perhaps, the most interesting DMR found in this study is the third DMR in Table 2. This DMR sits in the promotor region of *GSTT1* (glutathione *S*-transferases gene theta 1) on chromosome 22 (Fig. 4c). Polymorphisms in the *GST* genes are partially responsible for the variability in *GST* enzymatic activity across individuals. Maternal genetic variations (the null genotype or homozygous deletion) in *GSTT1* have been intensively associated with an increased risk of preterm delivery and low birthweight, alone [29, 30] or in combination with smoking

Table 3 MSigDB Pathways enriched by DMRs with nominal $p < 0.05$ from GREAT analysis

Binomial model						Hypergeometric model					
Term Name	Raw*p* value	*FDR*	Fold enrichment	Exp.	Obs. Gene Hits	Raw*p* value	*FDR*	Fold enrichment	Exp.	Obs.Gene Hits	TotalGenes
Antigen processing and presentation	1.33e−55	1.76e−52	12.28	6.27	77	3.55e−5	9.37e−3	2.10	13.79	29	80
Graft-versus-host disease	5.65e−53	3.73e−50	14.46	4.63	67	2.17e−6	9.56e−4	2.98	6.38	19	37
Type I diabetes mellitus	1.52e−50	6.72e−48	10.20	7.65	78	1.24e-7	1.63e−4	3.11	7.07	22	41
Allograft rejection	7.25e−50	2.40e−47	12.55	5.42	68	7.10e-7	4.69e−4	3.15	6.03	19	35
Viral myocarditis	4.92e−30	8.13e−28	5.13	15.02	77	9.64e-6	3.18e−3	2.30	11.72	27	68

[31–33]. The interaction between *GSTs* and smoking shows the involvement of epigenetic mechanism that links maternal behaviour and genetic susceptibility in contributing to adverse pregnancy outcomes. The association between *GST* genetic variation and PTB has been observed not only in the mother but also in the child [34]. In fact, Bustamante et al. [35] found that the child genotype is responsible for the effect after adjusting for maternal genotype. As our observation is based on PTB adults, our result is in line with their conclusion but from an epigenetic perspective. Most importantly, the latter suggests that environmental factors could also be involved in the association between *GSTT1* and PTB through the epigenetic mechanism. Taken together, both genetic and epigenetic variations in the child can be associated with PTB. The coherence between genetics and epigenetics here is sensible because DNA methylation at the promotor region turns the gene off, which is equivalent to a deletion or the null genotype of the gene.

As an extra effort, we explored the transcriptional profiles of the genes linked to significant DMRs. Gene expression data on two genes, *TAGLN3* and *GSTT1*, were available from the Agilent Human Gene Expression Microarray (v3) applied to the same discovery samples. After adjusting for covariates, no expression difference was found for *TAGLN3* between term birth and PTB ($p = 0.639$) while a borderline significance ($p = 0.059$) for the down-expression of *GSTT1* in PTB (Additional file 6: Figure S3). Although the expression of *GSTT1* can also be regulated by other mechanisms or influenced by deletion of the gene in PTB subjects, the reduced expression level in PTB group provides alternative evidence in support of DNA methylation analysis.

Among the three less significant DMRs in Table 2, the last one on chromosome 5 is replicated by a similar pattern in the old twins (Fig. 5f). The CpGs in this region are hypermethylated in the promotor region and gene body of *mir886*, a noncoding RNA repressed in cancer [36, 37]. The two DMRs on chromosome 6 display significant patterns (p values 2.55e–05 and 1.70e–05) in the replication samples but with opposite directions as compared to the discovery DMRs (hypomethylation in the discovery samples, and hypermethylation in the replication samples) which could possibly suggest age-dependent effects. The DMR located on chromosome 6 from bp 291,687 to 292,596 covers the promotor region of the *DUSP22* gene. Epigenetic alteration of this gene has been shown to mediate Alzheimer's disease [38] and dementia [39]. Interestingly, hypomethylation of the *DUSP22* promotor has been reported to correlate with duration of service in firefighters [40]. The observed epigenetic modification could result from exposure to complex mixtures of toxic substances from burning and overheated materials. Although the smoking status of mothers of our twins is not

available, the finding among the firefighters could resemble smoking-exposed foetuses. The DMR located from bp 41,068,646 to 41,068,752 on chromosome 6 is at the 3′ UTR of the *NFYA* (nuclear transcription factor Y) gene. As a transcription factor, *NFYA* binds to the CAAT box in promotors of many genes in eukaryotes and functions as a regulator of their overexpression in several types of cancer [41]. Note that the same gene has been found to be persistently hypermethylated by PTB in an epigenome-wide association study on both newborn and 18-year-old samples [14]. In brief, the genes covered by these less significant DMRs are implicated in neurodegenerative disorders and risk of cancer as well.

PTB newborns have immature immune systems with reduced innate and adaptive immune function [42]. It is interesting to see that four of the five pathways in Table 3 overlap with pathways deduced from genes linked to CpGs showing significant correlation in maternal and PTB fetal methylation [43], and that all the five pathways appeared in the enriched functional pathways from genes with copy number variations in common miscarriage [44]. Results from our biological pathway analysis reconfirm the importance of the immune system in PTB but in adult samples. Meanwhile the overlap in biological pathways could also suggest the broad involvement of immunity in labour complications in general. Most importantly, the immune implication of PTB could persist into adult life and even old ages. The high involvement of the immune system in PTB as revealed by region-based analysis can also be seen from the Manhattan plot for DMRs (Additional file 3: Figure S2) when compared with the Manhattan plot for single-CpG sites (Additional file 1: Figure S1). The former displays a clearer enrichment pattern of DMRs in the major histocompatibility complex (MHC) region on chromosome 6.

The fact that the significant DMRs were identified and replicated in independent and much older samples has a twofold significance. First, it reveals functional genes differentially regulated in association with PTB through epigenetic mechanism; the latter could serve to link PTB with maternal environmental exposure or lifestyle factors to provide clue for prevention of PTB. Second, and also most importantly, the altered DNA methylation patterns observed in our discovery young adults persist in old subjects of up to 80 years of age, suggesting that some of the PTB-associated epigenetic modifications can be long-lasting or perhaps persistent throughout the entire life. In summary, our genomic region-based analysis of the DNA methylome identified epigenetic fingerprints of premature birth in young adult subjects, consistently replicable in old adults. Functional annotation of the significant methylation patterns associated with PTB revealed genes involved in adverse pregnancy outcomes, in neurodevelopmental disorders and in cancer susceptibility, providing epigenetic evidence of long-term effects of early life events in support of the developmental origin of disease and health.

Finally, it should be kept in mind that our significant findings are based on twins. Even though findings from this study are highly relevant to PTB in general (e.g. the *GSTT1* gene), generalization of our results should be done with caution because the aetiology of PTB in twins could involve risk factors specific for twin pregnancies [45], such as uterine overdistention [46]. Further replication studies using twin and non-twin samples are warranted for validation, justification and generalization of our findings.

Conclusions

This study provides novel evidence for PTB-associated epigenetic regulation in important genes/pathways and meanwhile reveals that premature delivery, as an early life event, could be related to differential methylation regulation patterns observable in adults and even at high ages which could potentially mediate susceptibility to age-related diseases and adult health.

Abbreviations

CpG: Cytosine-phosphate-guanine; DMBR: Danish medical birth registry; DMP: Differentially methylated probe; DMR: Differentially methylated region; EDTA: Ethylene di-amine tetra acetic acid; EWAS: Epigenome-wide association study; FDR: False discovery rate; FWER: Family-wise error rate; GREAT: Genomic Regions Enrichment of Annotations Tool; MHC: Major histocompatibility complex; MSigDB: Molecular Signatures Database; SWAN: Subset-quantile Within Array Normalization; TSS: Transcription start site(s)

Acknowledgements

This study was supported by the Integrated research on Developmental determinants of Aging and Longevity (IDEAL), EU's FP7 project number: 259679 and by the DFF research project 1 from the Danish Council for Independent Research, Medical Sciences (DFF-FSS), project number: DFF – 6110-00114. The work of Shuxia Li was jointly supported by the Velux Foundation research grant number 000121540 and Novo Nordisk Foundation Medical and Natural Sciences Research Grant [grant number NNF13OC0007493].

Authors' contributions

QT, LC, KC and MF contributed to the conception and design. SL, QT, LC, MN, MS and ML contributed to the analysis and interpretation. QT and SL contributed to the drafting of the manuscript. All authors read and approved the final manuscript.

Competing interests

The authors declare that they have no competing interests in this work.

Author details

[1]Epidemiology and Biostatistics, Department of Public Health, Faculty of Health Science, University of Southern Denmark, J. B. Winsløws Vej 9B, DK-5000 Odense, Denmark. [2]Unit of Human Genetics, Department of Clinical Research, University of Southern Denmark, Odense, Denmark. [3]Department of Endocrinology, Odense University Hospital, Odense, Denmark. [4]Department of Clinical Genetics, Odense University Hospital, Odense, Denmark.

References

1. Chauhan SP, Scardo JA, Hayes E, Abuhamad AZ, Berghella V. Twins: prevalence, problems, and preterm births. Am J Obstet Gynecol. 2010; 203(4):305–15.
2. Luu TM, Katz SL, Leeson P, Thébaud B, Nuyt AM. Preterm birth: risk factor for early-onset chronic diseases. CMAJ. 2016;188:736–46.
3. Kerkhof GF, Breukhoven PE, Leunissen RW, Willemsen RH, Hokken-Koelega AC. Does preterm birth influence cardiovascular risk in early adulthood? J Pediatr. 2012;161:390–6.
4. Parkinson JR, Hyde MJ, Gale C, Santhakumaran S, Modi N. Preterm birth and the metabolic syndrome in adult life: a systematic review and meta-analysis. Pediatrics. 2013;131(4):e1240–63.
5. Fraser J, Walls M, McGuire W. Respiratory complications of preterm birth. BMJ. 2004;329:962–5.
6. Abbott A. Babies are increasingly surviving premature birth—but researchers are only beginning to understand the lasting consequences for their mental development. Nature. 2015;518:24–6.
7. Perera F, Herbstman J. Prenatal environmental exposures, epigenetics, and disease. Reprod Toxicol. 2011;31:363–73.
8. Ventura-Junca R, Herrera LM. Epigenetic alterations related to early-life stressful events. Acta Neuropsychiatr. 2012;24:255–65.
9. Vaiserman AM. Epigenetic programming by early-life stress: evidence from human populations. Dev Dyn. 2015;244:254–65.
10. Menon R, Conneely KN, Smith AK. DNA methylation: an epigenetic risk factor in preterm birth. Reprod Sci. 2012;19(1):6–13.
11. Maddalena P. Long term outcomes of preterm birth: the role of epigenetics. Newborn Infant Nurs Rev. 2013;13:137–9.
12. Parets SE, Bedient CE, Menon R, Smith AK. Preterm birth and its long-term effects: methylation to mechanisms. Biology (Basel). 2014;3:498–513.
13. Schroeder JW, Conneely KN, Cubells JC, Kilaru V, Newport DJ, Knight BT, Stowe ZN, Brennan PA, Krushkal J, Tylavsky FA, Taylor RN, Adkins RM, Smith

AK. Neonatal DNA methylation patterns associate with gestational age. Epigenetics. 2011;6:1498–504.

14. Cruickshank MN, Oshlack A, Theda C, Davis PG, Martino D, Sheehan P, Dai Y, Saffery R, Doyle LW, Craig JM. Analysis of epigenetic changes in survivors of preterm birth reveals the effect of gestational age and evidence for a long-term legacy. Genome Med. 2013;5(10):96.

15. Simpkin AJ, Suderman M, Gaunt TR, Lyttleton O, McArdle WL, Ring SM, Tilling K, Davey Smith G, Relton CL. Longitudinal analysis of DNA methylation associated with birth weight and gestational age. Hum Mol Genet. 2015;24:3752–63.

16. Sparrow S, Manning JR, Cartier J, Anblagan D, Bastin ME, Piyasena C, Pataky R, Moore EJ, Semple SI, Wilkinson AG, Evans M, Drake AJ, Boardman JP. Epigenomic profiling of preterm infants reveals DNA methylation differences at sites associated with neural function. Transl Psychiatry. 2016;6:e716.

17. Tan Q, Frost M, Heijmans BT, von Bornemann Hjelmborg J, Tobi EW, Christensen K, Christiansen L. Epigenetic signature of birth weight discordance in adult twins. BMC Genomics. 2014;15:1062.

18. Maksimovic J, Gordon L, Oshlack A. SWAN: subset-quantile within array normalization for illumina infinium HumanMethylation450 BeadChips. Genome Biol. 2012;13(6):R44.

19. Logue MW, Smith AK, Wolf EJ, Maniates H, Stone A, Schichman SA, McGlinchey RE, Milberg W, Miller MW. The correlation of methylation levels measured using Illumina 450K and EPIC BeadChips in blood samples. Epigenomics. 2017;9(11):1363–71.

20. Houseman EA, Accomando WP, Koestler DC, Christensen BC, Marsit CJ, Nelson HH, Wiencke JK, Kelsey KT. DNA methylation arrays as surrogate measures of cell mixture distribution. BMC Bioinformatics. 2012;13:86.

21. Benjamini Y, Hochberg Y. Controlling the false discovery rate: a practical and powerful approach to multiple testing. J R Statist Soc B. 1995;57:289–300.

22. Jaffe AE, Murakami P, Lee H, Leek JT, Fallin MD, Feinberg AP, Irizarry RA. Bump hunting to identify differentially methylated regions in epigenetic epidemiology studies. Int J Epidemiol. 2012;41(1):200–9.

23. McLean CY, Bristor D, Hiller M, Clarke SL, Schaar BT, Lowe CB, Wenger AM, Bejerano G. GREAT improves functional interpretation of cis-regulatory regions. Nat Biotechnol. 2010;28:495–501.

24. Hahne F, Ivanek R. Statistical genomics: methods and protocols. In: Mathé E, Davis S, editors. Chapter visualizing genomic data using Gviz and Bioconductor. New York: Springer New York; 2016. p. 335–51.

25. Chatterton Z, Hartley BJ, Seok MH, Mendelev N, Chen S, Milekic M, Rosoklija G, Stankov A, Trencevsja-Ivanovska I, Brennand K, Ge Y, Dwork AJ, Haghighi F. In utero exposure to maternal smoking is associated with DNA methylation alterations and reduced neuronal content in the developing fetal brain. Epigenetics Chromatin. 2017;10:4.

26. Ladd-Acosta C, Hansen KD, Briem E, Fallin MD, Kaufmann WE, Feinberg AP. Common DNA methylation alterations in multiple brain regions in autism. Mol Psychiatry. 2014;19:862–71.

27. Fan L, Jaquet V, Dodd PR, Chen W, Wilce PA. Molecular cloning and characterization of hNP22: a gene up-regulated in human alcoholic brain. J Neurochem. 2001;76:1275–81.

28. Ito M, Depaz I, Wilce P, Suzuki T, Niwa S, Matsumoto I. Expression of human neuronal protein 22, a novel cytoskeleton-associated protein, was decreased in the anterior cingulate cortex of schizophrenia. Neurosci Lett. 2005;378:125–30.

29. Parveen F, Faridi RM, Das V, Tripathi G, Agrawal S. Genetic association of phase I and phase II detoxification genes with recurrent miscarriages among north Indian women. Mol Hum Reprod. 2010;16:207–14.

30. Liu Y, Tang YB, Chen J, Huang ZX. Meta-analysis of GSTT1 null genotype and preterm delivery risk. Int J Clin Exp Med. 2014;7:1537–41.

31. Suter M, Abramovici A, Aagaard-Tillery K. Genetic and epigenetic influences associated with intrauterine growth restriction due to in utero tobacco exposure. Pediatr Endocrinol Rev. 2010;8:94–102.

32. Zheng X, Feingold E, Ryckman KK, Shaffer JR, Boyd HA, Feenstra B, Melbye M, Marazita ML, Murray JC, Cuenco KT. Association of maternal CNVs in GSTT1/GSTT2 with smoking, preterm delivery, and low birth weight. Front Genet. 2013;4:196.

33. Sheikh IA, Ahmad E, Jamal MS, Rehan M, Assidi M, Tayubi IA, AlBasri SF, Bajouh OS, Turki RF, Abuzenadah AM, Damanhouri GA, Beg MA, Al-Qahtani M. Spontaneous preterm birth and single nucleotide gene polymorphisms: a recent update. BMC Genomics. 2016;17(Suppl 9):759.

34. Nukui T, Day RD, Sims CS, Ness RB, Romkes M. Maternal/newborn GSTT1 null genotype contributes to risk of preterm, low birthweight infants. Pharmacogenetics. 2004;14:569–76.

35. Bustamante M, Danileviciute A, Espinosa A, Gonzalez JR, Subirana I, Cordier S, Chevrier C, Chatzi L, Grazuleviciene R, Sunyer J, Ibarluzea J, Ballester F, Villanueva CM, Nieuwenhuijsen M, Estivill X, Kogevinas M. Influence of fetal glutathione S-transferase copy number variants on adverse reproductive outcomes. BJOG. 2012;119:1141–6.

36. Cao J, Song Y, Bi N, Shen J, Liu W, Fan J, Sun G, Tong T, He J, Shi Y, Zhang X, Lu N, He Y, Zhang H, Ma K, Luo X, Lv L, Deng H, Cheng J, Zhu J, Wang L, Zhan Q. DNA methylation-mediated repression of miR-886-3p predicts poor outcome of human small cell lung cancer. Cancer Res. 2013;73:3326–35.

37. Lee K, Kunkeaw N, Jeon SH, Lee I, Johnson BH, Kang GY, Bang JY, Park HS, Leelayuwat C, Lee YS. Precursor miR-886, a novel noncoding RNA repressed in cancer, associates with PKR and modulates its activity. RNA. 2011;17: 1076–89.

38. Sanchez-Mut JV, Aso E, Heyn H, Matsuda T, Bock C, Ferrer I, Esteller M. Promoter hypermethylation of the phosphatase DUSP22 mediates PKA-dependent TAU phosphorylation and CREB activation in Alzheimer's disease. Hippocampus. 2014;24:363–8.

39. Delgado-Morales R, Esteller M. Opening up the DNA methylome of dementia. Mol Psychiatry. 2017;22:485–96.

40. Ouyang B, Baxter CS, Lam HM, Yeramaneni S, Levin L, Haynes E, Ho SM. Hypomethylation of dual specificity phosphatase 22 promoter correlates with duration of service in firefighters and is inducible by low-dose benzo[a]pyrene. J Occup Environ Med. 2012;54:774–80.

41. Dolfini D, Mantovani R. Targeting the Y/CCAAT box in cancer: YB-1 (YBX1) or NF-Y? Cell Death Differ. 2013;20:676–85.

42. Melville JM, Moss TJ. The immune consequences of preterm birth. Front Neurosci. 2013;7:79.

43. Parets SE, Conneely KN, Kilaru V, Menon R, Smith AK. DNA methylation provides insight into intergenerational risk for preterm birth in African Americans. Epigenetics. 2015;10:784–92.

44. Bagheri H, Mercier E, Qiao Y, Stephenson MD, Rajcan-Separovic E. Genomic characteristics of miscarriage copy number variants. Mol Hum Reprod. 2015; 21:655–61.

45. Aboulghar M, Islam Y. Twin and preterm labor: prediction and treatment. Cur Obstet Gynecol Rep. 2013;2:232–9.

46. Campbell S. Universal cervical-length screening and vaginal progesterone prevents early preterm births, reduces neonatal morbidity and is cost saving: doing nothing is no longer an option. Ultrasound Obstet Gynecol. 2011;38(1):1–9.

4

Vitamin C increases 5-hydroxymethylcytosine level and inhibits the growth of bladder cancer

Ding Peng[1,2,3,4,5] (iD), Guangzhe Ge[2,6], Yanqing Gong[1,3,4,5], Yonghao Zhan[1,3,4,5], Shiming He[1,3,4,5], Bao Guan[1,3,4,5], Yifan Li[1,3,4,5], Ziying Xu[2], Han Hao[1,3,4,5], Zhisong He[1,3,4,5], Gengyan Xiong[1,3,4,5], Cuijian Zhang[1,3,4,5], Yue Shi[2], Yuanyuan Zhou[2], Weimin Ci[2,6*], Xuesong Li[1,3,4,5*] and Liqun Zhou[1,3,4,5*]

Abstract

Background: 5-Hydroxymethylcytosine (5hmC) is converted from 5-methylcytosine (5mC) by a group of enzymes termed ten-eleven translocation (TET) family dioxygenases. The loss of 5hmC has been identified as a hallmark of most types of cancer and is related to tumorigenesis and progression. However, the role of 5hmC in bladder cancer is seldom investigated. Vitamin C was recently reported to induce the generation of 5hmC by acting as a cofactor for TET dioxygenases. In this study, we explored the role of 5hmC in bladder cancer and the therapeutic efficacy of vitamin C in increasing the 5hmC pattern.

Results: 5hmC was decreased in bladder cancer samples and was related to patient overall survival. Genome-wide mapping of 5hmC in tumor tissues and vitamin C-treated bladder cancer cells revealed that 5hmC loss was enriched in cancer-related genes and that vitamin C treatment increased 5hmC levels correspondingly. Vitamin C treatment shifted the transcriptome and inhibited the malignant phenotypes associated with bladder cancer cells in both in vitro cell lines and in vivo xenografts.

Conclusions: This study provided mechanistic insights regarding the 5hmC loss in bladder cancer and a rationale for exploring the therapeutic use of vitamin C as a potential epigenetic treatment for bladder cancer.

Keywords: Bladder cancer, 5-Hydroxymethylcytosine, Vitamin C, TET

Background

Bladder cancer is the most common cancer of the urogenital system, ranking sixth among all cancers and fourth in males [1, 2]. Despite the advancements in surgical techniques and chemotherapy, the outcome of bladder cancer is still poor, especially in patients with advanced and metastatic disease [3]. Therefore, there is a pressing need for novel biomarkers that can stratify the risk of mortality and provide potential therapeutic targets.

Alterations in DNA methylation are among the earliest and most common events in tumorigenesis [4]. Global loss and promoter-associated gains of DNA methylation

(5-methylcytosine, 5mC) have been considered to be the hallmarks of cancers [5–7]. Recently, 5-hydroxymethylcytosine (5hmC) was discovered as a transformed form of 5mC via ten-eleven translocation (TET) enzymes in the demethylation cycle [8]. In a number of cancers, 5hmC has been observed to be remarkably decreased and associated with tumorigenesis, progression, and outcomes [9–12].

Several studies have also reported the loss of 5hmC in bladder cancer [13, 14]. However, the genome-wide profile and role of 5hmC in bladder cancer tumorigenesis, progression, and outcome have been seldom investigated. Vitamin C is a co-substrate of Fe (II)-2-oxoglutarate-dependent dioxygenases, including TETs [15]. Recently, vitamin C was reported to block leukemia progression and promote differentiation by enhancing 5hmC formation [16, 17].

Here, we compared the 5hmC genome-wide profiles between normal bladder and bladder cancer tissues and

---

* Correspondence: ciwm@big.ac.cn; pineneedle@sina.com;
zhoulqmail@sina.com
[2]Key Laboratory of Genomic and Precision Medicine, Beijing Institute of Genomics, Chinese Academy of Sciences, Beijing 100101, China
[1]Department of Urology, Peking University First Hospital, Beijing 100034, China
Full list of author information is available at the end of the article

characterized the association between 5hmC and bladder cancer tumorigenesis, progression, and outcomes. We showed that vitamin C could increase 5hmC levels and inhibit malignant phenotypes in bladder cancer both in vitro and in vivo. Loss of 5hmC could be a novel biomarker and treatment target for bladder cancer.

Results

5hmC level is an independent molecular marker of bladder cancer

We first detected 5hmC levels in normal bladder and bladder cancer tissues by immunohistochemistry (IHC) staining with formalin-fixed, paraffin-embedded tissue sections. The clinicopathological characteristics of 135 patients with bladder urothelial carcinoma are shown in Table 1. Consistent with recent findings in other types of cancers, normal bladder tissues showed strong nuclear 5hmC staining ($n = 135$), whereas bladder cancer showed a partial or complete loss of 5hmC ($n = 135$) ($P < 0.05$, Fig. 1a, b; normal renal tissue was used as a positive control). The loss of 5hmC was also confirmed by anti-5hmC antibody-based dot blot assay in matched bladder cancer and normal bladder tissues (Fig. 1c). A Kaplan-Meier log-rank test revealed that patients with higher 5hmC levels had significantly longer overall survival than patients with lower 5hmC levels (Fig. 1d). Further, univariate and multivariate Cox proportional hazard regression analyses showed that the 5hmC level in tumor tissues independently provided predictive power and that lower 5hmC levels correlated with

Table 1 Clinicopathological characteristics of 135 patients with bladder urothelial carcinoma

Characteristics	Total $n = 135$
Age, years, median (IQR)	66 (56–74)
Gender	
female	23
male	112
Grade	
2	35
3	100
T stage	
Tis	3
T1	36
T2	39
T3	25
T4	32
N status	
Negative	110
Positive	25

IQR interquartile range

shorter overall survival, as reflected by the hazard ratio of 0.483 (Fig. 1e), suggesting that the loss of 5hmC is critical for bladder cancer progression. Meanwhile, a lower 5hmC level was also associated with a higher tumor stage and lymphatic metastasis (Table 2).

Genome-wide mapping of 5hmC in paired tumor and adjacent normal tissue

To explore whether 5hmC loss during bladder tumorigenesis was genome-wide or locus-specific, we used a hydroxymethylated DNA immunoprecipitation (hMeDIP) approach coupled with deep sequencing (hMeDIP-seq) to compare genome-wide changes in 5hmC between the normal bladder and bladder cancer tissue. We found that 5hmC is associated with gene-rich regions in the normal bladder genome and is relatively low in the bladder cancer genome (Fig. 2a). Importantly, we observed a significant decrease in 5hmC levels within the average gene and in the regions 2000 bp up- and downstream of the gene in bladder cancer tissue compared with normal bladder tissue (Fig. 2b). Using MACS software, we identified 27,565 5hmC peaks that were decreased in bladder cancer (FDR < 0.05), more than half of which were located either in exons (10.3%) or introns (58.9%) and 6.45% of which were located at the promoters (Fig. 2c). Using CEAS software, 27,565 5hmC peaks were mapped to 5843 genes. KEGG pathway enrichment and GO term analyses of the 5843 genes revealed that these genes are closely associated with various cancer-related pathways (Fig. 2d). As an example, the TIMP2 and ITIH5 genes showed decreased 5hmC in gene bodies in bladder cancer compared with the normal bladder samples, and hMeDip-qPCR/MeDip-qPCR verified the increase in 5hmC and a relative decrease in 5mC (Fig. 2e). Collectively, the loss of 5hmC occurred in multiple cancer-related genes during bladder carcinogenesis.

Increasing 5hmC by vitamin C can inhibit the malignant phenotype of bladder cancer cells

We next detected the 5hmC levels in normal and bladder cancer cell lines. According to dot blot assay, 5hmC content was relatively high in nonmalignant cells (primary urothelial cells Hum-u007 and immortalized normal cells SV-HUC-1) but was low in bladder cancer cells (Fig. 3a). To explore the molecular mechanisms underlying 5hmC loss in bladder cancer, we also measured the expression of 5hmC-related enzymes (TET1, TET2, TET3, IDH1, IDH2, and L2HGDH) and vitamin C transporters (SVCT1 and SVCT2) by RT-qPCR and found that the expression of TET2, L2HGDH, and vitamin C transporters (SVCT1 and SVCT2) were relatively decreased in all bladder cancer cell lines (Fig. 3b). Vitamin C is capable of increasing 5hmC by acting as a cofactor of TET proteins. We then treated several bladder

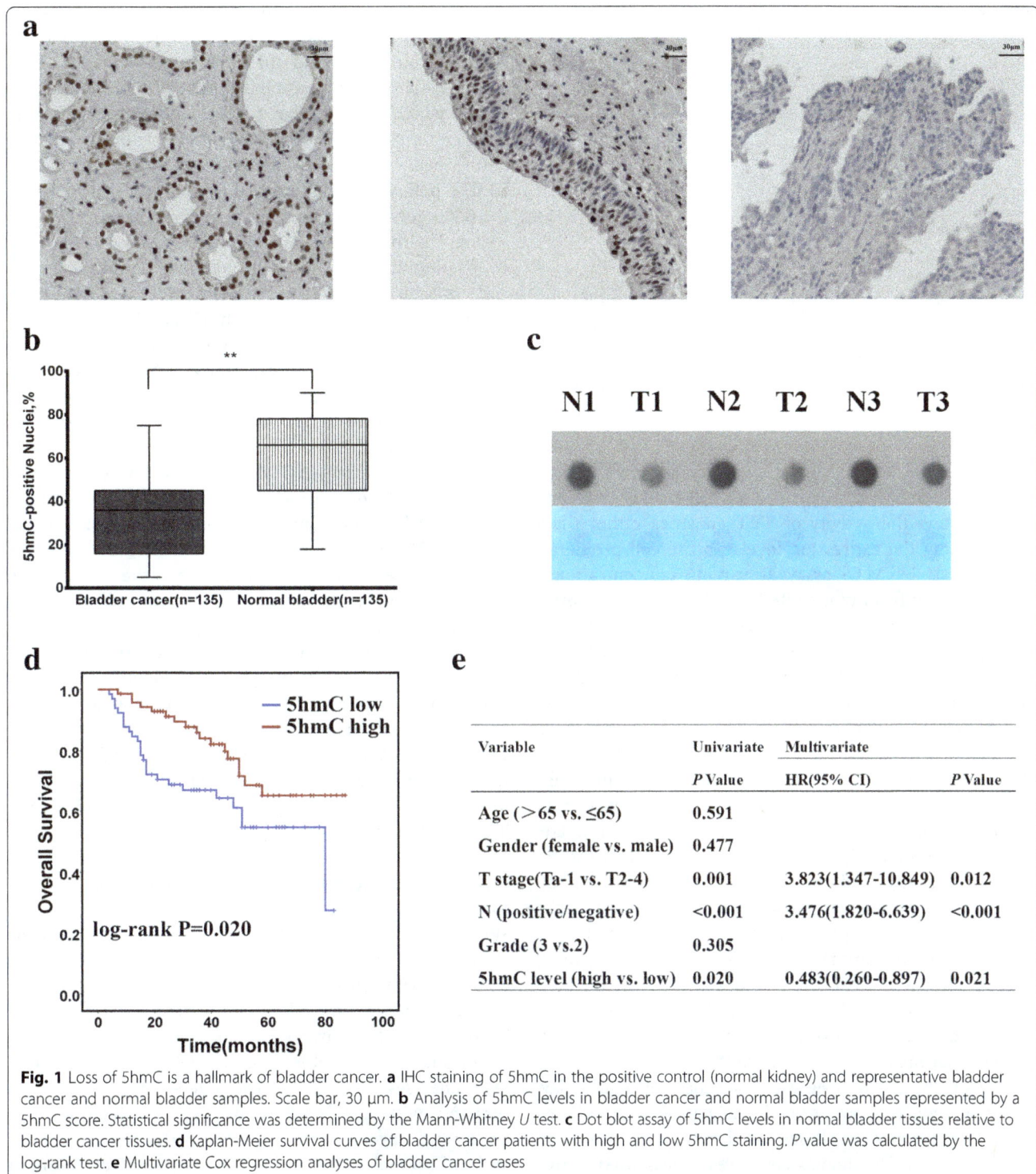

a

b

c

d

e

Variable	Univariate	Multivariate	
	P Value	HR(95% CI)	P Value
Age (>65 vs. ≤65)	0.591		
Gender (female vs. male)	0.477		
T stage(Ta-1 vs. T2-4)	0.001	3.823(1.347-10.849)	0.012
N (positive/negative)	<0.001	3.476(1.820-6.639)	<0.001
Grade (3 vs.2)	0.305		
5hmC level (high vs. low)	0.020	0.483(0.260-0.897)	0.021

Fig. 1 Loss of 5hmC is a hallmark of bladder cancer. **a** IHC staining of 5hmC in the positive control (normal kidney) and representative bladder cancer and normal bladder samples. Scale bar, 30 μm. **b** Analysis of 5hmC levels in bladder cancer and normal bladder samples represented by a 5hmC score. Statistical significance was determined by the Mann-Whitney U test. **c** Dot blot assay of 5hmC levels in normal bladder tissues relative to bladder cancer tissues. **d** Kaplan-Meier survival curves of bladder cancer patients with high and low 5hmC staining. P value was calculated by the log-rank test. **e** Multivariate Cox regression analyses of bladder cancer cases

cancer cell lines with vitamin C at varying concentrations and time periods. As a result, vitamin C increased the 5hmC levels in T24 cells in a time- and concentration-dependent manner (Fig. 3c). Meanwhile, global 5mC levels were slightly decreased (Fig. 3d). J82 and 5637 cells showed similar results (Additional file 1: Figure S1B and C). Moreover, we observed similar

effects with vitamin C, which increased 5hmC levels and inhibited cancer cell growth in renal cancer cells (Additional file 1: Figure S1D). We also measured relative TET1/2/3 expression levels after vitamin C treatment by RT-qPCR and found no significant changes (Additional file 2: Figure S2A). This result indicated that vitamin C increases 5hmC levels in bladder cancer cells

Table 2 Association between clinicopathological characteristics and 5hmC level of bladder urothelial carcinoma

Cohort characteristics	5hmc level		Chi-square test
	Low	High	P value
Grade			0.514
2	20	18	
3	45	52	
Age			0.412
< 65	27	34	
≥ 65	38	36	
T stage			0.010
Tis–T1	12	27	
T2–T4	53	43	
N stage			0.028
Negetive	47	62	
Positive	18	8	

by promoting the activity of TET enzymes rather than by increasing the expression levels. In the cell proliferation analysis by MTS assay at varying concentrations, vitamin C significantly inhibited bladder cancer cell proliferation at pharmacological concentrations (0.5 to 5 mM), although it was relatively less toxic to nonmalignant cells (Fig. 3e). High-dose vitamin C also induced significant apoptosis in T24 cells (Fig. 3f and Additional file 2: Figure S2B). Colony formation assays also demonstrated the inhibitory effects of vitamin C in bladder cancer cells relative to nonmalignant cells (Fig. 3g). It was reported that high-dose vitamin C can inhibit cancer cells by H_2O_2 production. To eliminate the influence of H_2O_2, we added 100 μg/ml catalase to block all H_2O_2 and found that the inhibition of high-dose vitamin C was partially rescued; however, vitamin C still had a suppression effect (Additional file 2: Figure S2C). In summary, high-dose vitamin C could directly induce growth arrest and apoptosis in bladder cancer cells, unlike low-dose vitamin C, which suppressed cancer cell growth in an H_2O_2-independent manner that included 5hmC restoration.

Additionally, an intraperitoneal injection of 2 g/kg/day vitamin C induced slower growth and a smaller tumor burden than saline in vivo without significant toxicity or weight loss (Fig. 4a–d). IHC staining also revealed increased 5hmC levels in the vitamin C treatment group (Fig. 4e). Collectively, our results support that vitamin C can increase 5hmC levels and block bladder cancer growth.

Vitamin C can re-establish the 5hmC landscape in bladder cancer cells

We next explored the re-established pattern of 5hmC with vitamin C treatment. T24 cells treated with

0.25 mM vitamin C or without treatment (control) were used to profile genome-wide 5hmC patterns by hMeDIP-seq. We found that vitamin C-treated bladder cancer cells showed re-establishment of the 5hmC landscape, which was similar to the landscape of normal bladder tissues (Fig. 5a). Using MACS software, 28,015 5hmC peaks and 6809 mapped genes were identified. KEGG pathway enrichment and GO term analyses of the 6809 genes revealed that these genes were closely associated with various cancer-related pathways (Fig. 5b). By overlapping the 5hmC profiles from normal tissues and vitamin C-treated T24 cells, we identified 2511 RefSeq genes with decreased 5hmC densities in bladder cancer tissue that were restored by vitamin C treatment in T24 cells. KEGG pathway and GO term analyses revealed that these genes were mainly associated with adhesion and cancer-related genes (Fig. 5c, d). As exemplified by the LATS2 and RND3 genes, vitamin C restored 5hmC levels in T24 cells; these levels were relatively low in bladder cancer cells compared with normal bladder cells, and 5mC showed an opposite trend (Fig. 5e). We further mapped these 28,015 5hmC peaks to different elements and found that the peaks were more enriched in the enhancers, exons, and promoters than in introns and intergenic regions (Fig. 5b). It was reported that 5hmC in the enhancer regions is associated with gene expression [18]. We identified 154 enhancers that overlapped with vitamin C-increased 5hmC peaks. IPA analysis of the 382 enhancer-assigned genes showed that the most significantly enriched pathways were cancer-related pathways, such as NRF2-mediated oxidative stress response, TNFR2 signaling, RhoA signaling, and IL-1 signaling.

Vitamin C treatment shifted the transcriptome of bladder cancer cells

We next examined the phenotypic changes in T24 cells at the global transcriptome level after treatment with 0.25 mM vitamin C. Using DEseq2, 1172 differentially expressed genes were identified, including 482 upregulated and 690 downregulated genes (Fig. 6a and Additional file 3: Table S1). KEGG pathway and GO term analyses showed that these genes were mainly associated with focal adhesion, DNA replication, cell cycle, and several cancer-related pathways (Fig. 6b, c and Additional file 4: Table S2). Gene set enrichment analysis (GSEA) analysis also showed an inhibitory effect on the cell cycle and DNA replication (Fig. 6d). Furthermore, among the 1172 genes, 503 genes overlapped with the 6809 restored 5hmC-related genes (Fig. 6e). KEGG pathway analysis of these 503 genes also showed enriched focal adhesion and several cancer-related pathways (Fig. 6f). We overlapped these 1172 genes with the genes that showed decreased

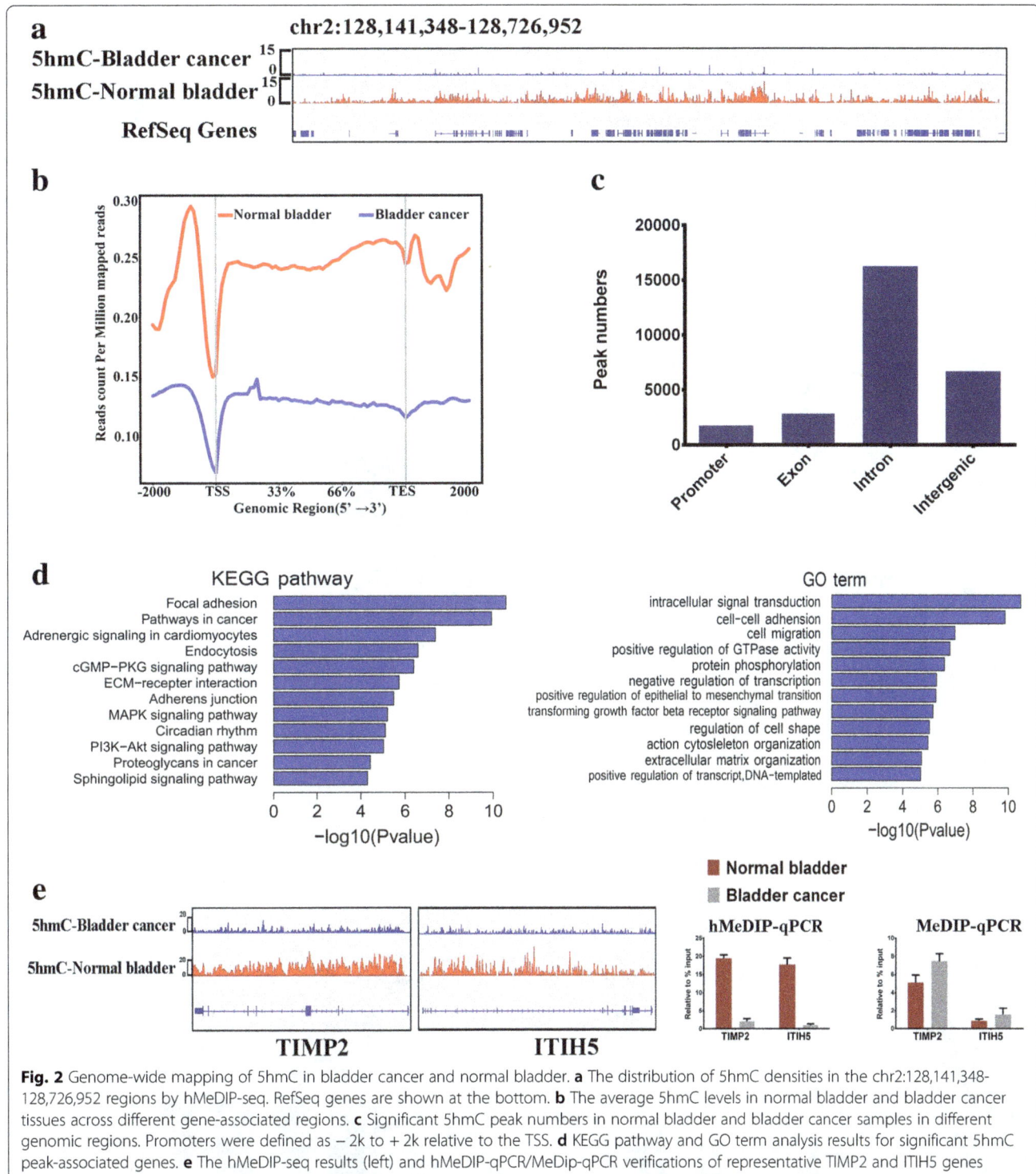

Fig. 2 Genome-wide mapping of 5hmC in bladder cancer and normal bladder. **a** The distribution of 5hmC densities in the chr2:128,141,348-128,726,952 regions by hMeDIP-seq. RefSeq genes are shown at the bottom. **b** The average 5hmC levels in normal bladder and bladder cancer tissues across different gene-associated regions. **c** Significant 5hmC peak numbers in normal bladder and bladder cancer samples in different genomic regions. Promoters were defined as − 2k to + 2k relative to the TSS. **d** KEGG pathway and GO term analysis results for significant 5hmC peak-associated genes. **e** The hMeDIP-seq results (left) and hMeDIP-qPCR/MeDip-qPCR verifications of representative TIMP2 and ITIH5 genes

5hmC in bladder cancer tissue, and 499 genes were identified as common to both sets. KEGG pathway analysis of these 499 genes also showed enriched focal adhesion and several cancer-related pathways (Additional file 2: Figure S2D). Furthermore, we intersected three sets of genes (genes with decreased 5hmC in bladder cancer tissue, genes with increased 5hmC after vitamin C treatment, and 1172 differently expressed genes) and found 265 overlapping genes. KEGG pathway analysis of these 265 genes showed enriched focal adhesion and several cancer-related pathways (Additional file 2: Figure S2E). Therefore, vitamin C treatment shifted the transcriptome of bladder cancer cells to inhibit malignant phenotypes.

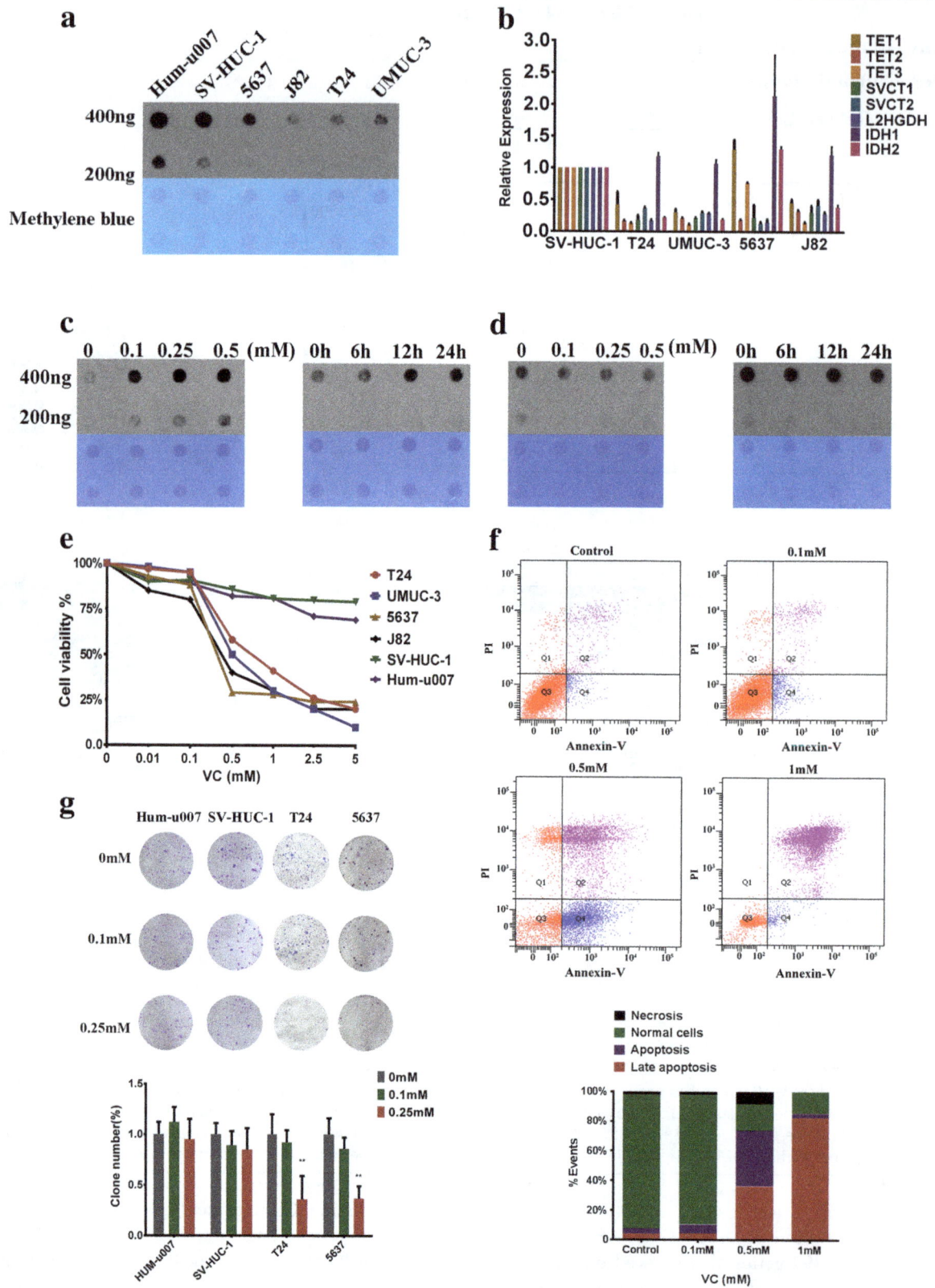

Fig. 3 (See legend on next page.)

(See figure on previous page.)
Fig. 3 Vitamin C treatment increases 5hmC levels and decreases malignant phenotypes in bladder cancer cells in vitro. **a** Dot blot assay of 5hmC levels in normal bladder and cancer cell lines. **b** The relative transcription levels measured by RT-qPCR of 5hmC-related genes and SVCTs in normal bladder and bladder cancer cells. **c** Dot blot assay of 5hmC levels of T24 cells at varying concentrations and time periods with vitamin C. **d** Dot blot assay of 5mC levels of T24 cells at varying concentrations and time periods with vitamin C. **e** MTS assay of cell viability for normal bladder and cancer cell lines at varying concentrations with vitamin C. **f** Apoptosis assay of T24 cells at varying concentrations with vitamin C. **g** Clone formation assay for normal bladder and cancer cell lines at varying concentrations with vitamin C. Statistical significance was determined by the Mann-Whitney U test

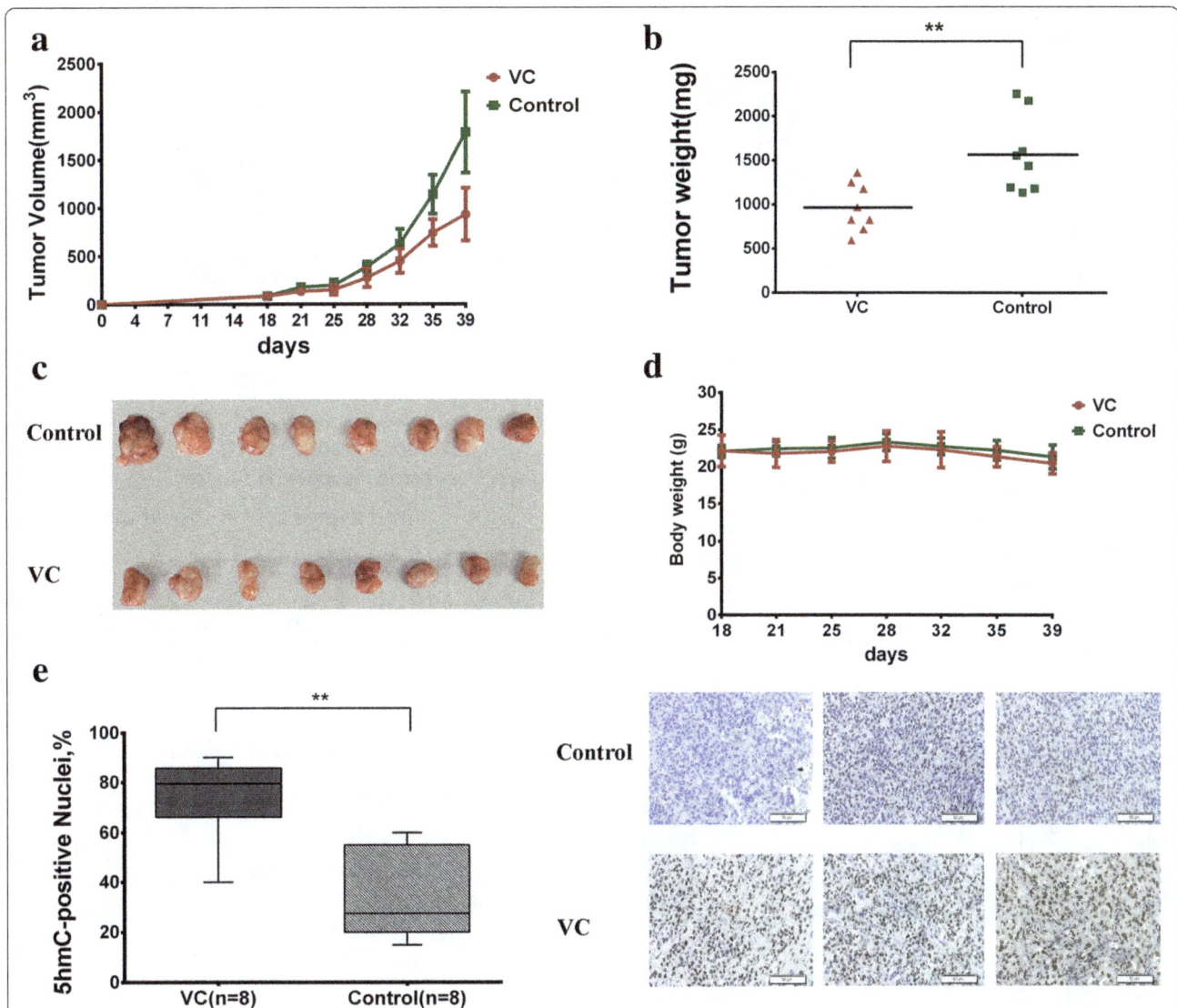

Fig. 4 Vitamin C treatment increases 5hmC levels and decreases malignant phenotypes in T24 cells in vivo. **a** Tumor growth curves of xenografts with T24 cells treated with vitamin C or placebo. Tumor volume is shown as the mean ± SD ($n = 8$ mice). **b** Tumor weights of the indicated xenografts at the endpoint (39 days) are shown as the mean ± SD ($n = 8$ mice). Statistical significance was determined by the Mann-Whitney U test. **c** Images of xenograft tissues in vitamin C in treated and control groups ($n = 8$). **d** The body weights of mice during treatment ($n = 8$ mice). **e** 5hmC score and representative IHC staining of xenograft tissues. Scale bar, 50 μm. Statistical significance was determined by the Mann-Whitney U test

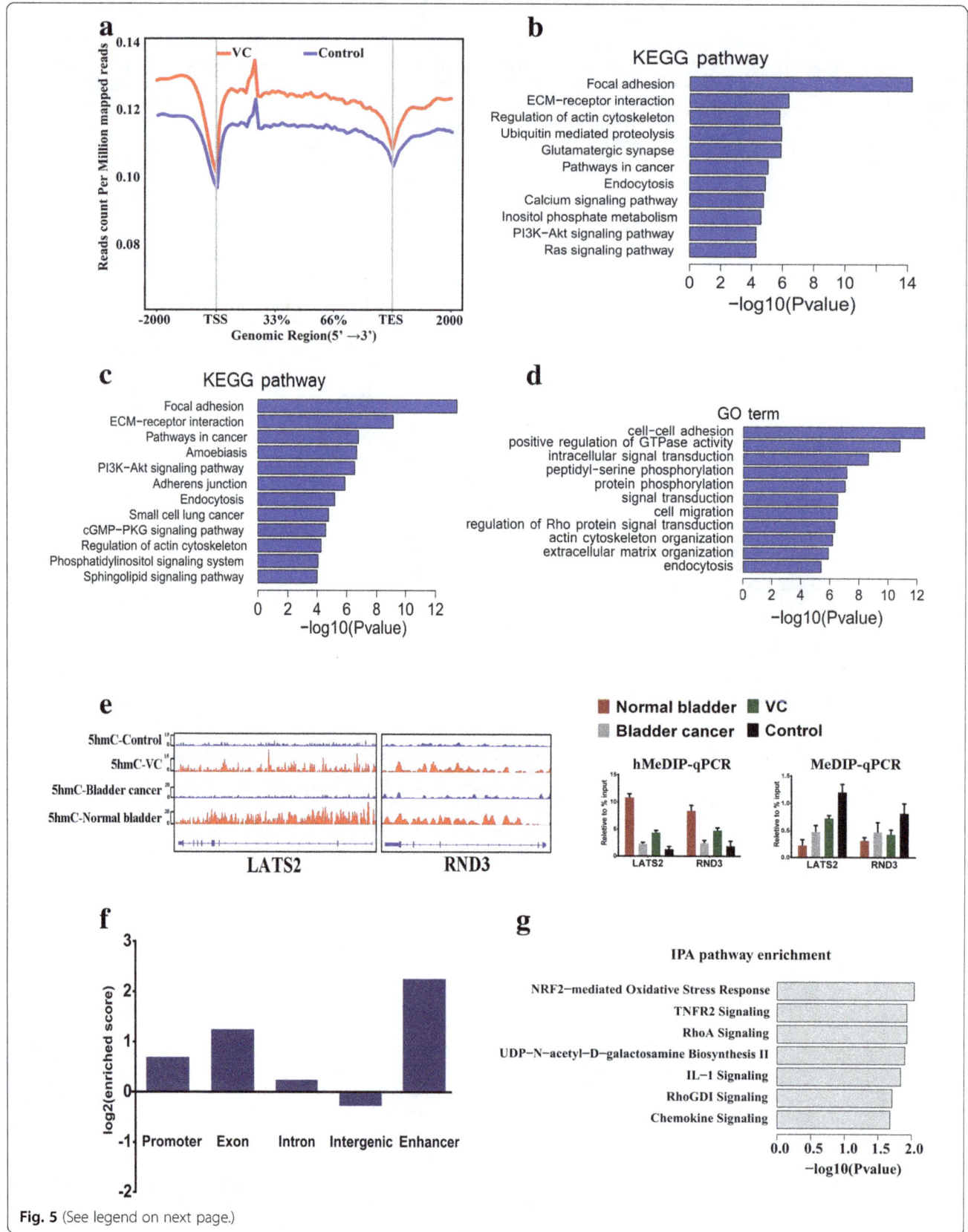

Fig. 5 (See legend on next page.)

(See figure on previous page.)
Fig. 5 Vitamin C treatment re-establishes the 5hmC landscape in the bladder cancer cell epigenome. **a** Average 5hmC levels in T24 cells treated with vitamin C or control across different gene-associated regions. **b** KEGG pathway analysis results for significantly elevated 5hmC peak-associated genes. **c** KEGG pathway analysis results for overlapping 5hmC peak-associated genes. **d** GO term analysis results for overlapping 5hmC peak-associated genes. **e** The hMeDIP-seq results and hMeDIP-qPCR/MeDip-qPCR verifications of representative overlapping LATS2 and RND3 genes. **f** The enrichment scores of vitamin C-restored 5hmC peaks in different genomic elements. **g** IPA pathway enrichment analysis for enhancer-assigned genes

Discussion

In this study, we illustrated the genome-wide profile of 5hmC loss in bladder cancer and the prognostic value of global 5hmC levels. Furthermore, we found that vitamin C increased 5hmC content and inhibited the malignant phenotypes associated with bladder cancer. Our results showed that the loss of 5hmC and 5hmC restoration by vitamin C were significantly associated with cancer-related genes.

5hmC was first discovered in the 1970s and has received renewed attention in the last decade for its involvement in the regulation of embryonic stem (ES) cell differentiation and nervous system development [19, 20]. The loss of 5hmC has been identified as a novel

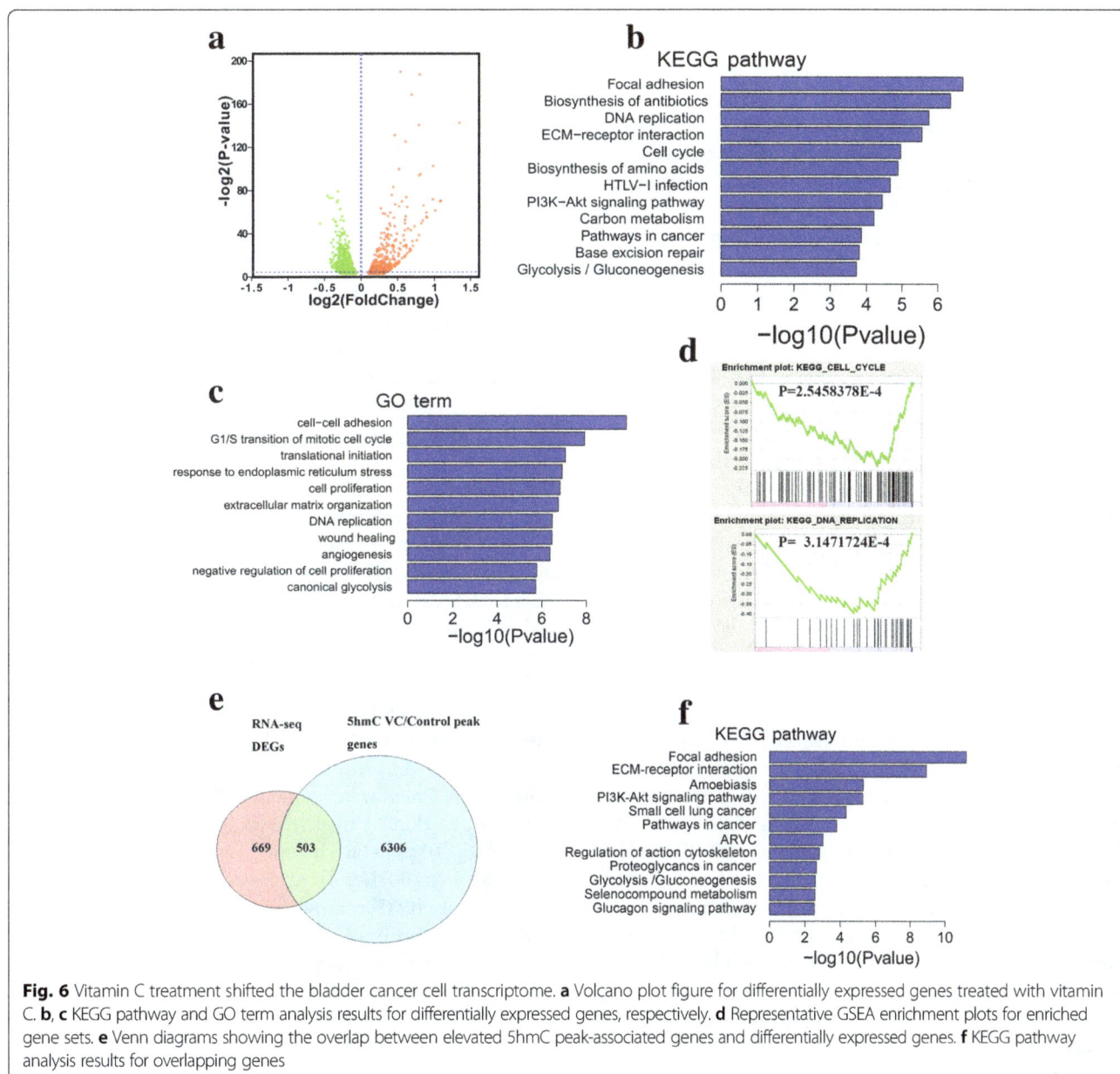

Fig. 6 Vitamin C treatment shifted the bladder cancer cell transcriptome. **a** Volcano plot figure for differentially expressed genes treated with vitamin C. **b, c** KEGG pathway and GO term analysis results for differentially expressed genes, respectively. **d** Representative GSEA enrichment plots for enriched gene sets. **e** Venn diagrams showing the overlap between elevated 5hmC peak-associated genes and differentially expressed genes. **f** KEGG pathway analysis results for overlapping genes

hallmark in most cancers [9–12]. In contrast to 5mC, 5hmC was found to be an important epigenetic mark of active genes and was mainly enriched in gene bodies [11]. These findings indicate that 5hmC might play an important role in tumorigenesis and progression. Various mechanisms may underlie 5hmC depletion in cancer, such as mutations in TETs and IDHs, which thus decrease the expression of TETs and IDHs [12, 21, 22]. Tumor hypoxia is also thought to be a reason for the loss of 5hmC by reducing TET activity [23]. Restoring 5hmC levels by overexpressing TET2 in melanoma cells, TET1 in breast cancer cells, and IDH1 in renal cancer cells demonstrated inhibitory effects in vitro and in vivo [11, 12, 24].

The inhibitory effects of vitamin C both in vitro and in vivo have been reported in several cancers [25–28]. A number of clinical experiments have been conducted in advanced cancer patients, and they revealed that vitamin C is a safe and well-tolerated micronutrient that can inhibit tumors [25, 26, 29]; however, the underlying therapeutic mechanism has remained largely undefined. One study suggested that vitamin C could inhibit nonsmall cell lung cancer (NSCLC) and glioblastoma (GBM) cells by increasing the levels of H_2O_2 and disrupting intracellular iron metabolism [26]. Other studies recently showed that vitamin C selectively killed KRAS and BRAF mutant colorectal cancer cells by targeting glyceraldehyde-3-phosphate dehydrogenase (GAPDH) [30].

As a cofactor, vitamin C can enhance the activity of Fe (II)-2-oxoglutarate dioxygenases, including TETs, leading to DNA demethylation [31]. Recent studies have shown that the suppression effects of vitamin C partly result from the demethylation caused by activating TET. In leukemia, vitamin C suppressed hematopoietic stem cell (HSC) frequency and leukemogenesis by promoting TET activity [16, 17]. Vitamin C restored 5hmC levels in melanoma and rebuilt the transcriptome in melanoma cells [28]. Another study also showed that vitamin C increased TET activity, leading to DNA demethylation in lymphoma cells independently of hydrogen peroxide [32]. Vitamin C also enhanced the antitumor effect of standard therapies. Vitamin C abrogated cetuximab resistance mediated by mutant KRAS in human colon cancer cells [33]. Another study reported that vitamin C enhanced the chemosensitivity of ovarian cancer and reduced the toxicity of chemotherapy [34]. Even at the physiological level, vitamin C also enhanced the effects of decitabine (5-aza-2'-deoxycytidine) in colorectal carcinoma, acute myeloid leukemia, breast carcinoma, and hepatocellular carcinoma cells [35]. Consistent with previous studies, we found that high-dose vitamin C could directly cause selective bladder cancer cell death and apoptosis in an H_2O_2-dependent manner and that low-dose vitamin C suppressed bladder cancer cell growth in an H_2O_2-independent manner that included 5hmC restoration.

In this study, we analyzed the transcriptome of bladder cancer cells after vitamin C treatment. However, the results of RNA-seq and hMeDip-seq did not fit very well. A total of 482 genes were upregulated, 690 genes were downregulated following vitamin C treatment, and 503 genes correlated with changes in 5hmC levels. The mechanisms of how these 5hmC changes alter gene expression and contribute to the decreased malignancy of bladder cancer cells remain unclear and require further examination in the future. We also found that the IC50 of vitamin C for different types of cancers was variable. In this study, the IC50 of vitamin C for bladder cancer was 0.5 mM, and the IC50 for renal cancer cells was above 1 mM. In a study by Christopher B Gustafson, the IC50 of vitamin C for melanoma cells was approximately 0.5 mM [28]. Chen et al. compared the cytotoxicity of vitamin C on different cancer cells and found that different cell lines have various sensitivities [25]. The underlying mechanism of the inhibitory effect of vitamin C on different types of cancers requires additional study.

Conclusions

Our results suggest that the loss of 5hmC is a novel hallmark of bladder cancer with prognostic and outcome significance. We also demonstrated that vitamin C treatment can decrease the malignant phenotypes of bladder cancer in vitro and in vivo by partially increasing the global content of 5hmC and consequently altering the transcriptome. These results suggest that vitamin C could be a potential epigenetic treatment for bladder cancer and perhaps other types of cancer.

Methods
Cell culture and treatment

SV-HUC-1 normal human urinary epithelial cells were obtained from ATCC and cultured in F-12K medium (Gibco, USA). Human normal bladder primary epithelial cells Hum-u007 (obtained from iCell Bioscience Inc., Shanghai) were cultured in n ICell Primary Keratinocyte Culture System (PriMed-iCell-010). Bladder cancer cell lines T24 and 5637 cells were cultured in RPMI-1640 medium (Gibco, USA), and UMUC-3 and J82 cells were cultured in MEM medium (Gibco, USA). All bladder cancer cell lines were obtained from the Institute of Urology at Peking University (Beijing, China). All media contained 10% fetal bovine serum (Gemini, USA), penicillin G (100 U/ml), and streptomycin (100 μg/ml) (Sigma-Aldrich, Germany). Cells were maintained as a monolayer culture at 37 °C in a humidified atmosphere containing 5% CO_2. After seeding on plates for 24 h, the cells were treated with vitamin C (L-ascorbic acid, A4034, Sigma-Aldrich, St Louis, MO, USA) at different concentrations for varying durations. Catalase was obtained from Sigma (C1345).

Immunohistochemistry

Surgical specimens were obtained from 135 patients diagnosed with bladder urothelial carcinoma at the Department of Urology, Peking University First Hospital, between 2010 and 2015. All patients signed informed consent, and the ethics committees of the Peking University First Hospital approved the protocol.

After fixing the tissues with 4% formalin and embedding them in paraffin wax, the tissues were cut into 5-μm sections using a microtome. The sections were deparaffinized in xylene and rehydrated with graded concentrations of alcohol. Subsequently, the slides were treated with 3% H_2O_2 to block endogenous peroxidase activity and were heated (95 °C) for 2.5 min in citrate buffer (10 mmol/l, pH 6.0) for antigen retrieval. To reduce nonspecific binding, 10% normal goat serum was applied. Subsequently, the slides were incubated with anti-5hmC antibody (Active Motif, USA, 39769, 1:10,000) at 4 °C overnight. A Power-Vision™ two-step histostaining reagent and 3,3-diaminobenzidine tetrahydrochloride substrate kit (ZSGB-Bio, China) were used to visualize the localization of the antigen according to the manufacturer's instructions.

The staining score of the 5hmC in tissues was evaluated by two independent pathologists by counting 5hmC-positive nuclei at 0~10%, 11~30%, 31~50%, and > 50% levels, and a positive rate ≥ 31% was defined as a high 5hmC level.

Dot blot

Genomic DNA was extracted from cultured cells using QIAamp DNA Mini Kits (Qiagen, Germany) according to the manufacturer's instructions. A Qubit Fluorometer (Life Technology, USA) was used to quantify the DNA concentration. DNA samples were diluted with 2 N NaOH and 10 mM Tris·Cl at pH 8.5 and then loaded onto a Hybond N+ nylon membrane (GE Health, USA) using a 96-well dot blot apparatus (Bio-Rad, USA). After baking at 80 °C for 60 min and being blocked with 5% nonfat milk for 1 h at room temperature, the membrane was incubated in anti-5hmC (Active Motif, 39769) and anti-5mC antibodies (ZYMO RESEARCH, #A3001-200) at 4 °C overnight and visualized by chemiluminescence. To ensure equal loading, the membrane was then stained with methylene blue.

hMeDIP-seq

One pair of bladder urothelial carcinoma and relative normal bladder tissues was used for hMeDip-seq. The sequencing libraries were prepared with 10 μg of genomic DNA ligated to PE adaptors (Illumina, USA), which was followed by 5hmC antibody capture for immunoprecipitation. The hydroxymethylated fragments were amplified with 10–12 cycles using adaptor-specific primers (Illumina, USA) and quantified on an Agilent 2100 Bioanalyser before cluster generation and sequencing on a HiSeq 3000 according to the manufacturer's protocols.

Identification of vitamin C-restored 5hmC peaks

Briefly, the reads were aligned to the hg19 human genome (bowtie2, default parameters) and de-duplicated; unique reads were kept. Significantly, enriched regions were determined using model-based analysis with the ChIP-Seq (MACS) package (v.2.1.0, default settings). GO term and KEGG pathway analyses were performed with the Database for Annotation, Visualization, and Integrated Discovery (DAVID) program.

Definition of enhancers

The enhancers in adult normal bladder tissue were identified using Roadmap H3K27ac CHIP-seq data (GSM1013133 and GSM1059457). The enhancer was assigned to the nearest gene within a distance of ~ 50 kb [36].

RT-qPCR

Total RNA was isolated from cell lines using the TRIzol reagent (Invitrogen, Thermo Fisher Scientific, Inc.). A total of 2 μg of RNA was reverse-transcribed into cDNA using M-MLV reverse transcriptase (Promega, USA) and oligo (dT) 15 (Promega, USA) as a primer. Quantitative PCR was performed using SYBR® FAST qPCR Kits (KAPA Biosystems, USA) in a final volume of 10 μl in the 7500 Fast Real-Time PCR System (Applied Biosystems, Thermo Fisher Scientific, Inc.). All primer pairs are shown in Table 3, and glyceraldehyde-3-phosphate dehydrogenase (GAPDH) served as the endogenous control. The expression of target mRNA was normalized to GAPDH according to the ΔΔCq method.

MTS cell viability assay, apoptosis assay, and colony formation assay

Cell viability assays were assessed using the CellTiter 96® AQ One Solution Reagent (Promega, USA) according to the manufacturer's instructions. An apoptosis assay was performed by FACS with Annexin V-FITC/PI staining. For colony formation assays, cells were seeded in 6-well plates at a density of 800 cells/well and cultured with different concentrations of vitamin C at 37 °C for 7 days.

Western blot analysis

Total protein of cell lines was prepared with ice-cold radioimmunoprecipitation assay buffer (Sigma-Aldrich; Merck Millipore) and quantified using BCA protein assay reagent (Pierce Chemical Co., Rockford, IL, USA). Equal amounts of proteins were separated by SDS-PAGE and transferred to a polyvinylidene fluoride membrane. After blocking for 1 h with 5% nonfat milk, the membranes were incubated overnight at 4 °C with Caspase-3 (Abcam, ab13847), Bcl-2 (Abcam, ab32124), Bcl-xl

Table 3 Primer pairs for real-time PCR

Genes	Sequence (5' to 3')	
GAPDH	Sense	GGTGAAGGTCGGAGTCAACG
	Antisense	TGGGTGGAATCATATTGGAACA
TET1	Sense	AATGGAAGCACTGTGGTTTG
	Antisense	ACATGGAGCTGCTCATCTTG
TET2	Sense	AATGGCAGCACATTGGTATG
	Antisense	AGCTTCCACACTCCCAAACT
TET3	Sense	GAGGAGCGGTATGGAGAGAA
	Antisense	AGTAGCTTCTCCTCCAGCGT
SVCT1	Sense	TCATCCTCCTCTCCCAGTACCT
	Antisense	AGAGCAGCCACACGGTCAT
SVCT2	Sense	TCTTTGTGCTTGGATTTTCGAT
	Antisense	ACGTTCAACACTTGATCGATTC
IDH1	Sense	TCCGTCACTTGGTGTGTAGG
	Antisense	GGCTTGTGAGTGGATGGGTA
IDH2	Sense	TGAACTGCCAGATAATACGGG
	Antisense	CTGACAGCCCCCACCTC
L2HGDH	Sense	TCAAAAATTCATCCCTGAAATTACT
	Antisense	CTACCAGATTTCCATCTCTATCCAG

(Abcam, ab32370), PARP (Abcam, ab191217), and beta-actin (Proteintech, 66009). After washing and incubating the membranes with secondary antibodies, signals were detected by applying ECL Western Blotting Detection Reagent (GE Healthcare Life Sciences).

Mice xenograft model

T24 cells (1×10^6 cells) were resuspended in 100 ml of PBS and subcutaneously injected into the axillary fossae in 4-week-old nude mice (BALB/c-nu). Tumor volume was calculated with the formula $V = 0.5\ ab^2$, where a is the longest tumor axis, and b is the shortest tumor axis. When the volume of the tumors reached approximately 150 mm^3, mice with tumors were intraperitoneally injected with vitamin C (2 g/kg/day) or saline. The animal protocol was approved by the animal ethics committee of Peking University First Hospital.

RNA-seq and gene set enrichment analysis

The KAPA Stranded RNA-seq Library Preparation Kit was used to construct RNA-seq libraries according to the manufacturer's instructions. Sequencing reads were aligned to the hg19 human genome using the Tophat program (tophat v2.1.1) with the default parameters. Total read counts for each protein-coding gene were extracted using HTSeq (HTSeq version 0.6.0) and then loaded into the R-package DEseq2 to calculate the differentially expressed genes with FDR < 0.05. GSEA was performed using C2 (curated gene sets) collections.

Statistical analysis

All data were evaluated with SPSS version 22.0 software (SPSS, Chicago, IL, USA). The Kaplan-Meier method and corresponding log-rank test were performed to determine the differences in postoperative survival rates. For univariate and multivariate analysis, the Cox regression method was used. Statistical significance was defined as *$P < 0.05$ and **$P < 0.01$.

Abbreviations

5hmC: 5-Hydroxymethylcytosine; 5mC: 5-Methylcytosine; hMeDIP: Hydroxymethylated DNA immunoprecipitation; IDH: Isocitrate dehydrogenases; IHC: Immunohistochemical staining; ITIH5: Inter-alpha-trypsin inhibitor heavy chain family member 5; LATS2: Large tumor suppressor kinase 2; MeDIP: Methylated DNA immunoprecipitation; RND3: Rho family GTPase 3; SVCT: Sodium-dependent vitamin C transporters; TET: Ten-eleven translocation family dioxygenases; TIMP2: TIMP metallopeptidase inhibitor 2

Funding

This study was supported by grants from the National Natural Science Foundation of China (Grant Number: 81672546 to LZ; 81772703 to YG; and 81422035 and 81672541 to WC), the Clinical Features Research of Capital (Z151100004015173 to LZ), the Capital Health Research and Development of Special (2016-1-4077 to LZ), CAS Strategic Priority Research Program (XDA16010102 to WC), and the National Basic Research Programme (2016YFC0900303 to WC).

Authors' contributions

The experiments were conceived and designed by WC, XL, and LZ. DP and GG conducted the experiments. YG, YZ, SH, BG, YL, ZX, HH, ZH, GX, CZ, YS, and YZ participated in the data collection. Bioinformatics and statistical analyses of hMeDIP-seq and RNA-seq were performed by DP and GG. The manuscript was written and reviewed by DP, WC, XL, and LZ. All authors read and approved the final manuscript.

Competing interests

The authors declare that they have no competing interests.

Author details

[1]Department of Urology, Peking University First Hospital, Beijing 100034, China. [2]Key Laboratory of Genomic and Precision Medicine, Beijing Institute of Genomics, Chinese Academy of Sciences, Beijing 100101, China. [3]Institute of Urology, Peking University, Beijing 100034, China. [4]National Urological Cancer Center, Beijing 100034, China. [5]Urogenital Diseases (Male) Molecular Diagnosis and Treatment Center, Peking University, Beijing 100034, China. [6]University of Chinese Academy of Sciences, Beijing 100049, China.

References

1. DeSantis CE, Lin CC, Mariotto AB, Siegel RL, Stein KD, Kramer JL, Alteri R, Robbins AS, Jemal A. Cancer treatment and survivorship statistics, 2014. CA Cancer J Clin. 2014;64:252–71.

2. Kamat AM, Hahn NM, Efstathiou JA, Lerner SP, Malmstrom PU, Choi W, Guo CC, Lotan Y, Kassouf W. Bladder cancer. Lancet. 2016;388:2796–810.

3. Alfred Witjes J, Lebret T, Compérat EM, Cowan NC, De Santis M, Bruins HM, Hernández V, Espinós EL, Dunn J, Rouanne M, et al. Updated 2016 EAU guidelines on muscle-invasive and metastatic bladder cancer. Eur Urol. 2017;71:462–75.

4. Baylin SB, Jones PA. A decade of exploring the cancer epigenome—biological and translational implications. Nat Rev Cancer. 2011;11:726–34.

5. Herman JG, Baylin SB. Gene silencing in cancer in association with promoter hypermethylation. N Engl J Med. 2003;349:2042–54.

6. Jones PA, Baylin SB. The fundamental role of epigenetic events in cancer. Nat Rev Genet. 2002;3:415–28.

7. Hanahan D, Weinberg RA. Hallmarks of cancer: the next generation. Cell. 2011;144:646–74.

8. Tahiliani M, Koh KP, Shen Y, Pastor WA, Bandukwala H, Brudno Y, Agarwal S, Iyer LM, Liu DR, Aravind L, et al. Conversion of 5-methylcytosine to 5-hydroxymethylcytosine in mammalian DNA by MLL partner TET1. Science. 2009;324:930–5.

9. Yang H, Liu Y, Bai F, Zhang JY, Ma SH, Liu J, Xu ZD, Zhu HG, Ling ZQ, Ye D, et al. Tumor development is associated with decrease of TET gene expression and 5-methylcytosine hydroxylation. Oncogene. 2013;32:663–9.

10. Jin SG, Jiang Y, Qiu R, Rauch TA, Wang Y, Schackert G, Krex D, Lu Q, Pfeifer GP. 5-hydroxymethylcytosine is strongly depleted in human cancers but its levels do not correlate with IDH1 mutations. Cancer Res. 2011;71:7360–5.

11. Hore TA, von Meyenn F, Ravichandran M, Bachman M, Ficz G, Oxley D, Santos F, Balasubramanian S, Jurkowski TP, Reik W. Retinol and ascorbate drive erasure of epigenetic memory and enhance reprogramming to naive pluripotency by complementary mechanisms. Proc Natl Acad Sci U S A. 2016;113:12202–7.

12. Lian CG, Xu Y, Ceol C, Wu F, Larson A, Dresser K, Xu W, Tan L, Hu Y, Zhan Q, et al. Loss of 5-hydroxymethylcytosine is an epigenetic hallmark of melanoma. Cell. 2012;150:1135–46.

13. Munari E, Chaux A, Vaghasia AM, Taheri D, Karram S, Bezerra SM, Gonzalez Roibon N, Nelson WG, Yegnasubramanian S, Netto GJ, et al. Global 5-hydroxymethylcytosine levels are profoundly reduced in multiple genitourinary malignancies. PLoS One. 2016;11:e0146302.

14. Li J, Xu Y, Zhang Z, Zhang M, Zhang Z, Zhang F, Li Q. Expression and clinical significance of 5hmC in bladder urothelial carcinoma. Chin J Cel Mol Immunol. 2016;32:232–5.

15. Cadet J, Wagner JR. TET enzymatic oxidation of 5-methylcytosine, 5-hydroxymethylcytosine and 5-formylcytosine. Mutat Res Genet toxicol Environ Mutagenesis. 2014;764-765:18–35.

16. Agathocleous M, Meacham CE, Burgess RJ, Piskounova E, Zhao Z, Crane GM, Cowin BL, Bruner E, Murphy MM, Chen W, et al. Ascorbate regulates haematopoietic stem cell function and leukaemogenesis. Nature. 2017;549:476.

17. Cimmino L, Dolgalev I, Wang Y, Yoshimi A, Martin GH, Wang J, Ng V, Xia B, Witkowski MT, Mitchell-Flack M, et al. Restoration of TET2 function blocks aberrant self-renewal and leukemia progression. Cell. 2017;170:1079–95.

18. Taylor SE, Li YH, Smeriglio P, Rath M, Wong WH, Bhutani N. Stable 5-hydroxymethylcytosine (5hmC) acquisition marks gene activation during Chondrogenic differentiation. J Bone Miner Res. 2016;31:524–34.

19. He XB, Kim M, Kim SY, Yi SH, Rhee YH, Kim T, Lee EH, Park CH, Dixit S, Harrison FE, et al. Vitamin C facilitates dopamine neuron differentiation in fetal midbrain through TET1- and JMJD3-dependent epigenetic control manner. Stem Cells. 2015;33:1320–32.

20. Blaschke K, Ebata KT, Karimi MM, Zepeda-Martinez JA, Goyal P, Mahapatra S, Tam A, Laird DJ, Hirst M, Rao A, et al. Vitamin C induces Tet-dependent DNA demethylation and a blastocyst-like state in ES cells. Nature. 2013;500:222–6.

21. Ko M, Huang Y, Jankowska AM, Pape UJ, Tahiliani M, Bandukwala HS, An J, Lamperti ED, Koh KP, Ganetzky R, et al. Impaired hydroxylation of 5-methylcytosine in myeloid cancers with mutant TET2. Nature. 2010;468:839–43.

22. Figueroa ME, Abdel-Wahab O, Lu C, Ward PS, Patel J, Shih A, Li Y, Bhagwat N, Vasanthakumar A, Fernandez HF, et al. Leukemic IDH1 and IDH2 mutations result in a hypermethylation phenotype, disrupt TET2 function, and impair hematopoietic differentiation. Cancer Cell. 2010;18:553–67.

23. Thienpont B, Steinbacher J, Zhao H, D'Anna F, Kuchnio A, Ploumakis A, Ghesquiere B, Van Dyck L, Boeckx B, Schoonjans L, et al. Tumour hypoxia causes DNA hypermethylation by reducing TET activity. Nature. 2016;537:6.

24. Hsu CH, Peng KL, Kang ML, Chen YR, Yang YC, Tsai CH, Chu CS, Jeng YM, Chen YT, Lin FM, et al. TET1 suppresses cancer invasion by activating the tissue inhibitors of metalloproteinases. Cell Rep. 2012;2:568–79.

25. Chen Q, Espey MG, Sun AY, Pooput C, Kirk KL, Krishna MC, Khosh DB, Drisko J, Levine M. Pharmacologic doses of ascorbate act as a prooxidant and decrease growth of aggressive tumor xenografts in mice. Proc Natl Acad Sci U S A. 2008;105:11105–9.

26. Schoenfeld JD, Sibenaller ZA, Mapuskar KA, Wagner BA, Cramer-Morales KL, Furqan M, Sandhu S, Carlisle TL, Smith MC, Abu Hejleh T, et al. O2- and H2O2-mediated disruption of Fe metabolism causes the differential susceptibility of NSCLC and GBM cancer cells to pharmacological ascorbate. Cancer Cell. 2017;31:487–500.

27. Miles SL, Fischer AP, Joshi SJ, Niles RM. Ascorbic acid and ascorbate-2-phosphate decrease HIF activity and malignant properties of human melanoma cells. BMC Cancer. 2015;15:867.

28. Gustafson CB, Yang C, Dickson KM, Shao H, Van Booven D, Harbour JW, Liu ZJ, Wang G. Epigenetic reprogramming of melanoma cells by vitamin C treatment. Clin Epigenetics. 2015;7:51.

29. Stephenson CM, Levin RD, Spector T, Lis CG. Phase I clinical trial to evaluate the safety, tolerability, and pharmacokinetics of high-dose intravenous ascorbic acid in patients with advanced cancer. Cancer Chemother Pharmacol. 2013;72:139–46.

30. Yun J, Mullarky E, Lu C, Bosch KN, Kavalier A, Rivera K, Roper J, Chio II, Giannopoulou EG, Rago C, et al. Vitamin C selectively kills KRAS and BRAF mutant colorectal cancer cells by targeting GAPDH. Science. 2015;350:1391–6.

31. Loenarz C, Schofield CJ. Expanding chemical biology of 2-oxoglutarate oxygenases. Nat Chem Biol. 2008;4:152–6.

32. Shenoy N, Bhagat T, Nieves E, Stenson M, Lawson J, Choudhary GS, Habermann T, Nowakowski G, Singh R, Wu X, et al. Upregulation of TET activity with ascorbic acid induces epigenetic modulation of lymphoma cells. Blood Cancer J. 2017;7:e587.

33. Jung SA, Lee DH, Moon JH, Hong SW, Shin JS, Hwang IY, Shin YJ, Kim JH, Gong EY, Kim SM, et al. L-ascorbic acid can abrogate SVCT2-dependent cetuximab resistance mediated by mutant KRAS in human colon cancer cells. Free Radic Biol Med. 2016;95:200–8.

34. Ma Y, Chapman J, Levine M, Polireddy K, Drisko J, Chen Q. High-dose parenteral ascorbate enhanced chemosensitivity of ovarian cancer and reduced toxicity of chemotherapy. Sci Transl Med. 2014;6:222ra18.

35. Liu M, Ohtani H, Zhou W, Orskov AD, Charlet J, Zhang YW, Shen H, Baylin SB, Liang G, Gronbaek K, et al. Vitamin C increases viral mimicry induced by 5-aza-2'-deoxycytidine. Proc Natl Acad Sci U S A. 2016;113:10238–44.

36. Chepelev I, Wei G, Wangsa D, Tang Q, Zhao K. Characterization of genome-wide enhancer-promoter interactions reveals co-expression of interacting genes and modes of higher order chromatin organization. Cell Res. 2012;22:490–503.

5

Epigenetic regulation of ID4 in breast cancer: tumor suppressor or oncogene?

Daniela Nasif[1†], Emanuel Campoy[3†], Sergio Laurito[2], Richard Branham[4], Guillermo Urrutia[1], María Roqué[2] and María T. Branham[1*] (iD)

Abstract

Background: Inhibitor of differentiation protein 4 (ID4) is a dominant negative regulator of the basic helix-loop-helix (bHLH) family of transcription factors. During tumorigenesis, ID4 may act as a tumor suppressor or as an oncogene in different tumor types. However, the role of ID4 in breast cancer is not clear where both an oncogenic and a tumor suppressor function have been attributed. Here, we hypothesize that ID4 behaves as both, but its role in breast differs according to the estrogen receptor (ER) status of the tumor.

Methods: ID4 expression was retrieved from TCGA database using UCSC Xena. Association between overall survival (OS) and ID4 was assessed using Kaplan–Meier plotter. Correlation between methylation and expression was analyzed using the MEXPRESS tool. In vitro experiments involved ectopic expression of ID4 in MCF-7, T47D, and MDA-MB231 breast cancer cell lines. Migration and colony formation capacity were assessed after transfection treatments. Gene expression was analyzed by ddPCR and methylation by MSP, MS-MLPA, or ddMSP.

Results: Data mining analysis revealed that ID4 expression is significantly lower in ER+ tumors with respect to ER− tumors or normal tissue. We also demonstrate that ID4 is significantly methylated in ER+ tumors. Kaplan–Meier analysis indicated that low ID4 expression levels were associated with poor overall survival in patients with FR+ tumors. In silico expression analysis indicated that ID4 was associated with the expression of key genes of the ER pathway only in ER+ tumors. In vitro experiments revealed that ID4 overexpression in ER+ cell lines resulted in decreased migration capacity and reduced number of colonies. ID4 overexpression induced a reduction in ER levels in ER+ cell lines, while estrogen deprivation with fulvestrant did not induce changes neither in ID4 methylation nor in ID4 expression.

Conclusions: We propose that ID4 is frequently silenced by promoter methylation in ER+ breast cancers and functions as a tumor suppressor gene in these tumors, probably due to its interaction with key genes of the ER pathway. Our present study contributes to the knowledge of the role of ID4 in breast cancer.

Keywords: ID4, Tumor suppressor, Breast cancer, Methylation

Background

Inhibitor of differentiation (ID) proteins 1, 2, 3, and 4 regulate the expression of genes by acting as dominant negative regulators of the basic helix-loop-helix (bHLH) transcription factors. ID proteins interact with the bHLH transcription factors and form heterodimers, inhibiting in this way their possible binding to DNA since ID proteins lack the basic DNA-binding domain [1]. During differentiation, the expression of ID proteins is downregulated in cells, and on the contrary, it is increased in stem cells [2]. In human tumors, an increased expression of ID proteins has been associated with reversion to an embryonic-like state, with loss of differentiation, increased migration, proliferation, and neo-angiogenesis [3]. However, discordant literature attributes opposite roles to ID proteins; for example, some studies have also recognized ID proteins as critical actors of antiproliferative signaling pathways in cancer [4]. So, it seems then that, according to the cellular context, ID proteins can

* Correspondence: mtbranham@mendoza-conicet.gob.ar; mbranham@fcm.uncu.edu.ar
†Daniela Nasif and Emanuel Campoy contributed equally to this work.
[1]IHEM, National University of Cuyo, CONICET, Mendoza, Argentina
Full list of author information is available at the end of the article

pursue divergent functions and act as oncoproteins or tumor suppressors [2].

ID4 is a member of this protein family and it has been shown to be highly expressed in neurons [5], osteoblasts [6], adipocytes [7], prostate epithelial cells [8], and testicular Sertoli cells [9]. In embryogenesis, ID4 is required for normal mammary [10] and prostate gland development [8]. In cancer, ID4 presents again divergent roles since it has been described to act as a tumor suppressor in prostate [11], lung [12], and gastric [13] tumors, and as an oncogene in ovarian cancer [14] and glioblastomas [15].

In breast cancer, the role of ID4 is not clear. Epigenetic silencing of ID4 (a characteristic mechanism to downregulate tumor suppressor genes during cancer progression) has been described in mammary columnar cell lesions, ductal carcinoma in situ, and invasive carcinomas [16]. In addition, the hypermethylation of ID4 promoter has been associated with an increased risk of lymph node metastasis [17]. Epigenetic silencing and gene expression downregulation are hallmarks of tumor suppressor gene function, since their absence allows the progress of a tumorigenic process. However, we and others have found the opposite role for ID4 in breast tumors. Increased ID4 expression has been informed in basal cell-like breast cancer [18], and we found increased expression and hypomethylation of its promoter in triple-negative breast cancer (TNBC) [19]. Moreover, increased ID4 expression has been associated with the ability of breast cancer cells to exhibit anchorage-independent growth [20]. Also, high ID4 expression in TNBC has been associated with BRCA1 down regulation and BRCAness phenotype [21, 22]. Therefore, enough evidence exists to conclude that ID4 can assume distinct roles in breast cancer, depending on the cellular context. We hypothesize that ID4 acts as both, tumor suppressor and oncogene, but its role will differ according to the ER status of the breast cancer cell. We have previously demonstrated that ID4 acts as an oncogene in ER-negative tumors. In this work, we hypothesize that ID4 may behave as a tumor suppressor in an ER+ cellular context.

Methods

Cell lines and cell culture

Human breast cancer cell lines MCF-7, T47D, and MDA-MB231, were kindly provided by Dr. Lanari from the IBYME Institute, Buenos Aires, Argentina and by Dr. Matias Sanchez, IMBECU Institute, Mendoza, Argentina, respectively. Cell lines were cultured in DMEM medium (Gibco by Life Technologies, Grand Island, NY, USA, # 1852779) supplemented with 10% fetal bovine serum (Internegocios S.A, Mercedes, BA, Argentina), 100 U/mL of penicillin, and 100 µg/mL streptomycin (Gibco by Life Technologies, Grand Island, NY, USA, #1796440). All cell lines were incubated at 37 °C in a humidified atmosphere containing 5% CO_2. For estrogen

depletion experiments, cells were cultured in phenol red-free RPMI supplemented with charcoal-stripped 10% fetal bovine serum for 1 week prior to drug treatment. After this time, fulvestrant 1 µM was added to the medium and cells were treated for 72 h.

Plasmids and transfections

The full-length human ID4 cloned into pCMV vector (pCMV-Id4) was a generous gift from Dr. Mark Israel. Transfection of 3 µg of pCMV-ID4 or 3 µg pGFP (as control vector) were performed with Lipofectamine 2000 (Invitrogen, Van Allen Way Carlsbad, CA, USA # 1828126) at 90% confluence according to the manufacturer's instructions. Transfection was monitored by fluorescence microscopy and after 48 h, it achieved a 70% efficiency. ID4 overexpression was confirmed by Western blot (Additional file 1: Figure S1). After transfection, different assays were performed as described below.

Migration assay

Forty-eight hours after transfection, the migration assay was started. Cells were serum-starved overnight before the scratch was produced; afterwards, the cells were maintained in a serum-reduced medium containing 0.5% FBS. Cell cultures were then scratched with a 200 µL sterile pipette tip and extensively washed with PBS to remove detached cells and debris. One cross was scratched in each well; then, images of the same area were taken at 24, 48, and 72 h. These were instantly center-imaged at × 4 magnification, using a T-2000 microscope equipment (Nikon, Tokyo, Japan).

Colony formation assay

After transfection, MCF7 and T47D cells were platted at a density of 1000 cells per well in six well plates and allowed to adhere overnight at 37 °C, 5% CO_2. The cells were allowed to grow until control treatment colonies reached > 50 cells per colony (approximately 12 days). Colonies were then fixed with glutaraldehyde for 30 min, stained with crystal violet 0.5% for 30 min and washed. Next, colony number was counted by using an automatized procedure with Image J software.

Methylation analysis

For MSP and droplet digital MSP (ddMSP) assays, DNA was firstly bisulfite-converted with the EZ DNA Methylation-Direct ™ Kit (Zymo RESEARCH, Irvine, California, USA). Primers used for MSP and ddMSP were specific for detection of the methylated and un-methylated status of the ID4 promoter. Primers were purchased from Integrated DNA Technologies (CA, USA). Forward primers for MSP covered the TATA box, E-box, and three CpG sites in the minimal promoter region (− 48 to + 32) [23]. The methylation-specific primer

set was as follows: forward, 5′-TTTTATAAATATAG
TTGCGCGGGC-3′; and reverse, 5′-GAAACTCCG
ACTAAACCCGAT-3′. The unmethylation-specific primer set was as follows: forward, 5′-TTT
TATAAATATAGTTGTGTGGTGG-3′; and reverse,
5′-TCA AAACTCCAACTAAACCCAAT-3′. The PCR
amplification reaction for MSP was performed in a
25 μl final volume and consisted of a 40-cycle program,
composed of 30s at 94 °C, 30 s at 58 °C, and 30 s at 72 °C,
followed by a 7 min final extension at 72 °C. Mg^{2+} concentration was 1.5 mM for methylated-specific and 2.5 mM
for unmethylated-specific primer sets. Primer concentration was 0.1 μM for methylated-specific and
0.4 μM for unmethylated-specific primer sets. PCR
products were resolved by 2% agarose gel electrophoresis and quantified by ImageJ software. ddPCR general specifications are described below.

The MS-MLPA assays were performed basically according to manufacturer's recommendations (MRC-Holland,
Amsterdam, The Netherlands, (www.mlpa.com). A CpG
site was considered to be methylated when the methylation dosage ratio between digested and undigested sample
was superior to the cut-off threshold of 8% [19].

Droplet digital PCR

Purified RNA was converted to cDNA using M-MLV
Reverse Transcriptase, and cDNA was diluted to 0.2 ng/μl
and stored at − 20 °C until use. For each assay, 5 μl of the
diluted sample (1 ng cDNA) was run using the Bio-Rad
EvaGreen master mix. For each assay, droplets were generated using Droplet Generation Oil for EvaGreen
(Bio-Rad) on the QX200 Droplet Generator (Bio-Rad)
according to the manufacture's protocol and adding the
specific primers for ER with the following sequence:
forward, 5′-CAGGACTCGGTGGATATGGT; and reverse, 5′-CCAGGGAAGCTACTGTTTGC. Droplets
were cycled on the C1000 Touch Thermal Cycler
(Bio-Rad) for 40 cycles, with a 58 °C annealing
temperature. Droplets were read using the QX200
Droplet Reader (Bio-Rad). Data was analyzed in Quan-
taSoft software (Bio-Rad). Each DNA sample was run
in three technical replicates and the mean was considered for further comparisons.

In silico data analysis

TCGA breast cancer data was obtained from the UCSC
Xena resource (http://xena.ucsc.edu/). For gene expression, the RNA-Seq (polyA+ Illumina HiSeq) data was
downloaded as log2 (norm_count+ 1) values. For methylation analysis, the Illumina Infinium Human Methylation 450 platform was retrieved. This platform
represents DNA methylation as beta values, which are
continuous variables between 0 and 1, representing the

ratio of the intensity of the methylated bead type to the
combined locus intensity.

Additionally, the MEXPRESS tool was used for
visualization and interpretation of the expression,
methylation, and clinical data available in TCGA
(http://mexpress.be/) [24]. Survival curves were estimated using the Kaplan–Meier plotter tool (http://
kmplot.com/analysis/). This tool uses an online database of published microarray datasets for breast, ovarian, lung, and gastric cancer, and it includes clinical
and gene expression data for 5143 breast cancer patients [25]. The analyses were performed using the Jet-
Set best probe set. Survival was also analyzed using the
breast cancer Miller cohort downloaded form (http://
xena.ucsc.edu/) [26].

The association between relative gene expression
values was performed by SVD (singular-value decomposition) as previously described [22]. The correlation coefficients between ID4 and each specific gene were
calculated by the standard statistical procedure described
by Wonnacott and Wonnacot (Introductory Statistics,
2nd ed., John Wiley, 1972, pp. 326–331). These statistical analyses were performed using MATLAB (Natick,
MA, USA). mRNA expression differences between
groups of breast cancers were assessed using unpaired
Student's t test and a one-way analysis of variance with
Bonferroni's post hoc analysis for comparison between
multiple groups.

ArrayExpress data

For ID4 expression analysis in MCF-7 control vs.
fulvestrant-treated cells, an in vitro model of MCF-7
cells treated with ER antagonists was retrieved from
ArrayExpress with the accession number E-MTAB-4426.
The intensity of ID4 probe (A_23_P59375) was compared between the following conditions: WT_CCS+ Fulv
vs. WT_CCS + DMSO [27].

Additional statistical analysis

Unless otherwise noted, all laboratory experiments were
realized a minimum of three separate times and statistical analysis were performed using Graph Pad Prism
software version 5. A Student's t test was used for comparison between two groups. Significance was defined as
a p value < 0.05.

Results

In silico analyses reveal that ID4 expression differs according to ER status in breast cancer

We first aimed to study the expression of ID4 across
breast tumors with different ER status. For this, we used
the IlluminaHiSeq_RNASeqV2 expression data from 780
breast tumors and 138 normal breast tissue samples from
the TCGA (The Cancer Genome Atlas) database. We

divided the tumor samples in two groups: ER+ ($n = 601$) and ER– ($n = 179$). As shown in Fig. 1a, ER+ breast tumors present a significant reduction in ID4 expression as compared to ER– tumors and to normal tissue ($p < 0.001$). Next, we performed a new analysis but, in this case, considering ID4 expression according to the PAM50 breast cancer molecular classification, i.e., luminal A, luminal B, normal-like, basal-like, and HER2-enriched. As shown in Fig. 1b, ID4

expression is significantly lower in luminal A ($n = 434$) and luminal B ($n = 194$) subtypes (both ER+) as compared with basal-like ($n = 142$) and normal-like breast tumors ($n = 119$) (both ER–) ($p < 0.001$). HER2-enriched subtype ($n = 66$) showed significantly lower levels of ID4 expression with respect to basal-like or normal-like tumors ($p < 0.001$). This observation could be confusing given that this subtype is often thought of as being ER– only. However, it should be taken into consideration that

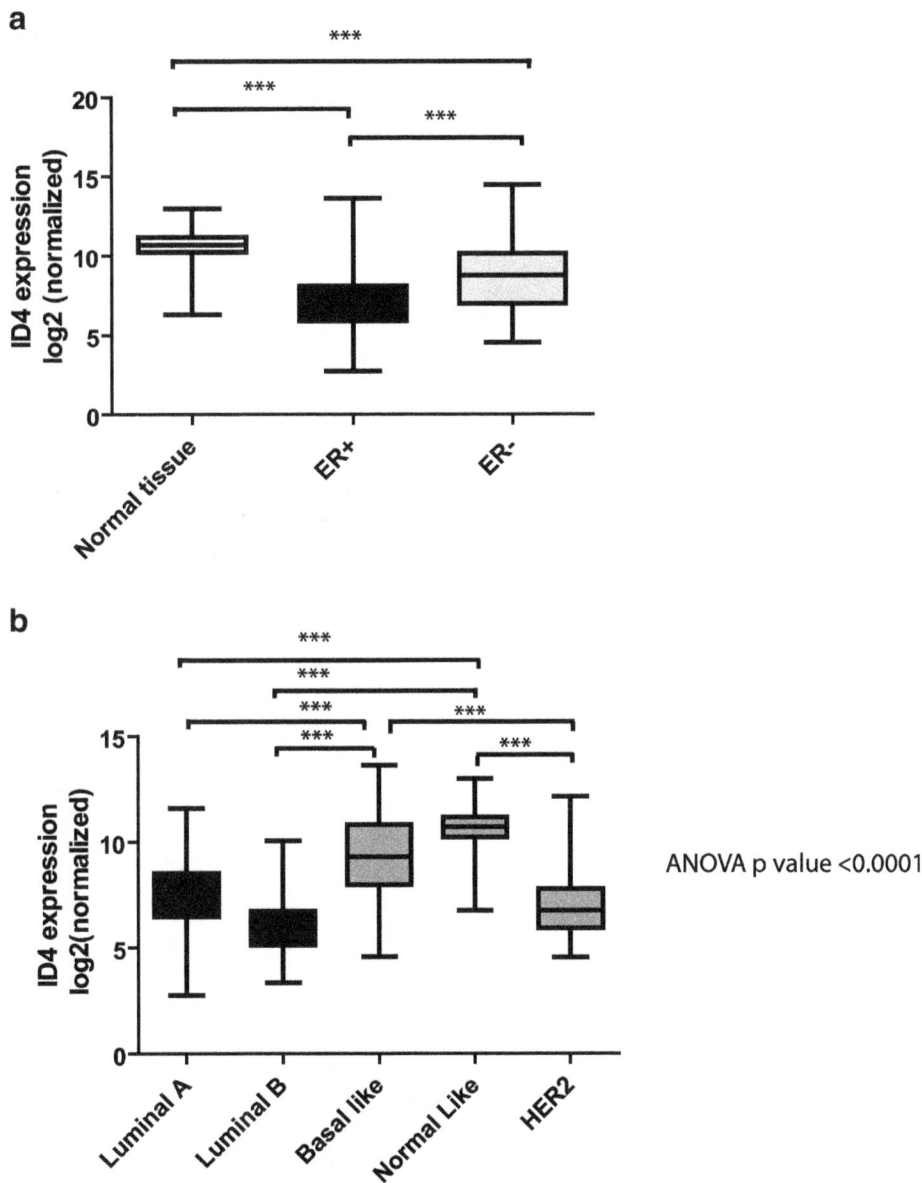

Fig. 1 Comparison of ID4 expression among different breast cancer subtypes. **a–b** The expression of ID4 is shown relative to **a** ER+ ($n = 601$) and ER– ($n = 179$) and normal tissue ($n = 114$), **b** PAM50 molecular subtypes: luminal a ($n = 434$), luminal b ($n = 194$), basal-like ($n = 142$), normal-like breast tumors ($n = 119$), and HER2-enriched ($n = 66$). The Student's t test was applied to evaluate differences in ID4 expression between two groups and one way analysis of variance (ANOVA) with Bonferroni's post hoc analysis to compare three or more groups. The bottom and top of the box represent the first and third quartiles of the data, respectively, and the band inside the box represents the median of the data. The lower and upper whiskers represent the lowest and highest data points of the data, respectively. As can be seen in panel **a** and **b**, ID4 expression is reduced in ER+ subgroups ***$p < 0.001$

the HER2-enriched subtype can include ER+ and ER− tumors as well. This mixed composition could explain lower levels of ID4 expression for this subtype.

Taken together, our results show that ID4 expression differs according to the ER status, and that its expression is significantly lower in ER+ breast tumors.

High ID4 expression is associated with better prognosis in ER+ breast tumors

To evaluate whether the expression level of ID4 could have any predictive value for breast cancer overall survival (OS), we used the online survival analysis software, Kaplan–Meier (KM) plotter [25]. This tool allowed us to study the expression of ID4 as dichotomized values in "high" or "low" according to the median expression of the gene. The relationship between ID4 expression and OS of 799 breast cancer patients was analyzed separating ER+ ($n = 548$) from ER− ($n = 251$) cases. As shown in Fig. 2a, among the patients with ER+ tumors, those with higher ID4 expression levels presented better probabilities of survival ($p < 0.001$); this result suggests that this group of patients with high ID4 expression levels have an active (not silenced) ID4 tumor suppressor gene. Remarkably this was not observed in ER− tumors (Fig. 2b) ($p = 0,49$). To confirm these results, we performed a Kaplan–Meier analysis using another database such as the Miller 2005 cohort. We analyzed OS in 213 ER+ breast cancer patients dividing ID4 values in high or low according to the median expression of the gene. As shown in Additional file 2: Figure S2 higher ID4 expression levels were associated with better probabilities of survival in line with Kaplan–Meier plotter results. Given that high ID4

expression was only beneficial in the ER+ group, we speculate that ID4 has a tumor suppressor role in these tumors.

ID4 expression is downregulated through methylation in ER+ breast tumors as assed by in silico analyses

Since ID4 expression has been shown to be principally regulated trough methylation [13, 17, 28], we asked if there are differences in the methylation levels of ID4 according to the ER status. To answer this question, we queried the MEXPRESS tool which allows the visualization and interpretation of the gene expression, the methylation and the clinical data available in TCGA [24]. As shown in Fig. 3, this tool permitted us to analyze the methylation of ID4 tested with 13 probes distributed in different regions of the gene (the localization of each probe is represented in the figure and the ones localized in the promoter region are highlighted in dark blue). As can be observed, the methylation values increase as tumors become ER+; this can also be observed in Additional file 3: Figure S3 for CpGs in the promoter of ID4. All the regions analyzed presented a negative correlation with respect to ID4 gene expression (Pearson's correlation coefficients for each probe are indicated on the right), suggesting that ID4 methylation silences gene expression.

Another interesting observation is that ER status and ID4 expression present an inverse correlation, where ID4 expression gradually diminishes (due to promoter methylation) as tumors become ER+ ($p < 0.0001$). The MEXPRESS tool also allowed us to visualize ID4 expression and methylation status according to PAM50 breast cancer molecular classification. As observed in Fig. 3 the methylation of ID4 increases (and ID4 expression decreases) in

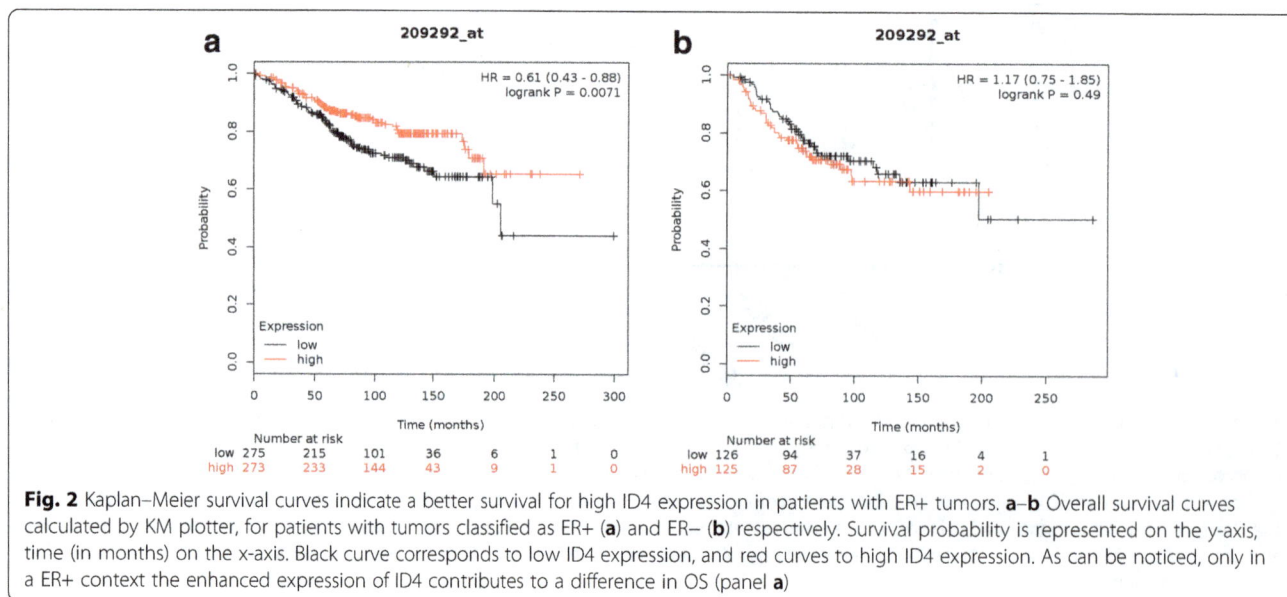

Fig. 2 Kaplan–Meier survival curves indicate a better survival for high ID4 expression in patients with ER+ tumors. **a–b** Overall survival curves calculated by KM plotter, for patients with tumors classified as ER+ (**a**) and ER− (**b**) respectively. Survival probability is represented on the y-axis, time (in months) on the x-axis. Black curve corresponds to low ID4 expression, and red curves to high ID4 expression. As can be noticed, only in a ER+ context the enhanced expression of ID4 contributes to a difference in OS (panel **a**)

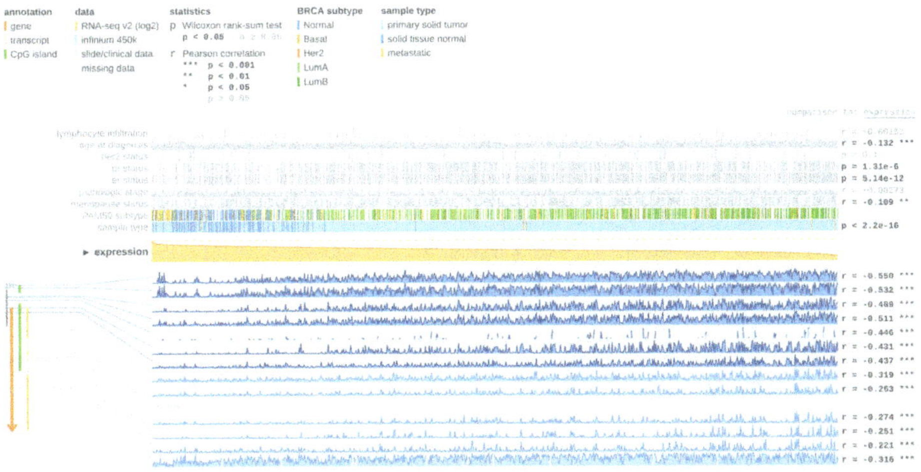

Fig. 3 ID4 expression and methylation status in breast cancer using MEXPRESS. At the top of the figure clinical TGCA data available is represented and ordered according to ID4 expression. At the right-hand side, the Pearson's correlation coefficient r and the p values for Wilcoxon rank-sum test are shown. ID4 expression is symbolized as the orange line in the center of the plot. The samples are ordered according to ID4 expression, with the highest expression on the left side and the lowest on the right. The blue lines (bottom right) represent the Infinium 450 k probes that are linked to ID4. The height of the blue lines indicates the beta value for the probe. The probes localized in the promoter region of the gene are highlighted in dark blue. ID4 gene and CpG islands (green lines) are represented on the left (bottom)

luminal A and luminal B subtypes (both ER+ and represented as green lines in Fig. 3) whereas methylation decreases (and expression increases) in basal-like and normal-like subtypes (both ER– and represented in Fig. 3 as yellow and blue lines respectively). Since aberrant DNA methylation of promoter regions is one of the mechanisms for the silencing of tumor suppressor genes in cancer, and because ID4 promoter is mostly methylated in ER+ tumors, we can again speculate that ID4 behaves principally as a tumor suppressor gene in these groups of breast tumors.

ID4 expression is associated to the expression of different genes according to ER status

We next expanded our analysis to investigate whether the expression of ID4 is associated with different genes according to the ER status. To test this, we used the singular-value decomposition (SVD) analysis and studied the expression of ID4 vs. the expression of 66 genes with different functions in breast cancer (Table 1) in 780 samples from TCGA database. SVD represents an appropriate tool for gene expression analysis in which the singular values are associated with the importance of each variable in the linear system. The SVD program we used for this analysis is not a commercial one, such as MATHLAB, because these programs sort the singular values after they are calculated, and as a consequence, one loses the correspondence between ID4 and the gene under study. Rather, we used a C++ program written by one of the authors that leaves the singular values unsorted and hence maintains this correspondence. To define the most relevant genes associated with ID4

expression, we selected the genes that were higher than the median for the 66 singular values; 15 of the 66 genes met this criterion, which differed depending on the ER status. In ER+ tumors, ID4 expression was associated with the expressions of FOXA1, GATA3, ESR1, CCND1, AKT1, and IGFR; whereas in ER– tumors, ID4 expression was associated with VEGF, JUN, and MKI67. Finally, shared association was found for CTNNB1, ERBB2, CTSD, KRT19, MMP2, and XBP1 (Fig. 4a).

Next, we focused on ER+ tumors to determine the type of correlation between ID4 and the specific genes of interest within this group. By calculation of the correlation coefficients, we found that ID4 expression is negatively correlated with the expression of FOXA1 ($r = -0.326$) ($p < 0.0001$), GATA3 ($r = -0.3515$) ($p < 0.0001$), ESR1 ($r = -0.333$) ($p < 0.0001$), CCND1($r = -0.19$) ($p < 0.0001$), AKT1 (-0.068) ($p = 0.094$), and IGFR (-0.065) ($p = 0.1$) (As shown in Fig. 4b). These negative correlations maintain their significance even when all the tumor cohorts (ER+ and ER–) are analyzed (Additional file 4: Figure S4). These results are particularly interesting given that some authors suggest that ID4 inhibits the expression of ESR1 and FOXA1 (through the interaction of ID4 with the promoter of these genes) in the developing mammary gland [29]. We hypothesize then that in an ER+ context, ID4 downregulation, trough methylation, disrupts the normal balance of important genes of the ER pathway.

Taken all together, from our in silico analyses, we can so far propose that in ER+ breast tumors, ID4 behaves as a tumor suppressor gene epigenetically regulated by DNA methylation.

Table 1 Genes involved with distinct functions in breast cancer

Gene symbol	Gene name	Molecular and cellular function
ABCB1 (MDR1)	ATP-binding cassette subfamily B member 1	Xenobiotic transport
ABCG2 (BCRP)	ATP-binding cassette subfamily G member 2	Xenobiotic transport
ADAM23	ADAM metallopeptidase domain 23	Proteolysis
AKT1	AKT serine/threonine kinase 1	Signal transduction (AKT and PI3 kinase signaling)
APC	Adenomatosis polyposis coli	Signal transduction (WNT signaling), cell adhesion, apoptosis, cell cycle, DNA damage, and repair
AR	Androgen receptor	Signal transduction (steroid receptor-mediated signaling) and transcription factor
ATM	ATM serine/threonine kinase	DNA damage and repair
BCL2	BCL2, apoptosis regulator	Signal transduction (hedgehog signaling), cell adhesion, apoptosis, and cell cycle
BIRC5	Baculoviral IAP repeat-containing	Signal transduction (Notch signaling)
BRCA1	Breast cancer 1	DNA damage and repair and signal transduction (steroid receptor-mediated signaling)
BRCA2	Breast cancer 2	DNA damage and repair
CCNA1	Cyclin A1	Cell cycle
CCND1	Cyclin D1	Cell cycle, DNA damage and repair, and signal transduction (hedgehog and WNT signaling)
CCND2	Cyclin D2	Cell cycle
CCNE1	Cyclin E1	Cell cycle and signal transduction (steroid receptor-mediated signaling)
CDH13	Cadherin 13	Cell adhesion and angiogenesis
CDK2	Cyclin-dependent kinase 2	Cell cycle
CDKN1A	Cyclin-dependent kinase inhibitor 1A	Cell cycle, DNA damage and repair, and apoptosis
CDKN1C	Cyclin-dependent kinase inhibitor 1AC	Cell cycle
CDKN2A	Cyclin-dependent kinase inhibitor 2A	Cell cycle, apoptosis, and cell adhesion
CST6	Cystatin E/M	Proteases
CTNNB1	Catenin beta 1	Signal transduction (steroid receptor-mediated signaling), epithelial to mesenchymal transition, angiogenesis, and cell adhesion
CTSD	Cathepsin D	Proteases
EGF	Epidermal growth factor	Angiogenesis
ERBB2	Erb-b2 receptor tyrosine kinase 2	Signal transduction (AKT/PI3K signaling), angiogenesis, and cell adhesion
ESR1	Estrogen receptor 1	Signal transduction (steroid receptor-mediated signaling) and transcription factor
ESR2	Estrogen receptor 2	Signal transduction (steroid receptor-mediated signaling) and transcription factor
FOXA1	Forkhead box A1	Transcription factor
GATA3	GATA-binding protein 3	Transcription factor
HIC1	HIC ZBTB transcriptional repressor 1	Transcription factor
ID1	Inhibitor of DNA binding 1	Angiogenesis and breast cancer metastasis to lung and breast cancer classification marker
IGF1	Insulin-like growth factor 1	Signal transduction (steroid receptor-mediated and AKT/PI3K signaling)
IGF1R	Insulin-like growth factor 1 receptor	Signal transduction (AKT/PI3K signaling)
IGFBP3	Insulin-like growth factor-binding protein 3	Signal transduction (glucocorticoid signaling)
IL6	Interleukin 6	Angiogenesis and apoptosis
JUN	Jun proto-oncogene	Angiogenesis, apoptosis, cell cycle, and transcription factor
KRT19	Keratin 19	Signal transduction (steroid receptor-mediated signaling)
MAPK1	Mitogen-activated protein kinase 1	Signal transduction (MAP kinase-mediated signaling) and DNA damage and repair
MAPK3	Mitogen-activated protein kinase 3	Signal transduction (MAP kinase-mediated signaling)
MAPK8	Mitogen-activated protein kinase 8	Signal transduction (MAP kinase-mediated signaling)
MGMT	O-6-methylguanine-DNA methyltransferase	DNA damage and repair
MKI67	Marker of proliferation Ki-67	Cell cycle
MLH1	MutL homolog 1	DNA damage and repair

Table 1 Genes involved with distinct functions in breast cancer *(Continued)*

Gene symbol	Gene name	Molecular and cellular function
MMP2	Matrix metallopeptidase 2	Proteases and breast cancer metastasis to lung and breast cancer classification marker
MMP9	Matrix metallopeptidase 9	Proteases
MYC	V-myc avian myelocytomatosis viral oncogene homolog	Cell cycle and transcription factor
NME1	NME/NM23 nucleoside diphosphate kinase 1	Signal transduction (glucocorticoid signaling) and apoptosis
NOTCH1	Notch 1	Signal transduction (Notch signaling) and angiogenesis
NR3C1	Nuclear receptor subfamily 3 group C member 1	Signal transduction (glucocorticoid signaling) and transcription factor
PGR	Progesterone receptor	Signal transduction (steroid receptor-mediated signaling) and transcription factor
PLAU	Plasminogen activator, urokinase	Angiogenesis and proteases
PRDM2	PR/SET domain 2	Transcription factor
PTEN	Phosphatase and tensin homolog	Signal transduction (AKT/PI3K signaling), angiogenesis, cell adhesion, and cell cycle
PYCARD	PYD and CARD domain-containing	Proteases
RARB	Retinoic acid receptor beta	Apoptosis and transcription factor
RASSF1	Ras-association domain family member 1	Cell cycle
RB1	RB transcriptional corepressor 1	Signal transduction (steroid receptor-mediated signaling), cell cycle, and transcription factor
SERPINE1	Serpin family E member 1	Angiogenesis
SFN	Stratifin	Apoptosis, cell cycle, and DNA damage and repair
SFRP1	Secreted frizzled-related protein	Signal transduction (WNT signaling) and apoptosis
SLIT2	Slit guidance ligand 2	Angiogenesis
THBS1	Thrombospondin 1	Angiogenesis and cell adhesion
TP53	Tumor protein p53	Apoptosis, cell cycle, DNA damage and repair, and transcription factor
TP73	Tumor protein p73	Apoptosis, DNA damage and repair, transcription factor, and signal transduction (MAP kinase signaling)
VEGFA	Vascular endothelial growth factor	Angiogenesis
XBP1	X-box binding protein 1	Transcription factor

Ectopic ID4 expression reduces aggressive phenotype only in ER+ breast cancer cell lines

Based on our in silico conclusions, we decided to extend our studies and measure tumoral behavior by modulating the expression of ID4 in cultured ER+ breast cancer cell lines. To accomplish this, we performed transfection experiments with an ID4 vector in MCF-7 and T47D cells. We have previously shown that both cell lines do not express ID4 due to promoter methylation. [22]. Next, we measured cell migration potential (by wound healing assays) and colony formation ability, two hallmarks of cancer cells. As shown in Fig. 5a, both cell lines transfected with ID4 presented a significant reduction in migration rate compared to cells transfected with the control vector ($p < 0.05$). Consistently, colony formation assay showed that ID4 overexpression in MCF-7 and T47D cells led to a significant decrease in the number of colonies when compared with cells transfected with the control vector ($p < 0.05$) (Fig. 5b).

To confirm that ID4 behaves as a tumor suppressor only in ER+ breast tumors, we tested the effect of ID4 overexpression in the ER− breast cancer cell line MDA-MB231. To accurately study the effect of ID4 in an ER− context, we first confirmed by ddPCR that the MDA-MB231 cell lines did not express ER. Next, we performed transfection experiments with the ID4 vector as previously described and tested cell migration potential (by wound healing assays). ID4 overexpression did not affect migration capacity of the MDA-MB231 cell lines (Fig. 6).

Taken together, the transfection assays suggest concordantly that the ectopic expression of ID4 is inducing a less aggressive phenotype only in ER+ cell lines, revealed by a decreased migration and a reduced ability to produce new colonies. These results are in line with a dual role of ID4 in breast cancer.

ID4 expression reduces ER levels in MCF-7 cells as assessed by ddPCR

As we mentioned previously, ID4 expression is associated with key genes of the ER pathway. Taking this observation

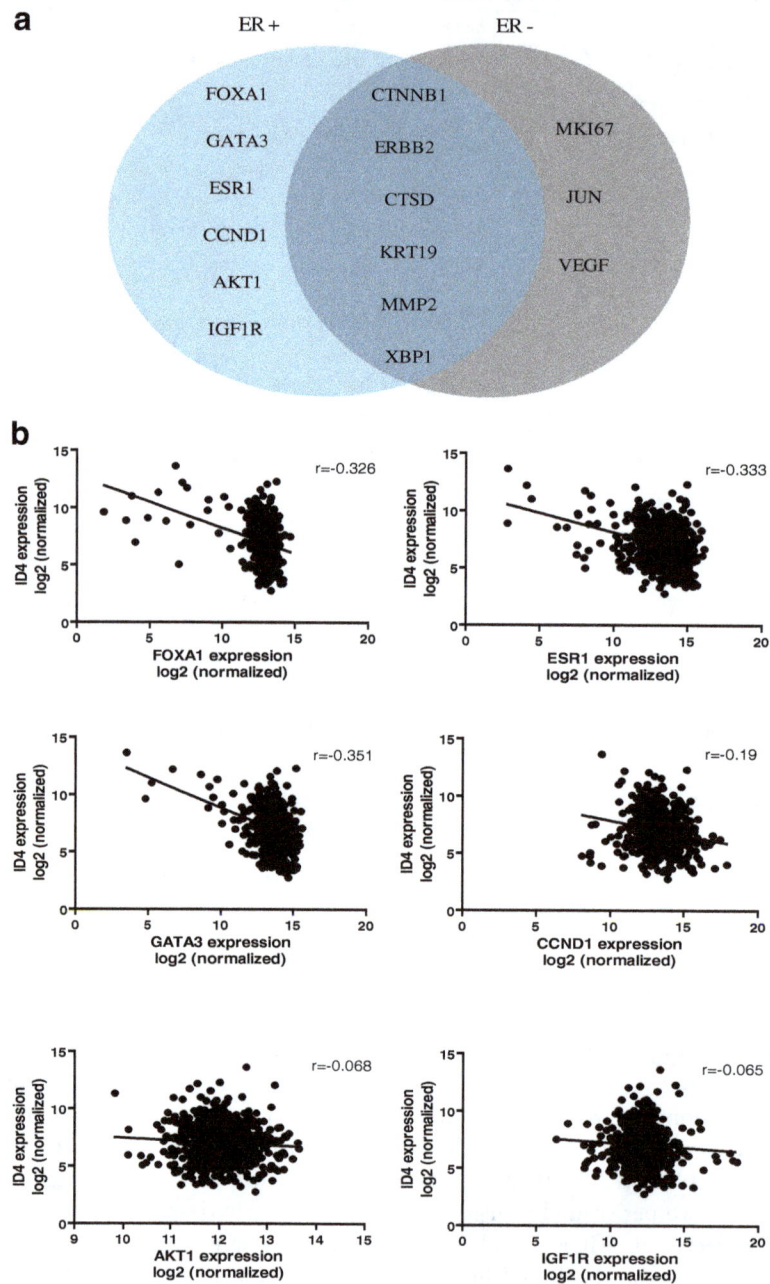

Fig. 4 Genes associated with ID4 expression. **a** Venn diagram representing the expression for genes significantly associated with the expression of ID4 in breast cancer as determined by SVD analysis. The figure depicts the genes significantly associated with ID4 in ER+ and ER− tumors and the overlap the genes with shared expression between the two groups. **b** Correlations between ID4 expression and the expression of FOXA1, ESR1, GATA3, CCND1, AKT, and IGF1R. Correlation values for each analysis are indicated on the right

into consideration, we decided to study the effect of ID4 overexpression on ER levels in an ER+ cell line. To test this, we transfected MCF-7 cells with the ID4-expressing plasmid. As control, cells were transfected with the GFP control vector. When obtaining total RNA from both experiments and measuring the expression level of ER by ddPCR, a significant difference could be observed. As

shown in Fig. 7, ID4 overexpression induced a significant reduction in ER levels of MCF-7 cells as compared to the same cells transfected with a control vector ($p < 0.01$).

Given that in ER+ breast, tumors ER levels are higher than in normal tissue, and these higher levels are associated with certain aggressive characteristics such as increased cell proliferation, and we speculate

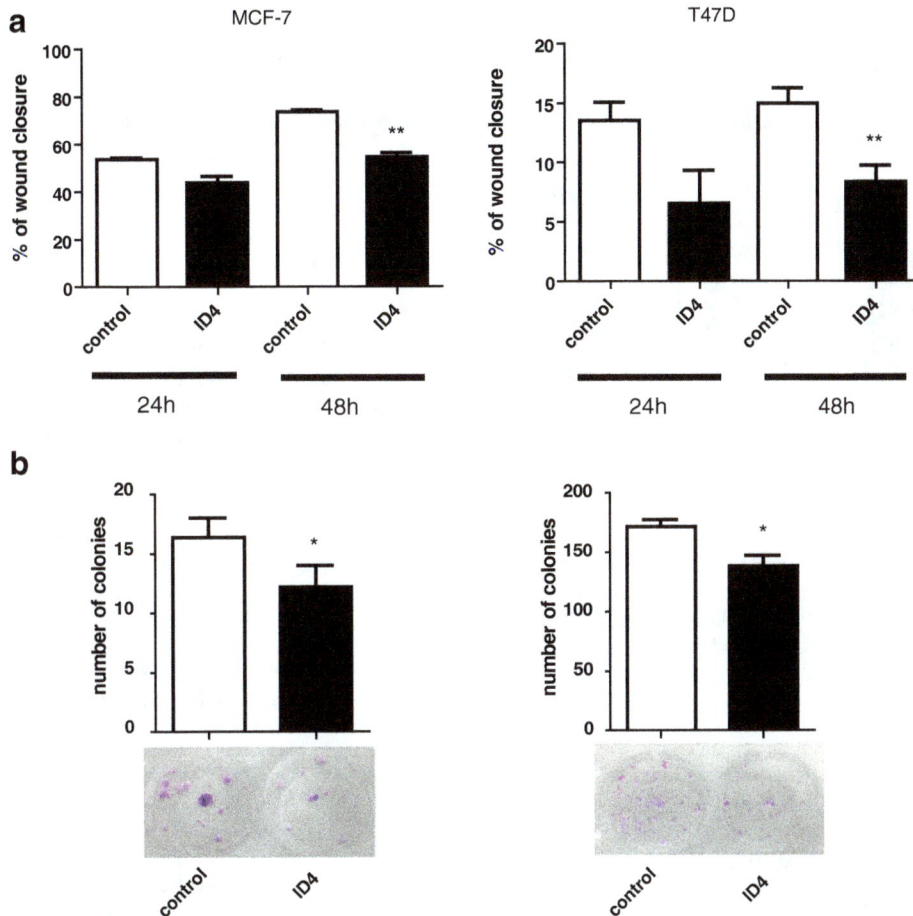

Fig. 5 Phenotypic changes associated with ectopic ID4 expression in breast cancer cell lines. **a** Bar graph presentation of wound healing assay comparisons. The effect of ectopic expression of ID4 was tested on cell migration ability in MCF-7 and T47D cell lines (left and right respectively). Columns represent the mean of at least three independent experiments. $*p < 0.05$ and $**p < 0.01$ in comparison with the control per Student's t test. For migration experiments, cells were maintained in a serum-reduced medium to inhibit the cells' ability to proliferate. **b** Colony formation assay was used to confirm the effect of ID4 expression in T47D and MCF-7 transfected either with ID4 or the control vector. Results are expressed as the mean $\pm$ SD of three independent experiments

that ID4 re-expression in ER+ cell lines reduces the ER levels perhaps to those of normal tissue and possibly exerts its tumor suppressor function trough ER regulation (Fig. 7).

ER levels do not affect methylation nor ID4 expression levels in MCF-7 cell lines

To study if there is a regulatory loop between ER and ID4, we next tested if estrogen deprivation affected the methylation status or the expression levels of ID4 in the ER+ cell line MCF-7. To test this, we first treated the cells with 1μM of the ER antagonist fulvestrant and measured ID4 methylation status by ddMSP and MS-MLPA. As shown in Fig. 8a, there was a slight reduction in the methylation levels of fulvestrant treated cells, but this difference was not statically significant ($p = 0.45$). To further analyze if

there were changes in the methylation status of other regions of ID4 promoter, we performed a MS-MLPA assay with the ME003 panel. This panel contains 27 probes two of which hybridize at different CpG sites from that tested by ddMSP. The MS-MLPA assay revealed that there was no significant difference in the methylation level between control and fulvestrant-treated cells in neither of the CpG sites tested (Additional file 5: Figure S5).

Since it has been shown that promoter methylation is the main mechanism that controls ID4 gene expression [13, 17, 28], we speculated (given our ddMSP and MS-MLPA results) that there was not going to be differences in ID4 gene expression after estrogen deprivation. To confirm this, we performed in silico analysis on a public data set of an in vitro model of MCF-7 cells treated with ER antagonists such as fulvestrant

a MDA-MB231

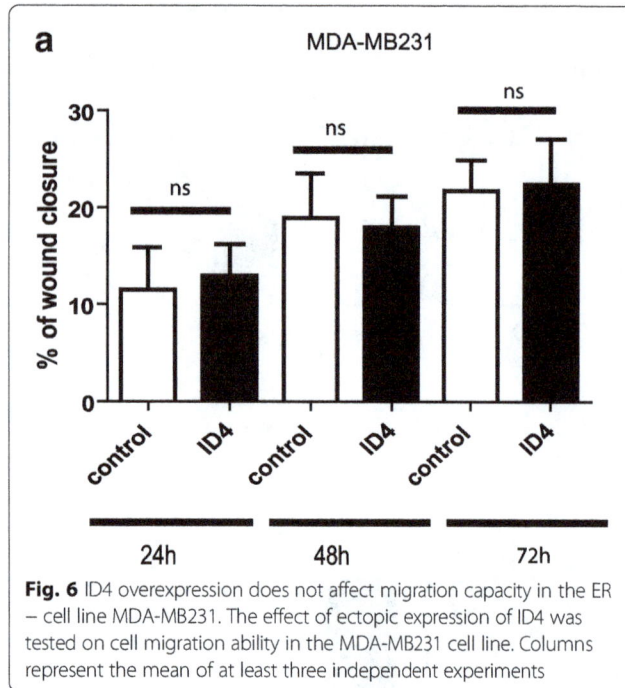

Fig. 6 ID4 overexpression does not affect migration capacity in the ER – cell line MDA-MB231. The effect of ectopic expression of ID4 was tested on cell migration ability in the MDA-MB231 cell line. Columns represent the mean of at least three independent experiments

(ArrayExpress accession number E-MTAB-4426), and as shown in Fig. 8b, there were no differences on ID4 gene expression between control and fulvestrant-treated cells.

Taken together, our results reveal that while ID4 reduces ER expression, estrogen levels do not affect neither ID4 methylation nor ID4 expression. These observations suggest that there seems not to be a regulation of estrogen towards ID4.

Discussion

Given a certain cellular context, ID proteins may follow divergent functions and act as tumor suppressors or as oncogenes [2]. Particularly, ID4 can act as a tumor suppressor and as an oncogene in different tumor types, e.g., prostate, gastric, glioblastomas, and colorectal tumors [1, 11, 13, 28–30]. In breast cancer, our group and others have previously shown that ID4 may behave as an oncogene in TNBC or basal-like breast tumors. Principally in ER– tumors, the role of ID4 has been linked to BRCA1 downregulation and BRCAness phenotype [21, 22, 31]. But other authors have shown that ID4 may also act as a tumors suppressor in breast cancer [17, 32], where there

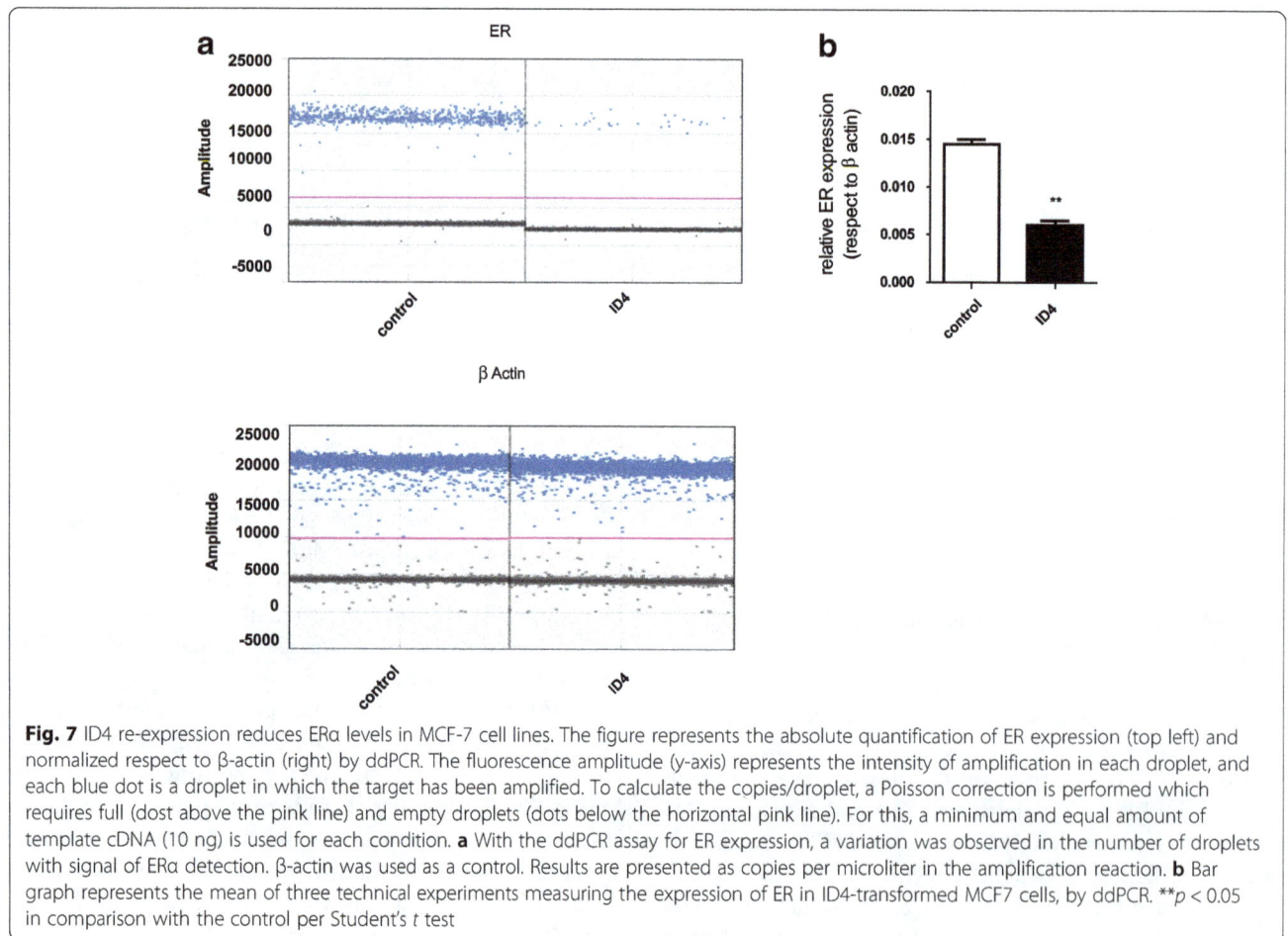

Fig. 7 ID4 re-expression reduces ERα levels in MCF-7 cell lines. The figure represents the absolute quantification of ER expression (top left) and normalized respect to β-actin (right) by ddPCR. The fluorescence amplitude (y-axis) represents the intensity of amplification in each droplet, and each blue dot is a droplet in which the target has been amplified. To calculate the copies/droplet, a Poisson correction is performed which requires full (dost above the pink line) and empty droplets (dots below the horizontal pink line). For this, a minimum and equal amount of template cDNA (10 ng) is used for each condition. **a** With the ddPCR assay for ER expression, a variation was observed in the number of droplets with signal of ERα detection. β-actin was used as a control. Results are presented as copies per microliter in the amplification reaction. **b** Bar graph represents the mean of three technical experiments measuring the expression of ER in ID4-transformed MCF7 cells, by ddPCR. **p < 0.05 in comparison with the control per Student's t test

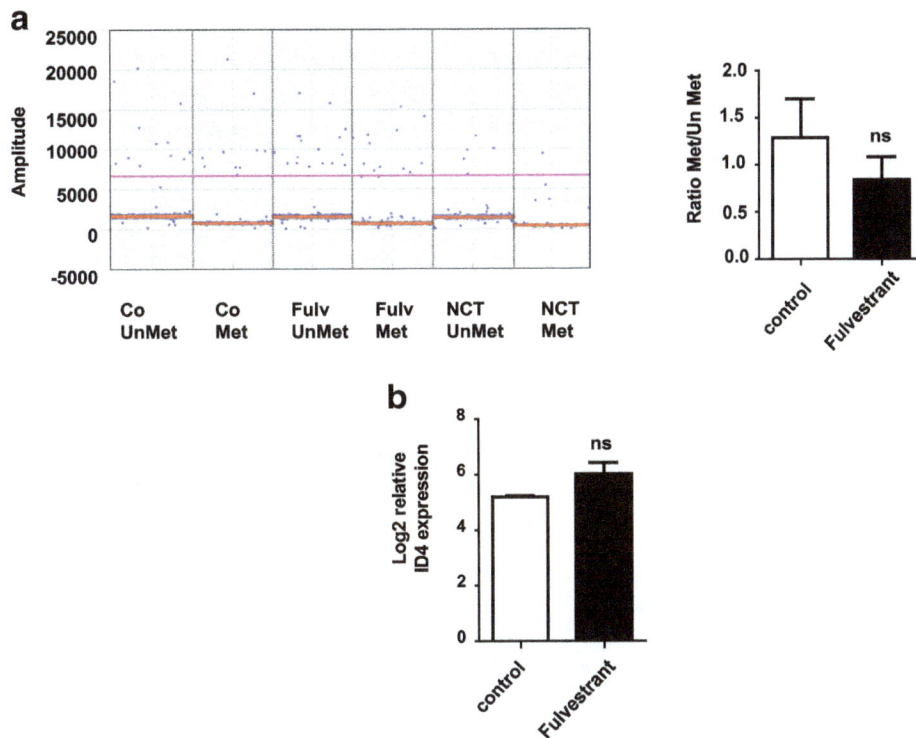

Fig. 8 Estrogen deprivation does not affect neither ID4 methylation nor ID4 expression. **a** Left, ddPCR assay for the detection of ID4-methylated status in control and fulvestrant-treated MCF-7 cells. Results are presented as copies per microliter in the amplification reaction. Right, bar graph represents the mean of three technical experiments measuring the methylated/unmethylated ratios of the control and experimental conditions. **b** ID4 probe (A_23_P59375) intensity was compared between control and fulvestrant-treated MCF-7 cells

seem to be controversial findings regarding the role of ID4. We hypothesize that ID4 behaves as both a tumor suppressor and an oncogene as well and that the difference in behavior varies according to the ER status of breast tumors.

In this report, we used two approaches to test our hypothesis: data mining analysis and in vitro experiments. Data mining analysis revealed that ID4 expression is significantly downregulated in ER+ breast tumors as compared with ER− tumors or normal tissue. We show here that ID4 is silenced in breast tumors through promoter methylation and that ID4 is methylated as tumors become ER+. Interestingly, ID4 expression is significantly higher in normal tissue with respect to breast tumors either they are ER+ or ER−. This could be indicating that ID4 expression is required for normal mammary function and that during a tumorigenic process (either ER+ or ER−), ID4's expression is reduced through methylation. Comparing ER+ with ER− tumors, the methylation levels are not the same. Therefore, there are different expression levels of ID4 between these tumor types and possibly different pathways are turned on or off according to differences in ID4 expression. Some authors suggest

that ID4 regulates linage commitment and forms part of a complex regulatory network with ERα and BRCA1 in the normal mammary gland [18]. Perhaps during mammary tumorigenesis, ID4 follows divergent pathways in ER+ and ER− tumors, affecting different cellular networks. Previously published work shows that specific binding of ID4 (as part of a larger complex) occurs at a region located 5.9 kb upstream of the ERα promoter [29]. Here, we show that ID4 re-expression in MCF-7 cells induced a significant reduction in ER α expression. We also demonstrate by in silico analysis that ID4 expression is associated with different genes according to ER status. In ER + tumors, ID4 expression was negatively correlated to the expression of key genes of the ER pathway such as FOXA1, GATA3, ESR1, and CCND1. Interestingly, all the four genes are involved in the ER pathway. An ID4 site has been identified 8.3 kb upstream of the FOXA1 transcription start site and perhaps forms part of a similar protein complex [29]. Taking these observations into consideration, we could speculate that in the normal mammary gland, ID4 is an important member of the ER pathway and when its expression is affected by methylation, and in ER+ tumors, the expression of important players of the ER pathway is disturbed.

The observation that the expression of ID4 associates with VEGF, JUN, and MKI67 in ER– tumors has not been previously described in breast cancer and it reveals that the involved pathways differ depending on the ER status.

We also evaluated the effect of ID4 expression on OS in breast cancer patients. We observed that in ER+ breast tumors, high ID4 expression was associated with better probabilities of survival. This was not observed among ER– tumors, where the expression of ID4 does not correlate with OS. It is worth mentioning, however, that in the basal-like subgroup of ER– tumors, the expression of ID4 did show a positive association with worst survival ($p = 0,043$). Even though we do not yet understand why this subgroup presents this behavior, it supports the hypothesis of a dual role for ID4 based on the ER status.

Finally, the putative tumor suppressor function of ID4 in ER+ breast cancer was verified by in vitro assays. ID4 overexpression induced phenotypic changes associated with a tumor suppressor role for this protein in ER + breast cancer cell lines. This was evidenced by reduced migration rates in both breast cancer cell lines analyzed. The reduction in migration could be related to the fact that we found ID4 associated with CCND1, which regulates migration and proliferation in breast cancer cells [33–35]; perhaps, these changes in migration are due to an interaction between ID4 and CCND1. This would not be the first case reporting an association between a member of the ID family with CCND1. For instance, Tobin et al. established that there exists a relationship between cyclin D1, ID1, and EMT in primary breast cancer [36]. Ours is the first report suggesting an association between ID4 and CCND1 in breast cancer. Further research should be conducted to confirm this data. Our observations that ectopic expression of ID4 also leads to a significant decrease in the number of colonies is also in line with a tumor suppressor role for this protein.

Conclusions

We propose that ID4 is frequently silenced by promoter methylation in ER+ breast cancers and functions as a tumor suppressor gene in these tumors, probably because of its negative interaction with key genes of the ER pathway. Our present study contributes to the knowledge of the role of ID4 in breast cancer.

Additional files

Additional file 1: Figure S1. qPCR and Western blot analysis of ID4 expression in control and transfected cells with ID4. (AI 1152 kb)

Additional file 2: Figure S2. Higher ID4 expression is associated with OS in ER+ tumors. Kaplan–Meier analysis of the Miller 2005 cohort evaluating OS in ER+ tumors. (AI 1076 kb)

Additional file 3: Figure S3. ID4 methylation values according to ER status. Box plot representation of β values of ID4 methylation at different sites in ID4 promoter. The bottom and top of the box represent the first and third quartiles of the data, respectively, and the band inside the box represents the median of the data. The lower and upper whiskers represent the lowest and highest data points of the data, respectively. ***$p < 0.001$. (AI 1193 kb)

Additional file 4: Figure S4. Genes associated with ID4 expression in ER+ and ER– tumors. Correlations between ID4 expression and the expression of FOXA1, ESR1, GATA3, CCND1, AKT, and IGF1R in the complete tumor cohort (ER+ and ER–). Correlation values for each analysis are indicates on the right. (AI 1561 kb)

Additional file 5: Figure S5. MS-MLPA analysis of ID4 status after fulvestrant treatment. MS-MLPA ME003 probemix was used to analyze ID4 status after estrogen deprivation in MCF7 cells. (AI 1416 kb)

Abbreviations

bHLH: Basic helix-loop-helix; ER: Estrogen receptor; ID: Inhibitor of differentiation; KM: Kaplan–Meier; OS: Overall survival; SVD: Singular-value decomposition; TCGA: The Cancer Genome Atlas

Funding

This work was supported in part by grants from the National Council for Scientific and Technical Research (CONICET, grant number PIP 112–201301-00693) and by the National Institute of Cancer ("Instituto Nacional del Cancer"), Argentina.

Authors' contributions

DN performed in vitro experiments, i.e., cellular transfection, and migration assays. EC performed cellular transfection, migration, and colony formation assays. SL and DN participated in droplet digital PCR experiments. RB performed computational and statistical analysis and revised the final manuscript. GU assisted in migration assays. MR made substantial contributions to the conception and design of the experiments and the manuscript. MTB conceived the study, participated in its design, and wrote the manuscript. All authors read and approved the final manuscript.

Author details

[1]IHEM, National University of Cuyo, CONICET, Mendoza, Argentina. [2]IHEM, Faculty of Exact and Natural Sciences, National University of Cuyo, CONICET, Mendoza, Argentina. [3]IHEM, CONICET, Facultad de Ciencias Médicas, National University of Cuyo, Mendoza, Argentina. [4]IANIGLA, CONICET, Mendoza, Argentina.

References

1. Patel D, Morton DJ, Carey J, Havrda MC, Chaudhary J. Inhibitor of differentiation 4 (ID4): from development to cancer. Biochim Biophys Acta Rev Cancer. 2015;1855:92–103.

2. Lasorella A, Benezra R, Iavarone A. The ID proteins: master regulators of cancer stem cells and tumour aggressiveness. Nat Rev Cancer. 2014;14:77–91.

3. Fontemaggi G, Dell'Orso S, Trisciuoglio D, Shay T, Melucci E, Fazi F, et al. The execution of the transcriptional axis mutant p53, E2F1 and ID4 promotes tumor neoangiogenesis. Nat Struct Mol Biol [Internet].2009; 16:1086–93.

4. Lasorella A, Uo T, Iavarone A. Id proteins at the cross-road of development and cancer. Oncogene [Internet]. 2001;20:8326–33.

5. Bedford L, Walker R, Kondo T, Van Crüchten I, King ER, Sablitzky F. Id4 is required for the correct timing of neural differentiation. Dev Biol. 2005;280: 386–95.

6. Tokuzawa Y, Yagi K, Yamashita Y, Nakachi Y, Nikaido I, Bono H, et al. Id4, a new candidate gene for senile osteoporosis, acts as a molecular switch promoting osteoblast differentiation. PLoS Genet. 2010;6:1–15.

7. Murad JM, Place CS, Ran C, SKN H, Watson NP, Kauppinen RA, et al. Inhibitor of DNA binding 4 (ID4) regulation of adipocyte differentiation and adipose tissue formation in mice. J Biol Chem. 2010;285:24164–73. Available from: http://www.pubmedcentral.nih.gov/articlerender.fcgi?artid=2911309&tool= pmcentrez&rendertype=abstract.

8. Sharma P, Knowell AE, Chinaranagari S, Komaragiri S, Nagappan P, Patel D, et al. Id4 deficiency attenuates prostate development and promotes PIN-like lesions by regulating androgen receptor activity and expression of NKX3.1 and PTEN. Mol Cancer. 2013;12:67. Available from: http://www.pubmedcentral.nih.gov/articlerender.fcgi?artid=3694449&tool= pmcentrez&rendertype=abstract.

9. Chaudhary J, Johnson J, Kim G, Skinner MK. Hormonal regulation and differential actions of the helix-loop-helix transcriptional inhibitors of differentiation (Id1, Id2, Id3, and Id4) in Sertoli cells. Endocrinology. 2001; 142:1727–36.

10. Dong J, Huang S, Caikovski M, Ji S, McGrath A, Custorio MG, et al. ID4 regulates mammary gland development by suppressing p38MAPK activity. Development. 2011;138:5247–56.

11. Vinarskaja A, Goering W, Ingenwerth M, Schulz WA. ID4 is frequently downregulated and partially hypermethylated in prostate cancer. World J Urol. 2012;30:319–25.

12. Castro M, Grau L, Puerta P, Gimenez L, Venditti J, Quadrelli S, et al. Multiplexed methylation profiles of tumor suppressor genes and clinical outcome in lung cancer. J Transl Med. 2010;8:86.

13. Chan ASW, Tsui WY, Chen X, Chu KM, Chan TL, Chan ASY, et al. Downregulation of ID4 by promoter hypermethylation in gastric adenocarcinoma. Oncogene. 2003;22:6946–53.

14. Ren Y, Cheung HW, von Maltzhan G, Agrawal A, Cowley GS, Weir BA, et al. Targeted tumor-penetrating siRNA nanocomplexes for credentialing the ovarian cancer oncogene ID4. Sci Transl Med. 2012;4:147ra112. Available from: http://stm.sciencemag.org/cgi/doi/10.1126/scitranslmed.3003778.

15. Martini M, Cenci T, D'Alessandris GQ, Cesarini V, Cocomazzi A, Ricci-Vitiani L, et al. Epigenetic silencing of Id4 identifies a glioblastoma subgroup with a better prognosis as a consequence of an inhibition of angiogenesis. Cancer. 2013;119:1004–12.

16. Verschuur-Maes AHJ, De Bruin PC, Van Diest PJ. Epigenetic progression of columnar cell lesions of the breast to invasive breast cancer. Breast Cancer Res Treat. 2012;136:705–15.

17. Noetzel E, Veeck J, Niederacher D, Galm O, Horn F, Hartmann A, et al. Promoter methylation-associated loss of ID4 expression is a marker of tumour recurrence in human breast cancer. BMC Cancer. 2008;8:154.

18. Junankar S, Baker LA, Roden DL, Nair R, Elsworth B, Gallego-Ortega D, et al. ID4 controls mammary stem cells and marks breast cancers with a stem cell-like phenotype. Nat Commun. 2015;6:6548. Available from: http://www.nature.com/doifinder/10.1038/ncomms7548.

19. Branham MT, Marzese DM, Laurito SR, Gago FE, Orozco JI, Tello OM, et al. Methylation profile of triple-negative breast carcinomas. Oncogene. 2012;1:e17.

20. Beger C, Pierce LN, Kruger M, Marcusson EG, Robbins JM, Welcsh P, et al. Identification of Id4 as a regulator of BRCA1 expression by using a ribozyme-library-based inverse genomics approach. Proc Natl Acad Sci U S A. 2001;98:130–5.

21. Wen YH, Ho A, Patil S, Akram M, Catalano J, Eaton A, et al. Id4 protein is highly expressed in triple-negative breast carcinomas: possible implications for BRCA1 downregulation. Breast Cancer Res Treat. 2012;135:93–102.

22. Branham MT, Campoy E, Laurito S, Branham R, Urrutia G, Orozco J, et al. Epigenetic regulation of ID4 in the determination of the BRCAness phenotype in breast cancer. Breast Cancer Res Treat. 2016;155:13–23.

23. Umetani N, Takeuchi H, Fujimoto A, Shinozaki M, Bilchik AJ, Hoon DSB. Epigenetic inactivation of ID4 in colorectal carcinomas correlates with poor differentiation and unfavorable prognosis. Clin Cancer Res. 2004;10:7475–83.

24. Koch A, De Meyer T, Jeschke J, Van Criekinge W. MEXPRESS: visualizing expression, DNA methylation and clinical TCGA data. BMC Genomics. 2015; 16:636. Available from: https://www.ncbi.nlm.nih.gov/pubmed/26306699.

25. Györffy B, Lanczky A, Eklund AC, Denkert C, Budczies J, Li Q, et al. An online survival analysis tool to rapidly assess the effect of 22,277 genes on breast cancer prognosis using microarray data of 1,809 patients. Breast Cancer Res Treat. 2010;155:725–31.

26. Miller LD, Smeds J, George J, Vega VB, Vergara L, Ploner A, et al. An expression signature for p53 status in human breast cancer predicts mutation status, transcriptional effects, and patient survival. Proc Natl Acad Sci. U S A. 2005;102:13550–5. Available from: http://www.ncbi.nlm.nih.gov/pubmed/16141321, http://www.pubmedcentral.nih.gov/articlerender.fcgi?artid=PMC1197273.

27. Thewes V, Simon R, Hlevnjak M, Schlotter M, Schroeter P, Schmidt K, et al. The branched-chain amino acid transaminase 1 sustains growth of antiestrogen-resistant and ERα-negative breast cancer. Oncogene. 2017;36:4124–34. Available from: http://www.nature.com/doifinder/10.1038/onc.2017.32.

28. Hagiwara K, Nagai H, Li Y, Ohashi H, Hotta T, Saito H. Frequent DNA methylation but not mutation of the ID4 gene in malignant lymphoma. J Clin Exp Hematop. 2007;47:15–8.

29. Best SA, Hutt KJ, Fu NY, Vaillant F, Liew SH, Hartley L, et al. Dual roles for Id4 in the regulation of estrogen signaling in the mammary gland and ovary. Development. 2014;141:3159–64. Available from: http://dev.biologists.org/content/141/16/3159.full.

30. Rahme GJ, Israel MA. Id4 suppresses MMP2-mediated invasion of glioblastoma-derived cells by direct inactivation of Twist1 function. Oncogene. 2015;34:53–62. Available from: http://www.nature.com/doifinder/10.1038/onc.2013.531.

31. Crippa E, Lusa L, De Cecco L, Marchesi E, Calin GA, Radice P, et al. miR-342 regulates BRCA1 expression through modulation of ID4 in breast cancer. PLoS One. 2014;9:e87039.

32. Umetani N, Mori T, Koyanagi K, Shinozaki M, Kim J, Giuliano AE, et al. Aberrant hypermethylation of ID4 gene promoter region increases risk of lymph node metastasis in T1 breast cancer. Oncogene. 2005;24:4721–7.

33. Gillett C, Smith P, Gregory W, Richards M, Millis R, Peters G, et al. Cyclin D1 and prognosis in human breast cancer. Int J Cancer. 1996;69:92–9. Available from: http://www.ncbi.nlm.nih.gov/pubmed/8608989.

34. Yang C, Chen L, Li C, Lynch MC, Brisken C, Schmidt EV. Cyclin D1 enhances the response to estrogen and progesterone by regulating progesterone receptor expression. Mol Cell Biol. 2010;30:3111–25. Available from: http://www.pubmedcentral.nih.gov/articlerender.fcgi?artid=2876668&tool= pmcentrez&rendertype=abstract.

35. Roy PG, Thompson AM. Cyclin D1 and breast cancer. Breast. 2006;15:718–27.

36. Tobin NP, Sims AH, Lundgren KL, Lehn S, Landberg G. Cyclin D1, Id1 and EMT in breast cancer. BMC Cancer. 2011;11:417. Available from: http://bmccancer.biomedcentral.com/articles/10.1186/1471-2407-11-417.

6

Retinoic acid-induced 2 (RAI2) is a novel tumor suppressor, and promoter region methylation of RAI2 is a poor prognostic marker in colorectal cancer

Wenji Yan[1,2], Kongming Wu[3], James G. Herman[4], Xiuduan Xu[1], Yunsheng Yang[1*], Guanghai Dai[2*] and Mingzhou Guo[1*] (iD)

Abstract

Background: Reduced expression of retinoic acid-induced 2 (RAI2) was found in breast cancer. The regulation and function of RAI2 in human colorectal cancer (CRC) remain unclear.

Methods: Eight CRC cell lines and 237 cases of primary CRC were analyzed. Methylation-specific PCR (MSP), flow cytometry, xenograft mouse model, and shRNA technique were employed.

Results: RAI2 was completely methylated in RKO, LOVO, and HCT116 cells; partially methylated in HT29 cells; and unmethylated in SW480, SW620, DLD1, and DKO cells. RAI2 was methylated in 53.6% (127/237) of primary colorectal cancer. Methylation of RAI2 was significantly associated with gender ($P < 0.001$), TNM stage ($P < 0.001$), and lymph node metastasis ($P < 0.001$). Analyzing by the Kaplan-Meier method, methylation of RAI2 was significantly associated with poor 5-year overall survival (OS) ($P = 0.0035$) and 5-year relapse-free survival (RFS) ($P = 0.0062$). According to Cox proportional hazards model analysis, RAI2 methylation was an independent poor prognostic marker for 5-year OS ($P = 0.002$) and poor 5-year RFS ($P = 0.022$). RAI2 suppressed cell proliferation, migration, and invasion and induced cell apoptosis in CRC. In addition, RAI2 inhibited AKT signaling in CRC cells and suppressed human CRC cell xenograft growth in mice.

Conclusion: RAI2 is frequently methylated in human CRC, and the expression of RAI2 is regulated by promoter region methylation. Methylation of RAI2 is an independent poor prognostic marker of CRC. RAI2 suppresses CRC cell growth both in vitro and in vivo. RAI2 suppresses CRC by inhibiting AKT signaling.

Keywords: RAI2, DNA methylation, Colorectal cancer, AKT signaling, 5-Aza-2′-deoxycytidine

Background

Colorectal cancer (CRC) is the third most common cancer and the fourth most common cause of cancer-related death globally, accounting for roughly 1.2 million new cases and 600,000 deaths per year [1, 2]. The notion that aberrant epigenetic changes are involved in cancer development is widely accepted [3, 4]. In cancer, it has been demonstrated that gene expression is largely perturbed by disrupting the epigenetic machinery [5]. The recognition of an epigenetic component in tumorigenesis, or the existence of a cancer "epigenome," has led to new opportunities for the understanding and detection, treatment, and prevention of cancer [6–8].

Retinoic acid (RA) plays an important role in development, adult hematopoiesis, and cell differentiation [9]. In fact, retinoid-based differentiation therapy of acute promyelocytic leukemia was one of the first successful examples of molecularly targeted treatment strategies [10]. The growth and differentiation of epithelial cells are strongly controlled by retinoid-activated genes. Retinoids

* Correspondence: sunny301ddc@126.com; guanghaidai@163.com; mzguo@hotmail.com
[1]Department of Gastroenterology and Hepatology, Chinese PLA General Hospital, #28 Fuxing Road, Beijing 100853, China
[2]Department of Oncology, Chinese PLA General Hospital, #28 Fuxing Road, Beijing 100853, China
Full list of author information is available at the end of the article

are currently used as chemotherapies against cancers of epithelial origin. CRC is highly influenced by diet; therefore, it stands to reason that direct contact with retinoids from supplemented diets or exogenous retinoids administered as medication may have chemotherapeutic effects on CRC tumors [11]. Our previous study found that epigenetic disruption of retinol-binding protein 1 (CRBP1) and retinoic acid receptor β2 (RARβ2) is a common event in human cancers, including CRC [12]. Retinoic acid-induced 2 (RAI2) is located in human chromosome Xp22.13 [13, 14], a region in which microdeletion has been identified in Nance-Horan syndrome (NHS). This chromosomal region mainly includes four genes: REPS2, NHS, SCML1, and RAI2 [14, 15]. By screening eight familial cases and one sporadic case, no mutations or polymorphic sequence alterations were identified within RAI2 gene, and RAI2 has been excluded as disease-causing in NHS by this study [16]. The expression of RAI2 has been reported to be reduced in breast cancer [17]. By analyzing The Human Protein Atlas, we found that RAI2 was highly expressed in normal human colonic tissue samples, and its expression levels were reduced in colorectal cancer samples. RAI2 was rarely mutated in CRC according to The Cancer Genome Atlas (TCGA) database analysis. The regulation and function of RAI2 in CRC remain to be elucidated. Therefore, in this study, we focused on the epigenetic regulation and function of RAI2 in human CRC.

Methods

Primary human colorectal cancer samples and cell lines

A total of 237 cases of primary colorectal cancer were surgically resected, and 15 cases of normal colorectal mucosa were collected from non-cancerous patients by biopsy under endoscopy. Among the 237 cancer samples, 32 cases of paraffin blocks were available with matched adjacent tissue. All tissues were collected from the Chinese PLA General Hospital according to the approved guidelines of the Chinese PLA General Hospital's Institutional Review Board. In addition, eight colorectal cancer cell lines (LOVO, SW480, HT29, RKO, HCT116, DLD1, SW620, and DKO) were included in this study. All colorectal cancer cell lines were previously established from primary colorectal cancer and maintained in 90% RPMI 1640 (Invitrogen, CA) supplemented with 10% fetal bovine serum. Cells were passaged 1:3 when total confluence (approximately 10^6 cells) was reached in a 75-cm^2 culture flask.

5-Aza-2'-deoxycytidine and MK2206 treatment

For methylation regulation analysis, colorectal cancer cell lines were split to low density (25% confluence) 12 h before treatment. Cells were treated with 5-aza-2'-deoxycytidine (DAC, Sigma, St. Louis, MO) at a concentration of 2 μM in the growth medium, which

was exchanged every 24 h for a total 96-h treatment. At the end of the treatment course, RNA was extracted. To evaluate the effect of RAI2 on AKT signaling, DLD1 cell knockdown of RAI2 by shRNA was then treated by MK2206 (MedChemExpress, Monmouth Junction, USA), an AKT inhibitor. Cells were treated by MK2206 at 1 μM for 24 h for further study.

RNA isolation and semi-quantitative RT-PCR

Total RNA was extracted using Trizol reagent; cDNA was synthesized according to the manufacturer's instructions (Invitrogen, CA, USA). Glyceraldehyde-3-phosphate dehydrogenase (GAPDH) was used as control. The RAI2 PCR primer sequences were as follows: 5'-GCGATTGC-GAGGCCAAGTG-3' (forward) and 5'-GGGCCTTCTT TACCAGGTCAG-3' (reverse). The GAPDH PCR primer sequences were as follows: 5'-GACCACAGTCCATGC-CATCAC-3' (forward) and 5'-GTCCACCACCCTGTTG CTGTA-3' (reverse). Each experiment was repeated for three times.

Bisulfite modification, methylation-specific PCR, and bisulfite sequencing

Methylation-specific PCR (MSP) and bisulfite sequence (BSSQ) primers were designed in the locations of CpG islands in the promoter region of RAI2 gene according to MethyPrimer (Fig. 1a, http://www.urogene.org/cgi-bin/ methprimer/methprimer.cgi). Genomic DNA from CRC cell lines and CRC tissue samples were prepared using the proteinase K method. Normal lymphocyte DNA was prepared from healthy donor blood lymphocytes by proteinase K method. Normal lymphocyte (NL) DNA was used as unmethylation control, and in vitro-methylated DNA (IVD) was used as methylation control. IVD was prepared using SssI methylase (New England Biolabs, Ipswich, USA) following the manufacturer's instructions. MSP primers were designed according to genomic sequences inside the CpG islands in the RAI2 gene promoter region. MSP was performed as described previously [18]. MSP primers were designed according to genomic sequences around the transcription start site (TSS) in the CpG islands of the RAI2 gene promoter region and synthesized to detect unmethylated (U) and methylated (M) alleles. MSP was performed using 2720 Thermal Cycler (Life Technologies, Carlsbad, USA), and cycle conditions were as follow: 95 °C 5 min for 1 cycle; 95 °C 30 s, 60 °C 30 s, and 72 °C 30 s for 35 cycles; and 72 °C 5 min for 1 cycle. BSSQ products were amplified by primers flanking the targeted regions including MSP products. BSSQ was performed as previously described [19]. Cycle conditions were as follows: 95 °C for 5 min for 1 cycle; 95 °C for 30 s, 55 °C for 30 s, and 72 °C for 40 s for 35 cycles; and 72 °C for 5 min for 1 cycle. MSP primers were designed as follows:

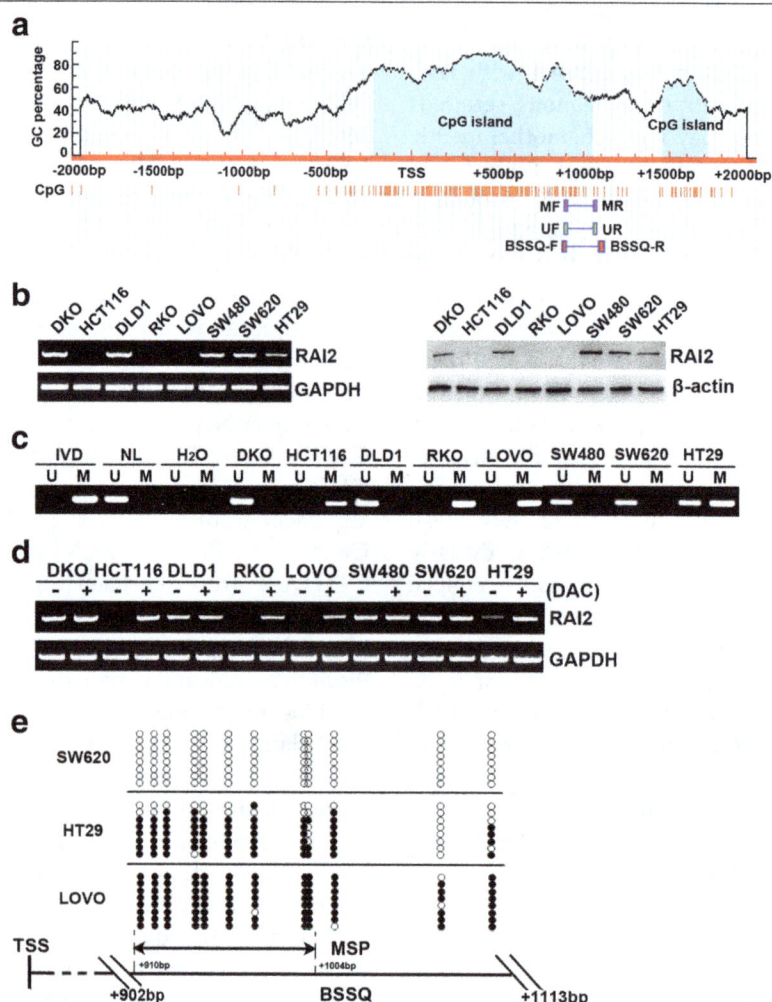

Fig. 1 Expression of RAI2 is inactivated by DNA methylation in colorectal cancer cell lines. **a** Schematic diagram of CpG islands in the RAI2 promoter region. MF, MSP forward primer; MR, MSP reverse primer; UF, unmethylation forward primer; UR, unmethylation reverse primer; BSSQ-F, bisulfite sequencing forward primer; BSSQ-R, bisulfite sequencing reverse primer. **b** Expression of RAI2 was analyzed by semi-quantitative RT-PCR and Western blot in colorectal cancer cell lines (DKO, HCT116, RKO, HT29, SW480, SW620, LOVO, and DLD1). **c** Methylation status of RAI2 detected by MSP in colorectal cancer cell lines. IVD, in vitro-methylated DNA; NL, normal lymphocyte DNA; M, methylated alleles; U, unmethylated alleles. **d** Expression of RAI2 was analyzed by RT-PCR in colorectal cancer cell lines in the absence or presence of 2 μmol/l DAC (+) for 96 h. **e** Bisulfite sequencing of RAI2 was performed in SW620, HT29, and LOVO cell lines. The region of CpG islands studied by MSP is indicated by a double-headed arrow spanning 95 bp. Filled circles represent methylated CpG sites within the RAI2 CpG islands, and open circles denote unmethylated CpG sites. Bisulfite sequencing focused on a 212-bp (+ 902 to + 1113 bp) CpG islands downstream of the RAI2 transcription start site

5′-TTATGTTAGGTATCGAGTAACGTTTTC-3′ (M-forward), 5′-CGAAAAAAAACAACAACTCCCTC CG-3′ (M-reverse), 5′-TGTTATGTTAGGTATTGAG TAATGTTTTT-3′ (U-forward), and 5′-CACAAAAA AAAACAATAACTCCCTCCA-3′ (U-reverse).

BSSQ primers encompassed a 212-bp region downstream of the RAI2 transcription start site (+ 902 to + 1113 bp) and included the region analyzed by MSP. BSSQ primers were designed as follows: 5′-GGGTTTTTTGTTATGT TAGGTAT-3′ (forward) and 5′-ATAAAATACCATTTCC CCACC-3′ (reverse).

Immunohistochemistry

IHC staining was performed on 4-μm thick serial sections derived from formalhyde-fixed paraffin blocks. Rabbit polyclonal antibody against RAI2 (Abcam, ST. Louis, MO) was diluted at 1:30. IHC was performed and evaluated as described previously [20].

Plasmid construction and transfection

The expression vectors for RAI2 were subcloned into Plenti6 lentivirus expression vector, and RAI2 expression lentiviral or empty vectors were packaged using

ViraPower™ Lentiviral Packaging Mix (Invitrogen, CA, USA) to infect RKO and LOVO cell lines to establish stable expression cells. The infected cells were selected by blasticidin (Invitrogen, 461,120) at a concentration of 10 μg/ml. Lipofectamine 3000 (Invitrogen, L3000015) was used for plasmid transfection. For transient transfection, RAI2 CDS region was cloned into the pcDNA3.1 (+) plasmid (Era Biotech, Shanghai, China). All constructs were confirmed by sequencing.

Knockdown of gene expression

Four shRNA molecules were designed to target all four transcripts of RAI2 and constructed into pGPU6/GFP/Neo vector (GenePharma, Shanghai, China). These shRNAs were then transfected into DLD1 cells according to the manufacturer's instructions. The target sequences in the RAI2 gene were as follows: shRNA-1 (5′-GCTGTGCTCC AGAATTTGTTT-3′), shRNA-2 (5′-GCCACACGGT-CATTAAGATGG-3′), shRNA-3 (5′-GGGAAGAGTC-CATGGGAAATG-3′), and shRNA-4 (5′-GAAATACACA TGCTCCCAATC-3′). The most effective construct, shRNA-2, was selected for the study.

Colony formation assay

Cells were seeded at 1000 cells per well in 6-well culture plates in triplicate. The complete growth medium conditioned with blasticidin at 2 μg/ml was exchanged every 48 h. After 2 weeks, the cells were fixed with 75% ethanol for 30 min and stained with 0.2% crystal violet (Beyotime, Nanjing, China) for visualization and counting. Each experiment was repeated for three times.

Cell viability detection

Cells were plated into 96-well plates at 1.5×10^3 cells/well, and the cell viability was measured by the MTT assay (KeyGEN Biotech, Nanjing, China) at 0, 24, 48, and 72 h. Absorbance was measured on a microplate reader (Thermo Multiskan MK3, MA, USA) at a wavelength of 490 nm. Each experiment was repeated for three times.

Flow cytometry

Staurosporine may induce apoptosis in cultured cells. To increase the sensitivity of apoptosis detection, RAI2 unexpressed and re-expressed RKO and LOVO cells were treated with staurosporine (STS) at 100 ng/ml for 24 h. DLD1 cells with or without RAI2 knocked down were treated with staurosporine (STS) at 120 ng/ml for 24 h. The cells were prepared using the Annexin V-FITC Apoptosis Detection Kit I (BD Biosciences, Franklin Lakes, NJ, USA) following the manufacturer's instructions and then sorted by FACS Calibur (BD Biosciences, Franklin Lakes, NJ, USA). Each experiment was repeated for three times.

Transwell migration assay and invasion assay

Cells were suspended in serum-free medium, seeded (1×10^5) into the upper chamber of an 8-μm pore size transwell apparatus (Corning, NY, USA) and incubated for 20 h. Cells that migrated to the lower surface of the membrane were stained with crystal violet and counted in three independent fields. For invasion analysis, cells (1×10^5) were placed into the upper chamber of a transwell apparatus coated with Matrigel (BD Biosciences, Franklin Lakes, NJ, USA) and incubated for 48 h. Cells that invaded into the lower membrane surface were stained with crystal violet and counted in three independent fields. Each experiment was repeated for three times.

Western blot

Protein preparation and Western blot were performed as described previously [20]. The antibodies for Western blot analysis were as follows: rabbit anti-RAI2 (Cell Signaling Technology, Danvers, MA,USA), rabbit anti-MMP2 (Abcam, Cambridge, UK), rabbit anti-MMP7 (Abcam, Cambridge, UK), rabbit anti-MMP9 (Abcam, Cambridge, UK), rabbit anti-caspase 3 (Abcam, Cambridge, UK), rabbit anti-cleaved caspase 3 (Abcam, Cambridge, UK), rabbit anti-AKT (Bioworld Technology, Beijing, China), mouse anti-phospho-AKT[ser473] (Cell Signaling Technology, Danvers, MA,USA), anti-E-cadherin (BD Biosciences, Franklin Lakes, NJ, USA), and anti-vimentin (Cell Signaling Technology, Danvers, MA,USA). Rabbit anti-actin (Cell Signaling Technology, Danvers, MA, USA) was used as a control. Each experiment was repeated for three times.

Xenograft mice model

Stably transfected RKO cell line with pLenti6 vector or pLenti6-RAI2 vector (3×10^6 cells in 0.15 ml phosphate-buffered saline) was injected subcutaneously into the dorsal right side of 4-week-old male Balb/c nude mice. Each group included five mice. Tumor volumes were measured every 3 days starting 7 days after implantation. Tumor volume was calculated according to the formula: $V = L \times W^2/2$, where V represents the volume (mm3), L represents the largest diameter (mm), and W represents the smallest diameter (mm). Mice were sacrificed on the 22nd day, and tumor weights were measured. All procedures were approved by the Animal Ethics Committee of the Chinese PLA General Hospital.

Statistical analysis

The RNA sequencing (RNA-Seq) data for RAI2 gene expression in the dataset of CRC and normal tissues were downloaded from Genotype-Tissue Expression (GTEx) database (https://www.gtexportal.org/home/datasets) and the Cancer Genome Atlas (TCGA) (http://xena.ucsc.edu/, 08/16/2016), respectively. Statistical analysis was performed using SPSS 17.0 software (SPSS, Chicago, IL). Chi-square or Fisher's exact tests were used to evaluate the relationship between methylation status and clinical pathological characteristics. The two-tailed independent samples t test was applied to determine the statistical significance of the differences between the two experimental groups. Survival rates were calculated by the Kaplan-Meier method, and the differences in survival curves were evaluated using the log-rank test. Cox proportional hazards models were fit to determine independent associations of RAI2 methylation with 5-year OS and 5-year relapse-free survival (RFS) outcomes. Two-sided tests were used to determine the significance, and $P < 0.05$ was considered to be statistically significant.

Results

RAI2 is silenced by promoter region hypermethylation in colorectal cancer cells

By analyzing The Human Protein Atlas, RAI2 was found to be highly expressed in normal human colonic tissue, and its expression was reduced in colorectal cancer samples (http://www.proteinatlas.org/ENSG00000131831). According to The Cancer Genome Atlas (TCGA) database analysis, in 224 cases of CRC samples, RAI2 was only mutated in three cases (https://cancergenome.nih.gov). To better understand the regulation of RAI2 expression in colorectal cancer, the levels of RAI2 expression were detected by semi-quantitative RT-PCR in eight colorectal cancer cell lines. RAI2 was highly expressed in SW480, SW620, DLD1, and DKO cells. Loss of RAI2 expression was detected in RKO, LOVO, and HCT116 cells, and reduced expression of RAI2 was found in HT29 cells (Fig. 1b). The expression of RAI2 was validated by Western blot in protein level in these cells (Fig. 1b).

RAI2 gene promoter region methylation was examined by MSP in these cell lines. Complete methylation was found in RKO, LOVO, and HCT116 cells; unmethylation was found in SW480, SW620, DLD1, and DKO cells, and partial methylation was found in HT29 cells (Fig. 1c). The promoter region methylation is correlated with loss of/reduced expression of RAI2 in colorectal cancer cells. To further validate whether the expression of RAI2 was regulated by promoter region methylation, colorectal cancer cells were treated with DAC, a demethylation agent. Restoration of RAI2 expression was induced by DAC in RKO, LOVO, and HCT116 cells, and increased expression of RAI2 was found in HT29 cells after DAC treatment. No expression changes were found in SW480, SW620, DLD1, and DKO cells after DAC treatment (Fig. 1d). These results suggest that the expression of RAI2 is regulated by promoter region methylation. To further validate the efficiency of MSP primers and the methylation density in the RAI2 promoter region, BSSQ technique was employed (Fig. 1e). Consistent with MSP results, complete methylation was found in LOVO cells, partial methylation was

seen in HT29 cells, and SW620 cells were completely unmethylated.

RAI2 is frequently methylated in primary colorectal cancer, and methylation of RAI2 is associated with poor prognosis

To explore the methylation status of RAI2 in colorectal cancer, 15 cases of normal colorectal mucosa and 237 cases of primary colorectal cancer samples were analyzed by MSP (Fig. 2a). Methylation was found in 53.6% (127/237) of the colorectal cancer samples, while all 15 cases of normal colorectal mucosa were unmethylated (Fig. 2a). As shown in Table 1, methylation of RAI2 was significantly associated with gender ($P < 0.001$), TNM stage ($P < 0.001$), and lymph node metastasis ($P < 0.001$). No association was found between RAI2 methylation and age, differentiation, tumor location, and size (all $P > 0.05$). Kaplan-Meier analysis indicated that methylation of RAI2 was significantly associated with poor 5-year overall survival (OS) ($P = 0.0035$, Fig. 2b) and 5-year relapse-free survival (RFS) ($P = 0.0062$, Fig. 2b). According to univariate analysis, RAI2 methylation, tumor differentiation, lymph node metastasis, and TNM stage were associated with both poor 5-year OS (all $P < 0.05$) and 5-year RFS (all $P < 0.05$, Table 2). By multivariate analysis, RAI2 methylation, tumor differentiation, and TNM stage were associated with both poor 5-year OS and 5-year RFS (all $P < 0.05$, Table 2). Age, gender, and lymph node metastasis were only associated with poor 5-year OS (all $P < 0.05$, Table 2). These results suggest that RAI2 methylation was an independent prognostic marker for poor 5-year OS ($P = 0.002$, Table 2) and 5-year RFS ($P = 0.022$, Table 2).

To explore the regulation of RAI2 expression in primary colorectal cancer, RAI2 expression was evaluated by immunohistochemistry (IHC) in 32 cases of matched colorectal cancer and adjacent tissue samples. The expression of RAI2 was reduced significantly in cancer tissue compared to the adjacent normal tissue ($P < 0.01$, Fig. 2c, d). Among the 19 cases of cancer samples that had loss of/reduced expression of RAI2, 12 cases were methylated (63.15%). In contrast, in 13 cases of cancer tissue samples that expressed RAI2, only 3 cases were methylated (23.1%). Loss/reduction of RAI2 expression was significantly associated with promoter region methylation in CRC ($P < 0.05$, Fig. 2d, bottom panel). These results suggest that the expression of RAI2 is regulated by promoter region methylation in human CRC.

To further validate our results, RAI2 mRNA expression and promoter region methylation data were extracted from Genotype-Tissue Expression (GTEx) and The Cancer Genome Atlas (TCGA) (http://xena.ucsc.edu/) databases. RAI2 expression data were obtained from RNA sequencing (RNA-Seq) in 383 cases of CRC samples and 50 cases of adjacent colorectal tissue

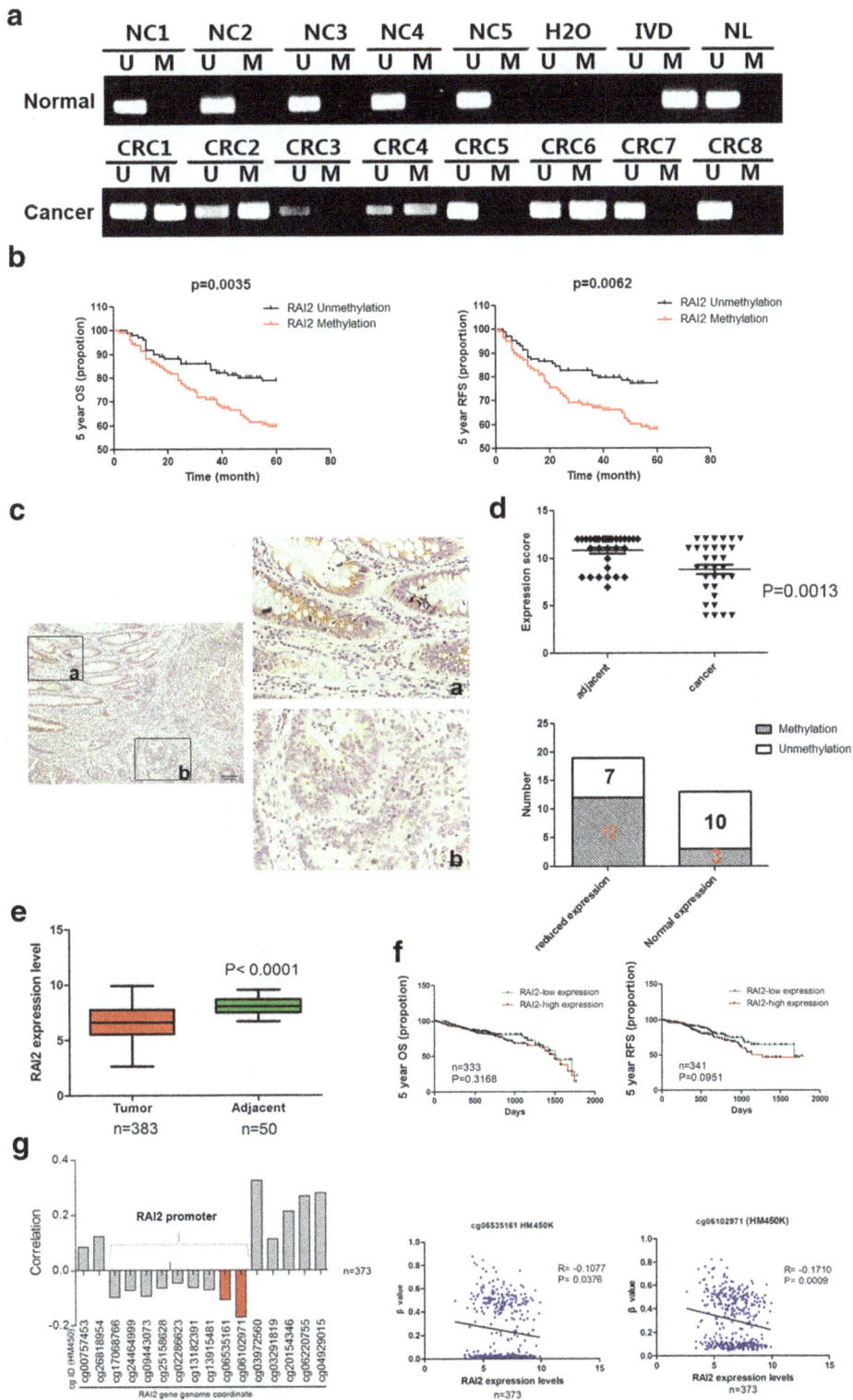

Fig. 2 (See legend on next page.)

(See figure on previous page.)

Fig. 2 Epigenetic inactivation of RAI2 in primary colorectal cancer. **a** Representative MSP results of RAI2 methylation status in normal colon mucosa (NC) and colorectal cancer tissues (CRC). **b** Kaplan-Meier curves show the association of 5-year overall survival (OS) rate and relapse-free survival (RFS) rate of colorectal cancer patients with the methylation status of RAI2. Black, RAI2-unmethylated colorectal cancer patients ($n = 110$, log-rank test); red, RAI2-methylated colorectal cancer patients ($n = 127$, log-rank test). **c** Representative images of RAI2 protein expression in colorectal cancer and adjacent non-tumor tissues determined by IHC (left images, ×100; right images, ×400). **d** RAI2 expression scores are shown as scatter plots; vertical bars represent the range of data. The expression levels of RAI2 were significantly different between adjacent tissue and colorectal cancer samples (**$P < 0.01$). The bar diagram shows the expression and DNA methylation status of RAI2 in different cancer samples. Reduced expression of RAI2 was significantly associated with promoter region methylation (**$P < 0.01$). **e** TCGA data and GTEx data show RAI2 mRNA expression levels in CRC tissues ($n = 383$) and normal colorectal mucosa ($n = 50$) according to RNA-Seq results. Box plots: the levels of RAI2 expression. Horizontal lines: counts of log2 (TPM + 1); TPM, transcripts per million (reads) (***$P < 0.001$). **f** RAI2 expression and 5-year OS ($n = 333$, log-rank test) and RFS ($n = 341$, log-rank test) from TCGA database for CRC. Kaplan-Meier curves show the association of 5-year OS and 5-year RFS of colorectal cancer patients with RAI2 mRNA expression. Green, RAI2 low-level expression colorectal cancer patients; red, RAI2 high-level expression colorectal cancer patients. **g** The correlation of methylation of 16 CpG sites around the promoter region and expression of RAI2 (upper panel), and the methylation status of the top three CpG sites (cg06102971, cg06535161) are correlated with loss/reduction of RAI2 expression in 373 cases of CRC (all $P < 0.05$).

Table 1 Clinical characteristics and RAI2 methylation status of 237 patients with colorectal cancer

Clinical parameter	RAI2 methylation status		P value
	Unmethylated ($n = 110$)	Methylated ($n = 127$)	
Gender			$P = 0.0000$***
Male	95	46	
Female	15	81	
Age (years)			$P = 0.5217$
≥ 50	87	96	
< 50	23	31	
Tumor location			$P = 0.2859$
Right-sided colon	29	28	
Left-sided colon	36	34	
Rectum	45	65	
Tumor size (cm)			$P = 0.4951$
< 5	61	76	
≥ 5	49	51	
TNM stage			$P = 0.0001$***
I–II	48	26	
III–IV	62	101	
Differentiation			$P = 0.0841$
Middle-high	84	84	
Low	26	43	
Lymph node metastasis			$P = 0.0000$***
Yes	59	101	
No	51	26	
Intravascular cancerous embolus			$P = 0.0901$
Yes	10	21	
No	100	106	

P values are obtained from the chi-squared test
Statistically significant *$P < 0.05$, **$P < 0.01$, ***$P < 0.001$

samples. The levels of RAI2 expression were significantly lower in CRC samples compared to adjacent normal colorectal mucosa samples ($P < 0.0001$, Fig. 2e), while no association was found between RAI2 mRNA expression and 5-year OS ($n = 333$, $P = 0.3168$, Fig. 2f) or 5-year RFS ($n = 341$, $P = 0.0951$, Fig. 2f) in this cohort. Methylation of RAI2 was analyzed by Illumina Infinium Human Methylation 450 (HM450) based on the methylation status of 16 CpGs in the promoter region. Available data were obtained from 373 cases of colorectal cancer samples for both RAI2 expression and methylation. The expression of RAI2 was inversely associated with promoter region methylation ($P < 0.05$; Fig. 2g). These data further support our results. Thus, methylation of RAI2 may serve as a detection and poor prognostic marker in CRC.

Restoration of RAI2 expression suppresses cell proliferation and induces cell apoptosis in CRC

Colony formation assays were performed to evaluate the effect of RAI2 on clonogenicity. The colony numbers were 233 ± 11 versus 164 ± 6 in RKO cells ($P < 0.001$) and 155 ± 6 versus 85 ± 5 in LOVO ($P < 0.001$) cells before and after the restoration of RAI2 expression, indicating a significant reduction in colony formation upon RAI2 re-expression (Fig. 3a). To further evaluate the effects of RAI2 on cell proliferation, cell viability was detected by MTT assays. The OD values were 2.13 ± 0.08 versus 1.49 ± 0.10 in RKO cells ($P < 0.001$) and 1.93 ± 0.130 versus 1.61 ± 0.08 in LOVO cells ($P < 0.05$) before and after re-expression of RAI2. The OD values were 1.650 ± 0.102 versus 2.239 ± 0.328 ($P < 0.05$) before and after knockdown of RAI2 in DLD1 cells. Cell viability decreased upon restoration of RAI2 expression in RKO and LOVO cells and increased after knockdown of RAI2 in DLD1 cells (Fig. 3b). These results suggest that RAI2 inhibits CRC cell proliferation.

The effects of RAI2 on cell cycle and apoptosis were analyzed by flow cytometry in human colorectal cancer cells. No significant differences in cell cycle phase

Table 2 Analysis of RAI2 methylation status with OS or RFS in colorectal cancer patients by Cox regression analysis

Variables	OS				RFS			
	Univariate analysis		Multivariate analysis		Univariate analysis		Multivariate analysis	
	HR (95% CI)	P	HR (95% CI)	P	HR (95% CI)	P	HR (95% CI)	P
RAI2 methylation	0.481	0.004**	0.405	0.002*	0.504	0.008**	0.512	0.022*
M vs U	(0.290–0.796)		(0.226–0.726)		(0.305–0.833)		(0.288–0.907)	
Age (years)	1.913	0.058	0.460	0.027*	1.187	0.567	0.790	0.440
≥ 50 vs < 50	(0.979–3.737)		(0.231–0.915)		(0.659–2.137)		(0.434–1.437)	
Gender	1.013	0.956	1.969	0.018*	1.029	0.907	1.576	0.101
Female vs male	(0.630–1.631)		(1.121–3.455)		(0.635–1.668)		(0.916–2.714)	
Tumor location	0.864	0.592	1.661	0.106	0.986	0.96	1.564	0.176
Distal colon or rectum vs proximal colon	(0.505–1.476)		(0.898–3.070)		(0.563–1.727)		(0.818–2.989)	
Tumor size	0.854	0.519	1.213	0.480	0.759	0.276	1.352	0.299
≥ 5 vs < 5 cm	(0.527–1.381)		(0.710–2.072)		(0.461–1.248)		(0.765–2.388)	
Differentiation	0.396	0.000***	0.460	0.002**	0.369	0.000***	0.449	0.001**
Low vs high/ middle	(0.247–0.634)		(0.283–0.748)		(0.229–0.597)		(0.274–0.735)	
TNM stage	0.262	0.000***	0.089	0.000***	0.237	0.000***	0.069	0.006**
III/IV vs I/II	(0.125–0.546)		(0.027–0.294)		(0.113–0.496)		(0.010–0.461)	
Pathologic N stage	0.418	0.006**	3.985	0.008**	0.283	0.000***	4.505	0.105
N1–2 vs N0	(0.224–0.778)		(1.439–11.034)		(0.140–0.570)		(0.732–27.731)	
Intravascular cancerous embolus	0.597	0.093	0.672	0.220	0.996	0.992	1.095	0.812
Yes vs no	(0.327–1.090)		(0.357–1.267)		(0.476–2.084)		(0.517–2.320)	

*$P < 0.05$, **$P < 0.01$, ***$P < 0.001$

distribution were found in RKO and LOVO cells before and after re-expression of RAI2 (all $P > 0.05$, data not shown). To increase the sensitivity of apoptosis detection, cultured cells were treated by STS. The ratios of apoptotic cells were $11.16 \pm 1.25\%$ versus $20.15 \pm 2.75\%$ in RKO cells ($P < 0.001$) and $28.92 \pm 2.78\%$ versus $38.12 \pm 0.87\%$ in LOVO cells ($P < 0.001$) before and after re-expression of RAI2 under the treatment of STS. The ratio of apoptotic cells increased significantly after re-expression of RAI2 ($P < 0.001$, Fig. 3c). In RAI2 highly expressed DLD1 cells, the ratio of apoptotic cells was $33.76 \pm 0.74\%$ before knockdown of RAI2 and $24.83 \pm 1.60\%$ after knockdown of RAI2 under STS treatment. The ratio of apoptotic cells decreased significantly ($P < 0.001$, Fig. 3c) after knockdown of RAI2 in DLD1 cells. As shown in Fig. 3d, the levels of cleaved caspase-3 increased after re-expression of RAI2 in RKO and LOVO cells and decreased after knockdown of RAI2 expression in DLD1 cells. The ratio of apoptotic cells was increased by RAI2 under STS treatment in CRC cells. The above results indicate that RAI2 induces apoptosis in CRC cells.

RAI2 suppresses cell migration and invasion by inhibiting AKT signaling in CRC

To investigate the role of RAI2 in cell migration and invasion, a transwell assay was employed in RKO and LOVO cells. In RKO cells, the numbers of migrated cells were

94 ± 9.64 and 55 ± 9.17 in the empty vector group and RAI2 re-expressed group for each microscopic field, respectively ($P < 0.001$, Fig. 4a). In LOVO cells, the numbers of migrated cells were 114.67 ± 5.51 and 47.33 ± 5.13 in the empty vector group and RAI2 re-expressed group for each microscopic field, respectively ($P < 0.001$, Fig. 4a). In RAI2 highly expressed DLD1 cells, the numbers of migrated cells for each microscopic field were 127.0 ± 18.08, 231.7 ± 56.50, and 85.67 ± 15.95 in the control group (shNC), shRAI2 knockdown group, and shRAI2 knockdown plus MK2206 treated group, respectively. The numbers of migrated cells were increased significantly in the shRAI2 knockdown group compared to the control group ($P < 0.05$, Fig. 4a). The numbers of migrated cells were reduced significantly after treatment with MK2206 in the shRAI2 knockdown group ($P < 0.01$, Fig. 4a).

Next, the transwell assay with Matrigel coating was employed to evaluate the effect of RAI2 on cell invasion. The numbers of invasive cells for each microscopic field were 187.3 ± 6.5 versus 59.7 ± 5.2 in RKO cells ($P < 0.01$, Fig. 4b) and 117.0 ± 11.2 versus 61.7 ± 5.3 in LOVO cells ($P < 0.01$, Fig. 4b) before and after the restoration of RAI2 expression. In RAI2 highly expressed DLD1 cells, the numbers of invasive cells for each microscopic field were 91.67 ± 10.41, 160.0 ± 10.39, and 86.33 ± 12.58 in the control group, shRAI2 knockdown group, and shRAI2 knockdown plus MK2206 treated group, respectively. The

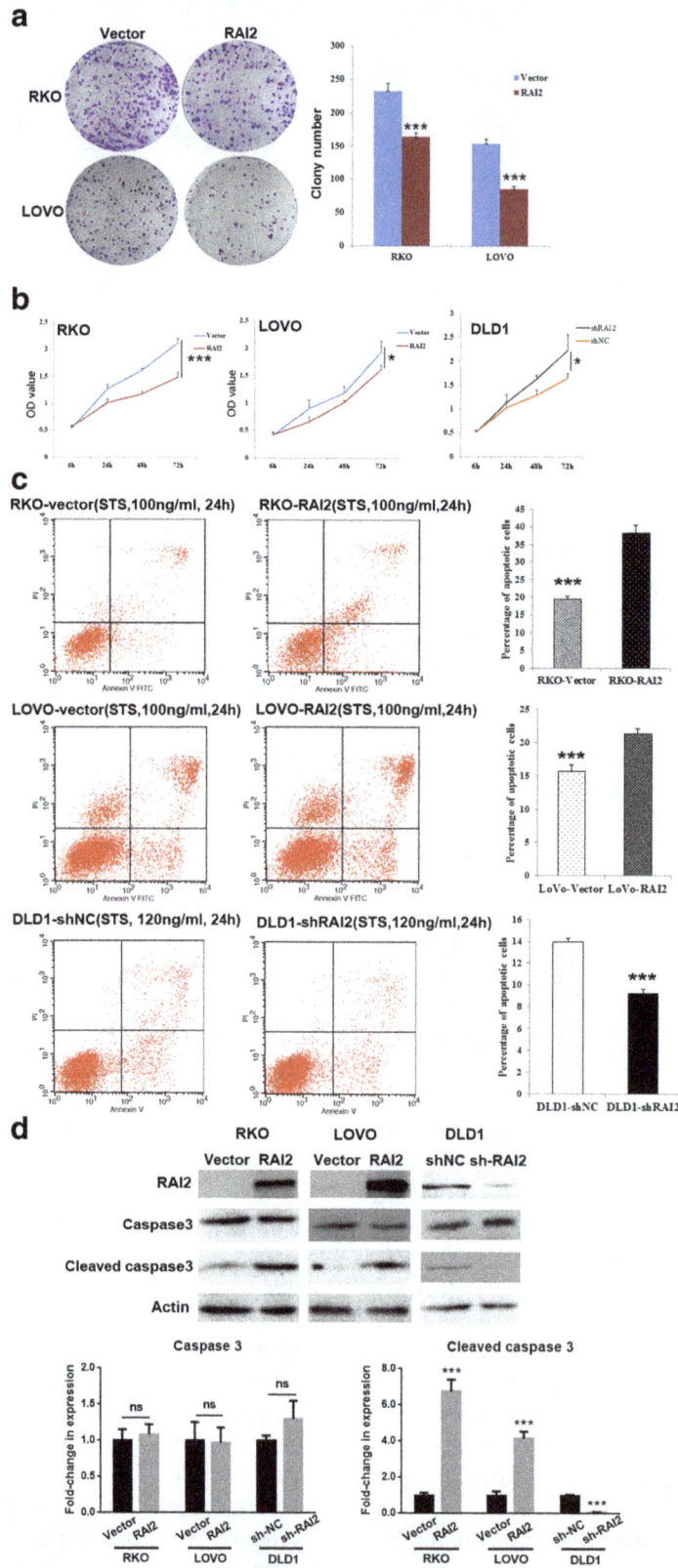

Fig. 3 (See legend on next page.)

(See figure on previous page.)
Fig. 3 The effect of RAI2 on cell proliferation and apoptosis in colorectal cancer cells. **a** The effects of RAI2 on colony formation in RKO and LOVO cell lines before and after the restoration of RAI2 expression. The experiment was repeated three times (***$P < 0.001$). **b** Growth curves demonstrate the effect of RAI2 on cell proliferation as measured by the MTT assay for 72 h in RKO and LOVO cell lines before and after the restoration of RAI2 expression, and in DLD1 cell line, before and after knockdown of RAI2. The experiment was repeated three times (***$P < 0.001$, *$P < 0.05$). **c** Upper and middle: percentage of apoptotic cells before and after the restoration of RAI2 expression in RKO and LOVO cells under the treatment of STS (100 ng/ml for 24 h). Down: percentage of apoptotic cells and before and after knockdown of RAI2 in DLD1 cells under the treatment of STS (120 ng/ml for 24 h). The experiment was repeated three times (***$P < 0.001$). **d** Expression levels of RAI2, caspase-3, and cleaved caspase-3 were detected by Western blot before and after the restoration of RAI2 expression in RKO and LOVO cells and before and after knockdown of RAI2 in DLD1 cells. Actin was used as a control.

numbers of invasive cells were increased significantly in the shRAI2 knockdown group compared to the control group ($P < 0.001$, Fig. 4b). The numbers of migrated cells were reduced significantly after treatment with MK2206 in the shRAI2 knockdown group ($P < 0.001$, Fig. 4b). These results suggest that cell migration and invasion were suppressed by RAI2 in CRC cells.

Epithelial-mesenchymal transition (EMT) is related to cancer invasion and metastasis [21, 22]. To explore the possible role of RAI2 in EMT, EMT-related markers, E-cadherin, and vimentin were examined by Western blot in RAI2 unexpressed and re-expressed RKO and LOVO cells. The expression of E-cadherin was upregulated, and the expression of vimentin was downregulated by RAI2 in RKO and LOVO cells (Fig. 4c). Metalloproteinases (MMPs) promote cancer cell invasion by degrading extracellular matrix (ECM) [23, 24]. Three representative MMP members, MMP-2, MMP-7, and MMP-9, have been reported to be highly expressed in invasive tumors [25–27]. As shown in Fig. 4c, the expression levels of MMP-2, MMP7, and MMP-9 were reduced after re-expression of RAI2 in RKO and LOVO cells. The expression levels of E-cadherin were reduced, and the levels of vimentin and MMPs were increased after knockdown of RAI2 in DLD1 cells (Fig. 4c). The levels of E-cadherin were increased, and the levels of vimentin and MMPs were decreased after treatment with MK2206 in shRAI2-treated DLD1 cells (Fig. 4c). These results suggest that RAI2 suppresses cell migration and invasion by inhibiting EMT in CRC. It has been reported that depletion of RAI2 activated the AKT signaling cascade in breast cancer [17]. In this study, we found that AKT protein phosphorylation at Ser473 decreased after re-expression of RAI2 in RKO and LOVO cells, phosphorylation of AKT increased after knockdown of RAI2 in RAI2 highly expressed DLD1 cells, and AKT inhibition reverted the phenotype induced by RAI2 depletion. Our results suggest that RAI2 suppresses cell migration and invasion by inhibiting AKT signaling in CRC (Fig. 4c).

RAI2 suppresses CRC cell xenograft growth in mice

To further explore the effects of RAI2 in CRC, a human colorectal cancer cell xenograft mouse model was employed. As shown in Fig. 5a–c, the average tumor volume was 105.09 ± 34.57 mm^3 in RAI2 expressed RKO cell xenografts, and the average tumor volume was 1428.26 ± 566.46 mm^3 in RAI2 unexpressed RKO cell xenografts. The tumor volume was significantly reduced after the restoration of RAI2 expression in RKO cells ($P < 0.01$). The tumor weight was 78.60 ± 66.83 mg in RAI2-expressed RKO cell xenografts and 606.00 ± 182.70 mg in RAI2-unexpressed RKO cell xenografts. The tumor weight was reduced significantly after the restoration of RAI2 expression in RKO cells ($P < 0.001$, Fig. 5d). The expression of MMP2 and MMP7 was inhibited by RAI2 in RKO cell xenografts Fig. 5e. These results suggest that RAI2 suppresses CRC cell tumor growth in vivo.

Discussion

There has only been one report addressing RAI2 in human cancers [17]. By using six publicly available datasets, the authors found that lower RAI2 transcript expression was associated with shortened OS in breast, lung, ovarian, and colonic cancer. In our study, according to the analysis using The Human Protein Atlas database, RAI2 was downregulated in human CRC, and based on the TCGA database, the RAI2 gene was rarely mutated in CRC. Then, we screened the expression of RAI2 in CRC cells and primary cancer samples. The loss of RAI2 expression was found frequently in CRC cells, and the expression of RAI2 was reduced significantly in cancer tissue compared to the adjacent normal tissue samples. These results suggest that RAI2 may be a tumor suppressor and diagnostic marker in CRC. RAI2 is rarely mutated in human CRC according to the TCGA database analyzing, while the expression of RAI2 was frequently lost/reduced in CRC cell lines and tissue samples. Thus, we explored the epigenetic regulation and function of RAI2 in human CRC. As our expectation, RAI2 was validated to be regulated by promoter region methylation in CRC. RAI2 was frequently methylated in human primary CRC, and methylation of RAI2 was significantly associated with female gender, TNM stage, and lymph node metastasis. There is no report about the association of RAI2 expression or methylation with gender. Werner et al. found that RAI2 expression was highest in the epithelial-like ER$^+$ cell lines, whereas its expression was lost in the mesenchymal-like and highly metastatic cell lines [17]. Interestingly, treatment with

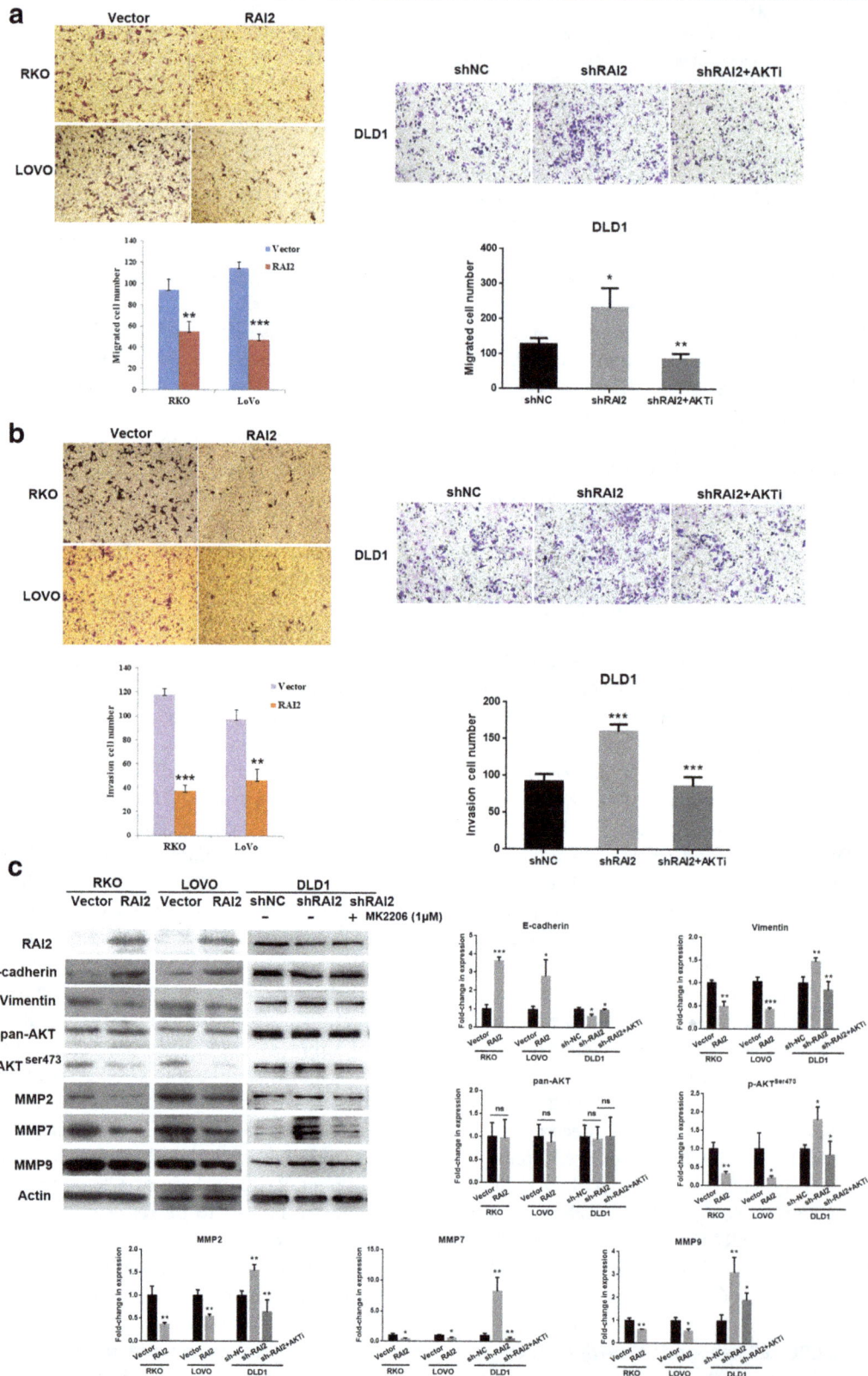

Fig. 4 (See legend on next page.)

(See figure on previous page.)
Fig. 4 The effect of RAI2 on colorectal cancer migration and invasion. **a** Migration assay results showing the number of migrated cells before and after the restoration of RAI2 expression in RKO and LOVO cells as well as in the control group (shNC), shRAI2 knockdown group, and shRAI2 knockdown plus MK2206 treated group (*$P < 0.05$, **$P < 0.01$). **b** Invasion assay results showing the number of invasive cells before and after re-expression of RAI2 in RKO and LOVO cells as well as in the control group (shNC), shRAI2 knockdown group, and shRAI2 knockdown plus MK2206 treated group (***$P < 0.001$). **c** The expression levels of E-cadherin, vimentin, pan-AKT, p-AKTser473, MMP-2, MMP-7, MMP-9, and actin (control) were detected by Western blot in RAI2 un-expressed and re-expressed RKO and LOVO cells as well as in the control group, shRAI2 knockdown group, and shRAI2 knockdown plus MK2206 treated group (ns, no significance, *$P < 0.05$, **$P < 0.01$, ***$P < 0.001$).

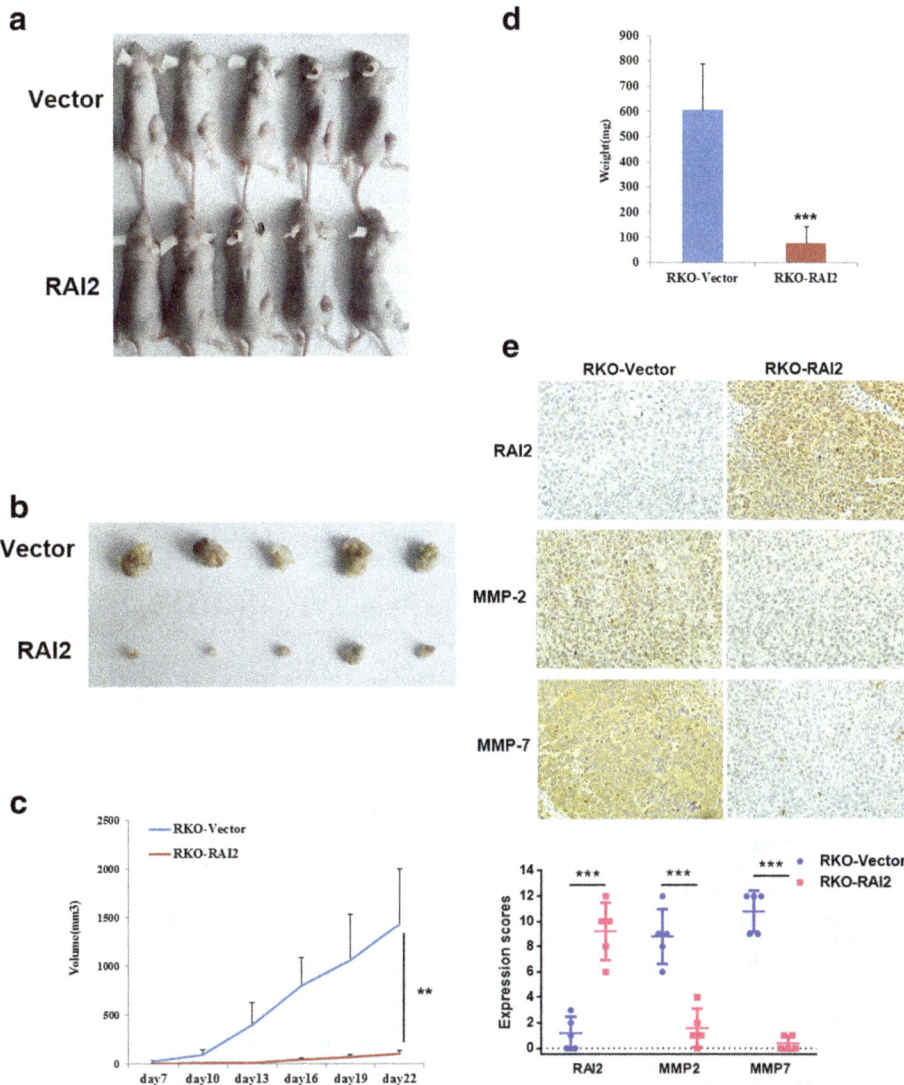

Fig. 5 The effect of RAI2 on colorectal cancer cell xenograft mice. **a**, **b** Representative pictures of xenograft tumors from RAI2-unexpressed (upper) and re-expressed RKO cells (lower). **c** Subcutaneous tumor growth curves in xenograft mice with or without RAI2 re-expression (**$P < 0.01$). **d** Histogram represents the average weight of xenograft tumors in RAI2 unexpressed and re-expressed groups (***$P < 0.001$). **e** IHC staining reveals the expression levels of RAI2, MMP2, and MMP7 in RAI2-unexpressed and RAI2 re-expressed-RKO cell xenografts (×400). The expression scores are shown below as scatterplots (***$P < 0.001$).

either ER antagonists or retinoic acid could induce RAI2 expression [17]. Therefore, it is important to further understand how retinoic acid and RAI2 influence estrogen signaling in the future [28]. RAI2 methylation may be related to CRC progression and metastasis. Further analysis suggested that methylation of RAI2 is significantly associated with poor 5-year overall survival and 5-year relapse-free survival (RFS). According to Cox proportional hazards model analysis, RAI2 methylation was an independent prognostic marker for poor 5-year OS and poor 5-year RFS. This is the first report on the epigenetic regulation of RAI2 and its clinical relevance in CRC. As DNA is very stable, it is much easier and more reproducible to detect DNA methylation than to detect the expression of mRNA and protein in human primary cancer. Thus, RAI2 methylation may serve as a prognostic marker in human CRC.

To further understand the role of RAI2 in CRC development, we analyzed the function of RAI2 both in vitro and in vivo. RAI2 suppressed CRC cell proliferation, migration, and invasion, as well as induced cell apoptosis. RAI2 inhibited the AKT signaling pathway in CRC cells and suppressed CRC cell xenograft growth. These results suggest that RAI2 is a tumor suppressor in human CRC, and methylation of RAI2 is a potential epigenetic therapeutic target.

Conclusion

RAI2 is frequently methylated in human CRC, and the expression of RAI2 is regulated by promoter region methylation. Methylation of RAI2 is significantly associated with poor 5-year OS and 5-year RFS, and it is an independent prognostic marker of poor 5-year OS and poor 5-year RFS. RAI2 suppresses CRC cell growth both in vitro and in vivo. RAI2 induces cell apoptosis and suppresses CRC cell migration and invasion. RAI2 may serve as a tumor suppressor by inhibiting the AKT signaling pathway in CRC.

Abbreviations

BSSQ: Bisulfite sequence; CRBP1: Retinol-binding protein 1; CRC: Colorectal cancer; DAC: 5-Aza-2′-deoxycytidine; ECM: Extracellular matrix; EMT: Epithelial-mesenchymal transition; GAPDH: Glyceraldehyde-3-phosphate dehydrogenase; GTEx: Genotype-Tissue Expression; HM450: Illumina Infinium Human Methylation 450; IHC: Immunohistochemistry; IVD: In vitro-methylated DNA; MMPs: Metalloproteinases; MSP: Methylation-specific PCR; NHS: Nance-Horan syndrome; NL: Normal lymphocyte DNA; OS: Overall survival; RA: Retinoic acid; RAI2: Retinoic acid-induced 2; RARβ2: Retinoic acid receptor β2; RFS: Relapse-free survival; RNA-Seq: RNA sequencing; STS: Staurosporine; TCGA: The Cancer Genome Atlas; TSS: Transcription start site

Acknowledgements
We thank Xiaomo Su and Qi Li for the experiment preparation.

Funding
This work was supported by grants from the National Key Research and Development Programme of China (2018YFA0208900, 2016YFC1303600), National Science Foundation of China (NSFC No. U1604281, 81672318, 81372286, 31671298), National Basic Research Program of China (973 Program No. 2012CB934002), National Key Scientific Instrument Special Programme of China (Grant No. 2011YQ03013405), and Beijing Science Foundation of China (BJSFC No. 7171008).

Authors' contributions
WY and XX performed the experiments and obtained the data. WY and MG wrote the manuscript. MG and KW made substantial contributions to the conception and design of the study. JGH, GD and YY provided manuscript and experimental advice and supervised the study. All authors read and approved the final manuscript.

Competing interests
The authors declare that they have no competing of interest.

Author details
[1]Department of Gastroenterology and Hepatology, Chinese PLA General Hospital, #28 Fuxing Road, Beijing 100853, China. [2]Department of Oncology, Chinese PLA General Hospital, #28 Fuxing Road, Beijing 100853, China. [3]Department of Oncology, Tongji Hospital of Tongji Medical College, Huazhong University of Science and Technology, Wuhan 430030, China. [4]The Hillman Cancer Center, University of Pittsburgh Cancer Institute, 5117 Centre Ave, Pittsburgh, Pennsylvania 15213, USA.

References
1. Brenner H, Kloor M, Pox CP. Colorectal cancer. Lancet. 2014;383:1490–502.
2. Arnold M, Sierra MS, Laversanne M, Soerjomataram I, Jemal A, Bray F. Global patterns and trends in colorectal cancer incidence and mortality. Gut. 2017; 66:683–91.
3. Moran S, Martinez-Cardus A, Boussios S, Esteller M. Precision medicine based on epigenomics: the paradigm of carcinoma of unknown primary. Nat Rev Clin Oncol. 2017;14(11):682–94.
4. Simo Riudalbas L, Esteller M. Targeting the histone orthography of cancer: drugs for writers, erasers and readers. Br J Pharmacol. 2015;172:2716–32.
5. Baylin SB, Jones PA. Epigenetic determinants of cancer. Cold Spring Harb Perspect Biol. 2016;8:a019505.
6. Yan W, Herman JG, Guo M. Epigenome-based personalized medicine in human cancer. Epigenomics. 2016;8:119–33.
7. Gao D, Herman JG, Guo M. The clinical value of aberrant epigenetic changes of DNA damage repair genes in human cancer. Oncotarget. 2016;7: 37331–46.
8. Yan W, Guo M. Epigenetics of colorectal cancer. Methods Mol Biol. 2015; 1238:405–24.
9. Canete A, Cano E, Munoz-Chapuli R, Carmona R. Role of vitamin A/retinoic acid in regulation of embryonic and adult hematopoiesis. Nutrients. 2017;9:E159.
10. Uray IP, Dmitrovsky E, Brown PH. Retinoids and rexinoids in cancer prevention: from laboratory to clinic. Semin Oncol. 2016;43:49–64.
11. Applegate CC, Lane MA. Role of retinoids in the prevention and treatment of colorectal cancer. World J Gastrointest Oncol. 2015;7:184–203.
12. Esteller M, Guo M, Moreno V, Peinado MA, Capella G, Galm O, et al. Hypermethylation-associated inactivation of the cellular retinol-binding-protein 1 gene in human cancer. Cancer Res. 2002;62:5902–5.
13. Walpole SM, Hiriyana KT, Nicolaou A, Bingham EL, Durham J, Vaudin M, et al. Identification and characterization of the human homologue (RAI2) of a mouse retinoic acid-induced gene in Xp22. Genomics. 1999;55:275–83.

14. Liao HM, Niu DM, Chen YJ, Fang JS, Chen SJ, Chen CH. Identification of a microdeletion at Xp22.13 in a Taiwanese family presenting with Nance-Horan syndrome. J Hum Genet. 2011;56:8–11.

15. Accogli A, Traverso M, Madia F, Bellini T, Vari MS, Pinto F, et al. A novel Xp22.13 microdeletion in Nance-Horan syndrome. Birth Defects Res. 2017; 109:866–8.

16. Walpole SM, Ronce N, Grayson C, Dessay B, Yates JR, Trump D, et al. Exclusion of RAI2 as the causative gene for Nance-Horan syndrome. Hum Genet. 1999;104:410–1.

17. Werner S, Brors B, Eick J, Marques E, Pogenberg V, Parret A, et al. Suppression of early hematogenous dissemination of human breast cancer cells to bone marrow by retinoic acid-induced 2. Cancer Discov. 2015;5: 506–19.

18. Herman JG, Graff JR, Myohanen S, Nelkin BD, Baylin SB, Methylation-specific PCR. A novel PCR assay for methylation status of CpG islands. Proc Natl Acad Sci USA. 1996;93:9821–6.

19. Jia Y, Yang Y, Liu S, Herman JG, Lu F, Guo M. SOX17 antagonizes WNT/beta-catenin signaling pathway in hepatocellular carcinoma. Epigenetics. 2010;5:743–9.

20. Yan W, Wu K, Herman JG, Brock MV, Fuks F, Yang L, et al. Epigenetic regulation of DACH1, a novel Wnt signaling component in colorectal cancer. Epigenetics. 2013;8:1373–83.

21. Huang B, Sun L, Cao J, Zhang Y, Wu Q, Zhang J, et al. Downregulation of the GnT-V gene inhibits metastasis and invasion of BGC823 gastric cancer cells. Oncol Rep. 2013;29:2392–400.

22. He L, Zhou X, Qu C, Hu L, Tang Y, Zhang Q, et al. Musashi2 predicts poor prognosis and invasion in hepatocellular carcinoma by driving epithelial-mesenchymal transition. J Cell Mol Med. 2014;18:49–58.

23. Visse R, Nagase H. Matrix metalloproteinases and tissue inhibitors of metalloproteinases: structure, function, and biochemistry. Circ Res. 2003;92:827–39.

24. Nagase H, Visse R, Murphy G. Structure and function of matrix metalloproteinases and TIMPs. Cardiovasc Res. 2006;69:562–73.

25. Fink K, Boratynski J. The role of metalloproteinases in modification of extracellular matrix in invasive tumor growth, metastasis and angiogenesis. Postepy Hig Med Dosw (Online). 2012;66:609–28.

26. Di Carlo A. Matrix metalloproteinase-2 and -9 in the sera and in the urine of human oncocytoma and renal cell carcinoma. Oncol Rep. 2012;28:1051–6.

27. Salem N, Kamal I, Al-Maghrabi J, Abuzenadah A, Peer-Zada AA, Qari Y, et al. High expression of matrix metalloproteinases: MMP-2 and MMP-9 predicts poor survival outcome in colorectal carcinoma. Future Oncol. 2016;12:323–31.

28. Esposito M, Kang Y. RAI2: linking retinoic acid signaling with metastasis suppression. Cancer Discov. 2015;5:466–8.

7

PRC2 targeting is a therapeutic strategy for EZ score defined high-risk multiple myeloma patients and overcome resistance to IMiDs

Laurie Herviou[2], Alboukadel Kassambara[1,2], Stéphanie Boireau[1,2], Nicolas Robert[1,2], Guilhem Requirand[1,2], Carsten Müller-Tidow[4], Laure Vincent[6], Anja Seckinger[4,5], Hartmut Goldschmidt[4,5], Guillaume Cartron[3,6,7], Dirk Hose[4,5], Giacomo Cavalli[2] and Jerome Moreaux[1,2,3,8]*

Abstract

Background: Multiple myeloma (MM) is a malignant plasma cell disease with a poor survival, characterized by the accumulation of myeloma cells (MMCs) within the bone marrow. Epigenetic modifications in MM are associated not only with cancer development and progression, but also with drug resistance.

Methods: We identified a significant upregulation of the polycomb repressive complex 2 (PRC2) core genes in MM cells in association with proliferation. We used EPZ-6438, a specific small molecule inhibitor of EZH2 methyltransferase activity, to evaluate its effects on MM cells phenotype and gene expression prolile.

Results: PRC2 targeting results in growth inhibition due to cell cycle arrest and apoptosis together with polycomb, DNA methylation, TP53, and RB1 target genes induction. Resistance to EZH2 inhibitor is mediated by DNA methylation of PRC2 target genes. We also demonstrate a synergistic effect of EPZ-6438 and lenalidomide, a conventional drug used for MM treatment, activating B cell transcription factors and tumor suppressor gene expression in concert with MYC repression. We establish a gene expression-based EZ score allowing to identify poor prognosis patients that could benefit from EZH2 inhibitor treatment.

Conclusions: These data suggest that PRC2 targeting in association with IMiDs could have a therapeutic interest in MM patients characterized by high EZ score values, reactivating B cell transcription factors, and tumor suppressor genes.

Keywords: PRC2, Multiple myeloma, Predictive score, Epigenetics

Background

Epigenetic events are key mechanisms in the regulation of cell fate and cell identity. DNA methylation, miRNA-associated gene repression, and histone modifications have been implicated in numerous diseases, including cancers and represent new therapeutic targets [1].

Gene expression regulation through polycomb-induced histone modifications is a well-studied mechanism. The polycomb repressive complex 2 (PRC2) contains three core subunits: EED (embryonic ectoderm development), SUZ12 (suppressor of zeste 12 homolog), and EZH2 (enhancer of zeste homolog 2). PRC2 represses gene transcription through tri-methylation of lysine 27 of histone 3 (H3K27me3) by its catalytic subunit EZH2.

EZH2 deregulation has been described in many cancer types, including hematological malignancies. Its overexpression or gain of function mutations lead to abnormal H3K27me3 accumulation, repressing tumor suppressor genes, such as cell cycle inhibitors, apoptotic activators, and senescence and differentiation factors [1].

Multiple myeloma (MM) is a neoplasia characterized by the accumulation of clonal plasma cells within the

* Correspondence: jerome.moreaux@igh.cnrs.fr; http://www.igh.cnrs.fr/
[1]Department of Biological Hematology, CHU Montpellier, Montpellier, France
[2]IGH, CNRS, Univ Montpellier, Montpellier, France
Full list of author information is available at the end of the article

bone marrow. Recent advances in treatment have led to an overall survival of intensively treated patients of 6–7 years and an event-free survival of 3–4 years [2]. However, patients invariably relapse after multiple lines of treatment, with shortened intervals between relapses, and finally become resistant to all treatments, resulting in loss of clinical control over the disease. MM is a genetically and clinically heterogeneous disease. Genome sequencing studies have revealed considerable heterogeneity and genomic instability, a complex mutational landscape and a branching pattern of clonal evolution [3, 4]. Epigenetic marks such as DNA methylation or histone posttranslational modifications are also involved in MM pathophysiology and drug resistance [5, 6].

Global gene expression profiling indicated that, while *EZH2* is upregulated, its target genes are downregulated in myeloma cells compared with normal plasma cells [7]. In human MM cell lines (HMCL), *EZH2* expression has been correlated with increased proliferation and an independence on growth factors [8]. Inhibition of EZH2 expression and activity is associated with HMCL growth inhibition [9, 10] and decreased tumor load in a mouse model of MM [7, 11]. One study shows that this effect is related to epithelial tumor suppressor gene upregulation [11]. However, the use of specific EZH2 inhibitors demonstrated that MM proliferation inhibition is time dependent and cell line specific, indicating that EZH2 does not play a universal and monotonous role in promoting MM [11]. Furthermore, the first genome-wide profiling of H3K27me3 and H3K4me3 in MM patient samples was recently published, showing a unique epigenetic profile of primary MM cells compared to normal bone marrow plasma cells [10]. EZH2 inhibition was associated with upregulation of microRNAs with potential tumor suppressor functions [12]. More recently, EZH2 overexpression was reported to be associated with poor outcome and dysregulation of proliferation [13]. These data underscore an oncogenic role of EZH2 in MM. EZH2 inhibitors are currently in phase 2 clinical development in relapsed or refractory non-Hodgkin lymphoma (NHL) and biomarkers are needed for patient selection since neither EZH2 mutations nor H3K27me3 levels are sufficient to predict NHL cell response to EZH2 inhibitors [1, 14].

Here, we identified that PRC2 core genes are overexpressed in MM cells in association with proliferation activation. Treatment of MM cells with EPZ-6438, a specific small molecule inhibitor of EZH2 methyltransferase activity, results in growth inhibition due to cell cycle arrest and apoptosis. Resistance to EZH2 inhibitor is mediated by DNA methylation of PRC2 target genes. We also observed a synergy between EPZ-6438 and lenalidomide, a conventional drug used for MM treatment. More interestingly, pretreatment of myeloma cells

with EPZ-6438 significantly re-sensitizes drug-resistant MM cells to lenalidomide. EPZ-6438/lenalidomide combination induced a significant transcriptional reprogramming of MM cells targeting major B and plasma cell transcription factors in association with MYC repression. RNA sequencing combined with H3K27me3 ChIP analyses allowed us to build an EZ GEP-based score that is able to predict HMCL and primary MM cell sensitivity to EZH2 inhibitors.

Methods

Human myeloma cell lines (HMCLs)

XG human myeloma cell lines were obtained as previously described [15]. JJN3 was kindly provided by Dr. Van Riet (Brussels, Belgium), JIM3 by Dr. MacLennan (Birmingham, UK), and MM1S by Dr. S. Rosen (Chicago, USA). AMO-1, LP1, L363, U266, OPM2, and SKMM2 were purchased from DSMZ (Braunsweig, Germany) and RPMI8226 from ATTC (Rockville, MD, USA). All HMCLs derived in our laboratory were cultured in the presence of recombinant IL-6. HMCLs were authenticated according to their short tandem repeat profiling and their gene expression profiling using Affymetrix U133 plus 2.0 microarrays deposited in the ArrayExpress public database under accession numbers E-TABM-937 and E-TABM-1088 [15].

Primary multiple myeloma cells

Bone marrow samples were collected after patients' written informed consent in accordance with the Declaration of Helsinki and institutional research board approval from Heidelberg and Montpellier University Hospital. Bone marrows were collected from 206 patients treated with high-dose Melphalan (HDM) and autologous stem cell transplantation (ASCT), and this cohort is termed "Heidelberg-Montpellier" (HM) cohort [16]. Patients' MMCs were purified using anti-CD138 MACS microbeads (Miltenyi Biotec, Bergisch Gladbach, Germany) and their gene expression profile (GEP) obtained using Affymetrix U133 plus 2.0 microarrays as described [17]. The CEL files and MAS5 files are available in the ArrayExpress public database (E-MTAB-372). The structural chromosomal aberrations, as well as numerical aberrations, were assayed by fluorescence in situ hybridization (iFISH). We also used publicly available Affymetrix GEP (Gene Expression Omnibus, accession number GSE2658) of a cohort of 345 purified MMC from previously untreated patients from the University of Arkansas for Medical Sciences (UAMS, Little Rock, AR, USA), termed in the following UAMS-TT2 cohort. These patients were treated with total therapy 2 including HDM and ASCT [18]. We also used Affymetrix data from total therapy 3 cohort (UAMS-TT3; $n = 158$; E-TABM-1138) [19] of 188 relapsed MM patients subsequently treated with bortezomib (GSE9782) from the study by Mulligan et al. [20].

EZH2 inhibition in primary MM cells

BM of patients presenting with previously untreated MM ($n = 7$) at the university hospital of Montpellier was obtained after patients' written informed consent in accordance with the Declaration of Helsinki and agreement of the Montpellier University Hospital Centre for Biological Resources (DC-2008-417). Mononuclear cells were treated with or without EPZ-6438 (370 nM or 1 μM) and/or lenalidomide (2 μM), and MMC cytotoxicity was evaluated using anti-CD138-phycoerythrin monoclonal antibody (Immunotech, Marseille, France) as described [6].

Cell growth assay

HMCLs were cultured for 15 days in RPMI 1640 medium, 10% FCS, and 2 ng/ml IL-6 (control medium) in the presence of EPZ-6438 (Selleckchem, Houston, TX, USA) and or decitabine. Cell concentration and viability were assessed using trypan blue dye exclusion test. The number of metabolic-active cells was also determined using intracellular ATP quantitation. For drug combination assay, HMCLs were cultured for 4 days in 96-well flat-bottom microtiter plates in RPMI 1640 medium, 10% FCS, and 2 ng/ml IL-6 (control medium) in the presence of lenalidomide. Cell growth was evaluated by quantifying intracellular ATP amount with a Cell Titer Glo Luminescent Assay (Promega, Madison, WI, USA) using a Centro LB 960 luminometer (Berthold Technologies, Bad Wildbad, Germany).

Global H3K27me3 and IKZF1 immunofluorescence

After deposition on slides using a Cytospin centrifuge, cells were fixed with 4% PFA, permeabilized with 0.5% Triton in PBS and saturated with 5% bovine milk in PBS. The rabbit anti-H3K27me3 (Active Motif, Rixensart, Belgium, #39156) and anti-IKZF1 (Santa Cruz Biotechnology, Heidelberg, Germany, H-100 sc-3039) antibodies were diluted 1/500 and 1/250 respectively in 5% bovine milk in PBS and deposited on cytospins for 60 min at room temperature. Slides were washed twice, and anti-rabbit alexa 555-conjugated antibodies (diluted 1/500 in 5% bovine milk in PBS) were added for 60 min at room temperature. Slides were washed and mounted with Vectashield and 1% DAPI. Images and fluorescence were captured with a ZEISS Axio Imager Z2 microscope (×63 objective) (Oberkochen, Germany) and analyzed with Omero (omero.mri.cnrs.fr) server and ImageJ software.

RNA sequencing

HMCLs were cultured for 4 days without or with 1 μM of EPZ6438. RNA samples were collected as previously described. The RNA sequencing (RNA-seq) library preparation was done with 150 ng of input RNA using the Illumina TruSeq Stranded mRNA Library Prep Kit. Paired-end RNA-seq were performed with Illumina NextSeq sequencing instrument (Helixio, Clermont-Ferrand, France). RNA-seq read pairs were mapped to the reference human GRCh37 genome using the STAR aligner [21]. All statistical analyses were performed with the statistics software R (version 3.2.3; available from https://www.r-project.org) and R packages developed by BioConductor project (available from https://www.bioconductor.org/) [22]. The expression level of each gene was summarized and normalized using DESeq2 R/Bioconductor package [23]. Differential expression analysis was performed using DESeq2 pipeline. P values were adjusted to control the global FDR across all comparisons with the default option of the DESeq2 package. Genes were considered differentially expressed if they had an adjusted P value of 0.05 and a fold change of 1.5. Pathway enrichment analyses were performed using online curated gene set collection on the Gene Set Enrichment Analysis software (http://software.broadinstitute.org/gsea/msigdb/index.jsp) [24, 25].

Gene expression profiling and statistical analyses

Gene expression data were normalized with the MAS5 algorithm and analyses processed with GenomicScape (http://www.genomicscape.com) [26] the R.2.10.1 and Bioconductor version 2.5 programs [22]. Gene set expression analysis (GSEA) was used to identify genes and pathways differentially expressed between populations. Univariate and multivariate analysis of genes prognostic for patients' survival was performed using the Cox proportional hazard model. Difference in overall survival between groups of patients was assayed with a log-rank test and survival curves plotted using the Kaplan-Meier method (Maxstat R package) [27]. The EZ score was built using our previously published methodologies [28]. EZ score is the sum of the Cox beta-coefficients of each of the 15 EPZ6438-deregulated genes with a prognostic value, weighted by ± 1 if the patient MMC signal for a given gene is above or below the Maxstat reference value of this gene (Table 1) [28].

Cell cycle analysis

HMCLs were cultured in 24-well, flat-bottomed microtiter plates at 10^5 cells per well in RPMI1640–10% FCS or X-VIVO 20 culture medium with or without IL-6 (3 ng/mL) and EPZ-6438 (Selleckchem). The cell cycle was assessed using DAPI staining (Sigma-Aldrich, Saint-Louis, MO, USA) and cells in the S phase using incubation with bromodeoxyuridine (BrdU) for 1 h and labeling with an anti-BrdU antibody (APC BrdU flow kit, BD Biosciences, San Jose, CA, USA) according to the manufacturer's instructions.

Table 1 EZ score genes

Probeset	Name	Maxstat_Cutpoint	Chisq	P value	Hazard_Ratio	Prognostic
210841_s_at	NRP2	702	4.3	0.038	1.6	Bad
204364_s_at	REEP1	226	13	0.00028	2	Bad
205551_at	SV2B	53	4.6	0.032	1.5	Bad
43511_s_at	ARRB1	293	3.9	0.047	0.61	Good
211802_x_at	CACNA1G	302	4.4	0.035	0.5	Good
1555480_a_at	FBLIM1	73	5.1	0.024	0.66	Good
207822_at	FGFR1	240	5	0.026	0.51	Good
1552477_a_at	IRF6	111	4.4	0.035	0.55	Good
227297_at	ITGA9	34	13	0.00029	0.51	Good
235560_at	NOVA2	85	3.9	0.049	0.67	Good
228140_s_at	PPP2R2C	131	5.8	0.016	0.55	Good
206628_at	SLC5A1	175	4.3	0.038	0.63	Good
212560_at	SORL1	29	9.1	0.0026	0.52	Good
1559956_at	SYT7	65	5.8	0.016	0.64	Good
213869_x_at	THY1	110	4.2	0.039	0.67	Good

Flow cytometry analysis

Cells were fixed for 10 min with Cytofix/Cytoperm (BD Biosciences, San Jose, CA, USA) at 4 °C. The overall expression of MYC, IKZF1, IRF4, and H3K27me3 was evaluated by incubating 10^5 cells with 5 μLof an alexa 647-conjugated mouse anti-H3K27me3 antibody (Cell Signaling, Danvers, MA, USA, 12158S), alexa 647-conjugated mouse anti-EZH2 antibody (BD Biosciences, 563491) PE-conjugated mouse anti-IKZF1 (BD Biosciences, 564476), rat anti-IRF4 (Biolegend, 646403), rabbit anti-MYC (Cell Signaling, #12189), or anti-Ki67 antibodies in phosphate-buffered saline (PBS) containing 2% FBS at 4 °C for 20 min.

For primary samples, cells were double stained with APC or PE-conjugated anti-CD138 (Beckman-Coulter, Brea, CA, USA). Flow cytometry analysis was done on a Fortessa flow cytometer (BD, Mountain View, CA, USA).

Study of apoptosis

HMCLs were cultured in 24-well, flat-bottomed microtiter plates at 10^5 cells per well in RPMI1640–10% FCS or X-VIVO 20 culture medium with or without IL-6 (3 ng/mL), EPZ-6438 (Selleckchem), and QVD. After 8 days of culture, cells were washed twice in PBS and apoptosis was assayed with PE-conjugated Annexin V labeling (BD Biosciences) using a Fortessa flow cytometer (BD).

H3K27me3-associated genes in MM patients

The list of H3K27me3 associated genes in MM patients was recovered from GEO GSE53215 and used for the development of the EZ score.

RT-qPCR

RNA was converted to cDNA using the Qiagen Quanti-Tect Reverse Transcription Kit (Qiagen, Hilden, Germany). The assays-on-demand primers and probes and the TaqMan Universal Master Mix were used according to the user's manual (Biosystems, Courtaboeuf, France). The measurement of gene expression was performed using the Roche LC480 Sequence Detection System. For each primer, serial dilutions of a standard cDNA were amplified to create a standard curve, and values of unknown samples were estimated relative to this standard curve in order to assess PCR efficiency. Ct values were obtained for *GAPDH* and the respective genes of interest during log phase of the cycle. Gene expression was normalized to that of *b2M* (dCt = Ct gene of interest–Ct *b2M*) and compared with the values obtained for a known positive control using the following formula: 100/2ddCt where ddCt = dCt unknown–dCt positive control.

Western blot

Cells were lysed in RIPA buffer (Cell Signaling Technology, Beverly, MA, USA) supplemented with 1 mM phenylmethylsulfonyl fluoride immediately before use. Lysates were separated by sodium dodecyl sulfate-polyacrylamide gel electrophoresis (10% gels) and transferred to nitrocellulose membranes using an iBlot® Gel Transfer Device (InVitrogen). Non-specific membrane sites were blocked by incubation at room temperature in 140 mM NaCl, 3 mM KCl, 25 mM Tris-HCl (pH 7.4), 0.1% Tween 20 (tris-buffered saline Tween-20), 5% non-fat milk for 2 h, and then immunoblotted with rabbit polyclonal antibodies against Ikaros (Santa Cruz Biotechnology, Dallas, TX, USA), cMyc

(Cell Signaling Technology), or IRF4 (Santa Cruz Biotechnology, Dallas, TX, USA). As a control for protein loading, a mouse monoclonal anti-β-actin antibody (Sigma-Aldrich) was used. The primary antibodies were visualized with peroxidase-conjugated goat anti-rabbit (Sigma-Aldrich) or goat anti-mouse (Jackson ImmunoResearch, West Grove, PA, USA) antibodies and an enhanced chemiluminescence detection system. Western blots were quantified by densitometry using the NIH ImageJ software (National Institutes of Health, Bethesda, MD, USA), and protein levels were normalized according to those of β-actin.

Chromatin immunoprecipitation followed by sequencing

Cells were cross-linked in formaldehyde at a final concentration of 1% for 8 min. All experiments reagents were included in the Auto iDeal ChIP-seq kit for Histones (Diagenode, Liege, Belgium). Sonication was performed using a Bioruptor Plus sonication devise (Diagenode, Liege, Belgium) under the optimal conditions to shear cross-linked DNA to fragments if 100–300 base pairs in length. ChIP was conducted with the IPStar Compact Automated System (Diagenode, Liege, Belgium). ChIP were performed starting from 1 million cells per IP, using the indirect method in 200 μL final volume. Crossed-linked DNA was incubated 13 h with the antibody (H3K27me3 catalog number C1540195 or H3K4me3 catalog number C15410003) and 3 h with the beads. After 5 min washes, eluates were recovered and reverse cross-linked for 4 h at 65 °C. Samples were treated for 1 h with RNAse at 37 °C, prior to DNA purification with the Auto IPure kit v2 (Diagenode, C03010010). Libraries were performed using NEBNext Ultra Library Prep Kit for Illumina (New England Biolabs). Sequencing was performed with Illumina NextSeq500 technology (Helixio, Clermont-Ferrand, France) using the following parameters: single-read, 50 bp, 40 million reads.

DNA methylation analysis

Methylation analysis was performed using the Illumina Infinium HumanMethylation450 BeadChip array (HM450K, Illumina Inc.). The microarray raw intensities were preprocessed using the R/Bioconductor package minfi [29].The methylated CpGs overlapping with genes promoter region were extracted using the R package GenomicFeatures [30] implemented in Bioconductor. A CpG is defined as highly methylated when the methylation beta level is above 0.8.

Results

PRC2 complex is overexpressed in malignant plasma cells in association with cell cycle deregulation

Using Affymetrix microarrays, we analyzed the expression of PRC2 core genes EZH2, SUZ12, and EED in

normal bone marrow plasma cells (BMPCs, $n = 5$), primary myeloma cells from patients (MMCs, $n = 206$), and human myeloma cell lines (HMCLs, $n = 26$). PRC2 core genes are significantly overexpressed in MM cells (Fig. 1a) and EZH2 expression is significantly correlated with SUZ12 and EED expression (Additional file 1: Figure S1). At the opposite, PRC1 core genes were significantly downregulated in MM cells compared to normal plasma cells underlining polycomb complex deregulation in MM (Additional file 1: Figure S2).

Investigating the prognostic value of EZH2, SUZ12, and EED expression in independent cohorts of previously untreated MM patients, using Maxstat R algorithm [31], only EZH2 expression was found to be associated with MM patient's outcome as recently reported [13] (Additional file 1: Figure S3). EZH2 is significantly overexpressed in patients with del17p and 1q21 gain (Additional file 1: Figure S4A and B). EZH2 expression is significantly correlated with MMC plasma cell labeling index (PCLI) in a cohort of 101 newly diagnosed patients ($P < 0.005$; Fig. 1b) underlining a link between PRC2 expression and deregulation of cell cycle in MM cells. Furthermore, GSEA analysis of patients with high EZH2 expression identified a significant enrichment for genes involved in cell cycle, upregulated in proliferating plasmablasts compared to mature BMPCs, and EZH2 targets ($P < 0.0001$) (Fig. 1c).

Altogether, these data underline that PRC2 complex is overexpressed in MMCs in association with a proliferative plasmablastic gene signature and a poor prognosis.

To investigate the therapeutic interest of PRC2 deregulation to target MM cells, XG1, XG12, XG19, LP1, XG25, and XG7 HMCLs were treated with clinically relevant doses of EZH2 inhibitor EPZ-6438 (370 nM and 1 μM) [14, 32]. EPZ-6438 treatment induced a significant decrease of global H3K27me3 in all the HMCLs tested ($P < 0.01$) (Additional file 1: Figures S5 and S6) and inhibited MM cell growth together with proliferation inhibition and apoptosis induction in 3 out of the 6 HMCLs tested (Fig. 2a and Additional file 1: Figure S7). The inhibitory effect appeared at day 6, suggesting that it is mediated by epigenetic reprogramming (Fig. 2a). EZH2 inhibitor induced apoptosis was partially rescued by the QVD pan-caspase inhibitor, suggesting a caspase-dependent mechanism (Additional file 1: Figure S7). LP1 and XG7 were more resistant to EZH2 inhibitor whereas XG25 HMCL was completely resistant. Primary MM cells co-cultured with their bone marrow microenvironment and recombinant IL-6 were also treated with EPZ-6438 as previously described [6]. EZH2 targeting significantly reduced the median number of viable myeloma cells by 35% ($P = 0.004$) in 9/17 patients whereas MM cells of 8 patients were not significantly affected by the EZH2 inhibitor (Fig. 2b and

PRC2 targeting is a therapeutic strategy for EZ score defined high-risk multiple myeloma patients...

79

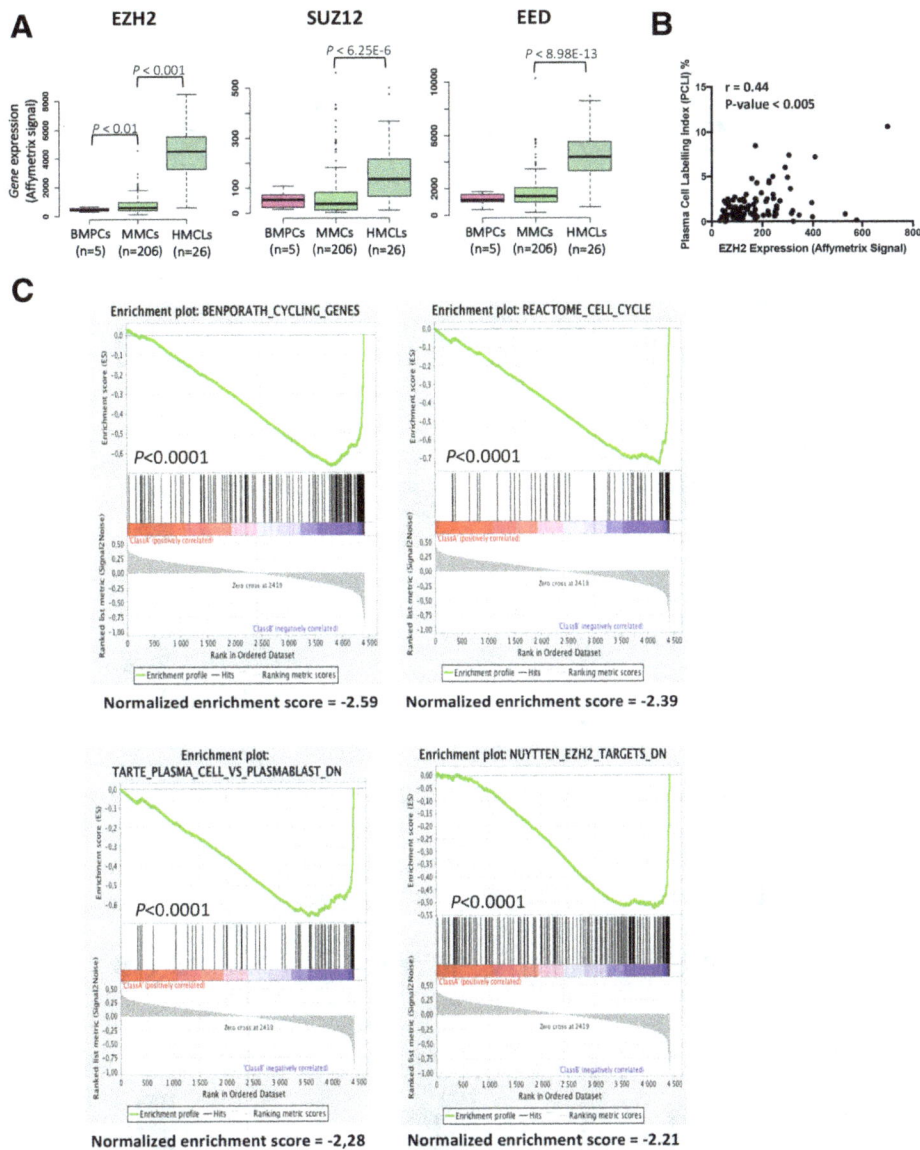

Fig. 1 PRC2 complex is deregulated in MM in association with cell proliferation. **a** EZH2, SUZ12, and EED gene expression in BMPCs, patients' MMCs, and HMCLs. Data are MAS5-normalized Affymetrix signals (U133 plus 2.0 microarrays). Statistical difference was assayed using a *t* test. **b** Correlation between EZH2 expression and malignant plasma cell labeling index. Plasma cell labeling index represents the percentage of malignant plasma cells in S phase of the cell cycle. It was investigated using Brdu incorporation and flow cytometry in 101 patients at diagnosis. **c** Top gene sets significantly associated with high EZH2 expression in MM using GSEA

Additional file 1: Figure S8). As described in HMCLs, EPZ-6438 induced a significant global H3K27me3 decrease in all the patients (Fig. 2c). The effect of EZH2 inhibitor was not correlated with EZH2 expression, H3K27me3 and levels in light of the 6 HMCLs and 17 primary MM samples tested. Moreover, UTX/JMJD3 demethylases mutation status did not seem to affect EPZ-6438 efficiency in the tested samples (Additional file 1: Figure S9 and Additional file 2: Table S1).

We therefore conclude that MM cell growth could be affected by PRC2 targeted therapy which presents a therapeutic interest in a subgroup of MM patients.

Genes deregulated by EZH2 targeted inhibition in myeloma cells

To better understand the molecular mechanisms associated with PRC2 deregulation in MM, six HMCLs were treated with 1 μM of EPZ-6438 for 4 days, and GEP were analyzed using RNA sequencing. Two hundred sixty-three genes are significantly upregulated in EPZ-6438-treated MMC compared to untreated cells (fold change ≥ 2, 1000 permutations, FDR < 0.05, Additional file 3: Table S2). Notably, no gene was significantly downregulated after EPZ-6438 treatment. EPZ-6438-regulated genes are significantly enriched in

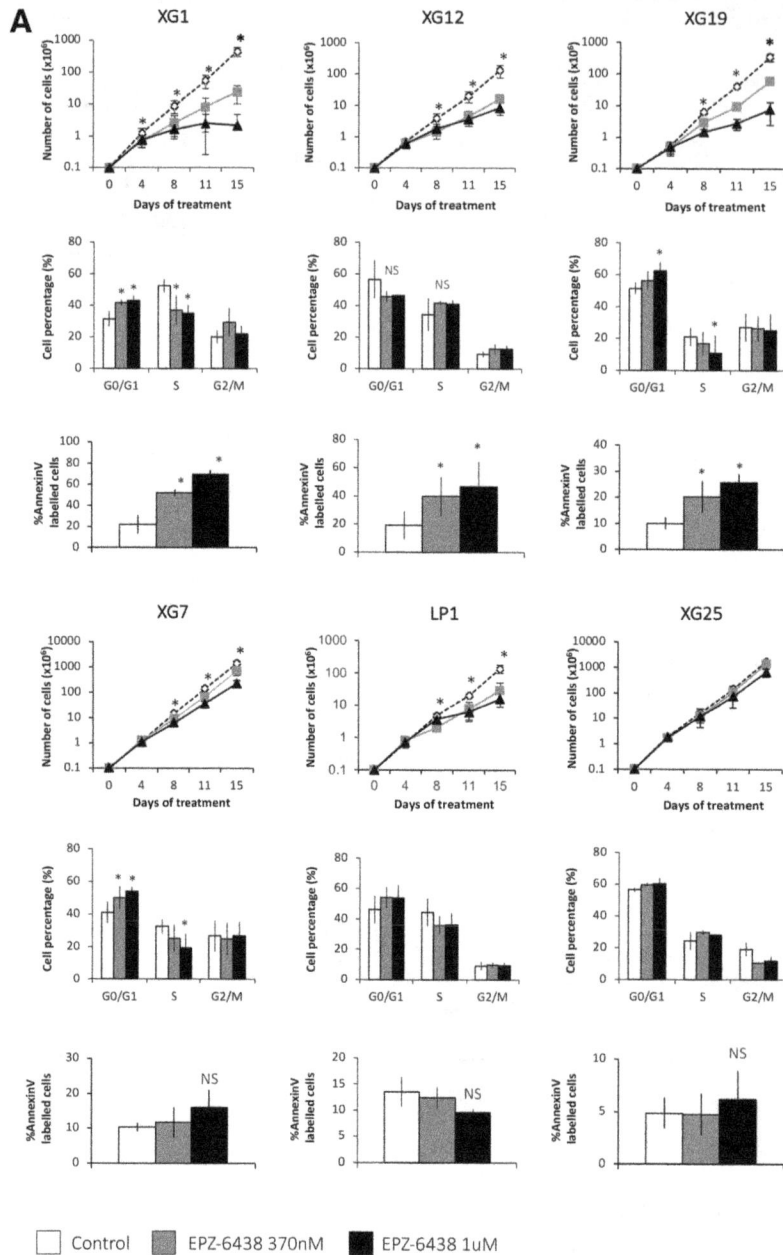

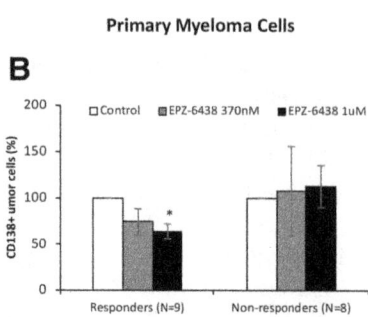

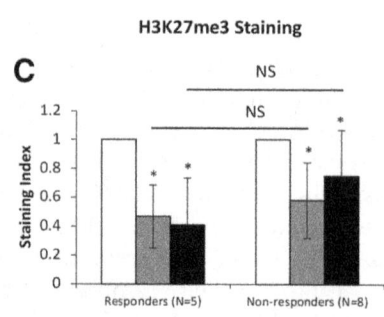

Fig. 2 (See legend on next page.)

(See figure on previous page.)
Fig. 2 EZH2 inhibition differentially affects MMCs survival. **a** EPZ-6438 treatment leads to MM cell growth inhibition and apoptosis induction. HMCLs were exposed to different doses of EPZ-6438 and cell viability was analyzed after 4, 8, 11, and 15 days. Cells were split, replated, and treated at each time points. Results are the mean absolute cumulated counts ± SD of viable myeloma cells of five independent experiments. Cell cycle of EPZ-6438-treated MM cell lines was analyzed by flow cytometry. Results are representative of four independent experiments. Apoptosis induction was analyzed with Annexin V PE staining by flow cytometry. The shown data are the mean values ± SD of four separate experiments. * indicates a significant difference compared to control cells using a Wilcoxon test for pairs ($P \leq 0.05$). **b** EZH2 inhibition induces mortality of primary MMCs from patients. At day 8 of culture, the viability and total cell counts were assessed, and the percentage of CD138 viable PC was determined by flow cytometry. Results are median values of the numbers of myeloma cells in the culture wells. **c** Global H3K27me3 status was also assessed by flow cytometry. Results are median values of the H3K27me3 staining index in CD138 viable PC. * indicates a significant difference compared to control cells using a Wilcoxon test for pairs ($P \leq 0.05$)

polycomb target genes, genes enriched in H3K27me3 histone mark, genes described to be associated with DNA methylation in MM, TP53, and RB1 target genes (Fig. 3a and Additional file 4: Table S3). Interestingly, a set of these genes is overexpressed in non-cycling mature normal plasma cells compared to proliferating plasmablasts (Fig. 3a and Additional file 4: Table S3). Among these 263 genes deregulated after EPZ-6438 treatment, 174 were also associated with H3K27me3 mark in XG7 HMCL including 160 bivalent genes characterized by H3K4me3 and H3K27me3 histone marks (Fig. 3b and Additional file 5: Table S4).

Resistance to EZH2 inhibitor is mediated by DNA methylation of PRC2 target genes

Since PRC2 target genes were associated with a significant enrichment of genes presenting DNA methylation in MM, we analyzed the methylation status at the promoter region of EZH2 inhibitor target genes using 450 k microarrays. Interestingly, 155 out the 263 EZH2 inhibitor target genes were associated with significant CpG methylation in their promoter (Fig. 3c). Furthermore, 111 of these 155 genes were also significantly upregulated after HMCL treatment with decitabine (ratio > 1.5) (Fig. 3d). A significant difference in CpG methylation status of EZH2 inhibitor target genes were identified between sensitive and resistant HMCLs ($P < 0.01$) (Fig. 3c). Interestingly, combination of a sublethal dose of decitabine (100 nM, IC10) with EPZ-6438 (1 μM) allowed to sensitize XG7 and XG25 EPZ-6438-resistant HMCLs. After 8 and 11 days of treatment, we observed a significant cell growth inhibition in both cell lines (67.4% and 62.4% respectively, $P < 0.01$ in XG7, and 72.2% and 85.2% respectively in XG25), compared to decitabine or EPZ-6438 used alone ($P < 0.05$) (Fig. 3e).

These data demonstrate that PRC2 target genes could be associated with DNA methylation underlying an overlap between epigenetic silencing mechanisms on potent key MM tumor suppressor genes.

PRC2 inhibition sensitizes myeloma cells to lenalidomide

We investigated whether EZH2 inhibition could enhance the anti-myeloma activity of melphalan, bortezomib, and lenalidomide treatment. EPZ-6438 pretreatment does not significantly enhance the effect of melphalan and bortezomib treatment on MMCs in vitro (data not shown). However, EPZ-6438 pretreatment significantly sensitized HMCLs to lenalidomide treatment. Treatment for 4 days with 1 μM of EPZ-6438 prior to lenalidomide treatment significantly enhanced toxicity on LP1 and XG19 HMCLs ($P < 0.05$) (Fig. 4a). Furthermore, EZH2 inhibition was able to overcome lenalidomide resistance in XG7 and XG25 cell lines (Fig. 4a). These data strongly suggest that combination of EZH2 inhibitor and IMiDs could be of therapeutic interest in MM.

These results were validated using primary MMCs from patients [6, 28]. The median percentage of viable MMCs was reduced of 43.4%, 26.9%, and 75.1% when cells were treated with lenalidomide, EPZ-6438, or the combination EPZ-6438/lenalidomide respectively ($P = 0.003$; $n = 5$) (Fig. 4b). Global H3K27me3 levels showed a tendency toward decrease under combination treatment, although the difference was not significant.

PRC2 targeting combined with Lenalidomide induced MM cell transcriptional reprogramming

Using RNA sequencing GEP data, we then compared MM cell lines treated by EPZ-6438, lenalidomide, or EPZ-6438/lenalidomide combination. Thirty-one genes were commonly upregulated by the EPZ-6438 and EPZ-6438/lenalidomide combination (Fig. 4c). Sixty-seven percent of the genes deregulated by lenalidomide in MM are also deregulated by the EPZ-6438/lenalidomide combination (Fig. 4c and Additional file 6: Table S6). Furthermore, EPZ-6438/lenalidomide induced a significantly higher deregulation of EPZ-6438 or lenalidomide target genes including PARP9, RGS1, DKK1, SEZ6L2, CAV2, ANTXR1, EMP1, and ANXA1 (ratio > 1.5, $P < 0.05$; Fig. 4d and Additional file 6: Table S6 and Additional file 7: Table S7).

Seventy-six percent of EPZ-6438/lenalidomide deregulated genes were not affected by EPZ-6438 or lenalidomide alone, suggesting that EZH2 inhibitor and IMiDs combination could modulate the expression of a specific set of genes. Among the 231 genes significantly upregulated uniquely after EPZ-6438/lenalidomide treatment,

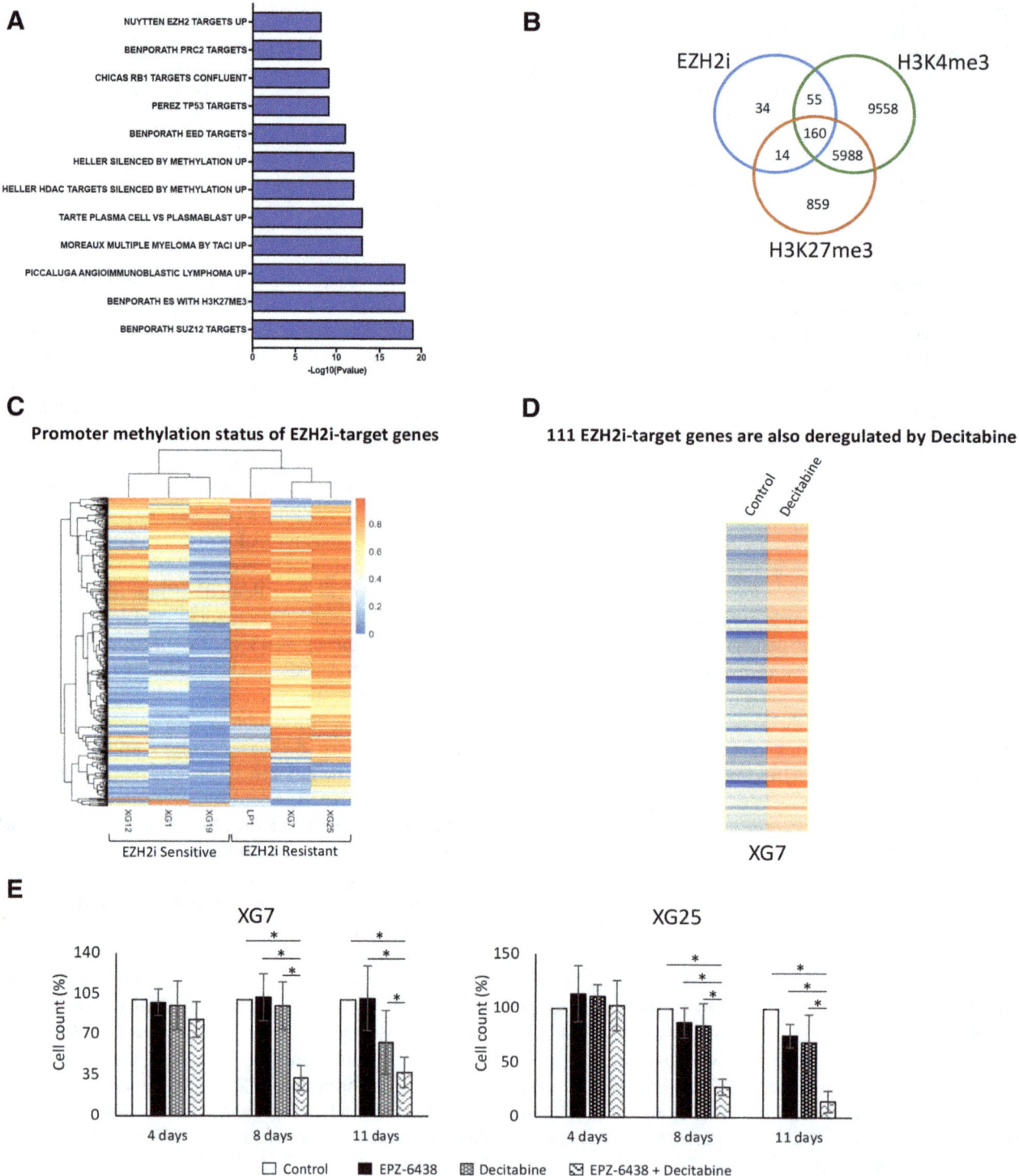

Fig. 3 EZH2i-target genes promoters are methylated in EPZ-6438-resistant cells. **a** Molecular signature of EZH2i-target genes in six HMCLs (XG1, XG12, XG19, XG7, LP1, and XG25) was investigated using GSEA Database (all curated gene sets), and relevant pathways were presented (FDR q value ≤ 0.05). **b** Venn diagram presenting EZH2i-target genes compared to genes associated with H3K27me3 or H3K4me3 in XG7 HMCL. **c** Methylation status of CpGs overlapping with PRC2 target genes promoter region in EZH2i sensitive and resistant myeloma cell lines. **d** Heatmap presenting 111 EZH2i-target genes that are deregulated by decitabine using Affymetrix U133 plus 2.0 microarrays. **e** HMCLs were exposed to 1 μM of EPZ-6438 and/or 100 nM of decitabine. Cell viability was analyzed by trypan blue assay after 4, 8, and 11 days of treatment. Results are the percentage ± SD of viable myeloma cells of three independent experiments. * indicates a significant difference compared to control using a Wilcoxon test for pairs ($P ≤ 0.05$)

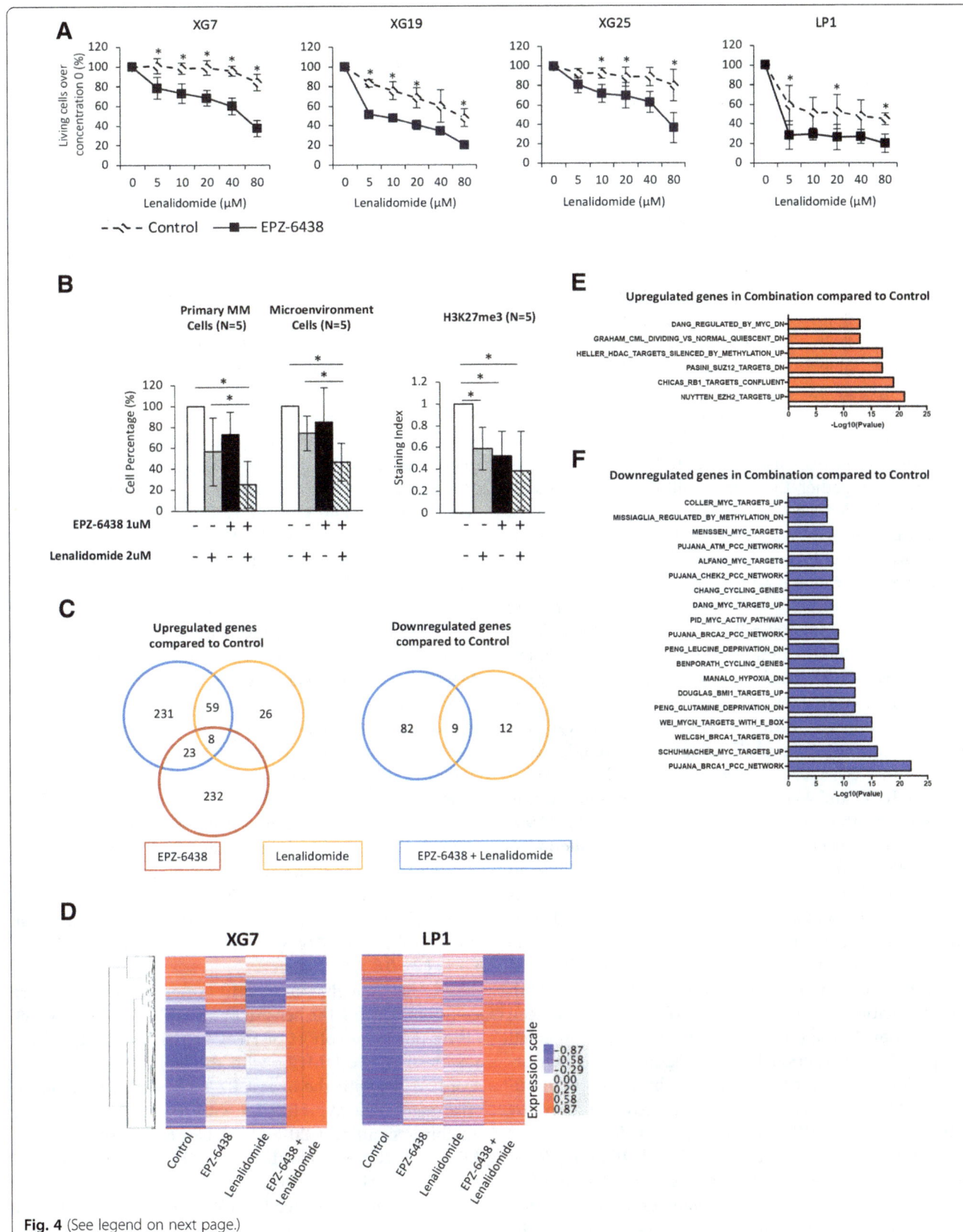

Fig. 4 (See legend on next page.)

(See figure on previous page.)
Fig. 4 EZH2 inhibition sensitizes HMCLs and primary MMCs to lenalidomide. **a** HMCLs were treated 4 days with 1 μM EPZ-6438 and then cultured 4 days with graded lenalidomide concentrations. Data are mean values ± standard deviation (SD) of five experiments. * indicates a significant difference compared to control cells using t test (P ≤ 0.05). **b** After a 4-day pre-treatment with EPZ-6438 (1 μM), mononuclear cells from five patients with MM were treated for 4 days with 2 μM lenalidomide. The viability and total cell counts were assessed, and the percentage of CD138 viable PC and non-malignant bone marrow cells was determined by flow cytometry. Results are median values of the numbers of myeloma cells in the culture wells. Results were compared with a Wilcoxon test for pairs. **c** EPZ-6438, lenalidomide, and EPZ-6438/lenalidomide combination deregulated genes in MM. XG7 and LP1 HMCLs were treated with 2 μM lenalidomide (2 days) with (combination) or without (lenalidomide) prior 4 days-treatment with 1 μM EPZ-6438. Venn diagram showing overlap of genes deregulated by EPZ-6438, lenalidomide, or EPZ-6438/lenalidomide combination. **d** Heatmaps of RNA-seq analysis presenting expression profiles of EPZ-6438, lenalidomide, or combination target genes in XG7 and LP1 HMCLs. **e, f** Molecular signature of EPZ-6438 and lenalidomide combination deregulated genes compared to control in XG7 and LP1 was investigated using GSEA Database (all curated gene sets), and relevant pathways were presented (FDR q value ≤ 0.05)

we found a significant enrichment of PRC2 and RB1 target genes, of genes downregulated by MYC, and genes silenced by DNA methylation (Fig. 4e and Additional file 8: Table S8). GSEA analysis of the 82 specifically downregulated genes by EPZ-6438/lenalidomide revealed a significant enrichment of MYC target genes in association with genes involved in proliferation and replicative stress response (Fig. 4f and Additional file 8: Table S8). Altogether, these data indicate that EPZ-6438/lenalidomide induced a significant upregulation of PRC2, RB1, and DNA methylation target genes in association with a significant downregulation of MYC target genes and cell proliferation gene program.

IMiDs promote Ikaros and Aiolos transcription factors binding to the E3 ubiquitin ligase cereblon (CRBN) leading to their ubiquitination and proteasomal degradation [33]. Ikaros and Aiolos degradation is associated with a downregulation of interferon regulatory factor 4 (IRF4) and MYC which, in turn, reduces MMCs survival [34]. Investigating the effect of EPZ-6438/lenalidomide combination in XG7 and LP1 MMCs, we found that Ikaros (IKZF1), IRF4, and MYC protein levels were significantly decreased by the combination treatment (65.5%, 63.9%, and 14.8% respectively) compared with lenalidomide (51.5%, 43% and 2.2%) or EPZ-6438 (45.2%, 38.7%, and 6.2%) alone (Fig. 5a). These data were validated by western blot and immunofluorescence (Additional file 1: Figures S10 and S11). Furthermore, EPZ-6438/lenalidomide combination strongly upregulated PAX5, BACH2, and BCL6 B cell transcription factors in association with downregulation of PRDM1 and IRF4 key plasma cell transcription factor (Fig. 5b). These data were validated by q-RT-PCR (Additional file 1: Figure S12). Interestingly, ChIP-seq analysis showed the bivalence of PAX5 gene. PAX5 expression could be directly regulated by EZH2 through H3K27me3 (Additional file 1: Figure S13). EPZ-6438/lenalidomide mediated transcriptional deregulation resulted in significant XG7 HMCL proliferation inhibition and quiescence induction characterized by a significant increase in the percentage of G0/G1 cells and ki67 negative cells together with E2F1 downregulation and CDKN1A induction (Fig. 5c–e).

EZ-GEP-based score allows to predict sensitivity of MMCs to EZH2 inhibitor treatment

Since the sensitivity of MMC to EZH2 inhibition is heterogeneous, we searched to define a biomarker allowing the identification of MM patients that could benefit from EZH2 inhibitor treatment. We built a GEP-based score (EZ score), using the prognostic information of 15 genes deregulated by EPZ-6438 and associated with H3K27me3 and a prognostic value in newly diagnosed MM patients (Fig. 6a and Additional file 9: TableS5). The EZ score is defined by the sum of the beta coefficients of the Cox model for each prognostic gene, weighted by − 1 according to the patient MMC signal above or below the probe set Maxstat value as previously described [16]. EZ score levels in normal, premalignant, or malignant plasma cells are displayed in Fig. 6b. MMCs of patients had a significantly higher EZ score than normal BMPCs or plasma cells from MGUS patients (P < 0.01). HMCLs present an even higher EZ score compared with primary MMCs (P < 0.001; Fig. 6b), demonstrating an association between EZ score and the progression of the disease.

Using patient's HM and UAMS-TT2 cohorts, the EZ score had prognostic value when used as a continuous variable or by splitting patients into two groups using the Maxstat R function [16]. The EZ score split patients in a high-risk group (EZ score > 0.686) and a low-risk group (EZ score < 0.686) in the HM and UAMS-TT2 cohorts (P < 0.0001) (Fig. 6c).

We then sought to identify whether the EZ score could predict for the sensitivity of HMCLs to EPZ-6438. Using our large cohort of HMCLs [15], we analyzed the response of five HMCLs with the highest EZ score and five HMCLs with the lowest EZ score to EZH2 inhibitor treatment. The five HMCLs with the highest EZ score exhibit a significant 20-fold median higher sensitivity to EPZ-6438 compared with the five HMCLs with low EZ score (P = 0.04) (Fig. 6d).

To determine whether the EZ score could predict the sensitivity of primary MMCs to EPZ-6438, we analyzed the correlation between its toxicity on MMCs and the EZ score value in a panel of 14 patients. Primary MMCs

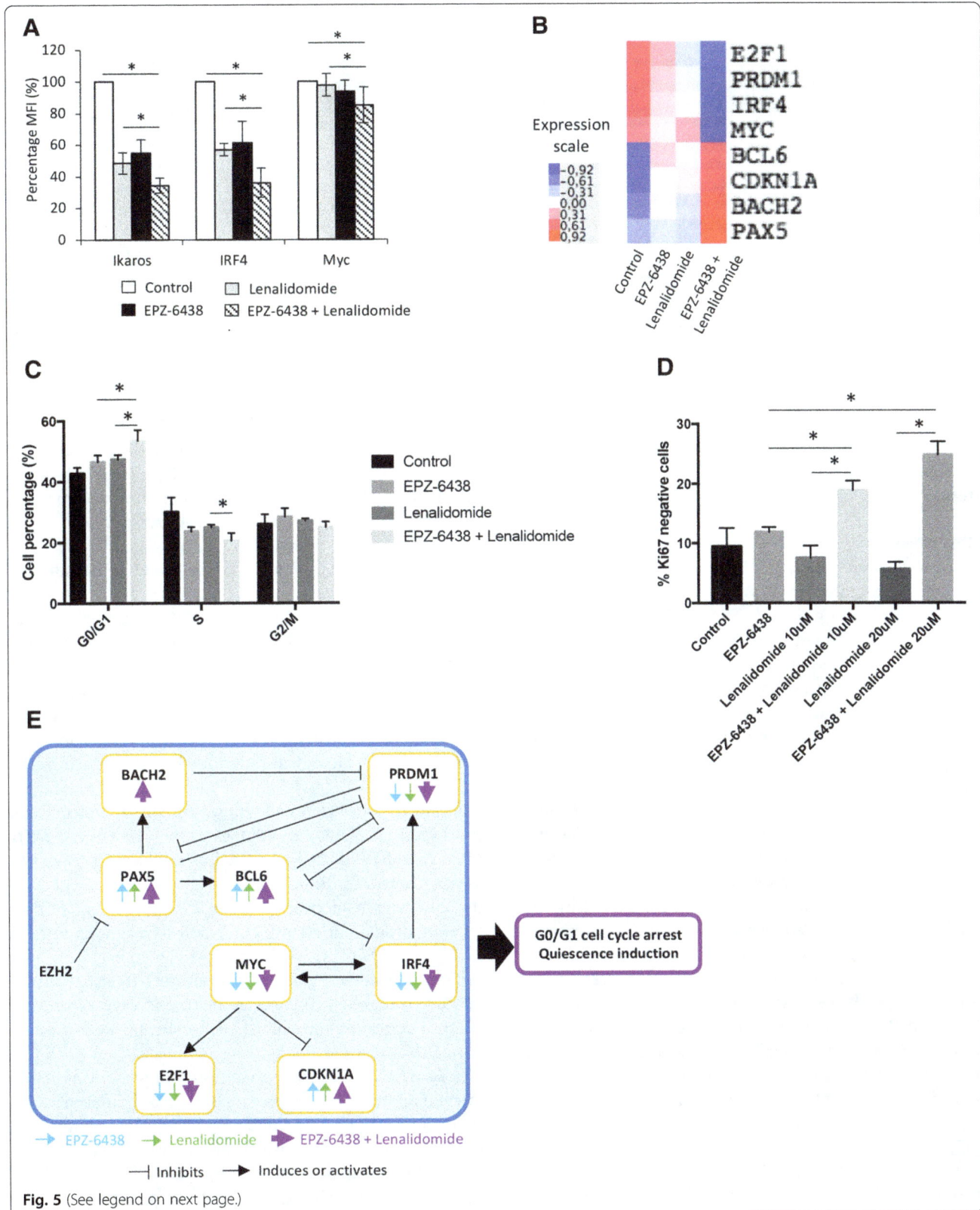

Fig. 5 (See legend on next page.)

(See figure on previous page.)
Fig. 5 EPZ-6438/lenalidomide combination targets key B cell transcription factors and induces MMCs quiescence. **a** The expression of Ikaros (IKZF1), c-Myc, and IRF4 of HMCLs was evaluated by flow cytometry in XG7 after EPZ-6438 (1 μM) and/or lenalidomide (2 μM) treatment using PE-conjugated anti-IKZF1, anti-MYC and anti-IRF4 mAb, and isotype matched PE-conjugated mAb. Data are mean values ± standard deviation of three experiments. **b** Heatmap presenting RNA-seq GEP expression of E2F1, PRDM1, IRF4, MYC, BCL6, CDKN1A, BACH2, and PAX5 in XG7 HMCL treated with EPZ-6438 (1 μM) and/or lenalidomide (2 μM). **c** XG7 cell cycle was analyzed, after EPZ-6438 (1 μM) and/or lenalidomide (2 μM) treatment, by flow cytometry using DAPI, BrdU incorporation, and labeling with an anti-BrdU antibody. Results are representative of four independent experiments. * indicates a significant difference compared to control cells using a paired t test ($P \leq 0.05$). **d** The percentage of Ki67 negative cells of EPZ-6438 and/or lenalidomide-treated XG7 HMCL was analyzed by flow cytometry using anti-Ki67 antibody. Data are the mean values ± SD of three separate experiments. * indicates a significant difference compared to control cells using a paired t test ($P \leq 0.05$). **e** Model of EPZ-6438/lenalidomide combination action in MMCs

were cultured together with their bone marrow environment, recombinant IL-6, and 1 μM of EPZ-6438 for 8 days. As identified in HMCLs, a significant correlation between EZ score and EZH2 inhibitor activity on primary MMCs was observed ($r = -0.68$; $P = 0.005$) (Fig. 6e). A high EZ score value is associated with a higher toxicity of EZH2 inhibitor in MMCs. The EZ score allows the identification of a subgroup of MM patients with a poor outcome that could benefit from EZH2 inhibitor treatment.

Discussion

Our results underline a significant deregulation of PRC1 and PRC2 complex in MM and extend recent studies which pointed out a role of EZH2 in MM biology [7–11, 13]. We demonstrated that PRC2 deregulation is associated with cell cycle deregulation and a proliferative plasmablastic gene expression signature. Our data suggest that PRC2 deregulation could support MM physiopathology, dissemination, and progression. EZH2 inhibitors have been reported to induce expression of miRNA and decrease expression of oncogenes [12, 35]. PRC2 targeting, using EZH2 inhibitor, represents a potent therapeutic strategy in a subgroup of MM patients resulting in a significant induction of polycomb target genes, genes associated with DNA methylation, TP53, and RB1 target genes. The analysis of genes deregulated by EED inhibitor or by knock down of other PRC2 component will be of interest to define the PRC2 specific target genes and the EZH2i unspecific targets. As reported in diffuse large B cell lymphoma [36], we found that H3K27me3 global levels are potently reduced after EPZ-6438 treatment in all HMCLs and primary MM samples tested. However, no link with EZH2 inhibitor sensitivity was identified. Even if UTX loss was recently reported to sensitize MM cell lines to EZH2 inhibition [35], neither EZH2 gene expression nor UTX mutation status was predictive of MM cell response to PRC2 targeting in our collection of MM cell lines representative of molecular heterogeneity or in the primary samples tested. However, analyses of a higher number of samples will be important to provide more significant conclusions. However, we identified a significant overlap

between H3K27me3 and DNA methylation of EPZ-6438 target genes in MM cells resistant to EZH2 inhibitor. These two epigenetic repression systems are mechanistically linked. Indeed, EZH2, as part of PRC2 complex, is required for its target gene promoter methylation [37]. These data underline that PRC2 target genes could comprise key MM tumor suppressor genes silenced by different epigenetic silencing. Interestingly, sublethal doses of DNMTi allow to sensitize EPZ-6438-resistant MM cell lines to EZH2 inhibitor. A major stake remains the identification of biomarkers that can quickly identify the subset patients who could benefit from EZH2 inhibitor treatment.

We developed an EZ score based on 15 EPZ-6438 target genes associated with H3K27me3 and prognostic value in primary MMCs. Our results demonstrate that the EZ score allows the identification of MM patients with a high EZ score value, an adverse prognosis and who could benefit from treatment with EZH2 inhibitors. The expression of 12 out of the 15 genes building the EZ score is associated with favorable outcome in MM. However, their biological functions in MM remain to be characterized.

Several of those genes are known tumor suppressors that are hypermethylated in solid cancers (CACNA1G, IRF6, ITGA9, and PPP2R2C) and used as biomarkers related to adverse outcome [38–51]. In MM, SORL1, a member of the low-density lipoprotein receptor family, is significantly hypermethylated at relapse compared to diagnosis in MM [52, 53]. SLC5A1 encodes a member of the sodium-dependent glucose transporter (SGLT) family. SLC5A1 is a good prognosis biomarker in cervical tumors. SLC5A1 activation through MAP17 increases ROS production [54].

FBLIM1 is a widely expressed protein presenting a role in cellular shape modulation, motility, and differentiation [55]. Interestingly, FBLIM1 expression is reduced in breast cancer and has also been shown to sensitize glioma cells to cisplatin-induced apoptosis [56, 57]. Members of beta-arrestin such as ARRB1 participate in the sensitization/desensitization of G-protein-coupled receptors. The loss of ARRB1 is related to a poor outcome in NSCLC patients [58]. ARRB1 can regulate apoptosis and DNA repair, and its overexpression induced DNA

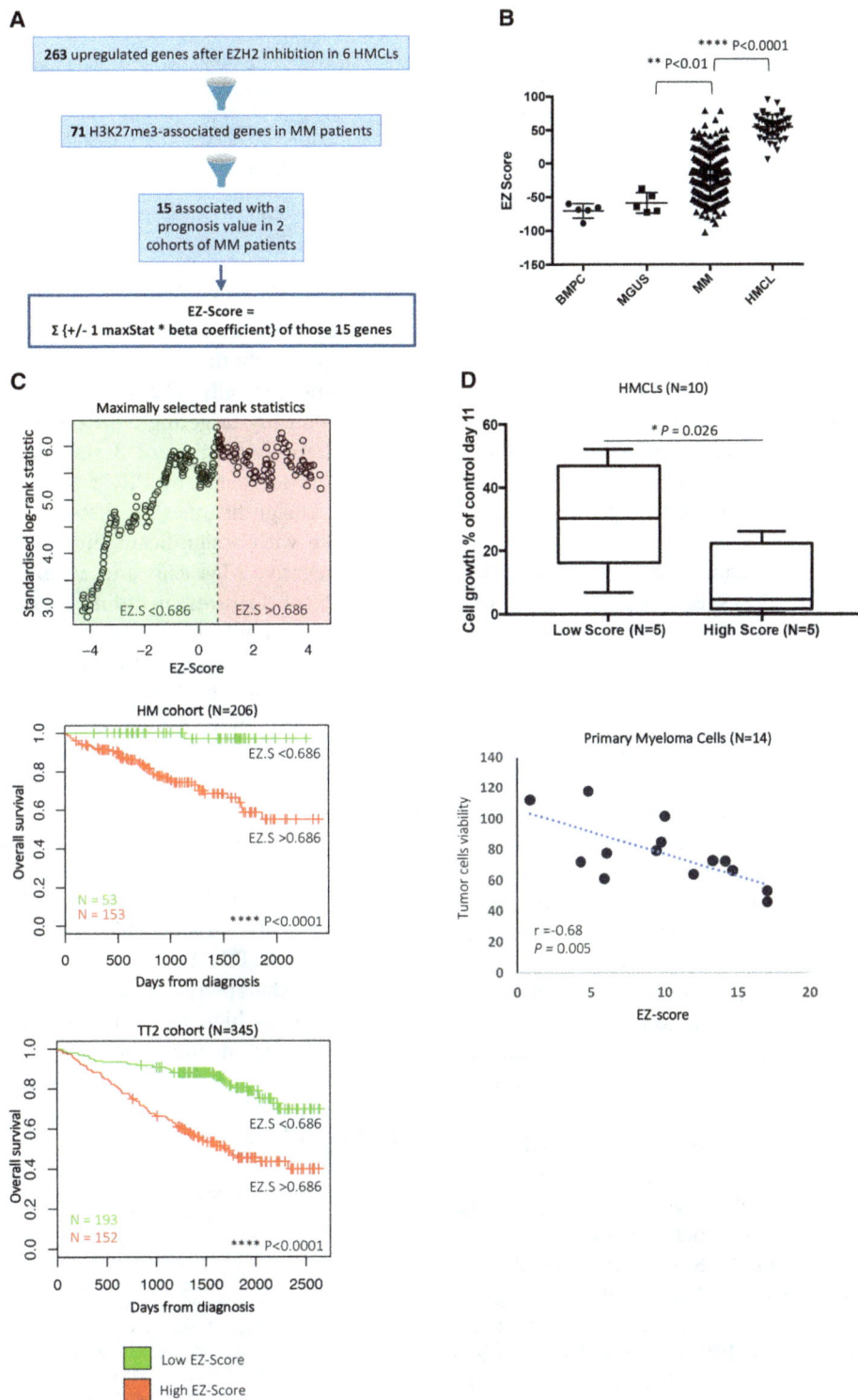

A

263 upregulated genes after EZH2 inhibition in 6 HMCLs

71 H3K27me3-associated genes in MM patients

15 associated with a prognosis value in 2 cohorts of MM patients

EZ-Score =
Σ {+/- 1 maxStat * beta coefficient} of those 15 genes

B

**** P<0.0001

** P<0.01

C

Maximally selected rank statistics

EZ.S <0.686   EZ.S >0.686

HM cohort (N=206)

EZ.S <0.686

EZ.S >0.686

N = 53
N = 153   **** P<0.0001

TT2 cohort (N=345)

EZ.S <0.686

EZ.S >0.686

N = 193
N = 152   **** P<0.0001

Low EZ-Score
High EZ-Score

D

HMCLs (N=10)

* P = 0.026

Low Score (N=5)   High Score (N=5)

Primary Myeloma Cells (N=14)

r = -0.68
P = 0.005

Fig. 6 (See legend on next page.)

(See figure on previous page.)

Fig. 6 EZ score can predict for sensitivity of poor prognosis MM patients to EZH2i. **a** Chart explaining the process of the EZ score creation. **b** EZ score in normal BMPCs ($N = 7$), in premalignant PCs of patients with MGUS ($N = 5$), in MMCs of patients ($N = 206$) and in HMCLs ($N = 40$). Results were compared with a Student's t test. **c** Prognostic value of the EZ score in MM. Patients of the HM cohort were ranked according to increased EZ score and a maximum difference in OS was obtained with EZ score of 0.686 splitting patients into high-risk ($N = 153$) and low-risk ($N = 53$) groups. EZ score also had a prognostic value of an independent cohort of 345 patients (UAMS-TT2 cohort). The parameters to compute the EZ score of patients of UAMS-TT2 cohort and the proportions delineating the two prognostic groups were those defined with HM cohort. **d** HMCLs with high EZ score ($N = 5$) exhibit significant higher EPZ-6438 sensitivity compared with HMCLs with low EZ score ($N = 5$). Data are mean values ± standard deviation of five experiments determined. **e** EZ score predicts for EPZ-6438 sensitivity of primary myeloma cells of patients. Mononuclear cells from tumor samples of 14 patients with MM were cultured for 8 days in the presence of IL-6 (2 ng/ml) with or without 1 μM EPZ-6438. At day 8 of culture, the count of viable MMCs was determined using CD138 staining by flow cytometry

damage in NSCLC cells [59]. THY1 (CD90) is a cell surface glycoprotein involved in cell adhesion and cell communication. In nasopharyngal carcinoma, THY1 is poorly expressed due to its promoter hypermethylation. THY1 overexpression in this cell type induces a G0/G1 cell cycle arrest [60]. These data emphasize that EZH2 inhibitor induces transcriptional activation of potential MM tumor suppressor genes.

Given that monotherapy remains inefficient in MM, a particular association of drugs is usually used to treat MM disease. Unfortunately, despite rising advances in drug development and patient care, MM patients often relapse [61, 62]. By combining EPZ-6438 with MM conventional drugs, we uncovered its synergistic activity with lenalidomide. Furthermore, pre-treatment of MMCs with EZH2 inhibitor was able to overcome lenalidomide resistance (Fig. 4). Transcriptome analysis of cells treated with EPZ-6438/lenalidomide showed a combination-specific deregulated set of genes enriched in GSEA signature related to MYC targeting and genes involved in proliferation and replicative stress response. Furthermore, PRC2 inhibition and most significantly EPZ-6438/lenalidomide combination upregulated PAX5, BACH2, and BCL6 B cell transcription factors. Recently, EZH2i have been shown to induce BCL6 expression in MM cell lines in association with cell death [35]. PAX5, BCL6, and BACH2 repress PRDM1 plasma cell transcription factor. PRDM1 is known to repress BCL6 and PAX5 [63–66], but epigenetic mechanisms may play a major role in B cell transcription factor silencing during plasma cell differentiation as underlined by the bivalent domain of PAX5, including H3K4me3 and H3K27me3 marks, identified in MM cells (Additional file 1: Figure S13). Accordingly, EPZ-6438/lenalidomide treatment resulted in downregulation of PRDM1 and IRF4 expression. By binding to cereblon (CRBN), the IMiD enhances Ikaros and Aiolos proteosomal degradation, thus leading to IRF4 and MYC downregulation [33]. These two factors have been shown to be critical for MMCs survival and disease progression [34]. Our data revealed that EPZ-6438 and lenalidomide combination interfere with MYC transcriptional activity and significantly decreased Ikaros, IRF4, and MYC expression

compared with lenalidomide alone. Finally, we discovered in this study that EZH2 inhibition and IMiDs activity act synergistically to alter gene transcription in MM cells, specifically targeting MM oncogenes and cell cycle genes. The deregulation of B and plasma cell transcription factors mediated by PRC2 targeting and IMiDs results in a significant shift between proliferation and quiescence with a significant increase in the percentage of ki67 negative MM cells and a significant induction of quiescent cell features including repression of E2F1 and higher level of p21 Cdk inhibitor [67–70]. Since MYC activates E2F expression and represses p21 [69], this reprogramming may be explained by the dual targeting of MYC-IRF4 axis by EPZ-6438/lenalidomide combination.

Conclusion

Altogether, our data demonstrate a deregulation of PRC profiles in MM cells contributing to malignant phenotype. The transcriptional deregulation mediated by PRC2 represent a therapeutic target in MM and a synergy was identified with IMiDs. PRC2 targeting in association with IMiDs could have a therapeutic interest in high-risk MM patients characterized by high EZ score values, reactivating B cell transcription factors and tumor suppressor genes.

Additional files

Additional file 1: Figure S1. EZH2 expression is correlated with EED and SUZ12 expression. Figure S2 PRC1 members are significantly downregulated in primary MM cells compared with normal bone marrow plasma cells. Figure S3 EZH2 is associated with a poor prognosis in MM. Figure S4 Association between EZH2 expression and patients' genetic abnormalities. Figure S5 EPZ-6438 leads to H3K27me3 loss in HMCLs. Figure S6 EPZ-6438 leads to H3K27me3 loss in HMCLs. Figure S7 EPZ-6438-induced apoptosis is partially rescued by QVD pan caspase inhibitor. Figure S8 EZH2 inhibition induces mortality of primary MM cells from patients. Figure S9 Correlation between EZH2 expression/H3K27m3 staining and drug response to EZH2 inhibitor in HMCLs and patients. Figure S10 IKZF1 protein level decreases after HMCLs were treated with EPZ-6438 and lenalidomide combination. Figure S11 Lenalidomide targets protein levels after treatment. Figure S12 B cell transcription factors mRNA expression after treatment. Figure S13 PAX5 is a bivalent gene in XG7 HMCL. (PDF 21322 kb)

Additional file 2: Table S1. HMCLs molecular characteristics (XLSX 15 kb)

Additional file 3: Table S2. EPZ-6438 regulated genes in HMCLs (XLSX 32 kb)

Additional file 4: Table S3. GSEA signature enrichment of the 264 EPZ-6438 target genes (XLSX 18 kb)

Additional file 5: Table S4. EZH2i target genes are mostly bivalent in XG7 HMCLs (XLSX 10 kb)

Additional file 6: Table S6. 67 Lenalidomide + combo upregulated genes (XLSX 17 kb)

Additional file 7: Table S7. 31 EPZ-6438 + combo upregulated genes (XLSX 11 kb)

Additional file 8: Table S8. Lenalidomide+EPZ-6438-regulated genes associated with GSEA signatures (XLSX 75 kb)

Additional file 9: Table S5. H3K27me3-associated and EPZ-6438-regulated genes (XLSX 12 kb)

Abbreviations
DNMTi: DNA methyltransferases inhibitor; EZH2: Enhancer of zeste homolog 2; EZH2i: EZH2 inhibitor; HMCL: Human myeloma cell line; IMiDs: Immunomodulatory drugs; MM: Multiple myeloma; MMC: Multiple myeloma cells; PRC: Polycomb repressive complex

Acknowledgements
We thank the Microarray Core Facility of IRMB, CHU Montpellier.

Funding
This work was supported by grants from French INCA (Institut National du Cancer) Institute (2012-109/087437 and PLBIO15-256), Languedoc Roussillon CRLR (R14026FF), LR-FEDER Hemodiag, Fondation de France (201400047510), ITMO Cancer (MM&TT), SIRIC Montpellier (INCa-DGOS-Inserm 6045), the German Federal Ministry of Education (BMBF) "CAMPSIMM" (01ES1103) and within the framework of the e:Med research and funding concept "CLIOM-MICS" (01ZX1309), and the Deutsche Forschungsgemeinschaft (SFB/TRR79; subproject B1). LH is supported by a grant from Labex EpiGenMed.

Authors' contributions
LH performed research and participated in the writing of the paper. GR, NR, and SB participated in the research. AK participated in GEP data analyses and bioinformatics. HG, AS, GCartron, LV, CMT, and DH participated in clinical data analysis and participated in the writing of the paper. GCavalli participated in the research and in the writing of the paper. JM supervised the research and the writing of the paper. All authors read and approved the final manuscript.

Competing interests
The authors declare that they have no competing interests.

Author details
[1]Department of Biological Hematology, CHU Montpellier, Montpellier, France. [2]IGH, CNRS, Univ Montpellier, Montpellier, France. [3]UFR de Médecine, Univ Montpellier, Montpellier, France. [4]Medizinische Klinik und Poliklinik V, Universitätsklinikum Heidelberg, Heidelberg, Germany. [5]Nationales Centrum für Tumorerkrankungen, Heidelberg, Germany. [6]Department of Clinical Hematology, CHU Montpellier, Montpellier, France. [7]UMR CNRS 5235, Univ Montpellier, Montpellier, France. [8]Laboratory for Monitoring Innovative Therapies, Department of Biological Hematology, Hôpital Saint-Eloi-CHRU de Montpellier, 80, av. Augustin Fliche, 34295 Montpellier, Cedex 5, France.

References
1. Herviou L, Cavalli G, Cartron G, Klein B, Moreaux J. EZH2 in normal hematopoiesis and hematological malignancies. Oncotarget. 2016;7:2284.
2. Barlogie B, Mitchell A, van Rhee F, Epstein J, Morgan GJ, Crowley J. Curing myeloma at last: defining criteria and providing the evidence. Blood. 2014; 124:3043–51.
3. Lohr JG, Stojanov P, Carter SL, Cruz-Gordillo P, Lawrence MS, Auclair D, et al. Widespread genetic heterogeneity in multiple myeloma: implications for targeted therapy. Cancer Cell. 2014;25:91–101.
4. Bolli N, Avet-Loiseau H, Wedge DC, Van Loo P, Alexandrov LB, Martincorena I, et al. Heterogeneity of genomic evolution and mutational profiles in multiple myeloma. Nat Commun. 2014;5. https://doi.org/10.1038/ncomms3997.
5. Delmore JE, Issa GC, Lemieux ME, Rahl PB, Shi J, Jacobs HM, et al. BET Bromodomain inhibition as a therapeutic strategy to target c-Myc. Cell. 2011;146:904–17.
6. Moreaux J, Reme T, Leonard W, Veyrune J-L, Requirand G, Goldschmidt H, et al. Gene expression-based prediction of myeloma cell sensitivity to histone deacetylase inhibitors. Br J Cancer. 2013;109:676–85.
7. Kalushkova A, Fryknäs M, Lemaire M, Fristedt C, Agarwal P, Eriksson M, et al. Polycomb target genes are silenced in multiple myeloma. PLoS One. 2010;5: e11483.
8. Croonquist PA, Van Ness B. The polycomb group protein enhancer of zeste homolog 2 (EZH2) is an oncogene that influences myeloma cell growth and the mutant ras phenotype. Oncogene. 2005;24:6269–80.
9. Zhao F, Chen Y, Li R, Liu Y, Wen L, Zhang C. Triptolide alters histone H3K9 and H3K27 methylation state and induces G0/G1 arrest and caspase-dependent apoptosis in multiple myeloma in vitro. Toxicology. 2010;267:70–9.
10. Agarwal P, Alzrigat M, Párraga AA, Enroth S, Singh U, Ungerstedt J, et al. Genome-wide profiling of histone H3 lysine 27 and lysine 4 trimethylation in multiple myeloma reveals the importance of polycomb gene targeting and highlights EZH2 as a potential therapeutic target. Oncotarget. 2016;7:6809.
11. Hernando H, Gelato KA, Lesche R, Beckmann G, Koehr S, Otto S, et al. EZH2 inhibition blocks multiple myeloma cell growth through upregulation of epithelial tumor suppressor genes. Mol Cancer Ther. 2016;15:287–98.
12. Alzrigat M, Párraga AA, Agarwal P, Zureigat H, Österborg A, Nahi H, et al. EZH2 inhibition in multiple myeloma downregulates myeloma associated oncogenes and upregulates microRNAs with potential tumor suppressor functions. OncoTarget. 2016. https://www.researchgate.net/profile/Mohammad_Alzrigat/publication/312021585_EZH2_inhibition_in_multiple_myeloma_downregulates_myeloma_associated_oncogenes_and_upregulates_microRNAs_with_potential_tumor_suppressor_functions/links/58694b7008ae8fce4917d807.pdf. Accessed 6 Apr 2017.
13. Pawlyn C, Bright MD, Buros AF, Stein CK, Walters Z, Aronson LI, et al. Overexpression of EZH2 in multiple myeloma is associated with poor prognosis and dysregulation of cell cycle control. Blood Cancer J. 2017;7:e549.
14. Kurmasheva RT, Sammons M, Favours E, Wu J, Kurmashev D, Cosmopoulos K, et al. Initial testing (stage 1) of tazemetostat (EPZ-6438), a novel EZH2 inhibitor, by the pediatric preclinical testing program: Kurmasheva et al. Pediatr Blood Cancer 2016. doi:https://doi.org/10.1002/pbc.26218.
15. Moreaux J, Klein B, Bataille R, Descamps G, Maiga S, Hose D, et al. A high-risk signature for patients with multiple myeloma established from the

molecular classification of human myeloma cell lines. Haematologica. 2011; 96:574–82.

16. Hose D, Reme T, Hielscher T, Moreaux J, Messner T, Seckinger A, et al. Proliferation is a central independent prognostic factor and target for personalized and risk-adapted treatment in multiple myeloma. Haematologica. 2011;96:87–95.

17. Hose D, Rème T, Meissner T, Moreaux J, Seckinger A, Lewis J, et al. Inhibition of aurora kinases for tailored risk-adapted treatment of multiple myeloma. Blood. 2009;113:4331–40.

18. Barlogie B. Total therapy 2 without thalidomide in comparison with total therapy 1: role of intensified induction and posttransplantation consolidation therapies. Blood. 2006;107:2633–8.

19. Pineda-Roman M, Zangari M, van Rhee F, Anaissie E, Szymonifka J, Hoering A, et al. VTD combination therapy with bortezomib–thalidomide– dexamethasone is highly effective in advanced and refractory multiple myeloma. Leukemia. 2008;22:1419–27.

20. Mulligan G, Mitsiades C, Bryant B, Zhan F, Chng WJ, Roels S, et al. Gene expression profiling and correlation with outcome in clinical trials of the proteasome inhibitor bortezomib. Blood. 2007;109:3177–88.

21. Dobin A, Davis CA, Schlesinger F, Drenkow J, Zaleski C, Jha S, et al. STAR: ultrafast universal RNA-seq aligner. Bioinformatics. 2013;29:15–21.

22. Gentleman RC, Carey VJ, Bates DM, Bolstad B, Dettling M, Dudoit S, et al. Bioconductor: open software development for computational biology and bioinformatics. Genome Biol. 2004;5:1.

23. Love MI, Huber W, Anders S. Moderated estimation of fold change and dispersion for RNA-seq data with DESeq2. Genome Biol. 2014;15. https://doi. org/10.1186/s13059-014-0550-8.

24. Liberzon A, Subramanian A, Pinchback R, Thorvaldsdottir H, Tamayo P, Mesirov JP. Molecular signatures database (MSigDB) 3.0. Bioinformatics. 2011;27:1739–40.

25. Subramanian A, Tamayo P, Mootha VK, Mukherjee S, Ebert BL, Gillette MA, et al. Gene set enrichment analysis: a knowledge-based approach for interpreting genome-wide expression profiles. Proc Natl Acad Sci. 2005;102: 15545–50.

26. Kassambara A, Rème T, Jourdan M, Fest T, Hose D, Tarte K, et al. GenomicScape: an easy-to-use web tool for gene expression data analysis. Application to investigate the molecular events in the differentiation of B cells into plasma cells. PLoS Comput Biol. 2015;11:e1004077.

27. Küffner R, Zach N, Norel R, Hawe J, Schoenfeld D, Wang L, et al. Crowdsourced analysis of clinical trial data to predict amyotrophic lateral sclerosis progression. Nat Biotechnol. 2014;33:51–7.

28. Moreaux J, Reme T, Leonard W, Veyrune J-L, Requirand G, Goldschmidt H, et al. Development of gene expression-based score to predict sensitivity of multiple myeloma cells to DNA methylation inhibitors. Mol Cancer Ther. 2012;11:2685–92.

29. Aryee MJ, Jaffe AE, Corrada-Bravo H, Ladd-Acosta C, Feinberg AP, Hansen KD, et al. Minfi: a flexible and comprehensive Bioconductor package for the analysis of Infinium DNA methylation microarrays. Bioinformatics. 2014;30:1363–9.

30. Lawrence M, Huber W, Pagès H, Aboyoun P, Carlson M, Gentleman R, et al. Software for computing and annotating genomic ranges. PLoS Comput Biol. 2013;9. https://doi.org/10.1371/journal.pcbi.1003118.

31. Hothorn T, Lausen B. On the exact distribution of maximally selected rank statistics. Comput Stat Data Anal. 2003;43:121–37.

32. Cummin TE, Araf S, Du M, Barrans S, Bentley MA, Clipson A, et al. Prognostic significance and correlation to gene expression profile of EZH2 mutations in diffuse large b-cell lymphoma (DLBL) in 2 large prospective studies. Hematol Oncol. 2017;35:158–9.

33. Guirguis AA, Ebert BL. Lenalidomide: deciphering mechanisms of action in myeloma, myelodysplastic syndrome and beyond. Curr Opin Cell Biol. 2015;37:61–7.

34. Bjorklund CC, Lu L, Kang J, Hagner PR, Havens CG, Amatangelo M, et al. Rate of CRL4CRBN substrate Ikaros and Aiolos degradation underlies differential activity of lenalidomide and pomalidomide in multiple myeloma cells by regulation of c-Myc and IRF4. Blood Cancer J. 2015;5:e354.

35. Ezponda T, Dupéré-Richer D, Will CM, Small EC, Varghese N, Patel T, et al. UTX/KDM6A loss enhances the malignant phenotype of multiple myeloma and sensitizes cells to EZH2 inhibition. Cell Rep. 2017;21:628–40.

36. Garapaty-Rao S, Nasveschuk C, Gagnon A, Chan EY, Sandy P, Busby J, et al. Identification of EZH2 and EZH1 small molecule inhibitors with selective impact on diffuse large B cell lymphoma cell growth. Chem Biol. 2013;20: 1329–39.

37. Viré E, Brenner C, Deplus R, Blanchon L, Fraga M, Didelot C, et al. The Polycomb group protein EZH2 directly controls DNA methylation. Nature. 2005;439:871–4.

38. Toyota M, Ho C, Ohe-Toyota M, Baylin SB, Issa J-PJ. Inactivation of CACNA1G, a T-type calcium channel gene, by aberrant methylation of its 5' CpG island in human tumors. Cancer Res. 1999;59:4535–41.

39. Cha Y, Kim K-J, Han S-W, Rhee YY, Bae JM, Wen X, et al. Adverse prognostic impact of the CpG island methylator phenotype in metastatic colorectal cancer. Br J Cancer. 2016;115:164–71.

40. Ohkubo T. T-type voltage-activated calcium channel Cav3.1, but not Cav3.2, is involved in the inhibition of proliferation and apoptosis in MCF-7 human breast cancer cells. Int J Oncol. 2012. https://doi.org/10.3892/ijo.2012.1422.

41. Cohen Y, Merhavi-Shoham E, Avraham RB, Frenkel S, Pe'er J, Goldenberg-Cohen N. Hypermethylation of CpG island loci of multiple tumor suppressor genes in retinoblastoma. Exp Eye Res. 2008;86:201–6.

42. Bailey CM, Abbott DE, Margaryan NV, Khalkhali-Ellis Z, Hendrix MJC. Interferon regulatory factor 6 promotes cell cycle arrest and is regulated by the proteasome in a cell cycle-dependent manner. Mol Cell Biol. 2008;28: 2235–43.

43. Zengin T, Ekinci B, Kucukkose C, Yalcin-Ozuysal O. IRF6 is involved in the regulation of cell proliferation and transformation in MCF10A cells downstream of notch signaling. PLoS One. 2015;10:e0132757.

44. Mostovich LA, Prudnikova TY, Kondratov AG, Loginova D, Vavilov PV, Rykova VI, et al. Integrin alpha9 (ITGA9) expression and epigenetic silencing in human breast tumors. Cell Adhes Migr. 2011;5:395–401.

45. Senchenko VN, Kisseljova NP, Ivanova TA, Dmitriev AA, Krasnov GS, Kudryavtseva AV, et al. Novel tumor suppressor candidates on chromosome 3 revealed by NotI-microarrays in cervical cancer. Epigenetics. 2013;8:409–20.

46. Nawaz I, Hu L-F, Du Z-M, Moumad K, Ignatyev I, Pavlova TV, et al. Integrin α9 gene promoter is hypermethylated and downregulated in nasopharyngeal carcinoma. Oncotarget. 2015;6:31493.

47. Mumby M. PP2A: unveiling a reluctant tumor suppressor. Cell. 2007;130:21–4.

48. Bluemn EG, Spencer ES, Mecham B, Gordon RR, Coleman I, Lewinshtein D, et al. PPP2R2C loss promotes castration-resistance and is associated with increased prostate Cancer-specific mortality. Mol Cancer Res. 2013;11:568–78.

49. Bi D, Ning H, Liu S, Que X, Ding K. miR-1301 promotes prostate cancer proliferation through directly targeting PPP2R2C. Biomed Pharmacother. 2016;81:25–30.

50. Wu A-H, Huang Y, Zhang L-Z, Tian G, Liao Q-Z, Chen S-L. MiR-572 prompted cell proliferation of human ovarian cancer cells by suppressing PPP2R2C expression. Biomed Pharmacother. 2016;77:92–7.

51. Fan Y, Chen L, Wang J, Yao Q, Wan J. Over expression of PPP2R2C inhibits human glioma cells growth through the suppression of mTOR pathway. FEBS Lett. 2013;587:3892–7.

52. Sugita Y, Ohwada C, Kawaguchi T, Muto T, Tsukamoto S, Takeda Y, et al. Prognostic impact of serum soluble LR11 in newly diagnosed diffuse large B-cell lymphoma: a multicenter prospective analysis. Clin Chim Acta. 2016; 463:47–52.

53. Krzeminski P, Corchete LA, García JL, López-Corral L, Fermiñán E, García EM, et al. Integrative analysis of DNA copy number, DNA methylation and gene expression in multiple myeloma reveals alterations related to relapse. Oncotarget. 2016. https://doi.org/10.18632/oncotarget.13025.

54. Guijarro MV, Leal JFM, Blanco-Aparicio C, Alonso S, Fominaya J, Lleonart M, et al. MAP17 enhances the malignant behavior of tumor cells through ROS increase. Carcinogenesis. 2007;28:2096–104.

55. Wu C. Migfilin and its binding partners: from cell biology to human diseases. J Cell Sci. 2005;118:659–64.

56. Fan J, Ou Y, Wu C, Yu C, Song Y, Zhan Q. Migfilin sensitizes cisplatin-induced apoptosis in human glioma cells in vitro. Acta Pharmacol Sin. 2012; 33:1301–10.

57. Gkretsi V, Papanikolaou V, Zacharia LC, Athanassiou E, Wu C, Tsezou A. Mitogen-inducible Gene-2 (MIG2) and migfilin expression is reduced in samples of human breast cancer. Anticancer Res. 2013;33:1977–81.

58. Ma H, Wang L, Zhang T, Shen H, Du J. Loss of β-arrestin1 expression predicts unfavorable prognosis for non-small cell lung cancer patients. Tumor Biol. 2016;37:1341–7.

59. Shen H, Wang L, Zhang J, Dong W, Zhang T, Ni Y, et al. ARRB1 enhances the chemosensitivity of lung cancer through the mediation of DNA damage response. Oncol Rep. 2016. https://doi.org/10.3892/or.2016.5337.

60. Kumar A, Bhanja A, Bhattacharyya J, Jaganathan BG. Multiple roles of CD90 in cancer. Tumor Biol. 2016;37:11611–22.

PRC2 targeting is a therapeutic strategy for EZ score defined high-risk multiple myeloma patients...

91

61. Cavo M, Rajkumar SV, Palumbo A, Moreau P, Orlowski R, Blade J, et al. International myeloma working group consensus approach to the treatment of multiple myeloma patients who are candidates for autologous stem cell transplantation. Blood. 2011;117:6063–73.

62. Anderson KC. The 39th David a. Karnofsky lecture: bench-to-bedside translation of targeted therapies in multiple myeloma. J Clin Oncol. 2012;30:445–52.

63. Méndez A, Mendoza L. A network model to describe the terminal differentiation of B cells. PLoS Comput Biol. 2016;12:e1004696.

64. Boi M, Zucca E, Inghirami G, Bertoni F. *PRDM1* /BLIMP1: a tumor suppressor gene in B and T cell lymphomas. Leuk Lymphoma. 2015;56:1223–8.

65. Alinikula J, Nera K-P, Junttila S, Lassila O. Alternate pathways for Bcl6-mediated regulation of B cell to plasma cell differentiation. Eur J Immunol. 2011;41:2404–13.

66. Inagaki Y, Hayakawa F, Hirano D, Kojima Y, Morishita T, Yasuda T, et al. PAX5 tyrosine phosphorylation by SYK co-operatively functions with its serine phosphorylation to cancel the PAX5-dependent repression of BLIMP1: a mechanism for antigen-triggered plasma cell differentiation. Biochem Biophys Res Commun. 2016;475:176–81.

67. Yao G. Modelling mammalian cellular quiescence. Interface Focus. 2014;4: 20130074.

68. Wu S, Cetinkaya C, Munoz-Alonso MJ, von der Lehr N, Bahram F, Beuger V, et al. Myc represses differentiation-induced p21CIP1 expression via Miz-1-dependent interaction with the p21 core promoter. Oncogene. 2003;22:351–60.

69. Bretones G, Delgado MD, León J. Myc and cell cycle control. Biochim Biophys Acta BBA - Gene Regul Mech. 2015;1849:506–16.

70. Fecteau J-F, Corral LG, Ghia EM, Gaidarova S, Futalan D, Bharati IS, et al. Lenalidomide inhibits the proliferation of CLL cells via a cereblon/p21WAF1/Cip1-dependent mechanism independent of functional p53. Blood. 2014; 124:1637–44.

8

Increased CD4+ T cell lineage commitment determined by CpG methylation correlates with better prognosis in urinary bladder cancer patients

Emma Ahlén Bergman[1][*] [iD], Ciputra Adijaya Hartana[1], Markus Johansson[2,3], Ludvig B. Linton[1], Sofia Berglund[1], Martin Hyllienmark[4], Christian Lundgren[1], Benny Holmström[5], Karin Palmqvist[6,3], Johan Hansson[7^], Farhood Alamdari[8], Ylva Huge[9], Firas Aljabery[9], Katrine Riklund[10], Malin E. Winerdal[1], David Krantz[1], A. Ali Zirakzadeh[1,3], Per Marits[1], Louise K. Sjöholm[11], Amir Sherif[3,10†] and Ola Winqvist[1†]

Abstract

Background: Urinary bladder cancer is a common malignancy worldwide. Environmental factors and chronic inflammation are correlated with the disease risk. Diagnosis is performed by transurethral resection of the bladder, and patients with muscle invasive disease preferably proceed to radical cystectomy, with or without neoadjuvant chemotherapy. The anti-tumour immune responses, known to be initiated in the tumour and draining lymph nodes, may play a major role in future treatment strategies. Thus, increasing the knowledge of tumour-associated immunological processes is important. Activated CD4+ T cells differentiate into four main separate lineages: Th1, Th2, Th17 and Treg, and they are recognized by their effector molecules IFN-γ, IL-13, IL-17A, and the transcription factor Foxp3, respectively. We have previously demonstrated signature CpG sites predictive for lineage commitment of these four major CD4+ T cell lineages. Here, we investigate the lineage commitment specifically in tumour, lymph nodes and blood and relate them to the disease stage and response to neoadjuvant chemotherapy.

Results: Blood, tumour and regional lymph nodes were obtained from patients at time of transurethral resection of the bladder and at radical cystectomy. Tumour-infiltrating CD4+ lymphocytes were significantly hypomethylated in all four investigated lineage loci compared to CD4+ lymphocytes in lymph nodes and blood (lymph nodes vs tumour-infiltrating lymphocytes: *IFNG* -4229 bp $p < 0.0001$, *IL13* -11 bp $p < 0.05$, *IL17A* -122 bp $p < 0.01$ and *FOXP3* -77 bp $p > 0.05$). Examination of individual lymph nodes displayed different methylation signatures, suggesting possible correlation with future survival. More advanced post-cystectomy tumour stages correlated significantly with increased methylation at the *IFNG* -4229 bp locus. Patients with complete response to neoadjuvant chemotherapy displayed significant hypomethylation in CD4+ T cells for all four investigated loci, most prominently in *IFNG* $p < 0.0001$. Neoadjuvant chemotherapy seemed to result in a relocation of Th1-committed CD4+ T cells from blood, presumably to the tumour, indicated by shifts in the methylation patterns, whereas no such shifts were seen for lineages corresponding to *IL13*, *IL17A* and *FOXP3*.

(Continued on next page)

* Correspondence: emma.ahlen.bergman@ki.se
†Amir Sherif and Ola Winqvist contributed equally to this work.
^Deceased
[1]Unit of Immunology and Allergy, Department of Medicine Solna, Karolinska Institutet, Karolinska University Hospital, Stockholm, Sweden
Full list of author information is available at the end of the article

(Continued from previous page)

Conclusion: Increased lineage commitment in CD4$^+$ T cells, as determined by demethylation in predictive CpG sites, is associated with lower post-cystectomy tumour stage, complete response to neoadjuvant chemotherapy and overall better outcome, suggesting epigenetic profiling of CD4$^+$ T cell lineages as a useful readout for clinical staging.

Keywords: DNA methylation, CD4-positive T lymphocytes, Urinary bladder neoplasms,

Background

Urinary bladder cancer (UBC) is the ninth most frequent cancer disease with 380,000 new cases diagnosed worldwide and about 150,000 deaths yearly [1, 2]. Environmental factors and life style seem to play an important role for tumour development. Chronic exposure to carcinogenic substances in the urine such as smoking-derived carcinogens, rubber and certain dyes may lead to cancer development [3]. In addition, infection with the trematode *Schistosoma haematobium* leads to chronic inflammation in the urinary bladder and development of squamous cell carcinoma [4]. Thus, chronic exposure to irritating substances, i.e. chemicals or pathogens, may lead to malignant transformation of cells and finally cancer development. Urothelial muscle invasive bladder cancer is diagnosed (defined as tumour stages T2-T4aN0M0), based on the pathologist's assessment of tumour obtained at transurethral resection of the bladder (TUR-B). Patients judged to be fit according to the Swedish national guidelines are treated with cisplatin-based neoadjuvant combination chemotherapy (NAC), prior to radical cystectomy (RC) typically MVAC (methotrexate, vinblastine, doxorubicin and cisplatin).

UBC development is highly associated with inflammation and immune cell infiltration, an association that provides a basis for immunotherapeutic strategies, such as intravesically administered BCG (Bacillus Calmette-Guerin vaccine) in treatment of high-risk non-muscle invasive bladder cancer (HR-NMIBC) [5]. We previously demonstrated that the presence of CD3$^+$ tumour-infiltrating T lymphocytes (TIL) is a positive prognostic factor for survival [6], supporting the importance of an anti-tumour T cell response. We have also demonstrated that the regional lymph nodes (LNs) contain lymphocytes that are reactive towards the tumour [7, 8], but that the inter-patient variation of responsiveness to autologous tumour antigen stimulus is highly variable.

The maturation process of T lymphocytes is localized in the thymus through a process of positive and negative selection resulting in CD4$^+$ MHC class II-restricted T cells and CD8$^+$ MHC class I-restricted T cells [9]. Upon encounter of intermediate affinity/concentration of self-peptides in the thymic medulla, naïve CD4$^+$ T cells are converted to Foxp3 stably expressing regulatory T cells (Treg). CD4$^+$ T cells emerging from the thymus pass into the periphery and circulate various tissues. Upon encountering their cognate antigen in a tumour setting, the pattern of their maturation and differentiation into separate CD4$^+$ T cell lineages will be decided by the combined signals from the antigen-presenting cells, tumour cells and stroma cells present in this distinct environment. The main CD4$^+$ T cell effector lineages are Th1, Th2 and Th17, as recognized by their production of effector cytokines IFN-γ, IL-13 and IL-17A, respectively [10]. Upon activation and proliferation, naïve T cells transform to differentiated effector cells with a stable phenotype that is difficult to reverse after five cell divisions [11, 12]. However, plasticity among committed T cell subpopulations have started to be explored [13–15]. Long-term epigenetic stability of a T cell phenotype can be evaluated using methylation markers at predictive CpG sites [16–19].

We and other groups have previously investigated the methylation status of the *IFNG* locus in CD4$^+$ T cells from LNs and tumours. We have also developed methods for investigating the *IL13*, *FOXP3* and *IL17A* loci to make a global CD4$^+$ T cell assessment regarding epigenetic commitment [17, 19–21].

Based on previous experiences and results, we performed a snapshot analysis of the in vivo epigenetic commitment of CD4$^+$ T cell populations in samples from patients with UBC, using DNA methylation pattern of epigenetic lineage markers for Th1, Th2, Th17 and Tregs predictive for assessing CD4$^+$ T cell subpopulation stability [19]. Further, we correlate our findings with clinical response to neoadjuvant chemotherapy and pathological tumour stage post-cystectomy.

Methods

Patient inclusion and clinical procedure

All patients were included in this study after giving their written and oral consent to participate, in accordance with the declaration of Helsinki. The study was approved by the local ethical committee (dnr: 2007/71-31, amendment 2017/190-32). Recruitment was performed between 2014 and 2017 from nine Swedish hospitals (Umeå University Hospital, Sundsvall Hospital, Västerås Central Hospital, Linköping University Hospital, Norrköping Hospital, Skellefteå Hospital and Gävle Hospital, Uppsala Akademiska University Hospital and Östersund County Hospital). The patients in the study were included either before TUR-B with suspected urinary bladder cancer, or before RC, after an established muscle invasive bladder cancer (MIBC) (tumour stages cT2-4aN0M0), as determined by pathologist's assessment of previously performed TUR-B. Patient characteristics are presented in Table 1. Tumour and blood samples were collected at TUR-B from 23 patients. Samples were also collected from 21 patients at RC, including blood, tumour draining sentinel lymph nodes (SN), non-draining lymph nodes (nSN) and, in cases with remaining tumour at this stage, tumour tissue. The method for sentinel node detection has previously been described [22]. From six patients, additional blood samples were obtained during NAC treatment (in-between NAC cycles). The total number of specimens was as follows: blood, $n = 48$; regional LN (both SN and nSN), $n = 76$; and tumour, $n = 22$. Not all specimens were analysed for every parameter, due to sample limitations.

Lymphocyte extraction

Peripheral blood mononuclear cells (PBMCs) from blood were extracted using Ficoll paque PLUS (GE Healthcare).

Tumour-infiltrating lymphocytes were extracted by cutting tumour tissue into small pieces and disassociating the dissected tumour pieces into single cells using a gentleMACS dissociator (Miltenyi Biotec). Samples were processed in GIBCO Aim V™ (Invitrogen) supplemented with collagenase/hyaluronidase (STEMCELL Technologies). Subsequently, the single cell suspension was strained through a 40-μm strainer to exclude remaining tumour cell aggregates and tissue debris.

Lymph nodes were gently homogenized by straining through a 40-μm strainer.

CD4$^+$ T lymphocyte purification

CD4$^+$ T lymphocytes from PBMC, lymph nodes and tumours were sorted in two steps: (1) pre-sorting of total CD3$^+$ cells was performed using EasySep Human CD3-positive selection kit II (STEMCELL Technologies). CD3$^+$ pre-sorted cells were then stained with anti-human CD4 (PerCp Cy5.5, BioLegend), anti-human CD8 (APC, BD Biosciences), anti-human CD56 (PE, BD Biosciences), anti-human CD45RA (V500, BD Biosciences) and anti-human C45RO (APC CY7 BioLegend). (2) CD4$^+$ cells were FACS-purified according to gating strategy presented in Fig. 1a using a BD FACSARIA I instrument (BD Biosciences). The purity of CD4$^+$ T lymphocytes was confirmed post-sorting and was consistently ≥ 95%. Analysis of flow cytometry data was performed using the FACS Diva software (BD Biosciences) and FlowJo (version 10, FlowJo LLC). Sorted cells were pelleted and stored in − 20 °C until further analysis.

Pyrosequencing of CD4$^+$ lymphocytes

DNA from CD4$^+$ cell pellets were extracted and bisulfite converted using EZ DNA methylation Direct kit (Zymo Research). The locus-specific pyrosequencing PCRs for *FOXP3*, *IFNG IL13* and *IL17A* were conducted using primers where one primer for each PCR reaction was

biotinylated (Thermo Scientific and Biomers.net) (Additional file 1: Table S1). The PCRs were performed using a Thermal cycler (Bio-Rad). The PCR product was immobilized using the PyroMark Q96 vacuum workstation (Qiagen). The sequencing reaction was performed on a Pyro Q96, using Pyromark Gold 96Q reagents (Qiagen) and PCR assay-specific sequencing primers (Additional file 1: Table S1). Analysis of the sequence data were performed by the Pyromark Q96 ID software (Qiagen) giving individual percentage for assayed CpGs. Graphic visualization of the four loci (Fig. 1b) was made using VISTA-point [23]. Histograms demonstrate species conservation between human and mouse, and circles below schematically demonstrate CpG sites in the specific region. The analysed signature CpG site is marked in red with their location, in base pairs, from transcription start site (TSS) indicated.

Cisplatin cultures

CD4$^+$ T lymphocytes were extracted from peripheral blood of healthy donors ($n = 4$) as described above. Cells were put in cultures at a concentration of 1×10^6 cells/ml in GIBCO Aim V™ medium, research grade (Invitrogen) supplemented with L-glutamine (Sigma-Aldrich). Cells were stimulated at day 0 or day 6, with 5 μg/ml plate bound αCD3 (BioLegend) and 2 μg/ml soluble αCD28 (BioLegend). Cisplatin (Hospira, Pfizer) was added on day 0 or day 6 of culture at a concentration of 25 μM (LD$_{50}$ [24], for subsequent ELISA) or 50 μM (for subsequent pyrosequencing). All cultures were incubated at 37 °C in 5% CO$_2$. Cells were harvested at day 12.

5-Methylcytosine ELISA

DNA from cultures exposed to 25 μM cisplatin was extracted using DNeasy blood and tissue kit (Qiagen). DNA quantity and quality were measured on a Nanodrop instrument (ThermoFisher Scientific), and 100 ng DNA/well was utilized to perform ELISA. 5-Methylcytosine (5mC) ELISA was conducted, and each sample was run in duplicate, using 5-mC DNA ELISA kit (ZYMO research) according to the manufacturer's instructions. Sample values were normalized against either day 0 untreated samples or day 12 samples without cisplatin treatment.

Statistical analysis

All statistical analysis was performed using GraphPad PRISM version 7.04. Non-parametric Mann-Whitney test, Kruskal-Wallis test and Friedmans test was used where applicable. Dunn's multiple comparisons test was employed when suitable. Statistical significance in graphs are shown as * if $p < 0.05$, ** if $p < 0.01$, *** if $p < 0.001$ and **** if $p < 0.0001$. Plots show mean with standard error of mean (SEM). No statistical calculations were made on data in Fig. 8a, c, d due to low sample number.

Table 1 Patients included in this study

No.	Age	Gender	Sampling	Clinical T-staging	pT stage	NAC	NAC response	LN	Tumor	Year
1	73	M	T	cTaG2	–	–	–	–	Tumour	2017
2	81	F	T, C	cT3	pT3	–	–	4	Tumour	2017
3	60	F	C	cT2	pTa-pTis	NAC	PR	2	–	2017
4	70	M	T	cTaG3	–	–	–	–	Tumour	2017
5	82	M	T	cT3	–	–	–	–	Tumour	2017
6	73	M	C	cT2	pTa-pTis	–	–	3	Tumour	2017
7	74	M	C	cT2	pT3	NAC	prog.	3	–	2017
8	62	M	C	cT2	pT0	NAC	CR	5	–	2017
9	73	M	C	cT2	pT3	NAC	prog.	4	–	2017
10	57	F	C	cT2	pT0	NAC	CR	9	Tumour	2017
11	70	M	C	cT2	pT1	NAC	PR	2	–	2017
12	68	M	T	cT1	–	–	–	–	Tumour	2017
13	68	M	C	cT2	pT0	NAC	CR	6	–	2017
14	73	M	T	cT2	–	–	–	–	Tumour	2017
15	61	F	T	cTaG2	–	–	–	–	Tumour	2017
16	75	M	C	cT2	pT0	NAC	CR	1	–	2017
17	70	F	T	cTaG2	–	–	–	–	Tumour	2017
18	73	F	T, post Ch	cT3	–	NAC	–	–	Tumour	2017
19	64	F	T, C	cT2	pT2	NAC	NR	4	Tumour	2017
20	71	M	C	cT2	pT2	NAC	NR	7	–	2017
21	77	M	T	cT1	–	–	–	–	Tumour	2017
22	72	M	T, post Ch	cT2	–	NAC	–	–	Tumour	2017
23	61	M	T	cT1 + CIS	–	–	–	–	Tumour	2017
24	68	M	C	cT2	pT0	NAC	CR	2	–	2017
25	79	F	T	cT2	–	–	–	–	Tumour	2017
26	74	M	T	cTaG2	–	–	–	–	Tumour	2017
27	67	M	C	cT2	pTa-pTis	NAC	PR	4	–	2017
28	67	F	T	cT2	–	NAC	–	–	Tumour	2017
29	79	M	T	cT1	–	–	–	–	Tumour	2017
30	84	F	T	Benign	–	–	–	–	Tumour	2017
31	71	M	C	cT2	pT0	NAC	CR	5	–	2017
32	75	M	T	cTaG2	–	–	–	–	Tumour	2017
33	69	F	T, post Ch	cT4a	–	–	–	–	–	2017
34	50	M	T, C post Ch	cT2	pT0	NAC	CR	4	–	2015
35	56	M	C	cT2	pT0	NAC	CR	3	–	2015
36	79	M	C	cT3	pT3	NAC	NR	4	–	2015
37	59	F	T	cT3	–	–	–	–	Tumour	2017
38	80	M	C	cT2	pT0	–	–	4	–	2017
39	60	M	T, C post Ch	cT3	–	NAC	prog.	–	–	2014
40	66	M	T, C post Ch	cT3	–	NAC	CR	–	–	2017

NAC was administered to indicated patients

Age, in years at time of inclusion; gender, *M* male, *F* female; sampling, *T* TUR-B, *C* radical cystectomy, *Ch* during chemo blood (post-chemo); NAC responder, *CR* complete responder, *NR* non-responder, *PR* partial responder, *prog.* progression; *LN*, number of lymph nodes obtained indicated, *Tumour*, specimens acquired from indicated patients. *Year*, years of intervention. –, no data/sample available

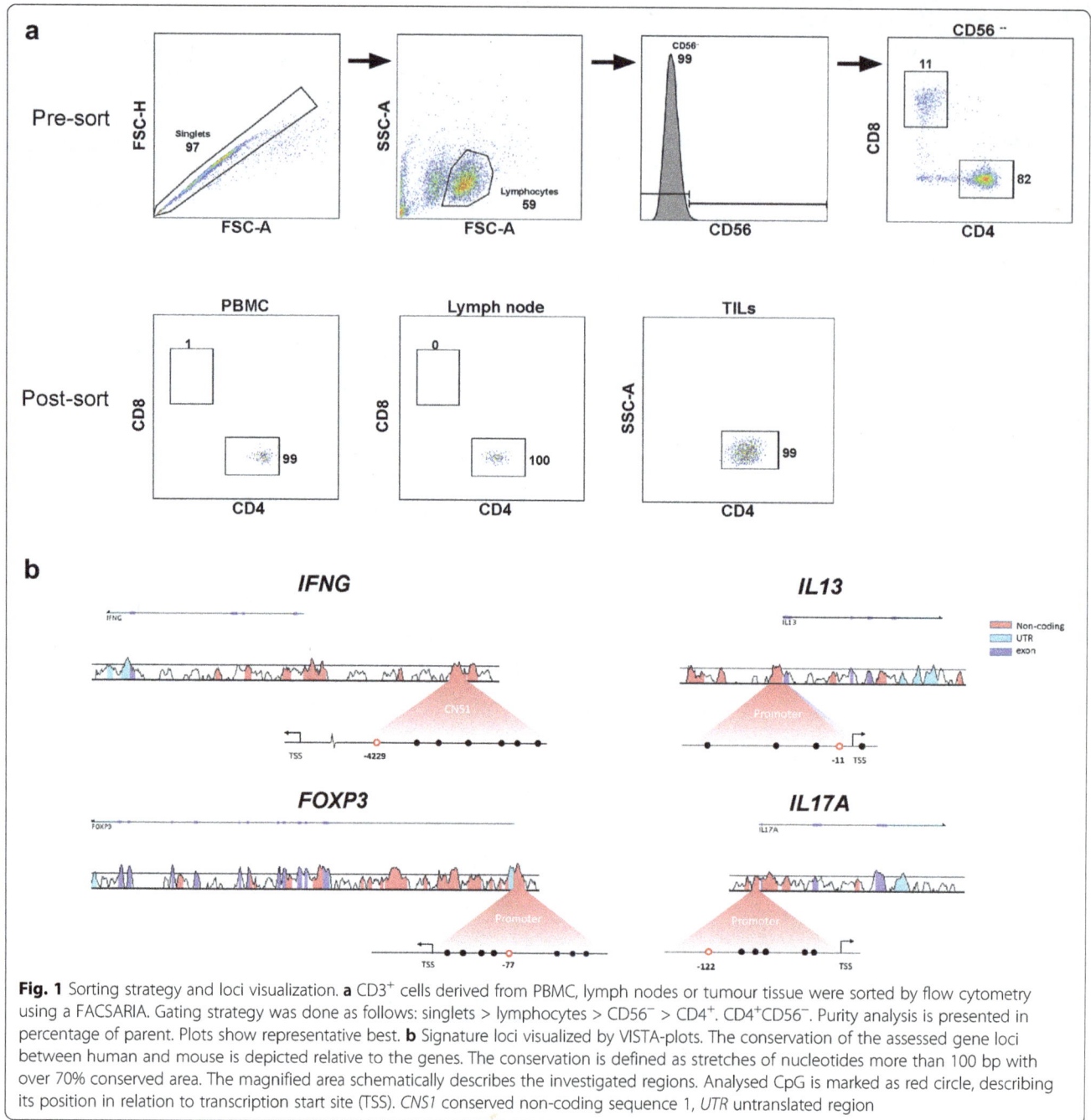

Fig. 1 Sorting strategy and loci visualization. **a** CD3+ cells derived from PBMC, lymph nodes or tumour tissue were sorted by flow cytometry using a FACSARIA. Gating strategy was done as follows: singlets > lymphocytes > CD56− > CD4+. CD4+CD56−. Purity analysis is presented in percentage of parent. Plots show representative best. **b** Signature loci visualized by VISTA-plots. The conservation of the assessed gene loci between human and mouse is depicted relative to the genes. The conservation is defined as stretches of nucleotides more than 100 bp with over 70% conserved area. The magnified area schematically describes the investigated regions. Analysed CpG is marked as red circle, describing its position in relation to transcription start site (TSS). *CNS1* conserved non-coding sequence 1, *UTR* untranslated region

Groups of data were consistently excluded from statistical analysis if $n = < 4$.

Results

Samples from patients with urinary bladder cancer, presented in Table 1, were analysed. Single cell suspensions from PBMC, tumour and lymph nodes were stained and sorted by flow cytometry (Fig. 1a). FACS analysis post-sorting demonstrated ≥ 95% purity (Fig. 1a). DNA was extracted and bisulfite converted for pyrosequencing and assessment of signature CpG sites for analysis of

lineage commitment to the Th1, Th2, Treg and Th17 lineages, using previously identified predictive sites in the corresponding genes *IFNG*, *IL13*, *FOXP3* and *IL17A* (Fig. 1b) [17, 19–21].

Evaluation of CD4+ T cell lineage commitment

The four selected loci were investigated in CD4+ T lymphocytes sorted from PBMCs, LNs and tumours obtained at TUR-B and RC. Comparisons of sentinel and non-sentinel lymph node data demonstrated no significant differences (data not shown), and thus, these specimens were analysed together as a group referred to as "lymph nodes" (LN) throughout the analysis. The *IFNG* locus methylation in the CpG position -4229 bp from transcription start site (TSS) (located in the conserved non-coding sequence 1 (CNS1)) (Fig. 1b) was used to assess the Th1-committed CD4+ T cells [20]. CD4+ T cells from TILs were significantly more demethylated in the *IFNG* locus compared to LN ($p < 0.0001$), whereas the methylation in LNs were higher compared to PBMC, suggesting an increased infiltration of Th1 IFN-γ producing CD4+ T cells into the tumour (Fig. 2a). With regard to Th2-committed CD4+ T cells, the *IL13* locus was evaluated at the signature CpG position -11 bp from TSS as previously demonstrated [21] (Fig. 1b). Again, we found a significantly decreased level of methylation in the *IL13* locus in TILs compared to lymph nodes ($p < 0.05$) (Fig. 2b). However, there were no significant changes when comparing CD4+ T cells derived from TILs with those from PBMCs. Interestingly, CD4+ T cells from LN demonstrated significantly increased methylation in the *IL13* locus compared with both PBMC ($p < 0.05$) and TILs ($p < 0.05$). CD4+ Tregs were assessed at the CpG -77 bp from TSS (Fig. 1b) in the *FOXP3* locus as previously described [17]. This signature CpG was significantly hypomethylated in CD4+ T cells from lymph nodes ($p < 0.05$)

and tumours ($p < 0.01$) compared to PBMC (Fig. 2c). Finally, Th17 cells were investigated at the *IL17A* signature locus at the CpG -122 bp from TSS (Fig. 1b) [19]. CD4+ T cells from tumours demonstrated significantly decreased methylation compared to LN ($p < 0.05$) and PBMCs ($p < 0.0001$) (Fig. 2d). No significant difference was seen when comparing CD4+ T cells from PBMC derived from either TUR-B or RC, rationalizing the equivalence between the samples obtained at the two time points (Additional file 2: Figure S2).

Analysis of lineage commitment at the time of TUR-B

Patient materials obtained at the time of TUR-B were analysed separately. CD4+ T cells purified from fresh TUR-B tumour resections did not demonstrate any difference in methylation profile in the *IFNG* locus compared to PBMCs ($p > 0.05$) (Fig. 3a). Neither was there any difference in the degree of methylation in the *IL13* locus (Fig. 3b). With regard to Tregs, the *FOXP3* signature locus was significantly demethylated in CD4+ T cells from the tumour compared to PBMCs ($p < 0.001$) (Fig. 3c). Finally, we found a decreased methylation of the *IL17A* locus in CD4+ T cells in the tumour compared to PBMCs ($p < 0.01$) (Fig. 3d). One patient (no.

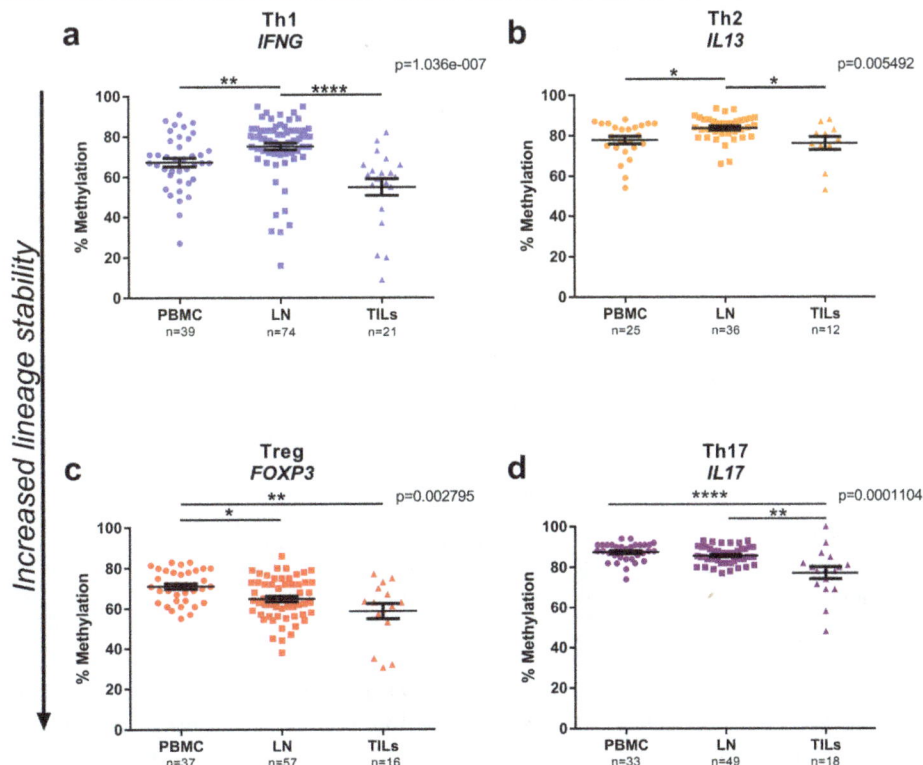

Fig. 2 CD4+ T cell lineage commitment in urinary bladder cancer. CD4+ T cells sorted from PBMC, LN and TILs were analysed by pyrosequencing at CD4+ T cell signature loci: **a** *IFNG* for Th1, **b** *IL13* for Th2, **c** *FOXP3* for Treg and **d** *IL17A* for Th17. *p* values stated in graphs are generated from Kruskal-Wallis test. *p* values from Dunn's multiple comparisons test are indicated as *$p < 0.05$, **$p < 0.01$, ***$p < 0.001$ and ****$p < 0.0001$. Plots show percentage of methylation for every specimen analysed (*n* stated on *x*-axis beneath sample type). Bars indicate mean with error bars displaying SEM. Downward arrow along *y*-axis illustrate increased lineage commitment, as a result of decreased methylation

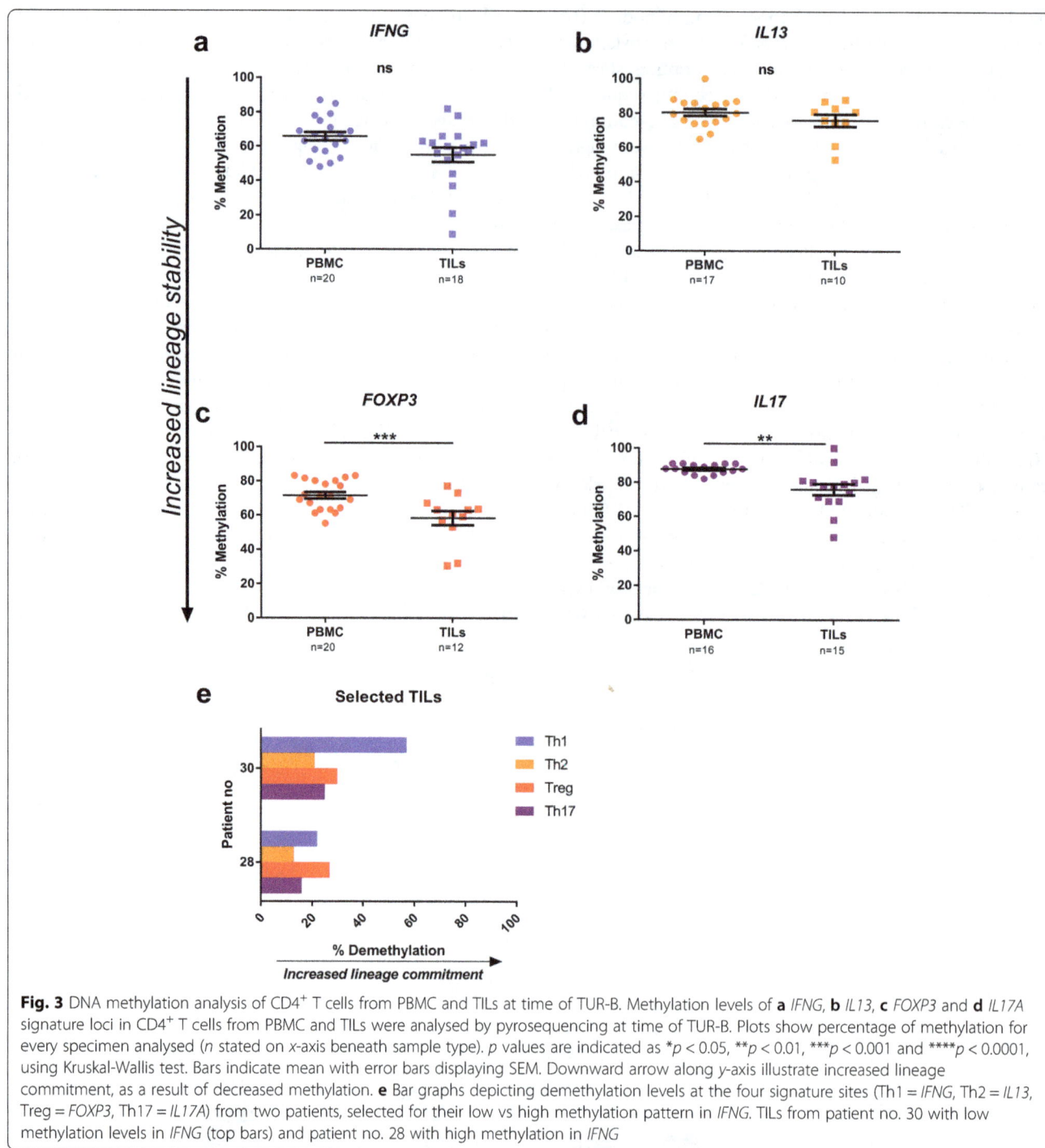

Fig. 3 DNA methylation analysis of CD4[+] T cells from PBMC and TILs at time of TUR-B. Methylation levels of **a** *IFNG*, **b** *IL13*, **c** *FOXP3* and **d** *IL17A* signature loci in CD4[+] T cells from PBMC and TILs were analysed by pyrosequencing at time of TUR-B. Plots show percentage of methylation for every specimen analysed (*n* stated on *x*-axis beneath sample type). *p* values are indicated as *$p < 0.05$, **$p < 0.01$, ***$p < 0.001$ and ****$p < 0.0001$, using Kruskal-Wallis test. Bars indicate mean with error bars displaying SEM. Downward arrow along *y*-axis illustrate increased lineage commitment, as a result of decreased methylation. **e** Bar graphs depicting demethylation levels at the four signature sites (Th1 = *IFNG*, Th2 = *IL13*, Treg = *FOXP3*, Th17 = *IL17A*) from two patients, selected for their low vs high methylation pattern in *IFNG*. TILs from patient no. 30 with low methylation levels in *IFNG* (top bars) and patient no. 28 with high methylation in *IFNG*

30), included at TUR-B had benign disease and was hence not included in the general data analysis. We examined the TILs from this patient and found the *IFNG* locus to be highly demethylated, whereas the three other loci were hypermethylated, suggesting a Th1 lineage commitment (Fig. 3e, top bars). For comparison, we examined TILs from a patient (no. 28) with hypermethylation at the *IFNG* locus (Fig. 3e bottom bars). This patient (cT stage

cT2a) displayed hypermethylation in all four loci, corresponding to an overall low lineage differentiation.

Analysis of lineage commitment at the time of cystectomy

CD4[+] T cells derived from samples obtained at the time of RC were analysed at the four signature loci. In LN, the methylation at the *IFNG* locus was significantly increased, compared to the corresponding cells from PBMC ($p < 0.05$) (Fig. 4a). Similarly, the level of methylation was increased at the *IL13* locus in lymph nodes compared to blood ($p < 0.05$) (Fig. 4b). No differences were seen in the methylation levels of *FOXP3* or *IL17A* loci between CD4+ T cells derived from PBMC and LN (Fig. 4c, d).

CD4+ T cells from five lymph nodes (indicated by red circles in Fig. 5a) were selected for their high (Fig. 5b) or low (Fig. 5c) methylation profiles at the *IFNG* locus and were individually investigated for all four signature loci. The two specimens with low methylation at the *IFNG* locus also demonstrated a demethylated pattern in the Treg locus, while no signs of Th2 and Th17 skewing were found: i.e. *IL13* and *IL17A* signature loci were almost completely methylated (Fig. 5c, patient no. 6 and 24). On the contrary, the samples demonstrating a high methylation pattern in the *IFNG* locus displayed more of a Treg/Th2 or Treg/Th17 commitment judged by the methylation profiles in signature loci (Fig. 5b, patient no. 7 and 2). One LN revealed low commitment for all four loci compared to the other four LNs investigated (Fig. 5b,

patient no. 20). The patients with LNs displaying low *IFNG* methylation, and therefore a Th1 signature, had a lower pathological tumour staging (pT stage), pTa-TisN1 (patient 6) and pT0 (patient 24) (Fig. 5c), although the former had a node metastasis (not included in specimens). The patients with LNs highly methylated at the *IFNG* locus had a more advanced disease stage, pT3aN2, pT3a and pT2a, respectively (patient, 7, 2 and 20) (Fig. 5b).

In order to epigenetically stage the collective immune response in a single patient (no. 6), the CD4+ T cell compartment in three individual LNs were analysed (Fig. 5d). LN1 demonstrated a Th1/Treg pattern, whereas the other two LNs (2 and 3) displayed different degrees of Treg/Th17 skewing, although still with a fraction of Th1commitment (Fig. 5d).

CD4+ T cells from LN are differentially committed when stratified over pT stage

The pT stage determined by histopathology following cystectomy is known to predict prognosis and to function as a surrogate marker for overall survival in MIBC patients undergoing NAC [25]. Complete response (CR), i.e.

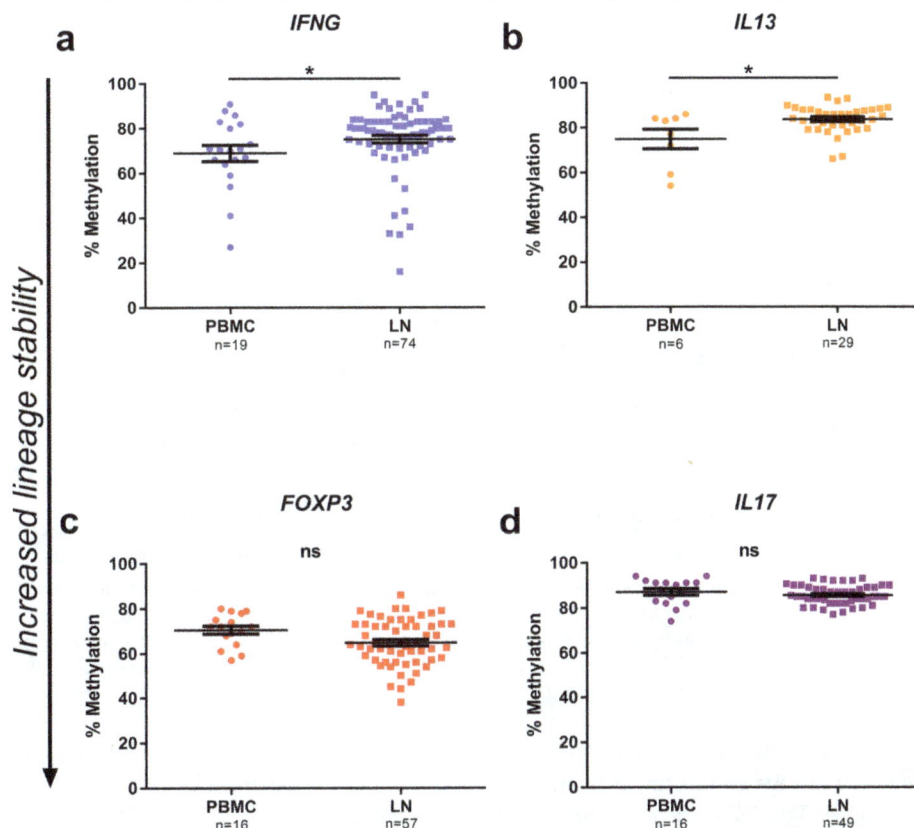

Fig. 4 Methylation analysis in specimens from radical cystectomy (RC). Methylation percentage in CD4+ T cells from PBMC and lymph nodes retrieved at time of RC. *IFNG* (**a**), *IL13* (**b**), *FOXP3* (**c**) and *IL17A* (**d**) were analysed. Plots show percentage of methylation for every specimen analysed (*n* stated on *x*-axis beneath sample type). *p* values are indicated as *$p < 0.05$, **$p < 0.01$, ***$p < 0.001$ and ****$p < 0.0001$, using Mann-Whitney test. Bars indicate mean with error bars displaying SEM. Downward arrow along *y*-axis illustrate increased lineage commitment, as a result of decreased methylation

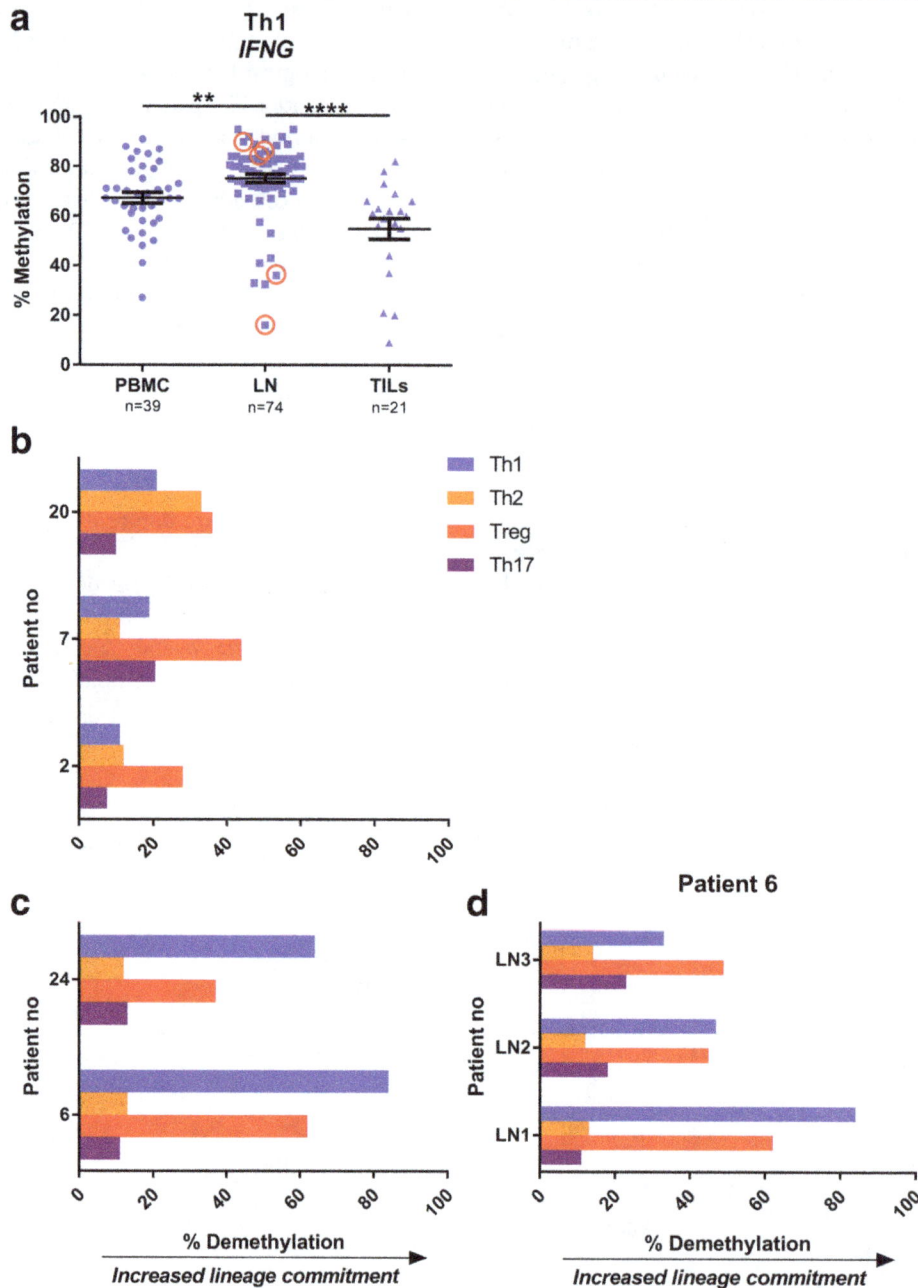

Fig. 5 Case studies of lymph nodes with low or high methylation in *IFNG* locus. **a** Same as Fig. 2a, with evaluated lymph nodes circled in red. **b–d** Bar graphs depicts percentage of demethylation levels at the four signature sites, representing increase in lineage commitment. Th1 = *IFNG*, Th2 = *IL13*, Treg = *FOXP3*, Th17 = *IL17A*. **b** LN from three patients with high *IFNG* methylation. **c** LNs from two patients with low *IFNG* methylation patterns. **d** Case study of three LNs from patient no. 6, chosen for a distinct *IFNG* demethylation in one node (from Fig. 5c, lower bars)

pT0N0M0 at RC, corresponds to an excellent long-term survival. We evaluated the lineage commitment in the four loci according to pT staging. The *IFNG* locus demonstrated a demethylated pattern in the primary tumours (at TUR-B) of pT0 patients (complete NAC-responders) and in non-invasive tumours (pTa-Tis) compared to in primary tumours with muscle invasive tumour outcomes post-RC (pT2) ($p < 0.0001$ resp. $p < 0.001$) (Fig. 6a). The methylation

was decreased in the perivesical infiltrating tumours (pT3) compared to the muscle invasive pT2 tumours ($p < 0.05$). In the *IL13* locus, the CD4$^+$ T cells demonstrated an increased methylation in muscle invasive pT2 tumours compared to the cells from patients with pT0 stage (Fig. 6b). Methylation levels at the *FOXP3* locus was increased in LN CD4$^+$ T cells from patient with muscle invasive pT2 compared to both non-muscle invasive pTa-Tis staged patients

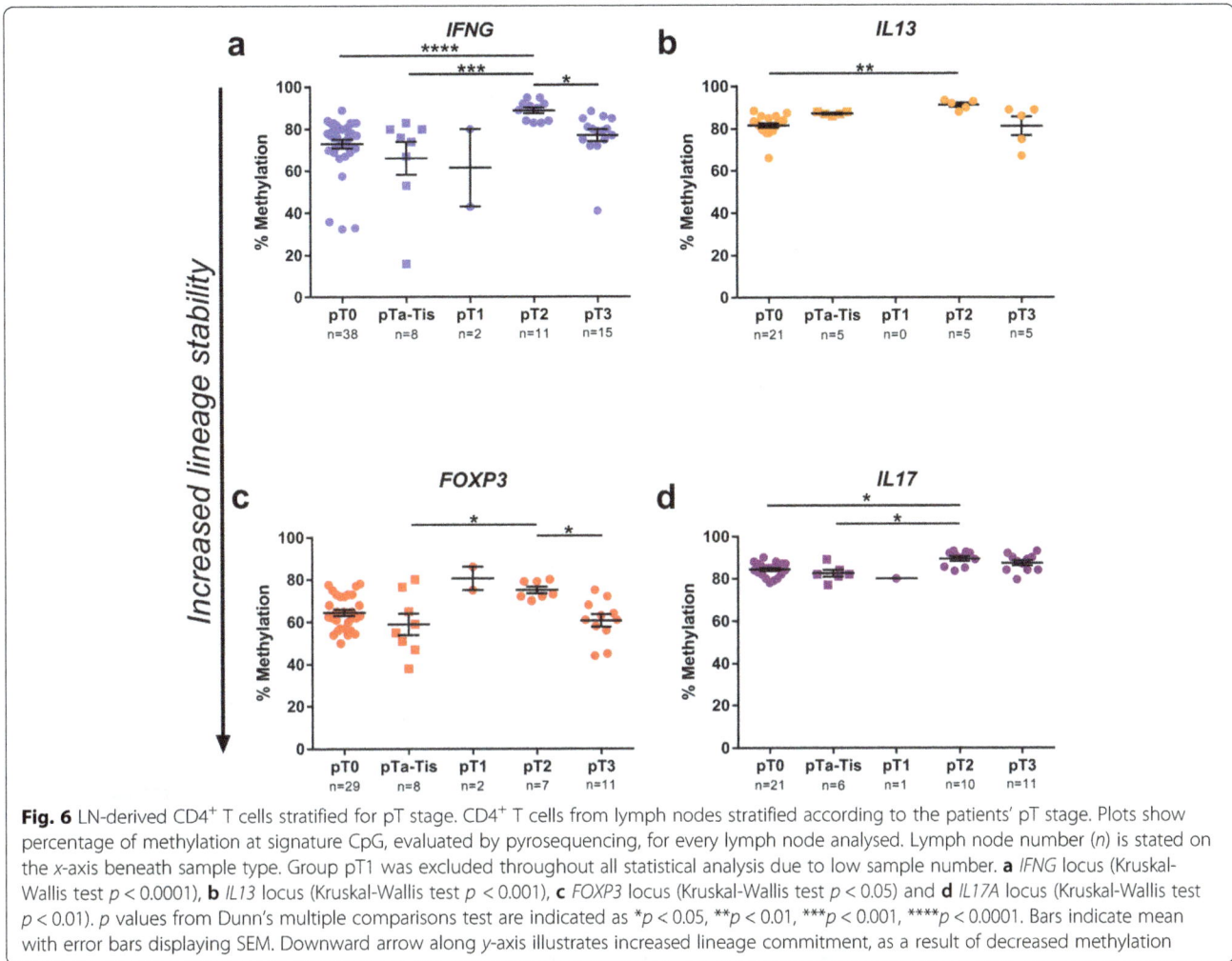

Fig. 6 LN-derived CD4$^+$ T cells stratified for pT stage. CD4$^+$ T cells from lymph nodes stratified according to the patients' pT stage. Plots show percentage of methylation at signature CpG, evaluated by pyrosequencing, for every lymph node analysed. Lymph node number (n) is stated on the x-axis beneath sample type. Group pT1 was excluded throughout all statistical analysis due to low sample number. **a** *IFNG* locus (Kruskal-Wallis test $p < 0.0001$), **b** *IL13* locus (Kruskal-Wallis test $p < 0.001$), **c** *FOXP3* locus (Kruskal-Wallis test $p < 0.05$) and **d** *IL17A* locus (Kruskal-Wallis test $p < 0.01$). p values from Dunn's multiple comparisons test are indicated as *$p < 0.05$, **$p < 0.01$, ***$p < 0.001$, ****$p < 0.0001$. Bars indicate mean with error bars displaying SEM. Downward arrow along y-axis illustrates increased lineage commitment, as a result of decreased methylation

and to the cells from patients with perivesical infiltrating tumours (pT3) ($p < 0.05$ for both) (Fig. 6c). In *IL17A*, the methylation was increased in LN-derived CD4$^+$ T cells from patients staged with pT2 compared to the pT0 as well as non-muscle invasive pTa-Tis staged patients ($p < 0.05$ for both) (Fig. 6d).

Methylation patterns in lymph nodes correspond with response to neoadjuvant chemotherapy

Patients were stratified according to their clinical response to NAC, and LN-derived CD4$^+$ T cells from patients with complete response (CR; pT0N0M0) and those with no response (NR; pT ≥ 2N0M0) were compared. Methylation was significantly lower in the group with CR compared to those with NR in all four loci, with the most pronounced difference in the *IFNG* locus (*IFNG* $p < 0.0001$, *IL13* $p < 0.0001$, *FOXP3* $p < 0.01$, *IL17A* $p < 0.001$) (Fig. 7a–d). When stratifying PBMC or LN samples according to their corresponding clinical T

stage, it revealed no significant differences (data not shown).

Th1 lineage affected during NAC treatment

Patients with MIBC, and in WHO class 0–1 health condition, are according to the national Swedish guidelines recommended to receive 3–4 cycles of cisplatin-based NAC prior to RC. Blood samples were obtained after first or second cycle of NAC therapy and CD4$^+$ T cells from PBMCs were extracted. Analysis of *IFNG* locus methylation at TUR-B, during NAC and at the time of RC demonstrated a temporary increase in the methylation status ($n = 3$) during NAC treatment (Fig. 8a). When comparing PBMC derived CD4$^+$ T lymphocytes from TUR-B with corresponding cells obtained during chemotherapy for an additional three patients, we found a tendency to increase methylation in the *IFNG* locus, however not significant (Fig. 8b). Interestingly, when investigating the *FOXP3* and *IL17A* loci at the same time

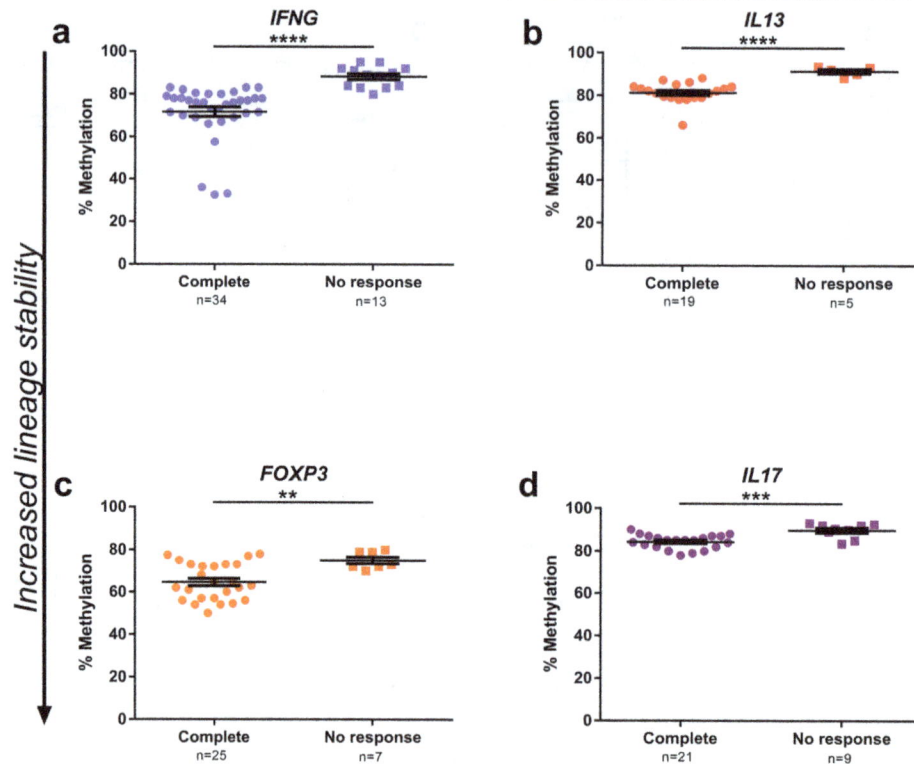

Fig. 7 Lymph nodes grouped according to NAC response. CD4⁺ T cells from lymph nodes sorted according to the patients' responses to neoadjuvant chemotherapy (NAC); complete response (CR; pT0N0M0) or no response (NR; pT2 or higher N0M0) Plots show percentage of methylation at signature CpG, evaluated by pyrosequencing, for every lymph node analysed. Lymph node number (n) stated on x-axis beneath sample type. **a** *IFNG* (number of patients: CR $n = 8$, NR $n = 3$). **b** *IL13* (number of patients: CR $n = 4$, NR $n = 2$). **c** *FOXP3* (number of patients: CR $n = 6$, NR $n = 2$). **d** *IL17A* (number of patients: *IL17A* CR $n = 6$ NR $n = 2$). Mann-Whitney test was used for the statistical analysis. p values are indicated as *$p < 0.05$, **$p < 0.01$, ***$p < 0.001$ and ****$p < 0.0001$. Bars indicate mean with error bars displaying SEM

points, no change in methylation status was noted (Fig. 8c, d). To investigate if the change in the *IFNG* locus methylation signature was altered due to a recruitment of naïve T cells into the circulation, we calculated the ratio between naïve CD45RA⁺CD45RO⁻ and memory CD45RO⁺ T cells. We found no significant difference in the CD45RA/CD45RO ratio or in the fraction of CD45RA single positive cells between TUR-B and cystectomy (after NAC) samples (Fig. 8e, f), suggesting that the hypermethylation of the *IFNG* locus is not due to an increased inflow of naïve CD4⁺ T cells into the circulation (Fig. 8a).

Cisplatin does not affect the DNA methylation

Cisplatin is the base of the neoadjuvant treatment, acting partly through cross binding of DNA (purine bases) [26, 27]. To investigate the possibility that cisplatin affects DNA methylation, in vitro cultures were established using CD4⁺ T lymphocytes from healthy donors ($n = 4$). 5mC ELISA showed no significant difference in the global methylation of cells treated with cisplatin (Additional file 3: Figure S1a). In addition, pyrosequencing of the *IFNG* locus revealed no significant

difference in the site-specific methylation (Additional file 3: Figure S1b).

Discussion

We here demonstrate that valuable information can be obtained by studying signature CpG methylation, indicating the degree of lineage commitment of CD4⁺ T cells in tissues from UBC patients. CD4⁺ T cell lineage commitment was found to be more pronounced in tumour-infiltrating lymphocytes (TILs) compared to PBMC and regional lymph nodes, indicating that differences in the tissue environments have a significant impact on CD4⁺ T cell destiny. In addition, we found correlations between increased lineage commitment of CD4⁺ T cells in LNs after neoadjuvant chemotherapy and an improved prognosis, indicating an important role for T cell immunity in the evolution of UBC towards more aggressive forms. To the best of our knowledge, this is the first time DNA methylation of CD4⁺ T cell lineage markers has been investigated in cells harvested from patients with UBC, and our data suggests that this type of investigation can contribute towards a deeper understanding of the role of the immune system in the UBC setting.

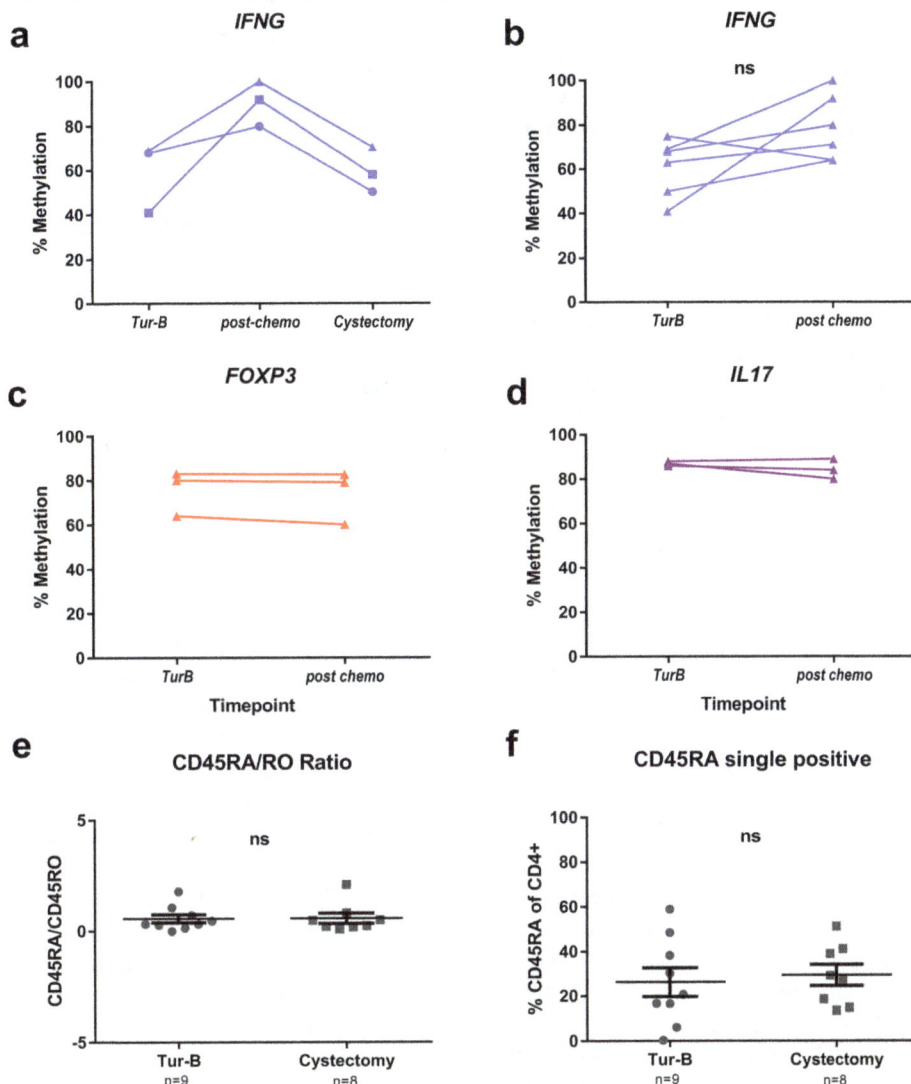

Fig. 8 Investigation of sample retrieved during NAC treatment. **a** Examination of *IFNG* locus in CD4$^+$ T cells from blood of three patients, taken at three time points: before (TUR-B), during (post-chemo) and after (cystectomy) neoadjuvant chemotherapy. **b** Methylation pattern in *IFNG* locus in paired samples from two time points, before (TUR-B) and during (post-chemo) NAC treatment ($n = 6$). Wilcoxon test was used for statistical analysis. **c** Methylation pattern in *FOXP3* locus in paired samples from two time points, before (TUR-B) and during (post-chemo) NAC treatment ($n = 3$). **d** Methylation pattern in *IL17A* locus in paired samples from two time points, before (TUR-B) and during (post-chemo) NAC treatment ($n = 3$). **e** CD45RA/RO protein expression ratio in PBMC derived CD4$^+$ T cells from TUR-B or cystectomy, as evaluated by flow cytometry. **f** Percentage of CD45RA$^+$ CD45RO$^-$ (single positive) CD4$^+$ T cells, determined by flow cytometry, at the two time points TUR-B and RC. **e**, **f** (n stated on x-axis beneath sample type) Bars show SEM

As a method, methylation analysis has advantages when compared to analysis of protein and mRNA expression. No stimulation of the cells is required in order to analyse the current methylation status; and thus, resting unmanipulated cells can be analysed for phenotype stability, with no risk of misinterpreting temporary, transient protein expression for stable effector lineages. This is a clear advantage when examining primary cells from clinical specimens since no tampering of the cells is needed. However, epigenetic status does not convey if the cells are active or resting, but rather indicate lineage commitment and effector capacity of the cells upon activation.

We demonstrate that TILs have a high degree of CD4$^+$ T cells with lineage commitment (Fig. 2), proposing an active immune response towards the tumour. The *IFNG*-committed Th1 compartment is the most prominent of the four T cell lineages examined here, indicating that Th1 is the major lineage response towards the tumour, which is in agreement with the literature [28]. Furthermore, the methylation pattern in the *IFNG* locus has the greatest variability, compared to the other three loci, in all investigated tissues, which we interpret as both intra- and inter-patient variation (Fig. 2). The Treg compartment was the only lineage with a gradual decrease in methylation, with the highest methylation in blood, through lymph nodes to the lowest methylation in tumour. This could be interpreted as an effect of the immune-stimulatory environment, where high proliferation rate leads to an increase in the Treg population [6]. In our patient samples, we assumed that a prolonged immune response towards the tumour would be present, and this seemed to lead to a co-commitment of several stable lineages, mainly Th1 and Tregs (Figs. 3 and 5b, c). It becomes evident, when individually examining the four lineages in separate samples, that the specimens low in *IFNG* methylation had a clear Th1/Treg profile in both TILs and LN (Figs. 3e top bars and 5c), whereas the highly methylated specimens inclined more towards a Th2 or Th17 profile (Figs. 3e bottom bars and 5b), or an overall low lineage commitment pattern (Fig. 5b, patient 2). Noteworthy, the specimen with the most prominent demethylation in *IFNG* locus had a benign tumour, suggesting a protective IFN-γ response limiting the progress of the tumour (Fig. 3c top bars).

When separating the material according to the two time points of intervention (TUR-B and RC), the CD4$^+$ T cells were found to display a higher degree of lineage commitment in TILs from the TUR-B (Fig. 3) compared to those from blood, while the LN CD4$^+$ T cells at the time of cystectomy showed less lineage commitment or no difference compared to their blood counterparts (Fig. 4). We suggest that this is due to the selective migration of activated T cells away from the LN towards the tumour.

Stratifying CD4$^+$ T cells from LNs according to the patients' pT stage revealed differences in methylation state relating to local tumour responses to NAC, which is correlated with disease progression. The level of committed hypomethylated CD4$^+$ T cells were increased in patients with low, non-muscle invasive pT stages as compared to those from patients with muscle invasive pT2 tumours (Fig. 6), which was most prominent in Th1 cells. These data suggest that an increase in committed Th1 effector cells in the tumour region is favourable for prognosis. Surprisingly, both Th1 and Treg commitment is increased in pT3, when the tumours have progressed to perivesical infiltration (a clear sign of a lack of response to NAC), perhaps suggesting that the balance between regulation and effector function has switched in the environment of more aggressive tumour cells.

The response to NAC in terms of histopathological tumour regression is a major positive prognostic factor for overall survival following radical cystectomy [25, 29]. Therefore, it was striking that the lineage commitment in LNs from patients with CR after NAC was significantly

higher than in those not responding as favourably (Fig. 7). Our group has also previously demonstrated that cisplatin-based NAC induces immune-stimulatory effects [24, 30] and the present findings are in line with that context.

The lack of paired patient samples from TUR-B and RC prevented us from investigating the methylation pattern in pre-treatment TILs from the patients who received NAC and correlate to subsequent NAC response in corresponding LNs. Instead, we examined the methylation pattern in paired blood samples, obtained during the course of NAC treatment. During the NAC treatment (post-chemo), PBMC-derived CD4$^+$ T cells demonstrated a tendency towards increased methylation in the *IFNG* locus (Fig. 8a, b) compared to paired blood samples acquired before NAC (at time of TUR-B) as well as after NAC (at time of RC). There was no indication of changes in *FOXP3*, *IL17A* or *IL13* methylation between these time points (Figs. 7c and 8d, data not shown). We further establish that the changes in DNA methylation are not a direct effect of cisplatin, by performing both a whole genome 5mC ELISA to ensure that this agent does not affect methylation on a global level, and an *IFNG* locus-specific analysis, for comparison with our data (Additional file 3: Figure S1). Since the CD45RA/CD45RO ratio between the two occasions of TUR-B and RC was not changed (Fig. 7e, f), we propose that the temporary increase of methylation in the *IFNG* locus is not due to the recruitment of naïve cells, but rather to the migration/relocation specifically of Th1 lineage-committed T cells towards the tumour environment. This hypothesis is also supported by the lack of effect on the other lineages (Fig. 7c, d, *IL13* data not shown). It has been demonstrated in various cancers that the tumour microenvironment expresses CXCL10 (IP-10), which leads to Th1-specific recruitment to the site mediated by the CXCL10 receptor CXCR3 expressed on Th1 cells. [31–33]. Thus, the changes in the proportion of Th1 cells specifically in different compartments may be based on their unique ability for tumour infiltration.

Our data indicates that NAC plays a role in activating and steering the immune system towards the tumour. It is tempting to speculate that patients with hypomethylation in the *IFNG* locus have better prognosis than those with hypermethylation. The short period of time from sample collection until present day prevents us from evaluating clinical parameters such as 5-year survival and relapse rates. However, histopathological response to NAC is a positive predictor of survival and, although a cause-and-effect relationship cannot be established, the data suggests that increased proportions of committed CD4$^+$ T cells in the tumour regional lymph nodes after NAC translates into a better outcome. Further characterization of the immune response during NAC treatment and a longer follow-up is needed to fully comprehend the significance of this interaction.

Conclusion

We found that patients with complete response to NAC treatment (CR) were hypomethylated in predictive CpG sites of CD4$^+$ T cell signature loci. In addition, hypomethylation of signature effector CD4$^+$ T cell loci were correlated with lower post-cystectomy tumour stage and overall better outcome, suggesting epigenetic staging of immune responses to be useful for clinical evaluation.

Abbreviations

CD4: Cluster of differentiation 4; CR: Complete response; FOXP3: Forkhead box P3; IFNG: Interferon gamma; IL13: Interleukin 13; IL17A: Interleukin 17A; LN: Lymph node; MIBC: Muscle invasive bladder cancer; NAC: Neoadjuvant chemotherapy; PBMC: Peripheral blood mononuclear cells; RC: Radical cystectomy; Th: T helper cell; TIL: Tumour-infiltrating lymphocyte; Treg: T regulatory cell; TUR-B: Transurethral resection of the bladder; UBC: Urinary bladder cancer

Acknowledgements

Research nurses Britt-Inger Dahlin and Kerstin Almroth (Department of Surgical and Perioperative Sciences, Urology and Andrology, Umeå University) were of great assistance in the work.

Funding

This paper was supported by the Swedish Cancer foundation, the Wallenberg foundation, the Swedish Medical Research Council, Regionala forskningsrådet i Uppsala-Örebroregionen (RFR in Uppsala-Örebro), the Swedish Research Council funding for clinical research in medicine (ALF) in Västerbotten, VLL, Sweden, the Cancer Research Foundation in Norrland, Umeå, Sweden, Stiftelsen Emil Anderssons fond för medicinsk forskning, Sundsvall, Sweden.

Authors' contributions

EAB designed and executed all the research and data analysis and wrote this article. CAH processed the clinical samples and contributed to the cell sorting, writing and making of the figures of this paper. MJ, BH, KP, JH, FA, YH, FA and KR evaluated, informed and included patients, collected and prepared clinical samples, and contributed with clinical information. KR also

had a senior responsibility for the protocol pertaining to technetium processing in sentinel node detection. LBL was involved in the original design of the method. MH evaluated the statistical analysis. SB, CL, MEW, DK and AAZ helped in the processing of the clinical material. SB and PM were involved in the clinical interpretations and writing of this paper. LKS oversaw the epigenetic methods and wrote the paper. AS compiled all the clinical data. AS and OW were the principal investigators of this research and major contributors of the writing of this article. All authors read and approved the final manuscript.

Competing interests

The authors declare that they have no competing interests.

Author details

[1]Unit of Immunology and Allergy, Department of Medicine Solna, Karolinska Institutet, Karolinska University Hospital, Stockholm, Sweden. [2]Department of Urology, Sundsvall Hospital, Sundsvall, Sweden. [3]Department of surgical and perioperative Sciences, Urology and Andrology, Umeå University, Umeå, Sweden. [4]TLA Targeted Immunotherapies AB, Stockholm, Sweden. [5]Department of Urology, Akademiska University Hospital, Uppsala, Sweden. [6]Department of Surgery, Urology Section, Östersund County Hospital, Östersund, Sweden. [7]Centre for Research and Development, Faculty of Medicine, Uppsala University, County Council of Gävleborg, Uppsala, Sweden. [8]Department of Urology, Västmanland Hospital, Västerås, Sweden. [9]Department of Clinical and Experimental Medicine, Division of Urology, Linköping University, Linköping, Sweden. [10]Department of Radiation Sciences, Diagnostic Radiology, Umeå University, Umeå, Sweden. [11]Center for Molecular Medicine, Department of Clinical Neuroscience, Karolinska Institutet, Stockholm, Sweden.

References

1. Malats N, Real FX. Epidemiology of bladder cancer. Hematol Oncol Clin North Am. 2015;29(2):177–89, vii.
2. Torre LA, et al. Global cancer statistics, 2012. CA Cancer J Clin. 2015;65(2):87–108.
3. Burger M, et al. Epidemiology and risk factors of urothelial bladder cancer. Eur Urol. 2013;63(2):234–41.
4. Murta-Nascimento C, et al. Epidemiology of urinary bladder cancer: from tumor development to patient's death. World J Urol. 2007;25(3):285–95.
5. Kawai K, et al. Bacillus Calmette-Guerin (BCG) immunotherapy for bladder cancer: current understanding and perspectives on engineered BCG vaccine. Cancer Sci. 2013;104(1):22–7.
6. Winerdal ME, et al. FOXP3 and survival in urinary bladder cancer. BJU Int. 2011;108(10):1672–8.
7. Marits P, et al. Sentinel node lymphocytes: tumour reactive lymphocytes identified intraoperatively for the use in immunotherapy of colon cancer. Br J Cancer. 2006;94(10):1478–84.
8. Marits P, et al. Detection of immune responses against urinary bladder cancer in sentinel lymph nodes. Eur Urol. 2006;49(1):59–70.
9. Starr TK, Jameson SC, Hogquist KA. Positive and negative selection of T cells. Annu Rev Immunol. 2003;21:139–76.
10. Zhu J, Yamane H, Paul WE. Differentiation of effector CD4 T cell populations (*). Annu Rev Immunol. 2010;28:445–89.
11. Murphy E, et al. Reversibility of T helper 1 and 2 populations is lost after long-term stimulation. J Exp Med. 1996;183(3):901–13.
12. Sornasse T, et al. Differentiation and stability of T helper 1 and 2 cells derived from naive human neonatal CD4+ T cells, analyzed at the single-cell level. J Exp Med. 1996;184(2):473–83.

13. Ahmadzadeh M, Farber DL. Functional plasticity of an antigen-specific memory CD4 T cell population. Proc Natl Acad Sci U S A. 2002;99(18):11802–7.

14. Sundrud MS, et al. Genetic reprogramming of primary human T cells reveals functional plasticity in Th cell differentiation. J Immunol. 2003;171(7):3542–9.

15. Murphy KM, Stockinger B. Effector T cell plasticity: flexibility in the face of changing circumstances. Nat Immunol. 2010;11(8):674–80.

16. Baron U, et al. DNA demethylation in the human FOXP3 locus discriminates regulatory T cells from activated FOXP3(+) conventional T cells. Eur J Immunol. 2007;37(9):2378–89.

17. Janson PC, et al. FOXP3 promoter demethylation reveals the committed Treg population in humans. PLoS One. 2008;3(2):e1612.

18. Lee GR, et al. T helper cell differentiation: regulation by cis elements and epigenetics. Immunity. 2006;24(4):369–79.

19. Janson PC, et al. Profiling of CD4+ T cells with epigenetic immune lineage analysis. J Immunol. 2011;186(1):92–102.

20. Janson PC, et al. CpG methylation of the IFNG gene as a mechanism to induce immunosuppression [correction of immunosupression] in tumor-infiltrating lymphocytes. J Immunol. 2008;181(4):2878–86.

21. Santangelo S, et al. DNA methylation changes at human Th2 cytokine genes coincide with DNase I hypersensitive site formation during CD4(+) T cell differentiation. J Immunol. 2002;169(4):1893–903.

22. Sherif A, et al. Lymphatic mapping and detection of sentinel nodes in patients with bladder cancer. J Urol. 2001;166(3):812–5.

23. Mayor C, et al. VISTA : visualizing global DNA sequence alignments of arbitrary length. Bioinformatics. 2000;16(11):1046–7.

24. Hu J, et al. The effects of chemotherapeutic drugs on human monocyte-derived dendritic cell differentiation and antigen presentation. Clin Exp Immunol. 2013;172(3):490–9.

25. Rosenblatt R, et al. Pathologic downstaging is a surrogate marker for efficacy and increased survival following neoadjuvant chemotherapy and radical cystectomy for muscle-invasive urothelial bladder cancer. Eur Urol. 2012;61(6):1229–38.

26. Pinto AL, Lippard SJ. Binding of the antitumor drug cis-diamminedichloroplatinum(II) (cisplatin) to DNA. Biochim Biophys Acta. 1985;780(3):167–80.

27. Eastman A. The formation, isolation and characterization of DNA adducts produced by anticancer platinum complexes. Pharmacol Ther. 1987;34(2):155–66.

28. Nishimura T, et al. The critical role of Th1-dominant immunity in tumor immunology. Cancer Chemother Pharmacol. 2000;46(Suppl):S52–61.

29. Witjes JA, et al. EAU guidelines on muscle-invasive and metastatic bladder cancer: summary of the 2013 guidelines. Eur Urol. 2014;65(4):778–92.

30. Zirakzadeh AA, et al. Doxorubicin enhances the capacity of B cells to activate T cells in urothelial urinary bladder cancer. Clin Immunol. 2017;176:63–70.

31. Sgadari C, et al. Interferon-inducible protein-10 identified as a mediator of tumor necrosis in vivo. Proc Natl Acad Sci U S A. 1996;93(24):13791–6.

32. Liu M, Guo S, Stiles JK. The emerging role of CXCL10 in cancer (Review). Oncol Lett. 2011;2(4):583–9.

33. Jiang Z, Xu Y, Cai S. CXCL10 expression and prognostic significance in stage II and III colorectal cancer. Mol Biol Rep. 2010;37(6):3029–36.

9

Multiomics analyses identified epigenetic modulation of the S100A gene family in Kawasaki disease and their significant involvement in neutrophil transendothelial migration

Lien-Hung Huang[1†], Ho-Chang Kuo[2,3†], Cheng-Tsung Pan[4], Yeong-Shin Lin[4,5], Ying-Hsien Huang[2,3] and Sung-Chou Li[1*] [iD]

Abstract

Background: Kawasaki disease (KD) is a prevalent pediatric disease worldwide and can cause coronary artery aneurysm as a severe complication. Typically, DNA methylation is thought to repress the expression of nearby genes. However, the cases in which DNA methylation promotes gene expression have been reported. In addition, globally, to what extent DNA methylation affects gene expression and how it contributes to the pathogenesis of KD are not yet well understood.

Methods: To address these important biological questions, we enrolled subjects, collected DNA and RNA samples from the subjects' total white blood cells, and performed DNA methylation (M450K) and gene expression (HTA 2.0) microarray assays.

Results: By analyzing the variation ratios of CpG beta values (methylation percentage) and gene expression intensities, we first concluded that the CpG markers close (− 1500 bp to + 500 bp) to the transcription start sites had higher variation ratios, reflecting significant regulation capacities. Next, we observed that, globally speaking, gene expression was modestly negatively correlated (correlation rho ≈ − 0.2) with the DNA methylation status of both upstream and downstream CpG markers in the promoter region. Third, we found that specific CpG markers were hypo-methylated in disease samples compared with healthy samples and hyper-methylated in convalescent samples compared with disease samples, promoting and repressing S100A genes' expressions, respectively. Finally, using an in vitro cell model, we demonstrated that S100A family proteins enhanced leukocyte transendothelial migration in KD.

Conclusions: This is the first study to integrate genome-wide DNA methylation with gene expression assays in KD and showed that the S100A family plays important roles in the pathogenesis of KD.

Keywords: Kawasaki disease, DNA methylation, CpG marker, Gene expression, Correlation, S100A gene family, Leukocyte transendothelial migration

* Correspondence: raymond.pinus@gmail.com
†Lien-Hung Huang and Ho-Chang Kuo contributed equally to this work.
[1]Genomics and Proteomics Core Laboratory, Department of Medical Research, Kaohsiung Chang Gung Memorial Hospital, 12th Floor, Children's Hospital, No.123, Dapi Rd, Niaosong District, Kaohsiung 83301, Taiwan
Full list of author information is available at the end of the article

Background

DNA methylation is a cellular activity at which the hydrogen atom on carbon 5 in the cytosine of CpG di-nucleotide (also called CpG marker) is replaced by a methyl group [1]. Through DNA methylation, gene activity can be silenced either by interfering with the binding of transcription factors or by interacting with the modification of histone protein [2].

Previous studies have demonstrated that abnormal DNA methylation led to gastric carcinogenesis by either hyper-methylating several tumor-suppressive miRNAs [3–5] or hypo-methylating onco-miR [6]. In addition, DNA methylation also regulated the erythropoiesis of embryonic stem cell [7], the pathogenesis of idiopathic pulmonary fibrosis [8], the neurodevelopment of the human hippocampus [9], and other processes. In addition to regulating disease pathogenesis, DNA methylation also performs long-term regulatory activities. Children suffered from early adversity, such as being raised in an orphanage, had higher global methylation patterns, and their neural-related genes were silenced by hyper-methylation [10]. Moreover, DNA methylation was also involved in nutritional control of the reproductive statuses of honeybees, as a result controlling the generation of workers or queens [11]. Through regulating the expressions of many critical genes, DNA methylation plays important roles not only in cellular activities but also in many human diseases. However, few DNA methylation-related studies have been conducted for Kawasaki disease.

Kawasaki disease (KD) is an acute systemic vasculitis disease, and it usually attacks children less than 5 years of age. The most severe complication of KD is coronary artery aneurysm (CAA), which affects approximately 20–25% of KD patients without timely treatment with intravenous immunoglobulin (IVIG) [12]. Therefore, KD is the major cause of acquired heart disease in children in developed countries [13]. The etiopathogenesis of KD may be attributed to the combined effects of genetics, immunity, and infection [14]. Although the exact etiology of KD is still unknown, predicting KD is possible with molecular markers [15]. To date, only few studies have focused on the regulation of DNA methylation in KD [16, 17]. However, these studies only conducted profiling of DNA methylation patterns, without further investigating whether the extent of DNA methylation affected the pathogenesis of KD. In addition, although considered to be negatively correlated with gene expression, DNA methylation of several CpG markers was reported to promote gene expressions [18, 19].

To answer these questions, we conducted a study in which we collected DNA and RNA samples from KD subjects, followed by combining the DNA methylation profiling data with the gene expression information for a systems biology perspective. Previous studies determined the correlations between DNA methylation and gene expression with CpG beta values (methylation percentages) and gene expression intensities [19]. In this study, we focused on the variation ratios of CpG beta values and the ones of gene expression intensities among different sets of samples. First, we identified modestly negative correlations between DNA methylation and gene expression regardless of whether the CpG markers were located upstream or downstream of the promoter regions. Second, we showed that the S100A gene family enhanced leukocyte transendothelial migration in KD with an in vitro cell model.

Results

Subject information

In this study, we enrolled 24 non-fever healthy control subjects (HC), 21 fever control subjects (FC, patients with fever but not diagnosed as KD or not having a KD history) and 18 KD patients. Blood samples from the KD patients were drawn both at the acute phase 1 day before IVIG treatment (KD1) and at the convalescent phase 3 weeks after IVIG treatment (KD3). Blood samples from the remaining subjects were drawn once. As shown in Additional file 1, 8 out of the 21 FC subjects suffered from acute sinusitis and 19.5 and 14.3% of the FC subject population had gastroenteritis and bronchopneumonia, respectively. No significant difference was observed in age ($p = 0.0536$, t test) or gender ($p = 1$, Fisher's exact test) between the 12 HC and 12 KD subjects whose samples were used for the Illumina Human-Methylation 450 BeadChip assays (M450 K). In addition, no significant difference was observed in age ($p = 0.1108$, t test) or gender ($p = 0.7$, Fisher's exact test) between the 18 HC and 18 KD subjects used for the Affymetrix GeneChip® Human Transcriptome Array 2.0 (HTA 2.0) assays. All of the KD patients met the diagnosis criteria of AHA 2004 [20].

DNA methylation variations among samples

From the total HC, KD1, and KD3 DNA samples, we selected 12 HC, 12 KD1, and 12 KD3 ones for bisulfite conversion, followed by M450K assays on the 36 bisulfite converted DNA samples (Additional file 1). The generated raw data was analyzed with Partek. First, we examined the overall methylation patterns of the three sets using a PCA plot. As shown in Fig. 1a, the three sets can be clearly distinguished in terms of their methylation patterns. The KD3 set was located distinct from the other two ones, whereas, the HC and KD1 sets slightly overlapped with each other. When the FDR < 0.05 and variation ratio > 1.1 criteria were specified, there were 12,209, 13,936, and 14,643 significant CpG markers among the KD1 vs. HC, KD3 vs. HC, and KD3 vs. KD1 comparisons (Table 1), respectively. These significant CpG markers formed a union of 25,984 CpG markers,

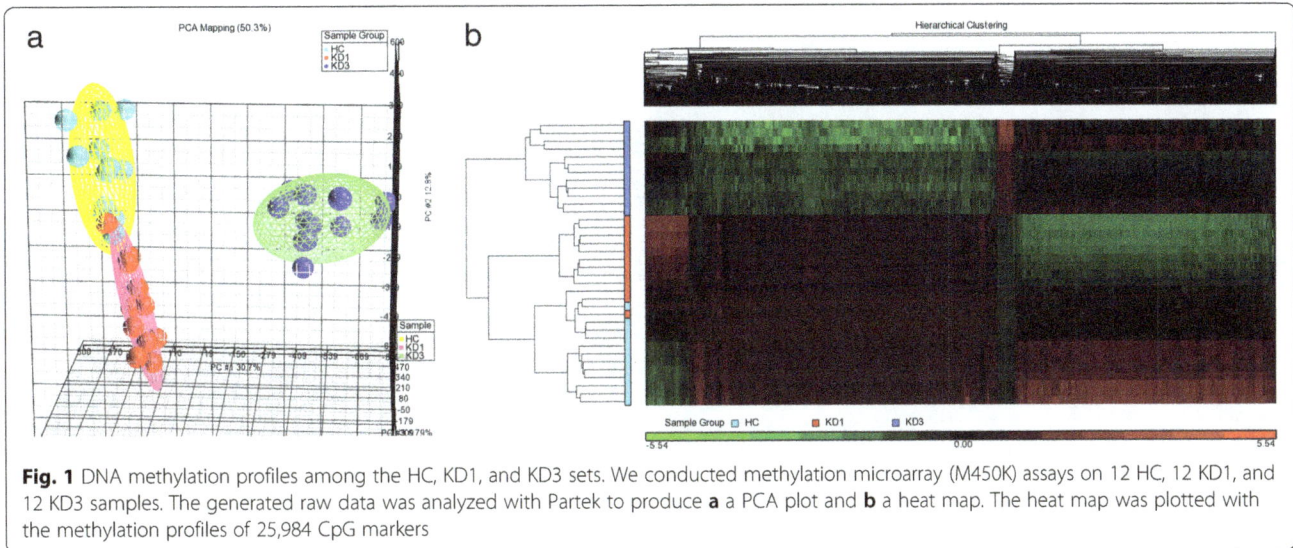

Fig. 1 DNA methylation profiles among the HC, KD1, and KD3 sets. We conducted methylation microarray (M450K) assays on 12 HC, 12 KD1, and 12 KD3 samples. The generated raw data was analyzed with Partek to produce **a** a PCA plot and **b** a heat map. The heat map was plotted with the methylation profiles of 25,984 CpG markers

and the heat map of which is demonstrated in Fig. 1b. Table 1 and Fig. 1b show that most of the significant CpG markers in the KD1 vs. HC comparison were hypo-methylated in the KD1 samples, reflecting hypo-methylation of CpG markers with the onset of KD.

The Manhattan plots of the three comparisons were also provided (Additional files 2, 3, and 4). Although the numbers of significant CpG markers in the three comparisons were almost equivalent (Table 1), the Manhattan plots showed that the KD3 vs. HC and KD3 vs. KD1 comparisons, both of which involved in the IVIG administration factor, had much lower p values and much more significant CpG markers. In our previous study, using M27K assays, we observed that IVIG administration had a much stronger impact on methylation variation than disease onset did [16]. Our current data also supported this finding.

Methylation variations of CpG markers within the putative promoter regions

Next, we investigated the methylation variations of CpG markers based on the distance to the transcription start sites (TSSs) of genes. Since a promoter is a rough and ambiguous region relative to the TSS of a gene, studies

have defined their putative promoter regions with different distances to the TSS [21, 22]. In this study, we adopted the default parameter of Partek and defined a promoter as the region ranging from − 5000 to 3000 of a transcript's TSS (RefSeq 41 annotation). Then, we mapped all significant CpG makers ($P < 0.05$) back to the promoters and marked their methylation variation ratios. According to Fig. 2, the densities of the significant CpG markers seemed to be higher within the − 1500 to 500 regions than the ones out of this region. To examine the densities of CpG markers within the promoters, we also mapped all CpG markers (both significant and non-significant) back to the promoters. As a result, we observed results similar to those shown in Fig. 2 (Additional file 5). Therefore, higher densities of CpG makers within the − 1500 to 500 regions were an intrinsic characteristic of the M450K microarray chip.

Figure 2a, c, e also shows that CpG markers within the − 1500 to 500 region tended to vary more than the rest CpG markers outside of this region. To investigate this issue, we divided the putative promoter region (− 5000 to 3000 bp) into three sub-regions as follows: the left (− 5000 to − 1500 bp), core (− 1500 to 500 bp), and right (500 to 3000 bp) sub-regions. As shown in Fig. 2b, d, f, consistently among the three comparisons, the CpG markers within the core regions significantly varied more than the ones within the two adjacent regions ($P < 2.2E−16$), implying that the CpG makers closer to the TSS of the transcript regulated gene expression more significantly.

Gene expression variations among samples

From the total HC, KD1, and KD3 RNA samples, we selected 18 HC, 18 KD1, and 18 KD3 ones to generate 3 HC, 3 KD1, and 3 KD3 evenly pooled samples. We then conducted the HTA 2.0 assays on the 9 pooled RNA

Table 1 Summary of significant CpG markers among the comparisons

Comparison	# all markers	# hyper markers	# hypo markers
KD1 vs. HC	12,209	1484	10,725
KD3 vs. HC	13,936	505	13,431
KD3 vs. KD1	14,643	4669	9974

Based on the criteria of an FDR < 0.05 and variation ratio > 1.1, we identified significant CpG markers among the three comparisons. Hyper marker and hypo marker denoted the significant hyper-methylated and hypo-methylated markers, respectively

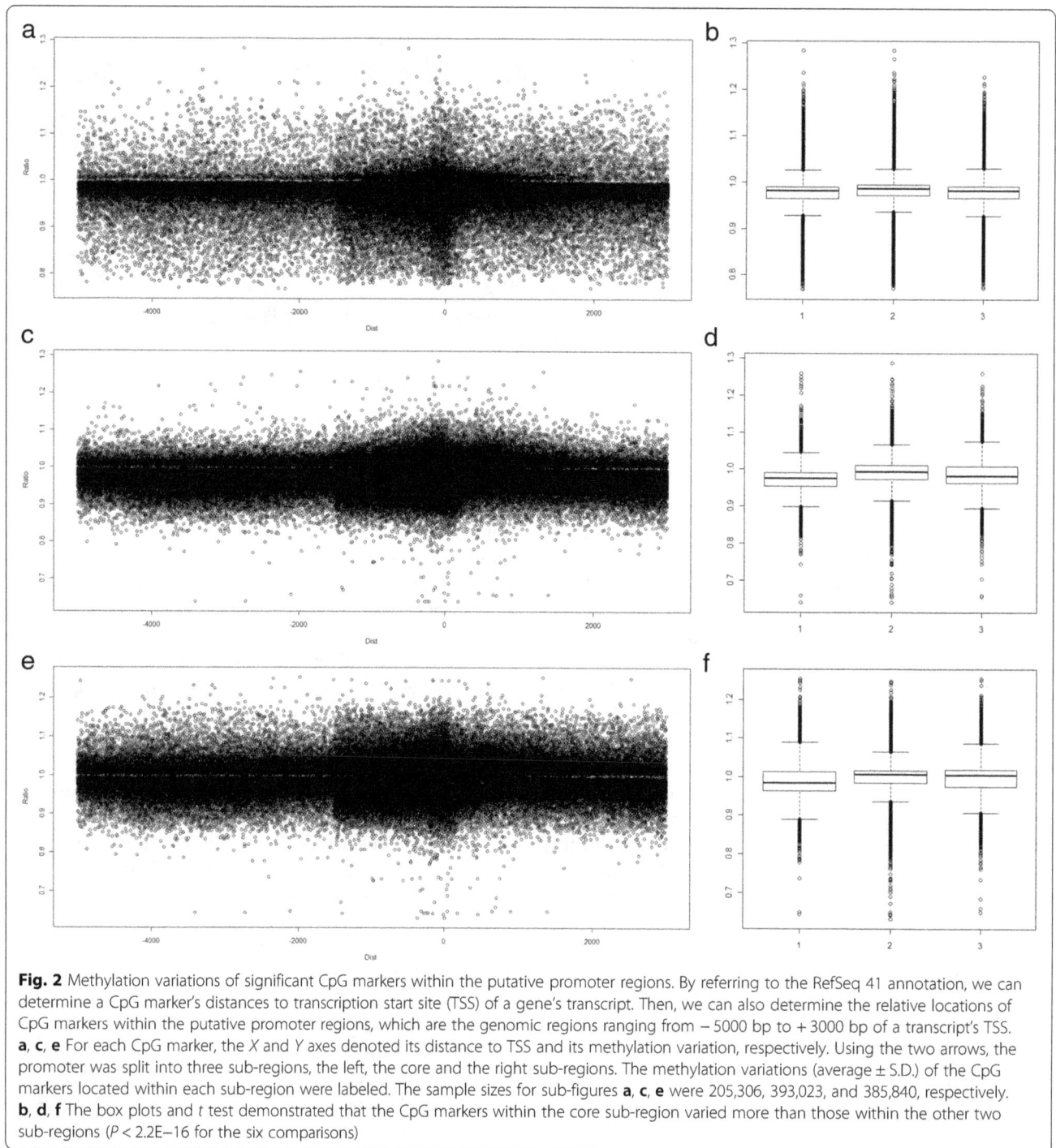

Fig. 2 Methylation variations of significant CpG markers within the putative promoter regions. By referring to the RefSeq 41 annotation, we can determine a CpG marker's distances to transcription start site (TSS) of a gene's transcript. Then, we can also determine the relative locations of CpG markers within the putative promoter regions, which are the genomic regions ranging from − 5000 bp to + 3000 bp of a transcript's TSS. **a**, **c**, **e** For each CpG marker, the *X* and *Y* axes denoted its distance to TSS and its methylation variation, respectively. Using the two arrows, the promoter was split into three sub-regions, the left, the core and the right sub-regions. The methylation variations (average ± S.D.) of the CpG markers located within each sub-region were labeled. The sample sizes for sub-figures **a**, **c**, **e** were 205,306, 393,023, and 385,840, respectively. **b**, **d**, **f** The box plots and *t* test demonstrated that the CpG markers within the core sub-region varied more than those within the other two sub-regions ($P < 2.2E−16$ for the six comparisons)

samples (Additional file 1). The generated raw data was analyzed with Partek. Like DNA methylation, we also examined the overall gene expression patterns of the three sets with a PCA plot. As shown in Fig. 3a, the distinguishability of the three sets based on the gene expression data was not as good as that based on the DNA methylation data, especially for the HC and KD3 sets. Table 2 shows only 10 significant genes ($P < 0.05$ and expression ratio > 1.5) in the KD3 vs. HC comparison, and the union of all significant genes comprised 936 genes. Using the 936 union genes, we drew a heat map (Fig. 3b), which demonstrated that the KD3 samples were hardly distinguishable from the HC ones based on the gene expression profiles.

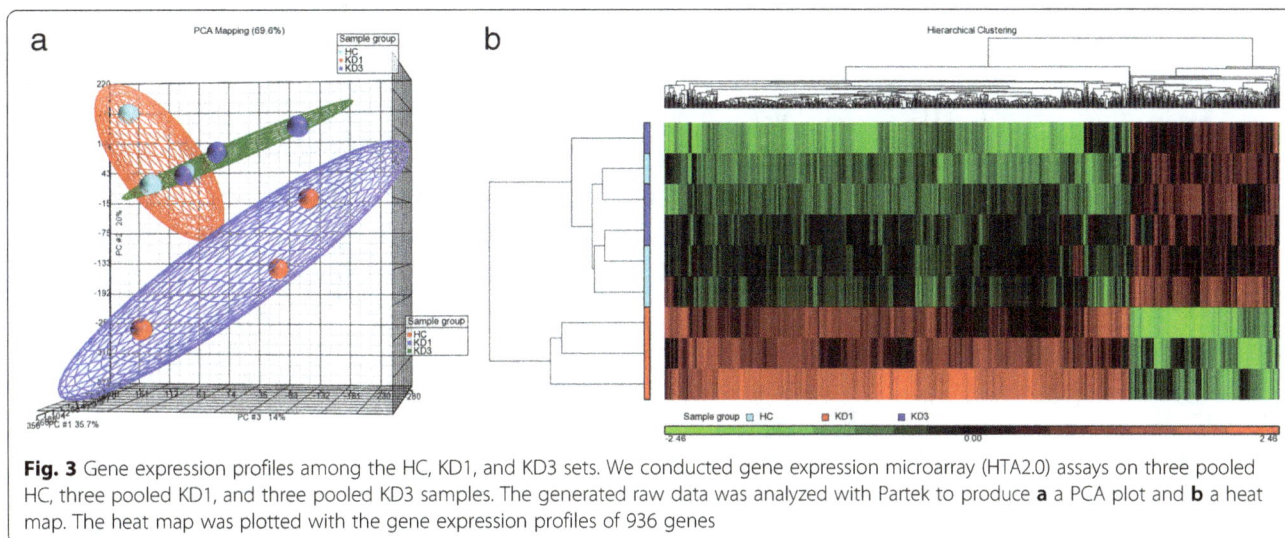

Fig. 3 Gene expression profiles among the HC, KD1, and KD3 sets. We conducted gene expression microarray (HTA2.0) assays on three pooled HC, three pooled KD1, and three pooled KD3 samples. The generated raw data was analyzed with Partek to produce **a** a PCA plot and **b** a heat map. The heat map was plotted with the gene expression profiles of 936 genes

Correlation between gene expression and DNA methylation

So far, we obtained both DNA methylation and gene expression data from the HC, KD1 and KD3 samples. DNA methylation was usually thought to be negatively correlated with gene expression. The higher the CpG marker was methylated, the less abundantly the gene was expressed. However, previous studies also found positive correlations, globally or specifically [18, 19]. In addition, few studies have attempted to investigate to what extent DNA methylation on CpG marker altered gene expression. In other words, what is the global correlation pattern between DNA methylation and gene expression?

To globally and comprehensively address this question, we first constructed regulation pairs of CpG markers and genes (see the "Methods" section), followed by tabulating the variation ratios of CpG markers and genes in each comparison, e.g., KD1 vs. HC. With this approach, we could calculate the correlation coefficient between the variation ratios of gene expression and CpG marker methylation, investigating to what extent DNA methylation repressed or activated gene expression.

We first constructed random regulation pairs of CpG markers and genes by randomly assigning one CpG marker and one gene into one pair without considering whether the marker was located within the putative promoter or

not. As shown in Additional file 6, the Spearman's rank correlation coefficients of the three comparisons (random column, sub-figure a, b and c) were almost zero, reflecting pretty low correlations. Then, we considered all regulation pairs of CpG markers and genes (both significant and non-significant). We also divided the regulation pairs of CpG markers and genes into two sets, based on their genomic positions being located upstream or downstream of the TSS. As shown in Additional file 6, the upstream, downstream, and both (union of the upstream and downstream sets) columns showed that Spearman's rho values were a little bit lower than those of the random column, reflecting slightly higher negative correlations.

Next, we considered only the significant CpG markers ($P < 0.05$) and the significant genes ($P < 0.05$). In other words, only significant CpG markers and genes were included to construct the regulation pairs of CpG markers and genes. As shown in Fig. 4, the upstream, downstream, and both columns showed much lower Spearman's rho values ($P = 0.0246$, paired t test) than the values in Additional file 6, reflecting stronger negative correlations between the three comparisons when only significant CpG markers and genes were considered.

Figure 2 shows that the CpG markers located within the core sub-regions of the putative promoters better regulated gene expression. So, we further performed similar analyses using only the CpG markers located within the core sub-regions (– 1500 to 500 bp). As a result, Fig. 5 shows that although not yet significant ($P = 0.0586$, paired t test) owing to the small sample size, 7 out of 9 comparisons (except for subfigures h and i) had stronger negative correlations than those shown in Fig. 4, which was consistent with the conclusion of Fig. 2 that the CpG makers closer to the TSSs of the transcripts better regulated gene expression.

Table 2 Summary of significant genes among the comparisons

Comparison	# all genes	# up genes	# down genes
KD1 vs. HC	678	495	183
KD3 vs. HC	10	1	9
KD3 vs. KD1	810	141	669

Based on the criteria of a $p < 0.05$ and variation ratio > 1.5, we tabulated the numbers of significant genes among the three comparisons. Up gene and down gene denoted the significant upregulated and downregulated genes, respectively

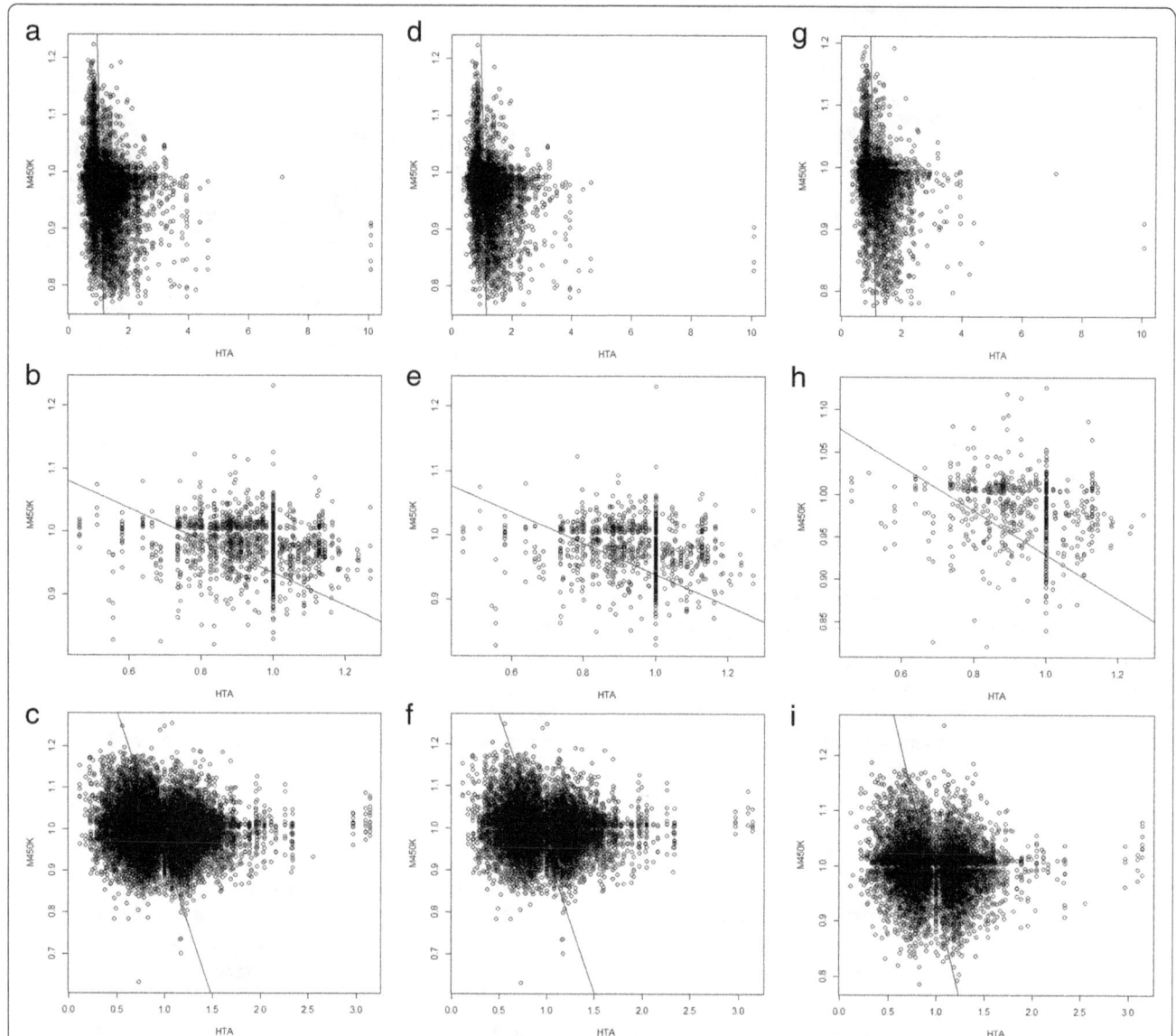

Fig. 4 The scatter plots of gene expression variations and DNA methylation variations for CpG markers located within the putative promoters. The X axis presented the gene expression variation determined with the HTA2.0 assay. The Y axis presented the DNA methylation variation determined with the M450K assay. Each dot denoted the regulation pair of one significant gene and one significant CpG marker; only those with a p value < 0.05 were concerned significant. For each comparison in each column, the Spearman's rank correlation coefficient (denoted as rho) was labeled. The correlation coefficient was calculated with the data from the full-length promoter (the Both column), in the − 5000 to − 1 bp region (the Upstream column) and the + 1 to + 3000 bp region (the Downstream column). The sample size for sub-figures **a** to **i** were in order: 28,776, 3903, 61,055, 18,068, 2318, 36,770, 10,698, 1575, and 24,285

In summary, no matter the CpG marker was located upstream or downstream of the transcript's TSS, globally speaking, DNA methylation and gene expression maintained a modestly negative correlation, at least in the KD cases in this study.

Perfect cases of negatively correlated genes and CpG markers

In this study, we collected samples from the healthy controls (HC), patients before disease treatment (KD1),

and patients after disease treatment (KD3). Therefore, we were interested in the variation profiles from HC to KD1 and from KD1 to KD3. In other words, we were interested in the genes or CpG markers that were upregulated from HC to KD1 and then downregulated from KD1 to KD3 (i.e., up-then-down cases). In addition, the down-then-up cases were also our targets. Figure 6 illustrates the perfect cases of negatively correlated genes and CpG markers. These perfect cases were composed of the up-then-down genes and the down-then-up CpG

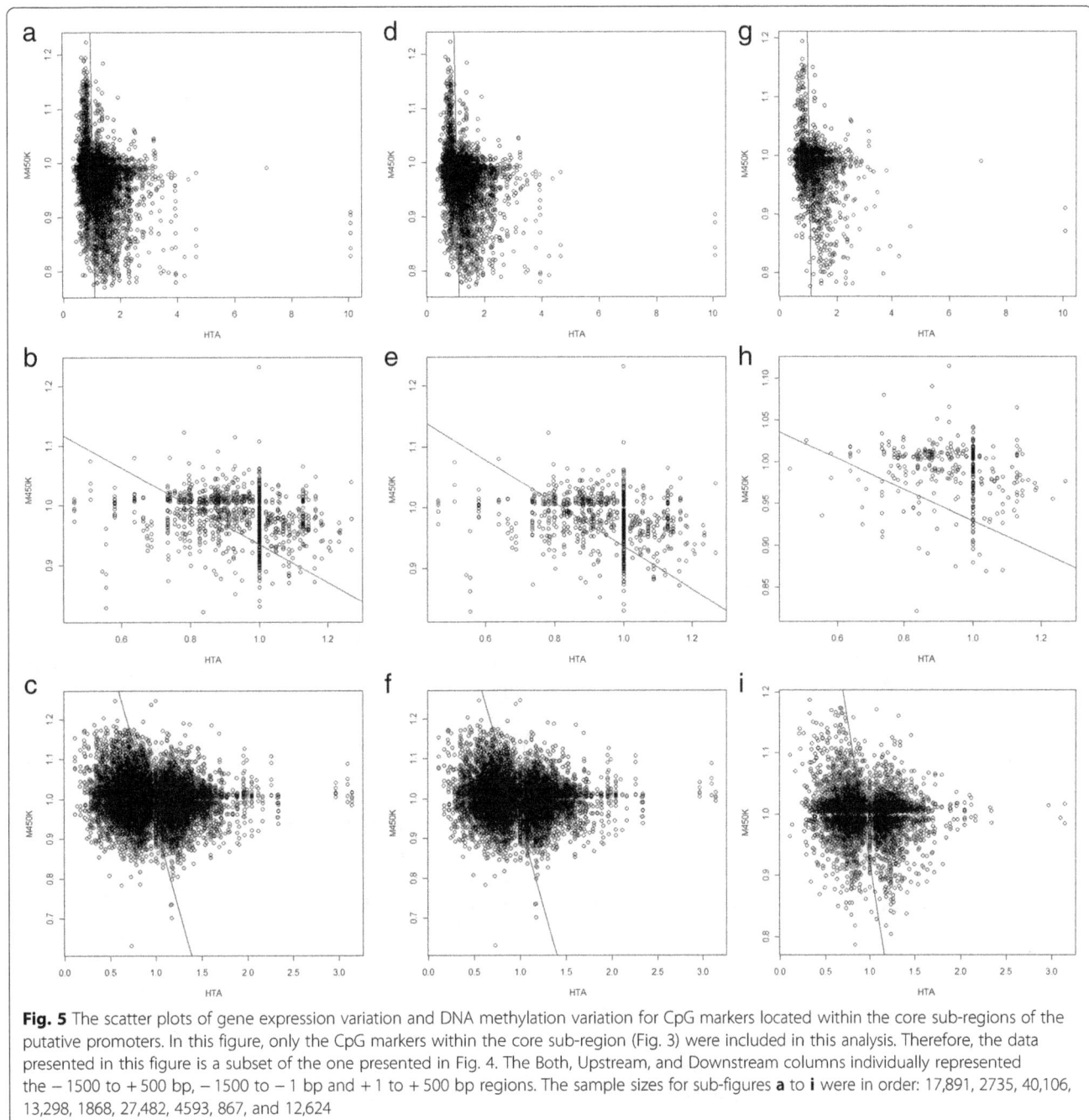

Fig. 5 The scatter plots of gene expression variation and DNA methylation variation for CpG markers located within the core sub-regions of the putative promoters. In this figure, only the CpG markers within the core sub-region (Fig. 3) were included in this analysis. Therefore, the data presented in this figure is a subset of the one presented in Fig. 4. The Both, Upstream, and Downstream columns individually represented the − 1500 to + 500 bp, − 1500 to − 1 bp and + 1 to + 500 bp regions. The sample sizes for sub-figures **a** to **i** were in order: 17,891, 2735, 40,106, 13,298, 1868, 27,482, 4593, 867, and 12,624

markers as well as the down-then-up genes and the up-then-down CpG markers.

Among the significant genes shown in Table 2, we identified 98 down-then-up and 440 up-then-down genes (Fig. 6). In addition, among the significant CpG markers in Table 1, we identified 3230 down-then-up and 818 up-then-down CpG markers, which were located at the promoters of 440 and 247 genes, respectively. Further intersection analyses generated 83 (80 + 3) perfect genes possessing negative correlation with CpG markers from HC to KD1 and from KD1

to KD3. Gene expression at the transcriptional level is regulated by many factors. These 83 genes were negatively correlated with DNA methylation on their promoter CpG markers not only in the HC to KD1 transition but also in the KD1 to KD3 transition. Therefore, they were the perfect targets for the further functional analysis.

The regulatory roles of the S100A gene family
We further conducted GO analysis on the 80 genes, and the result is shown in Additional file 7. After careful

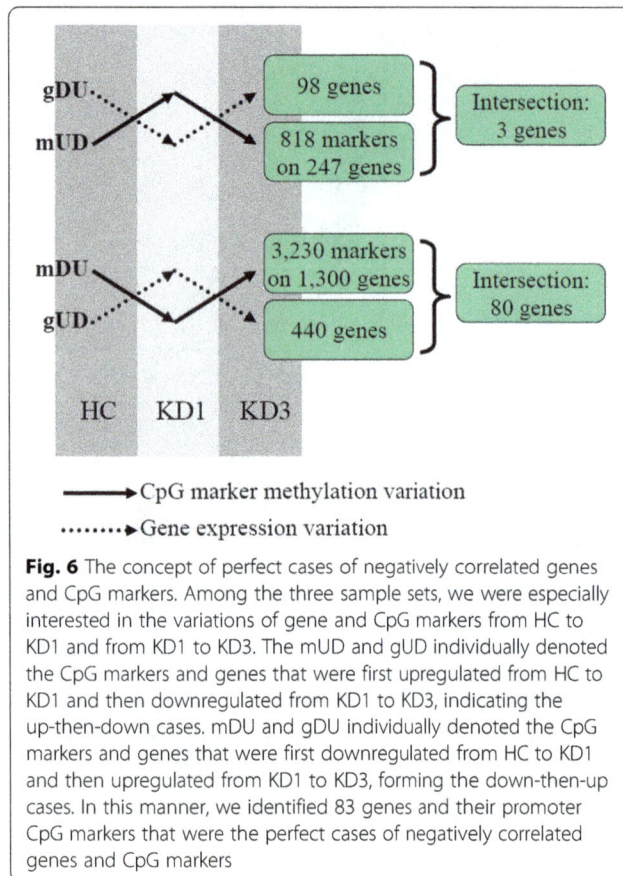

Fig. 6 The concept of perfect cases of negatively correlated genes and CpG markers. Among the three sample sets, we were especially interested in the variations of gene and CpG markers from HC to KD1 and from KD1 to KD3. The mUD and gUD individually denoted the CpG markers and genes that were first upregulated from HC to KD1 and then downregulated from KD1 to KD3, indicating the up-then-down cases. mDU and gDU individually denoted the CpG markers and genes that were first downregulated from HC to KD1 and then upregulated from KD1 to KD3, forming the down-then-up cases. In this manner, we identified 83 genes and their promoter CpG markers that were the perfect cases of negatively correlated genes and CpG markers

inspection, we found that four out of the 80 input genes, including S100A8, S100A9, S100A12, and FCER1G, were repetitively involved in the top five GO items in terms of *p* value. Therefore, we conducted qPCR assays on the four genes and succeeded in detecting the S100A gene family, namely S100A8, S100A9, and S100A12. Figure 7a illustrates five, four, and one CpG markers on the putative promoter regions of S100A8, S100A9, and S100A12, respectively. These CpG markers were all statistically significant and were all down-then-up cases. The qPCR assays also confirmed that the S100A genes were all the up-then-down cases (Fig. 7b). In summary, in the transitions from HC to KD1 and from KD1 to KD3, the CpG markers were negatively correlated with S100A gene expressions, demonstrating epigenomic regulation abilities.

We have demonstrated a global modestly negative correlation between DNA methylation and gene expression (Figs. 4 and 5). Here, we were also interested in to what extent these 10 CpG markers regulated the S100A genes. Using the $2^{-\Delta\Delta Ct}$ values (Fig. 7) determined with qPCR to replace the intensity values determined with HTA2.0, we conducted similar assays. We found that the rho value between S100A8 and its promoter CpG markers was − 0.4388. And, the rho values for S100A9 and A12

were − 0.3972 and − 0.4543, respectively. Therefore, the S100A genes and their promoter CpG markers were moderately negatively correlated, indicating stronger correlations than the global profiles.

S100A8 and S100A9 are inflammatory markers that are usually highly expressed in acute and chronic inflammation. They are expressed and secreted into the plasma by neutrophils and/or monocytes, performing cytokine-like functions in inflammation [23, 24]. S100A8 and S100A9 are also involved in the pathogenesis of many diseases. They were reported to predict cardiovascular events in humans [25], to promote reticulated thrombocytosis and atherogenesis in diabetes patients [26] and to trigger inflammation, apoptosis, and tissue injury in the kidney [27]. In addition, S100A8 and S100A9 were thought to be involved in neutrophil migration in inflammatory sites [28].

In addition to the conclusions drawn from the above studies, the top GO items were also involved in leukocyte migration, neutrophil migration, and neutrophil chemotaxis (Additional file 7). Moreover, S100A8, S100A9 and S100A12 were involved in all of these GO items. Therefore, we investigated whether these S100A genes regulated neutrophil transendothelial migration, which is the causes of vascular inflammation and coronary artery aneurysm (i.e., the complication of KD). For this purpose, we conducted an in vitro leukocyte transendothelial migration (LTEM) assay. We treated neutrophil cells with the recombinant S100A family proteins and examined whether S100A treatment enhanced neutrophil transendothelial migration (migrating from the upper chamber into the lower chamber, see the "Methods" section) with an in vitro cell model, in which neutrophil cells in the lower chamber were collected and counted with flow cytometry.

We first had non-treated neutrophil cells stained and analyzed with flow cytometry. As shown in Fig. 8a, we determined the target set of observed cells based on the specified FSC-A and SSC-A values. Then, using the same criteria, we selected the target set and counted the CD15$^+$ neutrophil cells. Figure 8b shows that, without S100A treatment, 595 CD15$^+$ neutrophil cells were counted. With S100A8/A9 complex, S100A9, and S100A12 treatment, 2687, 1370, and 1513 CD15$^+$ neutrophil cells were counted (Fig. 8c–e), respectively. By four independent assays, compared with that of the control treatment, S100A8/A9 complex, S100A9, and S100A12 treatment all significantly promoted neutrophil cells to penetrate the endothelial layer (Fig. 8f). The ANOVA *p* value was 0.0016, and the *p* values of the individual comparisons were all less than 0.01. In addition, no significant difference was observed between any two treatments.

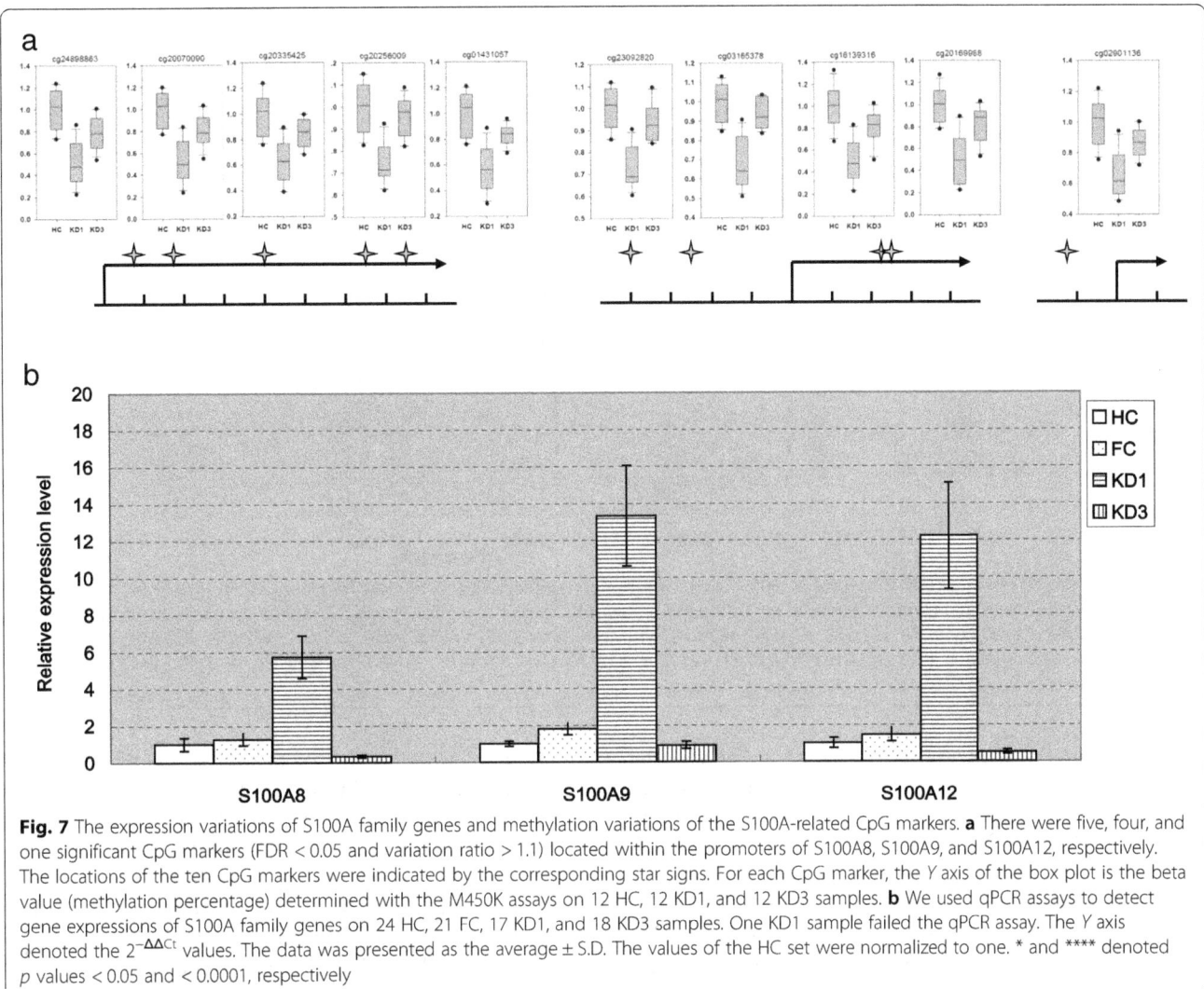

Fig. 7 The expression variations of S100A family genes and methylation variations of the S100A-related CpG markers. **a** There were five, four, and one significant CpG markers (FDR < 0.05 and variation ratio > 1.1) located within the promoters of S100A8, S100A9, and S100A12, respectively. The locations of the ten CpG markers were indicated by the corresponding star signs. For each CpG marker, the Y axis of the box plot is the beta value (methylation percentage) determined with the M450K assays on 12 HC, 12 KD1, and 12 KD3 samples. **b** We used qPCR assays to detect gene expressions of S100A family genes on 24 HC, 21 FC, 17 KD1, and 18 KD3 samples. One KD1 sample failed the qPCR assay. The Y axis denoted the $2^{-\Delta\Delta Ct}$ values. The data was presented as the average ± S.D. The values of the HC set were normalized to one. * and **** denoted p values < 0.05 and < 0.0001, respectively

Discussion

Intravenous immunoglobulin (IVIG) administration is the standard treatment for many autoimmune diseases, including idiopathic thrombocytopenic purpura, Guillain-Barré syndrome, dermatomyositis, and many others [29]. Although it is still a debate whether KD is an infectious or an autoimmune disease, IVIG is currently the most effective treatment for KD patients [13]. Based on the results from both the M27K [16] and M450K assays, IVIG administration may have a much stronger impact on DNA methylation than KD disease itself. In addition, the KD patients at the convalescent phase (KD3, 3 weeks after IVIG administration) recovered their health based on their gene expression profiles, with only 10 genes differentially expressed from the healthy control (HC) subjects. However, unlike the gene expression profiles, the DNA methylation profiles differed between the HC and KD3 sets. Actually, there are few chances to collect blood samples from KD patients without IVIG treatment at the convalescent phase.

Therefore, it is difficult to determine whether such long-term variations on DNA methylation are triggered by IVIG administration or by the intrinsic immune responses against KD.

Compared with the samples from the convalescent phase, S100A8, S100A9, and S100A12 were reported to keep higher expression levels in total leukocytes from KD patients at the acute phase [30]. Moreover, S100A12 was highly correlated with the response to IVIG treatment [31], reflecting its application for monitoring the KD status [32]. Some studies showed that inflammatory cytokines were regulated through an epigenetic mechanism [33]. Our data suggested that S100A8, S100A9, and S100A12 were also regulated in this manner in KD. In spite of the previous studies, the detailed mechanisms through which S100A genes regulate the pathogenesis of KD have not yet been well studied. And, our study bridges the gap, enhancing our understanding of S100A gene family on KD pathogenesis.

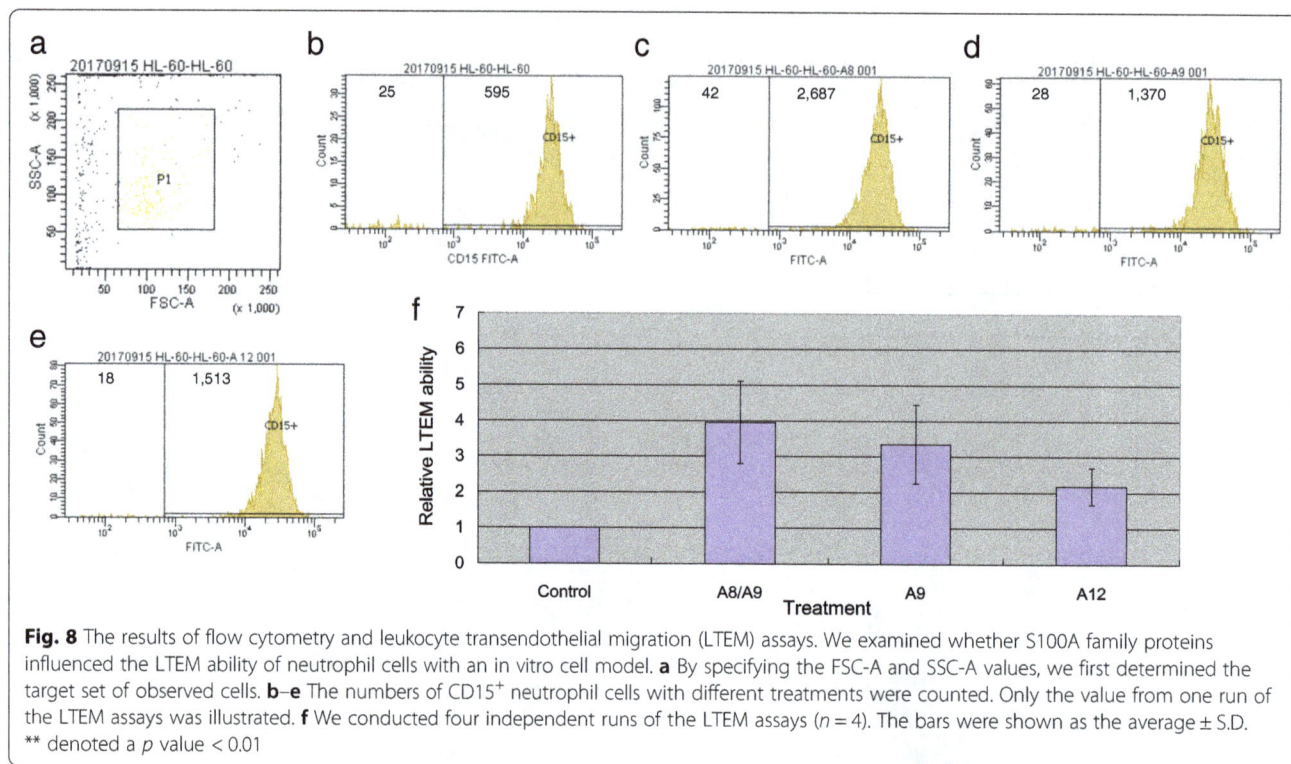

Fig. 8 The results of flow cytometry and leukocyte transendothelial migration (LTEM) assays. We examined whether S100A family proteins influenced the LTEM ability of neutrophil cells with an in vitro cell model. **a** By specifying the FSC-A and SSC-A values, we first determined the target set of observed cells. **b–e** The numbers of CD15$^+$ neutrophil cells with different treatments were counted. Only the value from one run of the LTEM assays was illustrated. **f** We conducted four independent runs of the LTEM assays ($n = 4$). The bars were shown as the average ± S.D. ** denoted a p value < 0.01

Coronary artery aneurysm (CAA) is a type of vascular inflammation and the most severe complication of KD. In this study, we used an in vitro cell model to demonstrate that S100A proteins enhanced the LTEM ability of neutrophil cells, implying the regulatory mechanism in KD pathogenesis. This study showed that LTEM assay may service as an in vitro vasculitis model for KD although, so far, there is no in vitro cell model specific for KD available. S100A8 and S100A9 form a heterodimer [24, 25], and the S100A8/A9 complex is commercially available; thus, we treated neutrophil cells with the A8/A9 complex. However, although it naturally functions as a heterodimer with A8, S100A9 alone also had the potential to enhance the LTEM ability of neutrophil cells.

In this study, we found that CpG markers within the core sub-region (– 1500 to 500 bp) tended to vary more than the rest CpG markers (Fig. 2), implying that the CpG makers closer to the TSS of the transcript regulated gene expression more significantly. Actually, promoter regions of genes usually carry many functional domains, e.g., transcription factor binding sites (TFBSs), responsible for transcriptional regulations. However, promoter is a rough and ambiguous region relative to the TSS of a gene. Although long genomic fragments were defined as putative promoter regions in studies [21, 22], the functional domains confirmed by experiment or selected for experiment were usually close to the TSSs [34–36]. Such phenomenon was also consistent with our finding in Fig. 5. In summary, since the target sites of transcription factor binding and histone

protein modification are close to the TSSs of genes, to perform the regulation abilities, the CpG markers close to the TSSs (– 1500 to 500 bp) tended to vary more.

The relationship between DNA methylation and gene expression may reflect the real immune response to a disease, although any part of the immune response cannot reflect the whole reaction. This study is the first to integrate a DNA methylation array with a gene expression one in KD and shows that S100A family plays important roles in the pathogenesis of KD.

Conclusion

Although DNA methylation usually represses gene expression, several cases in which DNA methylation plays promotion roles have also been reported. In addition, globally to what extent DNA methylation represses or promotes gene expression has seldom been discussed in previous studies and has never been discussed in relation to KD. In this study, by combining DNA methylation and gene expression data, we first concluded that the CpG markers close (– 1500 bp to + 500 bp) to the TSS varied more than those located far from the TSS did. Second, we identified global modestly negative correlations between DNA methylation and gene expression regardless of whether the CpG markers were located upstream or downstream of the promoter regions. Third, we found that the S100A gene family and their promoter CpG markers were perfect cases of negative correlations. Owing to disease onset (from HC to KD1), the CpG markers were hypo-methylated, which activated S100A genes' expressions. Owing to treatment (from KD1 to KD3), the CpG markers were hyper-methylated, which inactivated S100A genes' expressions. Finally, we proved that S100A family proteins enhanced leukocyte transendothelial migration in KD with an in vitro cell model.

Methods

Subject enrollment and sample collection

We enrolled volunteer subjects from Kaohsiung Chang Gung Memorial Hospital. This study was approved by the institutional ethics board (IRB number: 201700270A3C501) and all subjects or their guardians signed the informed consent form. Whole blood samples were collected from the subjects, followed by red blood cell (RBC) lysis with RBC lysis buffer to enrich total white blood cells (WBCs). Next, we used the QIAamp® DNA Blood Mini Kit (Qiagen, CA, USA) to extract DNA and the mirVana™ miRNA Isolation Kit (Ambion, CA, USA) to extract RNA following the manufacturer's protocols. The DNA and RNA concentrations were measured with the NanoDrop 2000 spectrophotometer (Thermo Scientific, MA, USA). All RNA samples passed the criterion of a RIN ≥ 7 assessed with the Agilent 2100 Bioanalyzer (Agilent, CA, USA).

DNA methylation microarray assay

The extracted DNA samples were bisulfite modified with EZ DNA Methylation-Lightning™ Kit (Zymo Research, Irvine, USA). Briefly, 0.5 μg of DNA was mixed with lightning conversion reagent, followed by the thermal-cycling condition: 98 °C for 8 min, 54 °C for 60 min, and held at 4 °C. Next, the DNA samples were loaded into spin column and mixed with M-binding buffer. After centrifuge, spin column was incubated with L-desulphonation buffer at room temperature. Finally, bisulfite-modified DNA was eluted using M-elution buffer and stock at − 80 °C. After bisulfite treatment, the bisulfite-converted DNA samples were subject to genome-wide screening on DNA methylation patterns with Illumina HumanMethylation450 (M450K) BeadChip microarray assay, able to determine the methylation percentages (called beta values) of approximately 450,000 CpG markers. The microarray assays passing the quality control criteria were then analyzed with Partek, a commercial software specific for microarray data analysis.

Gene expression microarray assay

The collected RNA samples were subject to microarray assay to determine gene expression profile. In this study, we adopted Affymetrix HTA 2.0 microarray chips for the profiling job. The RNA sample were first prepared with WT PLUS Reagent kit (Affymetrix) followed by hybridization on HTA 2.0 microarray chips. The raw data of HTA 2.0 chips were first subject to quality control examination as suggested by Affymetrix manuals. And, the chips passing the quality control criteria were then analyzed with Partek.

Mapping CpG markers and constructing the regulation pairs of CpG marker and gene

We mapped the CpG markers back to the human genome (hg19) and examined whether they were located within the putative promoter region, ranging from 5000 bp upstream to 3000 bp downstream (− 5000 to + 3000 bp) of mRNA's transcription start sites (TSSs) based on RefSeq 41 annotation. If so, this CpG marker was assumed to be regulating the gene, resulting in 618,621 unique regulation pairs of CpG markers and mRNAs.

Due to the existence of alternative splicing isoforms, one gene may have several mRNAs with different TSSs [37]. For example, the ABCC10 gene is located at chromosome 6 and has two alternative splicing isoforms, NM_001198934 and NM_033450, the TSSs of which are individually 43,395,292 and 43,399,489 bp. Owing to the varied TSSs and putative promoter regions, the CpG markers located at the upstream promoter of NM_001198934 could be located out of the promoter of NM_033450. Meanwhile, the CpG markers located at the downstream promoter of NM_001198934 could be located at the upstream promoter of NM_033450. Since we considered the differences in the upstream and downstream promoter regions, we enumerated all regulation pairs of CpG marker and mRNA. In addition, since we measured gene expression levels with a microarray and/or qPCR in this study, the term "mRNA" in the regulation pairs was replaced with the term "gene" for simplicity.

Real-time quantitative polymerase chain reaction

For the real-time PCR, 0.5 μg of total RNA was reverse transcribed into cDNA using the High-Capacity cDNA Reverse Transcription Kit (Applied Biosystems, CA, USA). Next, we performed real-time quantitative PCR using the Fast SYBR® Green Master Mix system and the StepOnePlus™ System (Applied Biosystems). The sequences of the primers used were as follows:

18S: forward primer (5′-GTAACCCGTTGAACCC CATT-3′) and reverse primer (5′-CCATCCAATCGGTA GTAGCG-3′); S100A8: forward primer (5′-ACCG AGTGTCCTCAGTA-3′) and reverse primer (5′-TCTT TGTGGCTTTCTTCATGG-3′); S100A9: forward primer (5′-AACACCTTCCACCAATACT-3′) and reverse primer (5′-GCCATCAGCATGATGAACT-3′); and S100A12: forward primer (5′-CTTACAAAGGAGCT TGCAAAC-3′) and reverse primer (5′-GGTGTGGTA ATGGGCAG-3′). The real-time PCR master mix was prepared as follows: 10 µl of 2X fast SYBR green master mix, 7 µl of nuclease-free water, 1 µl of cDNA, 1 µl of forward primer (10 µM), and 1 µl of reverse primer (10 µM). The default PCR thermal-cycling condition was as follows: 20 s at 95 °C and 40 cycles of 3 s at 95 °C and 30 s at 60 °C.

Cell culture and the leukocyte transendothelial migration assay

As suggested in a previous study, we used HL-60-like neutrophil cells to conduct the migration assay [38]. The HL-60 cells (BCRC No. 60027) were induced into neutrophil-like cells by culture in Iscove's modified Dulbecco's medium supplemented with 20% fetal bovine serum, 4 mM L-glutamine and 1.5 g/L of sodium bicarbonate at 37 °C in a humidified 95% air/5% CO_2 incubator. The cells were differentiated into neutrophil-like cells with the stimulus of 1.3% DMSO (Sigma-Aldrich, MO, USA). Primary human coronary endothelial cells (HCAEC, CC-2585, Clonetics, Lonza) were cultured in EBM-2 medium (CC-3156, Clonetics, Lonza) supplemented with EGM-2 MV SingleQuots (CC-4147, Clonetics, Lonza) which contains 5% FBS.

For the transendothelial migration assay, 2×10^5 HCAECs were first seeded into gelatin-coated 24-well hanging inserts (also called the upper chamber, 3 µm, PET, Merck, NJ, USA) for 24 h. Then, the inserts were put into 24-well culture plates (also called lower chamber). Neutrophil-like cells were first starved for 4 h and then cultured in serum-free culture medium with 10 g/ml of S100A8/A9 (8226-S8-050, R&D), 8 g/ml of S100A9 (9254-S9-050, R&D), or 4 g/ml of S100A12 (1052-ER-050, R&D) recombinant proteins for 24 h.

On the day of the migration assay, the S100A-treated neutrophil cells were washed with serum-free culture medium. Then, 1×10^5 cells were placed in the inserts, which were further moved into 24-well culture plates containing 600 µl of medium with 200 nM fMLP (Sigma-Aldrich, MO, USA) as a chemo-attractant. After 2 h of migration, the neutrophil cells penetrating the endothelial layer and migrating into the lower chamber were collected. The cells were washed with PBS and stained with CD15-FITC (340,703, BD), followed by analysis with the LSRII flow cytometer (BD Biosciences).

Additional files

Additional file 1: Demographic data. A total of 24 healthy control subjects (HC), 21 fever control subjects (FC), and 18 KD patients participated in this study. Each HC and FC subject contributed one tube of blood sample, whereas each KD patients contributed two tubes of blood samples, one at the acute phase before IVIG treatment (KD1) and one 3 weeks after IVIG treatment (KD3). (DOC 100 kb)

Additional file 2: Manhattan plot of p values in the KD1 vs HC comparison. We used a Manhattan plot to demonstrate the p values of

all CpG markers in the KD1 vs. HC comparison. In total, 482,421 CpG markers were plotted in this figure. (PNG 1154 kb)

Additional file 3: Manhattan plot of p values in the KD3 vs HC comparison. We used a Manhattan plot to demonstrate the p values of all CpG markers in the KD3 vs. HC comparison. In total, 482,421 CpG markers were plotted in this figure. (PNG 1025 kb)

Additional file 4: Manhattan plot of p values in the KD3 vs KD1 comparison. We used a Manhattan plot to demonstrate the p values of all CpG markers in the KD3 vs. KD1 comparison. In total, 482,421 CpG markers were plotted in this figure. (PNG 1078 kb)

Additional file 5: Methylation variations of all CpG markers within the putative promoter regions. By referring to the RefSeq 41 annotation, we can determine a CpG marker's distances to the transcription start site (TSS) of a gene' transcript. Then, we can also determine the relative locations of CpG markers within the putative promoter regions, which are the genomic regions ranging from the -5000 bp to $+3000$ bp of a transcript's TSS. (a, b, c) For each CpG marker, the X and Y axes denoted its methylation variation and its distance to the TSS, respectively. Using the two arrows, the promoter was split into three sub-regions, the left, the core, and the right sub-regions. The sample sizes for all sub-figures were 618,620, 618,553, and 618,553, respectively. (TIF 12711 kb)

Additional file 6: The scatter plots of all gene expression variations and all DNA methylation variations for CpG markers located within the putative promoters. Each dot denoted a regulation pair of one CpG marker and one gene, significant and non-significant. Since there were around 618,620 regulation pairs of CpG markers and genes in Additional file 5, we constructed the same number of random regulation pairs in the "Random" column. The sample sizes for the Both column were all 577,657; the sample sizes for Upstream column were all 347,878; the sample sizes for Downstream column were all 229,779. (TIF 785 kb)

Additional file 7: GO analysis results. We had the 80 genes analyzed with GO by mapping the genes to GO data set (Gene Ontology-Homo sapiens-2010-04-29). (XLS 344 kb)

Abbreviations

CAA: Coronary artery aneurysm; KD: Kawasaki disease; LTEM: Leukocyte trans-endothelium migration; TSS: Transcription start site

Acknowledgements

We thank the Genomics & Proteomics Core Laboratory, Department of Medical Research, Kaohsiung Chang Gung Memorial Hospital for technical supports. We thank Professor Wen-chang Lin for his valuable suggestions in this study.

Funding

This study was partly supported by the grants from the Ministry of Science and Technology, Taiwan (MOST 106-2311-B-182A-002 and MOST 105-2314-B-182 -050 -MY3) and Chang Gung Memorial Hospital (CMRPG8F0592, CMRPG8E0212, CORPG8F0012, CLRPG8G0591).

Authors' contributions

LHH, PHL, and YL conducted most of the experiments. HCK and YHH were responsible for the sample collection and microarray assays. CTP and YSL analyzed the data. SCL supervised this work. LHH and SCL wrote this manuscript. All authors read and approved the final manuscript.

Competing interests

The authors declare that they have no competing interests.

Author details

[1]Genomics and Proteomics Core Laboratory, Department of Medical Research, Kaohsiung Chang Gung Memorial Hospital, 12th Floor, Children's Hospital, No.123, Dapi Rd, Niaosong District, Kaohsiung 83301, Taiwan. [2]Department of Pediatrics, Kaohsiung Chang Gung Memorial Hospital and Chang Gung University College of Medicine, Kaohsiung, Taiwan. [3]Kawasaki Disease Center, Kaohsiung Chang Gung Memorial Hospital, Kaohsiung, Taiwan. [4]Institute of Bioinformatics and Systems Biology, National Chiao Tung University, Hsinchu, Taiwan. [5]Department of Biological Science and Technology, National Chiao Tung University, Hsinchu, Taiwan.

References

1. Moore LD, Le T, Fan G. DNA methylation and its basic function. Neuropsychopharmacology. 2013;38(1):23–38.
2. Irvine RA, Lin IG, Hsieh CL. DNA methylation has a local effect on transcription and histone acetylation. Mol Cell Biol. 2002;22(19):6689–96.
3. Chen WS, Leung CM, Pan HW, Hu LY, Li SC, Ho MR, Tsai KW. Silencing of miR-1-1 and miR-133a-2 cluster expression by DNA hypermethylation in colorectal cancer. Oncol Rep. 2012;28(3):1069–76.
4. Tsai KW, Liao YL, Wu CW, Hu LY, Li SC, Chan WC, Ho MR, Lai CH, Kao HW, Fang WL, et al. Aberrant hypermethylation of miR-9 genes in gastric cancer. Epigenetics. 2011;6(10):1189–97.
5. Tsai KW, Wu CW, Hu LY, Li SC, Liao YL, Lai CH, Kao HW, Fang WL, Huang KH, Chan WC, et al. Epigenetic regulation of miR-34b and miR-129 expression in gastric cancer. Int J Cancer. 2011;129(11):2600–10.
6. Tsai KW, Hu LY, Wu CW, Li SC, Lai CH, Kao HW, Fang WL, Lin WC. Epigenetic regulation of miR-196b expression in gastric cancer. Genes Chromosomes Cancer. 2010;49(11):969–80.
7. Liu Z, Feng Q, Sun P, Lu Y, Yang M, Zhang X, Jin X, Li Y, Lu SJ, Quan C. Genome-wide DNA methylation drives human embryonic stem cell erythropoiesis by remodeling gene expression dynamics. Epigenomics. 2017;9(12):1543–58.
8. Yang IV, Pedersen BS, Rabinovich E, Hennessy CE, Davidson EJ, Murphy E, Guardela BJ, Tedrow JR, Zhang Y, Singh MK, et al. Relationship of DNA methylation and gene expression in idiopathic pulmonary fibrosis. Am J Respir Crit Care Med. 2014;190(11):1263–72.
9. Schulz H, Ruppert AK, Herms S, Wolf C, Mirza-Schreiber N, Stegle O, Czamara D, Forstner AJ, Sivalingam S, Schoch S, et al. Genome-wide mapping of genetic determinants influencing DNA methylation and gene expression in human hippocampus. Nat Commun. 2017;8(1):1511.
10. Naumova OY, Lee M, Koposov R, Szyf M, Dozier M, Grigorenko EL. Differential patterns of whole-genome DNA methylation in institutionalized children and children raised by their biological parents. Dev Psychopathol. 2012;24(1):143–55.
11. Kucharski R, Maleszka J, Foret S, Maleszka R. Nutritional control of reproductive status in honeybees via DNA methylation. Science. 2008; 319(5871):1827–30.
12. Agarwal S, Agrawal DK. Kawasaki disease: etiopathogenesis and novel treatment strategies. Expert Rev Clin Immunol. 2017;13(3):247–58.
13. Burns JC, Glodé MP. Kawasaki syndrome. Lancet. 2004;364(9433):533–44.
14. Del Principe D, Pietraforte D, Gambardella L, Marchesi A, Tarissi de Jacobis I, Villani A, Malorni W, Straface E. Pathogenetic determinants in Kawasaki disease: the haematological point of view. J Cell Mol Med. 2017;21(4):632–9.
15. Kuo HC, Hsieh KS, Ming-Huey Guo M, Weng KP, Ger LP, Chan WC, Li SC. Next-generation sequencing identifies micro-RNA-based biomarker panel for Kawasaki disease. J Allergy Clin Immunol. 2016;138(4):1227–30.
16. Li SC, Chan WC, Huang YH, Guo MM, Yu HR, Huang FC, Kuo HC. Major methylation alterations on the CpG markers of inflammatory immune associated genes after IVIG treatment in Kawasaki disease. BMC Med Genet. 2016;9(Suppl 1):37.

17. Kuo HC, Chang JC, Yu HR, Wang CL, Lee CP, Huang LT, Yang KD. Identification of an association between genomic hypomethylation of FCGR2A and susceptibility to Kawasaki disease and intravenous immunoglobulin resistance by DNA methylation array. Arthritis Rheumatol. 2015;67(3):828–36.
18. Finegersh A, Kulich S, Guo T, Favorov AV, Fertig EJ, Danilova LV, Gaykalova DA, Califano JA, Duvvuri U. DNA methylation regulates TMEM16A/ANO1 expression through multiple CpG islands in head and neck squamous cell carcinoma. Sci Rep. 2017;7(1):15173.
19. Wagner JR, Busche S, Ge B, Kwan T, Pastinen T, Blanchette M. The relationship between DNA methylation, genetic and expression inter-individual variation in untransformed human fibroblasts. Genome Biol. 2014;15(2):R37.
20. Newburger JW, Takahashi M, Gerber MA, Gewitz MH, Tani LY, Burns JC, Shulman ST, Bolger AF, Ferrieri P, Baltimore RS, et al. Diagnosis, treatment, and long-term management of Kawasaki disease: a statement for health professionals from the Committee on Rheumatic Fever, Endocarditis and Kawasaki Disease, Council on Cardiovascular Disease in the Young, American Heart Association. Circulation. 2004;110(17):2747–71.
21. Megraw M, Baev V, Rusinov V, Jensen ST, Kalantidis K, Hatzigeorgiou AG. MicroRNA promoter element discovery in Arabidopsis. Rna. 2006;12(9):1612–9.
22. Wang X, Gu J, Zhang MQ, Li Y. Identification of phylogenetically conserved microRNA cis-regulatory elements across 12 Drosophila species. Bioinformatics. 2008;24(2):165–71.
23. Gebhardt C, Nemeth J, Angel P, Hess J. S100A8 and S100A9 in inflammation and cancer. Biochem Pharmacol. 2006;72(11):1622–31.
24. Donato R, Cannon BR, Sorci G, Riuzzi F, Hsu K, Weber DJ, Geczy CL. Functions of S100 proteins. Curr Mol Med. 2013;13(1):24–57.
25. Averill MM, Kerkhoff C, Bornfeldt KE. S100A8 and S100A9 in cardiovascular biology and disease. Arterioscler Thromb Vasc Biol. 2012;32(2):223–9.
26. Kraakman MJ, Lee MK, Al-Sharea A, Dragoljevic D, Barrett TJ, Montenont E, Basu D, Heywood S, Kammoun HL, Flynn M, et al. Neutrophil-derived S100 calcium-binding proteins A8/A9 promote reticulated thrombocytosis and atherogenesis in diabetes. J Clin Invest. 2017;127(6):2133–47.
27. Tan X, Zheng X, Huang Z, Lin J, Xie C, Lin Y. Involvement of S100A8/A9-TLR4-NLRP3 inflammasome pathway in contrast-induced acute kidney injury. Cell Physiol Biochem. 2017;43(1):209–22.
28. Ryckman C, Vandal K, Rouleau P, Talbot M, Tessier PA. Proinflammatory activities of S100: proteins S100A8, S100A9, and S100A8/A9 induce neutrophil chemotaxis and adhesion. J Immunol. 2003;170(6):3233–42.
29. Stangel M, Pul R. Basic principles of intravenous immunoglobulin (IVIg) treatment. J Neurol. 2006;253(Suppl 5):V18–24.
30. Ebihara T, Endo R, Kikuta H, Ishiguro N, Ma X, Shimazu M, Otoguro T, Kobayashi K. Differential gene expression of S100 protein family in leukocytes from patients with Kawasaki disease. Eur J Pediatr. 2005;164(7):427–31.
31. Ye F, Foell D, Hirono KI, Vogl T, Rui C, Yu X, Watanabe S, Watanabe K, Uese K, Hashimoto I, et al. Neutrophil-derived S100A12 is profoundly upregulated in the early stage of acute Kawasaki disease. Am J Cardiol. 2004;94(6):840–4.
32. Foell D, Ichida F, Vogl T, Yu X, Chen R, Miyawaki T, Sorg C, Roth J. S100A12 (EN-RAGE) in monitoring Kawasaki disease. Lancet. 2003;361(9365):1270–2.
33. Yasmin R, Siraj S, Hassan A, Khan AR, Abbasi R, Ahmad N. Epigenetic regulation of inflammatory cytokines and associated genes in human malignancies. Mediat Inflamm. 2015;2015:201703.
34. Gaspar C, Silva-Marrero JI, Salgado MC, Baanante IV, Meton I. Role of upstream stimulatory factor 2 in glutamate dehydrogenase gene transcription. J Mol Endocrinol. 2018;60(3):247–59.
35. Wang Y, Zhong T, Guo J, Li L, Zhang H, Wang L. Transcriptional regulation of pig GYS1 gene by glycogen synthase kinase 3beta (GSK3beta). Mol Cell Biochem. 2017;424(1–2):203–8.
36. Matsumoto M, Kogawa M, Wada S, Takayanagi H, Tsujimoto M, Katayama S, Hisatake K, Nogi Y. Essential role of p38 mitogen-activated protein kinase in cathepsin K gene expression during osteoclastogenesis through association of NFATc1 and PU.1. J Biol Chem. 2004;279(44):45969–79.
37. Tsai KW, Chang B, Pan CT, Lin WC, Chen TW, Li SC. Evaluation and application of the strand-specific protocol for next-generation sequencing. Biomed Res Int. 2015;2015:182389.
38. Walsh SW. Plasma from preeclamptic women stimulates transendothelial migration of neutrophils. Reprod Sci. 2009;16(3):320–5.

10

DNA methylation of imprinted genes at birth is associated with child weight status at birth, 1 year, and 3 years

Sarah Gonzalez-Nahm[1]* , Michelle A. Mendez[2], Sara E. Benjamin-Neelon[1], Susan K. Murphy[3], Vijaya K. Hogan[4], Diane L. Rowley[5] and Cathrine Hoyo[6]

Abstract

Background: This study assessed the associations between nine differentially methylated regions (DMRs) of imprinted genes in DNA derived from umbilical cord blood leukocytes in males and females and (1) birth weight for gestational age z score, (2) weight-for-length (WFL) z score at 1 year, and (3) body mass index (BMI) z score at 3 years.

Methods: We conducted multiple linear regression in $n = 567$ infants at birth, $n = 288$ children at 1 year, and $n = 294$ children at 3 years from the Newborn Epigenetics Study (NEST). We stratified by sex and adjusted for race/ethnicity, maternal education, maternal pre-pregnancy BMI, prenatal smoking, maternal age, gestational age, and paternal race. We also conducted analysis restricting to infants not born small for gestational age.

Results: We found an association between higher methylation of the sequences regulating paternally expressed gene 10 (*PEG10*) and anthropometric z scores at 1 year ($\beta = 0.84$; 95% CI = 0.34, 1.33; $p = 0.001$) and 3 years ($\beta = 1.03$; 95% CI = 0.37, 1.69; p value = 0.003) in males only. Higher methylation of the DMR regulating mesoderm-specific transcript (*MEST*) was associated with lower anthropometric z scores in females at 1 year ($\beta = -1.03$; 95% CI $-1.60, -0.45$; p value = 0.001) and 3 years ($\beta = -1.11$; 95% CI $-1.98, -0.24$; p value = 0.01). These associations persisted when we restricted to infants not born small for gestational age.

Conclusion: Our data support a sex-specific association between altered methylation and weight status in early life. These methylation marks can contribute to the compendium of epigenetically regulated regions detectable at birth, influencing obesity in childhood. Larger studies are required to confirm these findings.

Keywords: DNA methylation, Imprinted genes, Child weight

Background

Understanding factors that influence the risk of obesity in children is crucial to the development of new strategies for obesity prevention. Obesity in early childhood is a risk factor for obesity later in life [1–3] and for a number of chronic diseases in both childhood [4] and adulthood [5]. Birth weight has been associated with weight outcomes later in life, particularly for those who are on the extremes of the birth weight distribution [6–9]. Early identification of obesity or its risk factors will inform interventions to prevent the progression of obesity and its consequences later in life [10]. Consistent with the developmental origins of disease hypothesis, the intrauterine environment is hypothesized to influence an individual's later susceptibility for chronic diseases [11], including obesity [12, 13].

Epigenetic modifications have been proposed as a mechanism for the in utero origin of later obesity, and a growing literature has found supporting evidence [14–16]. DNA methylation is the most studied epigenetic mechanism in humans, due in part, to its stability. DNA methylation that controls the monoallelic expression of imprinted genes is established during gametogenesis and is stably maintained throughout somatic

* Correspondence: sarah.nahm@jhu.edu
[1]Department of Health, Behavior and Society, Johns Hopkins Bloomberg School of Public Health, 624 N Broadway, Baltimore, MD 21205, USA
Full list of author information is available at the end of the article

division [17–21] and therefore provides a stable "register" of early in utero exposures. A study of famine survivors found that adults who experienced famine in utero had hypo-methylation of the imprinted *IGF2* gene compared to their same sex siblings who had not experienced famine in utero [22]. The significance of this locus was reported to not have been replicated in this cohort using alternate techniques, including RRBS. However, this technique is generally biased toward CG-rich areas and may not have covered the specific and limited number of CpGs that comprise the IGF2 DMR. Additional genes, such as INSR and CPT1A, have also been identified in association with exposure to the Dutch famine [23]. Another study found that maternal nutrition, affected by striking seasonal variations in food intake in the Gambia, influenced methylation at *RBM46* [24]. A colorectal cancer study found that methylation status of the *IGF2/H19* imprinted locus of adult controls was maintained 3 years later [25]. Moreover, a study of NEST children between birth and age 1 year found similar results at the *IGF2/H19* locus [26].

Select imprinted genes have been identified as playing a role in the development of fetal over and undergrowth caused by imprinting defects. The IGF2 locus is used in clinical diagnostic settings to identify Beckwith-Wiedemann syndrome, which is characterized by overgrowth [27], and the H19 locus has been used in the diagnosis of Silver-Russell syndrome (SRS), which is characterized by undergrowth [28].

Although epigenetic data linking DNA methylation and childhood obesity has increased exponentially in the last 5 years [29, 30], few regions agnostically identified have been replicated. This could be in part due to differences in the ethnic composition; however, differences could also be due to the sex composition. At imprinted loci, weight has been associated with the *IGF2* locus. Studies have found a relationship between the *IGF2* domain and fetal growth [31–34] and children's body composition or weight [32, 35, 36]. Data with directional consistency in associations between additional differentially methylated regions (DMRs) and weight gain are required.

This study aims to assess the association between methylation at nine DMRs of imprinted genes and birth weight for gestational age (BW/GA) *z* score, weight-for-length (WFL) *z* score at 1 year, and BMI *z* score at 3 years. In this analysis, we include the following DMRs: *MEG3* and *MEG3-IG*, which are involved in regulating the delta-like 1 homolog/maternally expressed gene 3 imprinted domain on chromosome 14q32.2; *IGF2* and *H19*, which are involved in the imprinting of the insulin growth factor 2/*H19* domain on chromosome 11p15, which are located upstream of the imprinted promoters of *IGF2* and at the imprinting control region for the *IGF2/H19* imprinted domain near the *H19* promoter,

respectively; *PLAGL1* at the pleiomorphic adenoma gene-like 1 locus at 6q24.2; *MEST* at the mesoderm-specific transcript promoter at 7q32.2; *NNAT* at the neuronatin locus at 20q11.23; *PEG3* at the paternally expressed gene 3 promoter region at 19q13.43; and *PEG10* at the epsilon sarcoglycan and paternally expressed gene 10 promoter region at 7q21.3. We selected these regions for their association with infant and child growth [32, 34, 37], chronic disease [22, 38], and parental obesity [39].

Methods
Study sample and data collection
We included data from mothers and children in the Newborn Epigenetic Study (NEST). We have described recruitment and enrollment strategies in detail elsewhere [40]. Briefly, between 2009 and 2011, we recruited women from five prenatal clinics and obstetric facilities in Durham, North Carolina. Eligibility criteria included being at least 18 years of age and intention to use one of the qualifying obstetric facilities for delivery. We excluded women if they planned to relinquish custody of the child or planned to move away from the area in the following 3 years. We obtained written informed consent from all participating women. Upon enrollment, mothers completed questionnaires providing information on sociodemographic factors, lifestyle characteristics, and anthropometrics. At delivery, study personnel abstracted birth outcomes from medical records and infant cord blood specimens were obtained to assess offspring methylation. At 1 year, we collected data on child anthropometrics, feeding, and lifestyle. This study was approved by the Institutional Review Board at Duke University Medical Center.

Of the 1700 enrolled, we excluded 396 women for reasons including miscarriage, refusing further participation, moving away from the area, or delivering at a hospital not included in the study. We analyzed DNA methylation data for the first 600 infants in the study. Infants with analyzed DNA methylation were not significantly different than infants whose DNA methylation had been analyzed with respect to race, maternal education, maternal smoking status, maternal pre-pregnancy BMI, maternal age, or weight at age 1 (data not shown).

Among infants with DNA methylation data, birth weight and length measurements were available for 594. At age 1, we used available weight and length measurements for 306 infants, and at age 3, we used available weight and height measurements for 314 children. We calculated BW/GA *z* scores using an international standard [41]. We classified infants with BW/GA below the 10th percentile as small for gestational age (SGA). We calculated WFL *z* scores at age 1 year using WHO standards for children's exact age [42]. We then calculated

BMI z scores at age 3 years using CDC standards [43]. We excluded 7 children with a WFL z score greater than 5 or less than -5 at age 1 year, and 11 children with a BMI z score greater than 5 or less than -5. In addition, we excluded infants with possible growth disorders or imprinting defects; therefore, we excluded from analysis infants with DNA methylation values ± 4 standard deviations from the mean ($n = 6$). The current study includes children with available DNA methylation data at birth on at least one of the nine DMRs of interest, and who had plausible length and weight measurements at birth ($n = 576$), age 1 ($n = 288$), or age 3 ($n = 294$). Plausible weight and length was defined as a measurement that fell within the SD limits set for the combined WFL or BMI and that clearly was not a transcript error (e.g., birth weight being copied onto 1-year weight). In addition, we conducted supplemental analysis on 166 children who had non-missing anthropometric values at birth and age 1 and 3 years to assess directional consistency over time.

DNA methylation

Specimen collection and DNA methylation methods have been described in detail elsewhere [26]. Briefly, we collected infant cord blood specimens at birth. We collected samples in EDTA-containing vacutainer tubes and centrifuged using standard protocols to allow for collection of plasma and buffy coat, with buffy coat used for DNA extraction (Qiagen; Valencia, CA). We stored specimens at $-80\ °C$ until the time of analysis. We extracted DNA using Puregene reagents according to the manufacturer's protocol (Qiagen) and assessed quantity and quality using a Nanodrop 1000 Spectrophotometer (Thermo Scientific; Wilmington, DE).

We modified infant genomic DNA (800 ng) by treatment with sodium bisulfite using the EZ DNA Methylation kit (Zymo Research; Irvine, CA). Bisulfite treatment of denatured DNA converts all unmethylated cytosines to uracils, leaving methylated cytosines unchanged, allowing for quantitative measurement of cytosine methylation status. We performed pyrosequencing using a PyroMark Q96 MD pyrosequencer (Qiagen). Pyrosequencing assay design, genomic coordinates, assay conditions, and assay validation are described in detail elsewhere [33]. Briefly, we designed assays to query established imprinted gene DMRs using the PyroMark Assay Design Software (Qiagen). We optimized PCR conditions to produce a single, robust amplification product. We used defined mixtures of fully methylated and unmethylated control DNAs to show a linear increase in detection of methylation values as the level of input DNA methylation increased (Pearson r is 0.99 for all DMRs). Once we defined optimal conditions, we analyzed each DMR using the same amount of input DNA from each specimen (40 ng, assuming complete

recovery following bisulfite modification of 800 ng DNA). We determined percentage of methylation for each CpG cytosine using Pyro Q-CpG software (Qiagen). We performed pyrosequencing assays in duplicate for all specimens whose values fell more than two SD above or below the means, in which case we used the average of the two runs. The values obtained represent the mean methylation for the CpG sites contained within the sequence being analyzed (Additional file 1: Figure S1).

Statistical analysis

We calculated frequencies and means of sociodemographic variables and conducted multiple linear regression to test the association between DNA methylation and early anthropometric outcomes. We determined covariates a priori based on directed acyclic graphs (DAG). We chose sex as a potential effect measure modifier (EMM), as DNA methylation has been previously shown to vary by sex [44, 45]. We tested the following covariates as potential confounders: maternal education (less than a college degree/college degree or greater), maternal gestational diabetes (yes/no), maternal pre-pregnancy BMI, maternal smoking at any time during pregnancy (yes/no), gestational weight gain, parity (primiparous, multiparous), maternal age at delivery, gestational age, paternal race, maternal race, and date of length and weight measurements relative to child's birthday. We tested potential confounders in the model one at a time and kept variables if they changed the estimate by more than 10%. Final models included maternal race, maternal education, maternal pre-pregnancy BMI, maternal smoking, maternal age, gestational age, and paternal race. As infants who are SGA may have different growth patterns compared to infants who are average for gestational age, we conducted supplemental analysis to determine the effect of excluding infants who were SGA. We also conducted supplemental analysis including maternal alcohol consumption during pregnancy as a covariate, and an additional supplemental analysis, in which we stratified by race/ethnicity to determine possible effect measure modification.

Previously reported Cronbach's alpha for correlations among methylation values from all CpGs measured at each DMR was > 0.89 [40]; therefore, we used mean DNA methylation values for each DMR. DNA methylation was assessed in tertiles (low, moderate, high), as both higher and lower levels of methylation have been associated with health outcomes, depending on the DMR [39, 40]. Given the expected 50% methylation of imprinted genes, we used the mid tertile of methylation as the referent category. Thus, results represent the child z scores associated with high or low methylation compared to "moderate" methylation. We conducted all statistical analysis using SAS 9.4 (SAS Institute, Inc., Cary, NC).

Among infants, 37.0% of mothers were African American, 28.3% were White/Caucasian, and 34.7% were of other races/ethnicities including Hispanic and Asian/Pacific Islander (Table 1). For the 1-year sample, 37.9% of mothers were African American, 30.2% were White, and 31.9% were "other" race. For the 3-year sample, 39.4% of mothers were African American, 28.3% were White, and 32.3% were of other races and ethnicities. In all samples, the majority of women in the study completed less than a college degree (70.8% for newborns, 66.4% for age 1 year, and 68.4% for age 3 years) and reported not smoking at any point during pregnancy (83, 85.5, and 85.3% for newborns, age 1, and age 3, respectively). Approximately half of the newborn sample reported some sort of alcohol consumption in early pregnancy (50.9%). The mean (SD) maternal age for women in the birth sample was 28 years ($\pm$ 5.7). Mothers in the 1-year sample were on average 28.0 ($\pm$ 5.8) years, and those in the 3-year sample were on average 28.1 ($\pm$ 5.8) years. The mean maternal pre-pregnancy BMI for women in the birth weight sample was 27.4 ($\pm$ 7.2), BMI for mothers in the 1-year sample was 28.0, and BMI for mothers in the 3-year sample was 28.1 ($\pm$ 5.8) years. The mean gestational age for the sample at birth was 38.7 (1.7) weeks. The mean birthweight of infants in the sample was 3304 g ($\pm$ 540). There were no significant differences in the study sample demographic makeup between children or mothers in the newborn, age 1 year, or age 3 year samples (data not shown). However, women were more likely to be college educated in the sample of 166

Table 1 Sociodemographic characteristics of study sample

	Newborn	1 year	3 years	Complete cases
Birth weight (grams), mean (SD)	3304.2 (540.3)	–	–	3279.8 (621.1)
Child BMI (kg), mean (SD)	–		16.4 (2.1)	16.4 (1.9)
Birth weight for gestational age z score, mean (SD)	– 0.09 (1.0)	–	–	– 0.01 (0.9)
BMI z score, mean (SD)	–	–	0.15 (1.3)	0.20 (1.5)
Weight-for-length z score, mean (SD)	–	0.83 (1.9)	–	0.78 (1.3)
Race, N (%)				
Black	213 (37)	109 (37.9)	117 (39.4)	66 (39.8)
White	163 (28.3)	87 (30.2)	84 (28.3)	44 (26.5)
Other	200 (34.7)	92 (31.9)	96 (32.3)	56 (33.7)
Maternal education, N (%)				
Less than HS	175 (32.1)	86 (30.1)	87 (29.9)	48 (29.1)
Completed high school	211 (38.7)	104 (36.3)	112 (38.5)	61 (37.0)
Completed college	159 (29.2)	96 (33.6)	92 (31.6)	56 (33.9)
Missing	31	2	6	1
Maternal smoking, N (%)				
Yes	91 (17)	41 (14.5)	42 (14.7)	23 (14.2)
No	445 (83)	242 (85.5)	243 (85.3)	139 (85.8)
Missing	40	5	12	4
Maternal alcohol consumption, N (%)				
Yes	179 (50.9)	105 (54.4)	98 (51.0)	63 (57.3)
No	173 (49.1)	88 (45.6)	94 (49.0)	64 (42.7)
Missing	224	95	104	56
Maternal age, mean (SD)	27.8 (5.8)	28.0 (5.8)	28.1 (5.8)	27.9 (5.6)
Maternal pre-pregnancy BMI, mean (SD)	27.6 (7.2)	27.1 (6.6)	27.4 (6.9)	27.2 (6.6)
Gestational age	38.7 (1.7)	38.5 (2.0)	38.6 (1.9)	38.7 (2.1)
Infant sex, N (%)				
Male	299 (52.1)	149 (51.7)	152 (51.2)	86 (51.8)
Female	275 (47.9)	139 (48.3)	145 (48.8)	80 (48.2)

complete cases, in which children had anthropometric data for all 3 time points.

Results

Birth weight and DNA methylation by sex

In girls, we observed a statistically significant association between high methylation at MEST and greater birth weight for gestational age ($\beta = 0.45$; 95% CI 0.12, 0.78; p value 0.007; data not shown). However, this association did not persist after adjustment. We observed no statistically significant associations between methylation and birth weight for gestational age z scores in boys.

Weight-for-length z scores at 1 year and DNA methylation by sex

After adjustment (Table 2), we observed an association between high PEG10 DMR methylation and greater WFL z scores at 1 year in boys ($\beta = 0.84$; 95% CI 0.34, 1.33; p value = 0.001). Alternatively, low methylation at IGF2 DMR was associated with a lower WFL z score at 1 year in boys ($\beta = -0.63$; 95% CI -1.16, -0.10; p value = 0.02). In girls, both low and high methylation at the PLAGL1 DMR (low: $\beta = 0.72$; 95% CI 1.19, -0.25; p value = 0.003; high: $\beta = -0.81$; 95% CI -1.29, -0.33; p value = 0.0001) and the MEST DMR (low: $\beta = -0.99$; 95% CI -1.59, -0.39; p value = 0.002; high: $\beta = -1.03$; 95% CI -1.60, -0.45;

Table 2 Adjusted results of the association between DNA methylation at birth and birth weight for gestational age z scores, BMI z scores at age 1 and age 3

	Birth weight for gestational age		WFL age 1		BMI age 3	
	Boys	Girls	Boys	Girls	Boys	Girls
	β (95% CI)	β (95% CI)	β (95% CI)	β (95% CI)	β (95% CI)	β (95% CI)
MEG3						
Low	0.09 (− 0.23, 0.40)	0.10 (− 0.22, 0.42)	− 0.67 (− 1.23, − 0.11)	− 0.16 (− 0.70, 0.38)	0.11 (− 0.58, 0.80)	− 0.21 (− 1.04, 0.61)
High	− 0.05 (− 0.35, 0.26)	− 0.26 (− 0.56, 0.04)	− 0.79 (− 1.37, − 0.21)	− 0.08 (− 0.58, 0.42)	0.05 (− 0.64, 0.74)	− 0.29 (− 1.10, 0.52)
PLAGL1						
Low	0.20 (− 0.08, 0.49)	0.24 (− 0.06, 0.54)	0.02 (− 0.50, 0.53)	− 0.72** (− 1.19, − 0.25)	0.12 (− 0.53, 0.76)	0.39 (− 1.40, 1.19)
High	0.13 (− 0.16, 0.43)	0.14 (− 0.16, 0.44)	0.52 (− 0.003, 1.04)	− 0.81** (− 1.29, − 0.33)	0.31 (− 0.32, 0.93)	− 0.07 (− 0.81, 0.67)
PEG10						
Low	− 0.10 (− 0.39, 0.20)	0.31 (− 0.003, 0.63)	0.20 (− 0.31, 0.71)	− 0.03 (− 0.59, 0.52)	0.32 (− 0.32, 0.95)	0.14 (− 0.70, 0.97)
High	0.01 (− 0.31, 0.32)	0.09 (− 0.24, 0.43)	0.84** (0.34, 1.33)	0.03 (− 0.51, 0.58)	1.03** (0.37, 1.69)	0.04 (− 0.82, 0.89)
IGF2						
Low	− 0.15 (− 0.46, 0.16)	0.40 (0.08, 0.72)	− 0.63* (− 1.16, − 0.10)	0.24 (− 0.28, 0.75)	− 0.12 (− 0.76, 0.52)	− 0.10 (− 0.87, 0.66)
High	0.06 (− 0.26, 0.38)	0.21 (− 0.11, 0.53)	− 0.21 (− 0.73, 0.31)	− 0.03 (− 0.53, 0.48)	− 0.14 (− 0.80, 0.52)	− 0.61 (− 1.39, 0.18)
MEST						
Low	0.04 (− 0.27, 0.34)	0.21 (− 0.12, 0.34)	0.07 (− 0.47, 0.61)	− 0.99** (− 1.59, − 0.39)	0.26 (− 0.43, 0.94)	− 0.41 (− 1.28, 0.45)
High	− 0.04 (− 0.26, 0.38)	0.38 (0.04, 0.72)	0.32 (− 0.23, 0.86)	− 1.03** (− 1.60, − 0.45)	0.08 (− 0.63, 0.79)	− 1.11* (− 1.98, − 0.24)
MEG3-IG						
Low	− 0.01 (− 0.31, 0.34)	− 0.07 (− 0.41, 0.27)	0.09 (− 0.47, 0.65)	− 0.56 (− 1.13, 0.02)	− 0.24 (− 0.92, 0.45)	− 0.62 (− 1.44, 0.21)
High	− 0.31 (− 0.66, 0.05)	− 0.08 (− 0.42, 0.26)	− 0.44 (− 1.00, 0.12)	− 0.30 (− 0.83, 0.23)	− 0.10 (− 0.87, 0.67)	− 0.80 (− 1.68, 0.08)
H19						
Low	0.29 (−0.04, 0.62)	0.04 (− 0.26, 0.35)	0.26 (− 0.29, 0.80)	− 0.13 (− 0.63, 0.37)	0.24 (− 0.48, 0.96)	0.09 (− 0.73, 0.90)
High	0.03 (− 0.30, 0.36)	0.22 (− 0.09, 0.54)	0.29 (− 0.25, 0.82)	− 0.51 (− 1.02, 0.01)	0.39 (− 0.30, 1.09)	0.34 (− 0.50, 1.19)
NNAT						
Low	− 0.06 (− 0.40, 0.28)	− 0.07 (− 0.41, 0.28)	− 0.28 (− 0.89, 0.34)	0.24 (− 0.25, 0.72)	− 0.26 (− 1.00, 0.48)	1.52** (0.69, 2.34)
High	− 0.07 (− 0.42, 0.27)	0.16 (− 0.18, 0.50)	− 0.10 (− 0.69, 0.48)	0.26 (− 0.26, 0.79)	− 0.14 (− 0.82, 0.54)	0.55 (− 0.27, 1.37)
PEG3						
Low	0.09 (− 0.19, 0.38)	− 0.09 (− 0.41, 0.23)	− 0.15 (− 0.72, 0.42)	− 0.29 (− 0.84, 0.26)	0.41 (− 0.23, 1.05)	− 0.95* (− 1.80, − 0.10)
High	0.06 (− 0.25, 0.38)	− 0.15 (− 0.48, 0.18)	− 0.20 (− 0.76, 0.37)	− 0.48 (− 1.02, 0.06)	− 0.18 (− 0.91, 0.55)	− 0.46 (− 1.35, 0.44)

Adjusted for maternal and paternal race, maternal education, maternal smoking, maternal pre-pregnancy BMI, maternal age, and gestational age. DNA methylation measured in tertiles, comparing low and high methylation to moderate methylation

*$p < 0.05$. **Statistically significant after Bonferroni correction ($p < 0.006$)

p value = 0.001) were associated with lower WFL z scores at age 1 year after adjustment (Fig. 1).

BMI z scores at 3 years and DNA methylation by sex

At age 3 years, the association between high methylation at the *PEG10* DMR and greater anthropometric z score persisted after adjustment in boys (β = 1.03; 95% CI 0.37, 1.69; p value 0.003). In girls, the association between high methylation at the *MEST* DMR and lower anthropometric z score also persisted after adjustment (β = − 1.11; 95%CI − 1.98, − 0.24; p value 0.01). In addition, we observed an association between low methylation at the *PEG3* DMR and lower BMI z score at 3 years after adjustment in girls (β = − 0.95; 95% CI − 1.80, − 0.10; p value = 0.03).

Analysis excluding SGA infants

When excluding SGA infants (n = 69 at birth, n = 31 at 1 year, n = 27 at 3 years), additional associations emerged at the *MEST* DMR at birth and the *MEG3*, *H19*, and *NNAT* DMRs at 1 year of age (data not shown). High methylation at the *MEST* DMR was associated with a greater BW/GA z score in girls (β = 0.32; 95% CI 0.009, 0.63; p value = 0.04). At 1 year, high and low methylation at the *MEG3* DMR were associated with a lower WFL z score in boys (low: β = − 0.81; 95% CI − 1.44, − 0.18; p value = 0.01; high: β = − 0.91; 95% CI − 1.57, − 0.25; p value = 0.008). In girls, high methylation at the *H19* DMR was also associated with a lower WFL z score (β = − 0.58; 95% CI − 1.15, − 0.008; p value = 0.047), and lower methylation at the *NNAT* DMR was associated with a greater WFL z score (β = 0.63; 95% CI 0.13, 1.13; p value = 0.02). All other associations, with the exception of the association between

low methylation at the *IGF2* DMR and a lower WFL z score at 1 year, persisted after exclusion of SGA infants.

Analysis including maternal alcohol consumption as a covariate

We conducted additional analyses, in which we included maternal alcohol consumption during early pregnancy as a covariate. We found that all associations between methylation and WFL z scores at 1 year remained statistically significant compared to our main analysis (data not shown). Additionally, we observed an association between low IGF2 methylation and greater birth weight for gestational age z score in girls (β = 0.53; 95% CI 0.13, 0.93; p value = 0.01) and an association between both low and high *MEST* DMR methylation and lower BMI z scores at 3 years in girls (low: β = − 1.31; 95% CI − 2.46, − 0.15; p value = 0.03; high: β = − 1.40; 95% CI − 2.51, − 0.29; p value = 0.01).

Analysis stratified by race/ethnicity

Additionally, we conducted supplemental stratified analyses to see if there were differences by race/ethnicity, as previous studies have found differential methylation in association with race/ethnicity. The only statistically significant association we observed was between low methylation at the *MEST* DMR and greater birth weight for gestational z scores among Blacks (β = 0.54; 95% CI 0.09, 0.99; p value = 0.02—data not shown). At year 1, we found an association between high *PEG10* DMR methylation and greater WFL z scores among Blacks and Whites (Blacks: β = 0.69; 95% CI 0.12, 1.27; p value = 0.02; Whites: β = 0.66; 95% CI 0.11, 1.21; p value = 0.02). We also found an association between high *MEG3*-IG DMR methylation

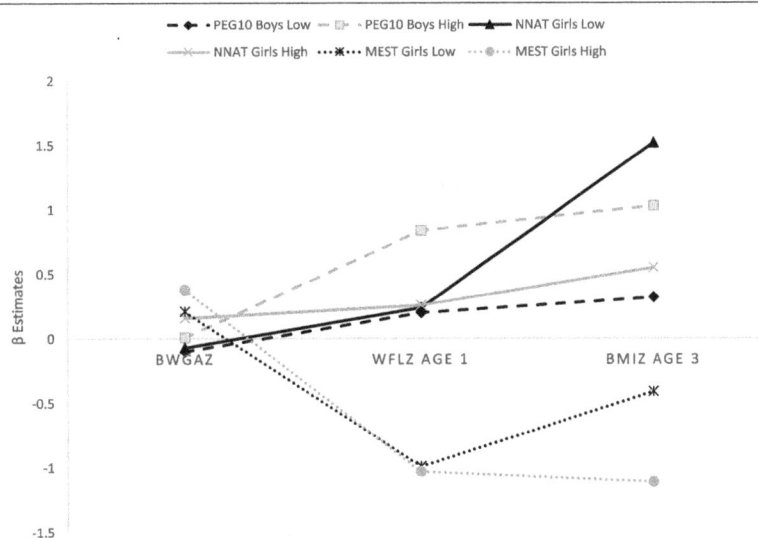

Fig. 1 Association between select DMR methylation and BW/GA z scores, WFL z scores age 1 year, and BMI z scores age 3 years. Comparison of girls vs. boys at *PEG10*, *NNAT*, and *MEST* DMRs

and lower WFL z scores among Whites ($\beta = -0.64$; 95% CI -1.25, -0.03; p value = 0.04). At 3 years, we found an association between low $MEG3$-IG DMR methylation and lower BMI z scores among Blacks ($\beta = -0.76$; 95% CI -1.48, -0.05; p value = 0.04). An association was also observed between low $NNAT$ DMR methylation and greater BMI z scores among Blacks ($\beta = 0.99$; 95% CI 0.14, 1.84; p value = 0.02).

Complete case analysis

Supplemental analysis on the 166 infants ($n = 15$ SGA children) who had non-missing anthropometric data for all 3 time points showed directional consistency in all associations. However, not all associations remained statistically significant in the smaller sample (Table 3). In girls, the association between high methylation at the $PLAGL1$ DMR and lower WFL z scores remained statistically significant ($\beta = -0.82$; 95% CI -1.51, -0.12; p value = 0.02), as did the associations between low and high methylation at the $MEST$ DMR and WFL z scores (low: $\beta = -1.18$; 95% CI -2.04, -32; p value = 0.009; high: $\beta = -1.57$; 95% CI -2.4, -0.73; p value = 0.0004). At 3 years in boys, the association between high $PEG10$ DMR methylation and greater BMI z scores remained statistically significant ($\beta = 1.25$; 95% CI 0.38, 2.12; p value = 0.006). In girls, the association between lower $PEG3$ DMR methylation and lower BMI z scores at 3 years also remained statistically significant ($\beta = -1.30$; 95% CI -2.34, 0.26; p value = 0.02). Notably, additional statistically significant associations were observed

Table 3 Supplemental analysis: complete cases: adjusted regression of DNA methylation at birth and anthropometric z scores

| | BW/GA | | WFL z scores 1 year | | BMI z scores 3 years | |
| | Boys | Girls | Boys | Girls | Boys | Girls |
	β (95% CI)	β (95% CI)	β (95% CI)	β (95% CI)	β (95% CI)	β (95% CI)
MEG3						
Low	0.46 (−0.08, 0.10)	0.23 (−0.43, 0.85)	−0.73 (−1.56, 0.09)	0.01 (−0.69, 0.71)	−0.22 (−1.26, 0.83)	0.24 (−0.79, 1.27)
High	0.04 (−0.53, 0.60)	−0.02 (−0.68, 0.63)	−0.87 (−1.73, 0.00)	0.47 (−0.25, 1.18)	−0.10 (−1.20, 0.99)	−0.17 (−1.22, 0.87)
PLAGL1						
Low	0.20 (−0.29, 0.70)	0.30 (−0.30, 0.89)	−0.13 (−0.89, 0.64)	−0.46 (−1.17, 0.25)	0.07 (−0.82, 0.97)	−0.04 (−1.01, 0.94)
High	0.26 (−0.24, 0.76)	0.13 (−0.44, 0.71)	0.22 (−0.53, 0.97)	−0.82* (−1.51, −0.12)	0.82 (−0.06, 1.70)	0.05 (−0.90, 1.00)
PEG10						
Low	−0.35 (−0.86, 0.16)	0.40 (−0.21, 1.00)	0.06 (−0.77, 0.88)	0.11 (−0.69, 0.90)	0.53 (−0.39, 1.46)	0.54 (−0.47, 1.56)
High	0.03 (−0.44, 0.50)	0.63* (0.07, 1.19)	0.65 (−0.12, 1.42)	0.01 (−0.73, 0.74)	1.25* (0.38, 2.12)	0.64 (−0.31, 1.58)
IGF2						
Low	−0.46 (−1.02, 0.10)	0.21 (−0.37, 0.78)	−0.51 (−1.27, 0.25)	0.30 (−0.46, 1.06)	−0.40 (−1.35, 0.55)	0.40 (−0.58, 1.38)
High	−0.17 (−0.70, 0.36)	0.58* (0.03, 1.12)	−0.02 (−0.73, 0.68)	−0.28 (−0.99, 0.43)	−0.36 (−1.25, 0.53)	−0.25 (−1.17, 0.66)
MEST						
Low	0.41 (−0.13, 0.95)	−0.17 (−0.85, 0.50)	0.20 (−0.58, 0.99)	−1.18* (−2.03, −0.32)	0.03 (−0.98, 1.05)	−0.36 (−1.57, 0.86)
High	−0.05 (−0.56, 0.47)	0.62 (−0.04, 1.28)	0.38 (−0.37, 1.12)	−1.57** (−2.41, −0.74)	−0.14 (−1.11, 0.82)	−1.09 (−2.27, 0.08)
MEG3-IG						
Low	−0.10 (−0.59, 0.39)	−0.58 (−1.30, 0.13)	−0.22 (−0.98, 0.55)	−0.14 (−1.03, 0.75)	−0.60 (−1.56, 0.36)	−0.15 (−1.08, 0.78)
High	−0.77* (−1.29, −0.24)	−0.10 (−0.77, 0.56)	−0.70 (−1.52, 0.12)	−0.16 (−0.98, 0.67)	−0.19 (−1.22, 0.83)	−0.59 (−1.46, 0.27)
H19						
Low	0.21 (−0.32, 0.73)	−0.28 (−0.86, 0.31)	−0.001 (−0.77, 0.77)	0.24 (−0.53, 1.01)	0.53 (−0.39, 1.46)	0.06 (−0.97, 1.06)
High	0.01 (−0.52, 0.53)	0.23 (−0.33, 0.79)	−0.001 (−0.75, 0.75)	−0.41 (−1.13, 0.32)	0.45 (−0.45, 1.35)	−0.08 (−1.05, 0.89)
NNAT						
Low	0.07 (−0.48, 0.61)	−0.41 (−1.02, 0.20)	−0.89* (−1.68, −0.09)	0.47 (−0.18, 1.13)	−0.59 (−1.60, 0.42)	1.12* (0.09, 2.15)
High	−0.26 (−0.76, 0.24)	0.39 (−0.30, 1.08)	−0.53 (−1.27, 0.22)	0.39 (−0.34, 1.12)	−0.31 (−1.25, 0.63)	0.24 (−0.91, 1.38)
PEG3						
Low	0.03 (−0.52, 0.58)	0.16 (−0.46, 0.78)	−0.22 (−1.07, 0.62)	0.00 (−0.81, 0.81)	0.46 (−0.48, 1.40)	−1.30* (−2.34, −0.25)
High	0.06 (−0.54, 0.65)	0.42 (−0.20, 1.04)	−0.26 (−1.17, 0.66)	−0.30 (−1.12, 0.52)	−0.31 (−1.33, 0.71)	−0.86 (−1.91, 0.20)

Adjusted for maternal and paternal race, maternal education, maternal smoking, maternal pre-pregnancy BMI, maternal age, and gestational age. DNA methylation measured in tertiles, comparing low and high methylation to moderate methylation
*$p < 0.05$. **Statistically significant after Bonferroni correction ($p < 0.006$)

between high methylation at the *MEG3*-IG DMR and lower birth weight for gestational age z scores in boys ($\beta = -0.77$; 95% CI -1.30, -0.24; p value = 0.005) and between high methylation at the *IGF2* and *PEG10* DMRs and greater birth weight for gestational age z scores in girls (*IGF2*: $\beta = 0.58$; 95% CI 0.03, 1.12; p value = 0.04; *PEG10*: $\beta = 0.63$; 95% CI 0.07, 1.20; p value = 0.03).

Discussion

In these analyses, we examined DNA methylation of nine regulatory regions at birth and anthropometric measures at birth and age 1 and 3 years. No DMR showed a consistent association between methylation and anthropometric z scores at all 3 time points explored. Our key findings were that high methylation of the sequences regulating the *PEG10* DMR at birth was associated with a higher age 1-year WFL z score and 3-year BMI z score in boys, low methylation at the *NNAT* DMR was associated with higher BMI z scores at age 3 in girls, and high methylation was associated with lower WFL z scores at 1 year and BMI z scores at 3 years. These associations persisted after excluding SGA infants. Additional findings included associations between methylation at the *PLAGL1* DMR and WFL z scores in girls at age 1, as well as an association at the *IGF2* DMR at age 1 among boys. At age 3, we also observed an association between methylation at the *PEG3* DMR and BMI z scores in girls. These results suggest that methylation of imprinted genes at birth is associated with anthropometric measures at ages 1 and 3 years, with the *PEG10* and *NNAT* DMRs potentially indicating an early risk for obesity, and *MEST* potentially indicating a lower risk for obesity.

This study adds to a growing body of epidemiologic evidence on early postnatal growth associated with DNA methylation at birth and suggests that DNA methylation at multiple DMRs may be associated with WFL z score at age 1 year and BMI z score at age 3 years. *PLAGL1*, *MEST*, *NNAT*, and *PEG10* have been associated with obesity or weight in previous literature. Paternal obesity has been previously associated with reduced *PEG10* transcription in mouse placentas [46]. Our results indicating a higher level of *PEG10* methylation is associated with a greater BMI z score show a similar pattern. Previous literature has also shown a possible association between increased *MEST* expression and inhibition of adipogenesis [47]. The results of this study echo these findings, as boys with higher than average methylation levels had lower BMI z scores. Methylation at the *MEST*, *NNAT*, and *PEG10* DMRs has also been previously associated with paternal obesity [39], and small and large for gestational age [48, 49]. In addition, the *NNAT* gene has been associated with severe obesity in childhood and adulthood [50]. Higher methylation at *PLAGL1* has also

been associated with maternal obesity [39], and fetal and postnatal growth [37]. A previous study found a positive correlation between *PLAGL1* methylation and BMI z scores at age 1 year. *PLAGL1* is thought to be an imprint control region [51]; however, the implications of this in relation to a potential role in the risk of early obesity are not yet clear. More research is needed to gain a better understanding of the relationship between child BMI and methylation at these DMRs. Previous literature has supported the role of the *IGF2* DMR in fetal growth [31–34] and birth weight [32, 52], as well as infant weight gain [32, 36] and child adiposity [35]. We observed an association between *IGF2* methylation and lower BMI z scores; however, this association was not seen at birth or age 3 years.

We observed sex-specific differences in the associations between DNA methylation at birth and anthropometric z scores at ages 1 and 3 years. Sex-specific methylation has been previously observed in relation to nutrition and other environmental exposures [44, 45, 53], as well as in relation to outcomes, such as small for gestational age [54]. However, these studies did not find sex-specific differences in methylation in *PEG10*, *NNAT*, or *MEST*. This study also adds to the growing literature on sex-specific DNA methylation.

We conducted additional analysis to explore the influence of infants who are SGA, as their growth patterns may differ from those of infants who are not SGA, and found that SGA may be associated with DNA methylation. No associations between methylation and BW/GA z scores remained significant after SGA exclusion, suggesting that SGA may have been driving these associations. We also found that associations between *PEG3* and BMI z scores at both ages 1 and 3 years became statistically significant after exclusion of SGA infants. This suggests that perhaps the association between *PEG3* methylation and SGA is in the opposite direction of the association between *PEG3* methylation and BMI z scores for non-SGA infants, thus attenuating the original association. However, a cautious interpretation is warranted, as exclusion of SGA infants also decreased the statistical power, which may have led to unstable estimates. Additional supplemental analysis including only the 166 infants who had non-missing anthropometric values at all 3 time points showed that many of our associations remained statistically significant, including our key findings at the *PEG10* and *NNAT* DMRs. This suggests that these associations were not related to differences in the samples at each time point. Additional associations emerged as statistically significant at *MEST*, *IGF2*, *PEG10*, and *NNAT*; however, these results must be interpreted with caution, as the analysis was underpowered. Similarly, the results of the supplemental analysis including maternal alcohol consumption and the analysis stratified by race/ethnicity should be interpreted with caution, as our sample size was greatly reduced, and estimates may be underpowered.

The direction of the association between higher methylation at *MEST* and *z* scores changed from positive to negative from birth to ages 1 and 3. The reasons for this are unclear; however, it is possible that the modest increase in BW/GA *z* scores at birth, which we found to be associated with a higher level of methylation at *MEST*, is also associated with a greater likelihood of becoming lean as the child grows and becomes more mobile. *MEST* expression has been previously associated with obesity in mice [55]; however, a study in humans found *MEST* to possibly inhibit adipogenesis [47].

This study benefits from an ethnically diverse cohort, and prospectively collected data at multiple time points. This facilitates a better understanding of the timing of methylation with regard to our outcome of interest, weight gain. In addition, the use of BMI *z* scores provides widely accepted estimate of adiposity that accounts for a child's age. However, it is not without limitations. Our study only included nine DMRs of imprinted genes. Although these genes were chosen because they have been linked to growth or chronic disease, it is possible that important genes have been left out of this study. In addition, our study's small sample size may have limited our ability to see statistically significant differences associated with DNA methylation among our population. Although our analyses were hypothesis driven, multiple testing is a limitation in this study, as it may increase the possibility that our results are observed by chance. However, many associations remained (*PEG10, MEST, PLAGL1, NNAT*) even after the stringent Bonferroni correction. A final limitation was the use of weight status instead of weight gain. Much of the literature has pointed to weight gain in the first year of life as being associated with later obesity [8]; however, there is some literature indicating high weight status in early childhood as a risk factor for later obesity [56]. It is unclear whether or not these findings are related to later obesity.

In addition, the results of this study show differences in anthropometric *z* scores in association with DNA methylation that is either lower or higher than the "average" methylation of our study sample. Notably, the actual change in continuous methylation associated with our results is likely small (approximately 1%). However, even a 1% change in methylation has been previously shown to result in a doubling or halving of gene expression at these imprint regulatory regions [45]. Not assessing DNA methylation continuously may be a limitation of our study, as it creates a challenge in comparing our results to those of other studies. However, we believe the results presented in this study may be meaningful for public health, as it provides a range of methylation values that may be associated with anthropometric, and possibly even adiposity.

Conclusions

In summary, our study findings suggest that DNA methylation of the *PLAGL1, MEST, PEG10, and NNAT* DMRs at birth is associated with BMI *z* scores in early childhood and varies by sex. Longitudinal assessment of DNA methylation in these DMRs at older age time points is needed to determine whether or not methylation at these DMRs is associated with obesity later in life. Determining the associations between DNA methylation and early obesity risk is important, as DNA methylation of regulatory regions may serve as markers for the assessment of early obesity risk. However, gaining a better understanding of the exposures that affect methylation at these regions is also important, as exposures that modify methylation of regions that are associated with obesity risk may be a good target for early obesity prevention efforts.

Abbreviations
BMI: Body mass index; BW/GA: Birth weight for gestational age; DMR: Differentially methylated region; IGF2: Insulin-like growth factor 2; MEG3: Maternally expressed gene 3; MEG3-IG: Maternally expressed gene 3—intergenic; MEST: Mesoderm-specific transcript; NNAT: Neuronatin; PEG10: Paternally expressed gene 10; PEG3: Paternally expressed gene 3; PLAGL1: Pleiomorphic adenoma gene-like 1; SGA: Small for gestational age; WFL: Weight-for-length

Acknowledgements
We thank the NEST participants for their generous contributions to the study and Carole Grenier for her excellent technical assistance.

Funding
This research was supported in part by the National Institutes of Health, grant numbers R01ES016772, P30ES025128, R01DK094841, and P01ES022831, and USEPA grant RD-83543701.

Authors' contributions
SKM and CH developed the study design. SKM and ZH generated the methylation data. SGN initiated the research question and hypothesis, conducted statistical analysis, and wrote the manuscript. MAM, SBN, SKM, VKH, DLR, and CH reviewed and edited the manuscript. All authors have read and approved the manuscript.

Competing interests
The authors declare that they have no competing interests.

Author details

[1]Department of Health, Behavior and Society, Johns Hopkins Bloomberg School of Public Health, 624 N Broadway, Baltimore, MD 21205, USA. [2]Department of Nutrition, Gillings School of Global Public Health, University of North Carolina at Chapel Hill, Chapel Hill, NC, USA. [3]Department of Obstetrics and Gynecology, Duke University Medical Center, Durham, NC, USA. [4]W.K. Kellogg Foundation, Battle Creek, MI, USA. [5]Department of Maternal and Child Health, Gillings School of Global Public Health, University of North Carolina at Chapel Hill, Chapel Hill, NC, USA. [6]Department of Biological Sciences, North Carolina State University, Raleigh, NC, USA.

References

1. Monasta L, Batty GD, Cattaneo A, et al. Early-life determinants of overweight and obesity: a review of systematic reviews. Obes Rev. 2010;11(10):695–708.
2. Rooney BL, Mathiason MA, Schauberger CW. Predictors of obesity in childhood, adolescence, and adulthood in a birth cohort. Matern Child Health J. 2011;15(8):1166–75.
3. Skilton MR, Marks GB, Ayer JG, et al. Weight gain in infancy and vascular risk factors in later childhood. Pediatrics. 2013;131(6):e1821–8.
4. Freedman DS, Dietz WH, Srinivasan SR, Berenson GS. The relation of overweight to cardiovascular risk factors among children and adolescents: the Bogalusa Heart Study. Pediatrics. 1999;103:1172-85.
5. Dietz WH. Health consequences of obesity in youth: childhood predictors of adult disease. Pediatrics. 1998;101:518–25.
6. Yu ZB, Han SP, Zhu GZ, et al. Birth weight and subsequent risk of obesity: a systematic review and meta-analysis. Obes Rev. 2011;12(7):525–42.
7. Gallo P, Cioffi L, Limauro R, et al. SGA children in pediatric primary care : what is the best choice, large or small ? A 10-year prospective longitudinal study. Global Pediatric Health. 2016;3(194):1–7.
8. Baidal JAW, Locks LM, Cheng ER, Blake-lamb TL, Perkins ME, Taveras EM. Risk factors for childhood obesity in the first 1,000 days. Am J Prev Med. 2016; 50(6):761–79.
9. Vidal AC, Overcash F, Murphy SK, et al. Associations between birth and one year anthropometric measurements and IGF2 and IGF2R genetic variants in African American and Caucasian American infants. Journal of Pediatric Genetics. 2013;2:119–27.
10. Dietz WH. Critical periods in childhood for the development of obesity. Am J Clin Nutr. 1994;1:1–5.
11. Barker DJP. The fetal and infant origins of adult disease the womb may be more important than the home. BMJ. 1990;301(156):1990–0.
12. Gluckman PD, Hanson MA, Cooper C, Thornburg KL. Effect of in utero and early-life conditions on adult health and disease. N Engl J Med. 2008;359(1):61–73.
13. Langley-Evans SC. Developmental programming of health and disease. Proc Nutr Soc. 2006;65(1):97–105.
14. Dolinoy DC, Weidman JR, Ra W, Jirtle RL. Maternal genistein alters coat color and protects Avy mouse offspring from obesity by modifying the fetal epigenome. Environ Health Perspect. 2006;114(4):567–72.
15. Godfrey KM, Sheppard A, Gluckman PD, et al. Epigenetic gene promoter methylation at birth is associated with child's later adiposity. Diabetes. 2011; 60(5):1528–34.
16. Plagemann A, Roepke K, Harder T, et al. Epigenetic malprogramming of the insulin receptor promoter due to developmental overfeeding. J Perinat Med. 2010;38(4):393–400.
17. Heijmans BT, Tobi EW, Lumey LH, Slagboom PE. The epigenome: archive of the prenatal environment. Epigenetics. 2009;4(8):526–31.
18. Ja H, Surani MA. DNA methylation dynamics during the mammalian life cycle. Philosophical transactions of the Royal Society of London Series B, Biological sciences. 2013;368(1609):20110328.
19. Reik W, Walter J. Genomic imprinting: parental influence on the genome. Nature Reviews. 2001;2(January):21–32.
20. Gluckman PD, Hanson MA, Low FM. The role of developmental plasticity and epigenetics in human health. Birth Defects Research Part C. 2011;93(1):12–8.
21. Dolinoy DC, Weidman JR, Jirtle RL. Epigenetic gene regulation: linking early developmental environment to adult disease. Reprod Toxicol. 2007;23:297–307.

22. Heijmans BT, Tobi EW, Stein AD, et al. Persistent epigenetic differences associated with prenatal exposure to famine in humans. Proc Natl Acad Sci U S A. 2008;105:17046–9.
23. Tobi EW, Goeman JJ, Monajemi R, et al. DNA methylation signatures link prenatal famine exposure to growth and metabolism. Nat Commun. 2014;5:5592.
24. Dominguez-Salas P, Moore SE, Baker MS, et al. Maternal nutrition at conception modulates DNA methylation of human metastable epialleles. Nat Commun. 2014;5:1–7.
25. Cruz-Correa M, Zhao R, Oviedo M, et al. Temporal stability and age-related prevalence of loss of imprinting of the insulin-like growth factor-2 gene. Epigenetics. 2009;4(2):114–8.
26. Murphy SK, Huang Z, Hoyo C. Differentially methylated regions of imprinted genes in prenatal, perinatal and postnatal human tissues. PLoS One. 2012; 7(7):e40924.
27. Hoovers JM, Kalikin LM, Johnson LA, et al. Multiple genetic loci within 11p15 defined by Beckwith-Wiedemann syndrome rearrangement breakpoints and subchromosomal. Proc Natl Acad Sci USA. 1995;92:12456–60.
28. Bliek J, Terhal P, van den Bogaard M-J, et al. Hypomethylation of the H19 gene causes not only Silver-Russell syndrome (SRS) but also isolated asymmetry or an SRS-like phenotype. Am J Hum Genet. 2006;78(4):604–14.
29. Pan H, Wu Y, Chen L, et al. HIF3A association with adiposity: the story begins before birth. Epigenomics. 2015;7(6):937–50.
30. Huang RC, Garratt ES, Pan H, et al. Genome-wide methylation analysis identifies differentially methylated CpG loci associated with severe obesity in childhood. Epigenetics. 2015;10(11):995–1005.
31. Kadakia R, Josefson J. The relationship of insulin-like growth factor 2 to fetal growth and adiposity. Hormone Res Paediatr. 2016;85:75–82.
32. Bouwland-Both MI, van Mil NH, Stolk L, et al. DNA methylation of IGF2DMR and H19 is associated with fetal and infant growth: the generation R study. PLoS One. 2013;8(12):e81731.
33. Su R, Wang C, Feng H, et al. Alteration in expression and methylation of IGF2/H19 in placenta and umbilical cord blood are associated with macrosomia exposed to intrauterine hyperglycemia. PLoS One. 2016;11(2): e0148399.
34. St-pierre J, Hivert M-f, Perron P, et al. IGF2 DNA methylation is a modulator of newborn ' s fetal growth and development. Epigenetics. 2012;7(10):1125–32.
35. Huang R-C, Galati JC, Burrows S, et al. DNA methylation of the IGF2/H19 imprinting control region and adiposity distribution in young adults. Clin Epigenetics. 2012;4(1):21.
36. Perkins E, Murphy SK, Murtha AP, et al. Insulin-like growth factor 2/H19 methylation at birth and risk of overweight and obesity in children. J Pediatr. 2012;161(1):31–9.
37. Azzi S, Sas TCJ, Koudou Y, et al. Degree of methylation of ZAC1 (PLAGL1) is associated with prenatal and post-natal growth in healthy infants of the EDEN mother child cohort. Epigenetics. 2014;9(3):338–45.
38. Kameswaran V, Bramswig NC, McKenna LB, et al. Epigenetic regulation of the DLK1-MEG3 microRNA cluster in human type 2 diabetic islets. Cell Metab. 2014;19(1):135–45.
39. Soubry A, Murphy SK, Wang F, et al. Newborns of obese parents have altered DNA methylation patterns at imprinted genes. Int J Obes. 2015; 39(4):650–7.

40. Liu Y, Murphy SK, Murtha AP, et al. Depression in pregnancy, infant birth weight and DNA methylation of imprint regulatory elements. Epigenetics. 2012;7(7):735–46.

41. Villar J, Ismail LC, Victora CG, et al. International standards for newborn weight , length , and head circumference by gestational age and sex : the Newborn Cross-Sectional Study of the INTERGROWTH-21 st Project. Lancet. 2014;384:857–68.

42. World Health Organization. The WHO Growth Standards. http://www.who.int/childgrowth/standards/en/. Accessed Sept 10, 2016.

43. Centers for Disease Control and Prevention. A SAS program for the 2000 CDC Growth Charts (ages 0 to <20 years). 2016; http://www.cdc.gov/nccdphp/dnpao/growthcharts/resources/sas.htm. Accessed Sept 10, 2016.

44. Tobi EW, Lumey LH, Talens RP, et al. DNA methylation differences after exposure to prenatal famine are common and timing- and sex-specific. Hum Mol Genet. 2009;18(21):4046–53.

45. Murphy SK, Adigun A, Huang Z, et al. Gender-specific methylation differences in relation to prenatal exposure to cigarette smoke. Gene. 2012; 494(1):36–43.

46. Mitchell M, Strick R, Strissel PL, et al. Gene expression and epigenetic aberrations in F1-placentas fathered by obese males. Mol Reprod Dev. 2017; 84(November 2016):316–28.

47. Karbiener M, Glantschnig C, Pisani DF, et al. Mesoderm-specific transcript (MEST) is a negative regulator of human adipocyte differentiation. Int J Obes. 2015;39(12):1733–41.

48. Kappil MA, Green BB, Armstrong DA, et al. Placental expression profile of imprinted genes impacts birth weight. Epigenetics. 2015;10(9):842–9.

49. Lim AL, Ng S, Ching S, et al. Epigenetic state and expression of imprinted genes in umbilical cord correlates with growth parameters in human pregnancy. J Med Genet. 2012;49:689–97.

50. Vrang N, Meyre D, Froguel P, et al. The imprinted gene neuronatin is regulated by metabolic status and associated with obesity. Obesity (Silver Spring, Md). 2010;18(7):1289–96.

51. Arima T, Ra D, Arney KL, et al. A conserved imprinting control region at the HYMAI/ZAC domain is implicated in transient neonatal diabetes mellitus. Hum Mol Genet. 2001;10(14):1475–83.

52. Ong KK, Loos RJF. Rapid infancy weight gain and subsequent obesity: systematic reviews and hopeful suggestions. Acta Paediatr. 2006;95(8):904–8.

53. Gonzalez-Nahm S, Mendez MA, Robinson WR, et al. Low maternal adherence to a Mediterranean diet is associated with increase in methylation at the MEG3-IG differentially methylated region in female infants. Environmental Epigenetics. 2017;3(March):1–10.

54. Qian Y, Huang X, Liang H, et al. Effects of maternal folic acid supplementation on gene methylation and being small for gestational age. J Hum Nutr Diet. 2016;29:643–51.

55. Voigt A, Ribot J, Sabater G, Palou A, Bonet ML, Klaus S. Identification of Mest/Peg1 gene expression as a predictive biomarker of adipose tissue expansion sensitive to dietary anti-obesity interventions. Genes Nutr. 2015;10(5):27.

56. Evensen E, Emaus N, Kokkvoll A, Wilsgaard T, Furberg AS, Skeie G. The relation between birthweight, childhood body mass index, and overweight and obesity in late adolescence: a longitudinal cohort study from Norway, the Tromso study, Fit Futures. BMJ Open. 2017;7(6):e015576.

11

Genome-wide analysis of DNA methylation in bronchial washings

Sang-Won Um[1†], Yujin Kim[2†], Bo Bin Lee[2], Dongho Kim[2], Kyung-Jong Lee[1], Hong Kwan Kim[3], Joungho Han[4], Hojoong Kim[1], Young Mog Shim[3] and Duk-Hwan Kim[2,5*] (ID)

Abstract

Background: The objective of this study was to discover DNA methylation biomarkers for detecting non-small lung cancer (NSCLC) in bronchial washings and understanding the association between DNA methylation and smoking cessation.

Methods: DNA methylation was analyzed in bronchial washing samples from 70 NSCLCs and 53 hospital-based controls using Illumina HumanMethylation450K BeadChip. Methylation levels in these bronchial washings were compared to those in 897 primary lung tissues of The Cancer Genome Atlas (TCGA) data.

Results: Twenty-four CpGs ($p < 1.03E-07$) were significantly methylated in bronchial washings from 70 NSCLC patients compared to those from 53 controls. The CpGs also had significant methylation in the TCGA cohort. The 123 participants were divided into a training set ($N = 82$) and a test set ($N = 41$) to build a classification model. Logistic regression model showed the best performance for classification of lung cancer in bronchial washing samples: the sensitivity and specificity of a marker panel consisting of seven CpGs in *TFAP2A*, *TBX15*, *PHF11*, *TOX2*, *PRR15*, *PDGFRA*, and *HOXA11* genes were 87.0 and 83.3% in the test set, respectively. The area under the curve (AUC) was equal to 0.87 (95% confidence interval = 0.73–0.96, $p < 0.001$). Methylation levels of two CpGs in *RUNX3* and *MIR196A1* genes were inversely associated with duration of smoking cessation in the controls, but not in NSCLCs, after adjusting for pack-years of smoking.

Conclusions: The present study suggests that NSCLC may be detected by analyzing methylation changes of seven CpGs in bronchial washings. Furthermore, smoking cessation may lead to decreased DNA methylation in nonmalignant bronchial epithelial cells in a gene-specific manner.

Keywords: Hypermethylation, Lung cancer, Smoking, Bronchial washing, Epigenome

Background

Lung cancer is the most common cause of cancer deaths worldwide. Despite recent advances in the diagnosis and treatment for lung cancer, prognosis of patients remains very poor. The overall 5-year survival rate of lung cancer has improved slightly from 12 to 16% over the past 30 years [1]. Such poor prognosis is largely due to occult metastatic dissemination of tumor cells, which occurs in more than half of all patients at the time of diagnosis. The majority of patients undergoing curative surgical resection at an early stage have achieved long-term survival. Overall 5-year survival rate for patients with surgically resected stage IA, stage IB, and stage II non-small cell lung cancers (NSCLCs) has been reported to be 83, 69, and 48%, respectively [2]. Accordingly, it is imperative to develop efficient diagnostic tools that can identify lung cancer at an early stage so that curative treatment is feasible.

De novo methylation of CpG islands at the promoter region of tumor suppressor genes is usually associated with transcriptional silencing of a gene. It is one of the most common epigenetic modifications in lung cancer. Aberrant methylation of CpG loci in bronchial washings

---

* Correspondence: dukhwan.kim@samsung.com
†Equal contributors
2Department of Molecular Cell Biology, Samsung Biomedical Research Institute, Sungkyunkwan University School of Medicine, Suwon 440-746, South Korea
5Samsung Medical Center, Research Institute for Future Medicine, #50 Ilwon-dong, Kangnam-gu, Professor Rm #5, Seoul 135-710, South Korea
Full list of author information is available at the end of the article

could become a powerful tool for early diagnosis of lung cancer. To discover aberrant methylation that occur at an early stage of lung cancer, several groups have analyzed methylation statuses of multiple CpG loci in bronchial aspirate or sputum from both lung cancer patients and healthy individuals [3–9]. Epigenetic studies of human cancer have recently shifted from candidate gene analyses toward epigenome-wide analysis with rapid technological advances. However, most studies on bronchial aspirate were restricted to a few candidate CpG loci with inadequate genome coverage.

Cigarette smoke is a well-known environmental modifier of DNA methylation [10]. It modulates DNA methylation by the following these mechanisms: (i) recruiting DNA methyltransferase 1 (DNMT1) to damage sites during DNA repair; (ii) altering nuclear protein levels and activity of DNA-binding factors such as SP1; or (iii) inhibiting GSK3β function and attenuating DNMT1 degradation [11–13]. Recently, several groups have reported a reversibility of methylation change after smoking cessation in peripheral blood samples. Ambatipudi et al. [14] have reported that methylation levels at smoking-related CpG sites are reversible after smoking cessation, although changes in DNA methylation of specific genes can remain for up to 22 years after quitting smoking. Guida et al. [15] have also reported that some methylated CpGs can revert back to levels present in never-smokers after a certain time since smoking cessation.

In this study, we analyzed DNA methylation at the genome level to discover a panel of CpGs for the detection of NSCLC in bronchial washings and investigated the effect of smoking cessation on reversion of methylated DNA to normal levels.

Methods

Study population

A total of 123 patients (70 non-small cell lung cancers [NSCLCs] and 53 hospital-based controls with benign lung disease) who were admitted for fiberoptic bronchoscopy or for curative surgical resection at Samsung Medical Center in Seoul, Korea, between March 2010 and November 2015 participated in this study. NSCLC patients underwent surgery as well as bronchoscopy. Controls were recruited from patients with benign lung diseases such as actinomycosis, anthracofibrosis, bronchiolitis, pneumonia, or tuberculosis. Patients with benign lung tumors such as localized organizing pneumonia or hamartoma were excluded from this study. This is because methylation profiling of these diseases is not well known yet which can lead to misclassification. Small-cell lung cancer was also excluded from this study for comparison with The Cancer Genome Atlas (TCGA) methylation profiling. Stage IIIB and IV NSCLCs were excluded because this study was aimed to identify biomarkers for detecting NSCLC at early stages.

Bronchial washings were obtained through bronchoscopy with written informed consent from all participants. The control group received bronchoscopy to confirm the diagnosis. Bronchial washing samples were analyzed cytologically for the presence of malignant cells. All lung cancer patients were diagnosed with early-stage lung cancer which was pathologically proven. They underwent curative resection. Information on sociodemographic characteristics was obtained through an interviewer-administered questionnaire. Individuals who were clinically negative for cancer at the time of bronchoscopy without having abnormal findings on their chest radiograph or chest computerized tomography (CT) were included in the hospital-based control group. This study was approved by the Institutional Review Board (IRB #: 2010-07-204) of Samsung Medical Center. All cases of NSCLC were classified based on the guideline of tumor-node-metastasis (TNM) staging system introduced by the American Joint Committee on Cancer [16].

Bronchoscopy

Flexible fiberoptic bronchoscopy (Olympus, Tokyo, Japan) and sample preparation were performed as described previously [4]. Bronchial washing was performed by instilling 10 mL of sterile normal saline when the bronchoscope (Olympus, Tokyo, Japan) was located at the segmental bronchi of the pulmonary lobe. Bronchial washing samples were mixed with 100 mg of N-acetylcysteine for 10 min to disrupt disulfide bond in mucoproteins and stored at – 20 °C until use.

Genome-wide methylation analysis

Genomic DNA was extracted from bronchial washing specimens using a QIAamp DNA Blood Mini Kit (Qiagen, Valencia, CA, USA) according to the manufacturer's instructions, followed by quality control using a UV spectrophotometer (Pharmacia Biotech, Cambridge, England). Double-stranded DNA in solution was quantitated using PicoGreen™ double-stranded DNA quantitation kit (Molecular Probes, Eugene, OR, USA) on a SpectraMax Gemini UV spectrometer (Molecular Devices, Sunnyvale, CA, USA). Bisulfite treatment of genomic DNA was performed using Zymo EZ DNA Methylation Kit (Zymo Research, Orange, CA, USA). Genome-wide DNA methylation levels were measured using Infinium HumanMethylation450 BeadChip (Illumina, Inc) according to the manufacturer's instructions. β value ranging from 0 (no methylation) to 1 (100% methylation) was measured as the ratio of signal intensity of methylated alleles to the sum of methylated and unmethylated signal intensity of alleles at each CpG site.

Pyrosequencing

Methylation levels obtained by 450K array were validated by pyrosequencing a cg27364741 locus at the promoter region of *OTX1* gene using QIAGEN's PyroMark Q24 systems. Biotinylated PCR primer sets for amplification of the locus were purchased from Qiagen (Cat no. PM00616336).

Feature selection for predicting lung cancer

Preprocessing of 450K array data was conducted using wateRmelon [17] and ran on R programming language. After preprocessing, candidate CpGs for NSCLC prediction were selected in the following order: (i) identifying differentially methylated CpGs; (ii) removing age-related methylation; (iii) performing gene set enrichment analysis; (iv) selecting features; and (v) testing model performance. Gene set enrichment analysis was performed using DAVID (http://david.abcc.ncifcrf.gov/). Annotation clusters with EASE score (a modified Fisher's exact p value) below 1.0E–5 were selected as candidate clusters for model building. Any candidate CpG that was significantly correlated in the same cluster was removed from model building.

Statistical analysis

T test (or Wilcoxon rank-sum test) and chi-square test (or Fisher's exact test) were used to analyze continuous and categorical variables, respectively. Pearson's (or Spearman's) rank correlation coefficient was used to analyze correlations between two continuous variables. Linear regression analysis was performed to analyze the effect of smoking cessation on DNA methylation after adjusting for potential confounding factors such as pack-years of smoking. Multiple logistic regression analysis was performed to discover methylated CpGs associated with the development of NSCLC after controlling for age, sex, and smoking status. Statistical analysis was conducted using R software (version 3.1.1). Diagnostic performance of the model was measured using a receiver operating characteristic (ROC) curve, which was created with MedCalc statistical software (version 16.8).

Results

Methylation levels of 450K array in bronchial washings were slightly inflated

Assay quality of 450K array was tested by comparing measured DNA methylation levels with levels of predefined subsets (0, 33, 66, and 100%) that were prepared by mixing fully methylated and unmethylated human control DNA (Qiagen, Hilden, Germany). Methylation levels of predefined subsets were similarly reproduced by 450K array (Additional file 1: Figure S1A). β values from 450K array were further confirmed using pyrosequencing (Additional file 1: Figure S1B). A cg27364741 locus at *OTX1* gene that was significantly methylated in bronchial washing showed higher methylation in the 450K array than that in pyrosequencing, suggesting background signal of the 450K array (Additional file 1: Figure S1C).

Data from the 450K array were quantile normalized using the wateRmelon R package. Samples were first filtered using the "pfilter" function from the wateRmelon package. Samples having 1% of CpG sites with a detection p value > 0.05, CpG sites containing a beadcount < 3 in 5% of samples, and CpG sites with a detection p value > 0.05 in 1% of samples were removed. Data preprocessing including background noise removal and type I/type II probes bias correction was conducted using the "dasen" function from the package. A total of 2046 (0.42%) of 485,577 CpGs were filtered out.

Identification of differentially methylated CpGs in bronchial washing

Clinicopathological characteristics of 53 hospital-based controls and 70 NSCLC patients are described in Additional file 2: Table S1. Average ages of controls and cases were 55 and 64 years, respectively. This difference in age was statistically significant ($p < 0.0001$). The proportion of women was significantly higher in controls than that in cases (45 vs. 26%, $p = 0.02$). The control group had more never-smokers than the case group (55 vs. 29%, $p = 0.007$). This required age- and sex-matched controls with absence of significant differences in smoking. However, we could not match controls by age and sex due to low statistical power. Instead, we stratified these data into cases and controls and analyzed age- and smoking-related methylation separately for cases and controls as different cohorts. To identify differentially methylated CpGs in bronchial washings from 70 cases and 53 controls, we transformed the β values of methylation level into log scale ($\log2[\beta/(1-\beta)]$) because the distribution of β values did not follow a normal distribution (Shapiro-Wilk test, $p < 0.05$). It was negatively skewed in 450K data from bronchial washing samples. Fifty-eight CpGs with p value less than or equal to 1.03E–07 (Bonferroni significance threshold) in two-sided Student's t test were identified from 483,531 CpGs. We selected 31 (Additional file 3: Table S2) out of these 58 CpGs after removing 27 CpGs with a maximum β value greater than 0.3 in 53 control samples because background signal in the control DNA of 0% methylation was mostly below $\beta = 0.3$. Finally, we applied multiple logistic regression analysis to find CpGs related to lung cancer after adjusting confounding factors such as age, sex, and the pack-years of smoking. Twenty-four CpGs were found to be significantly methylated in bronchial washing from lung cancer patients than those from healthy individuals. Of the 31 CpGs, the 7 CpGs that were not statistically significant in multiple logistic regression were as follows: SLC15A3 and 6 CpGs (*HOXA9, EVX1, HIST1H2BK, EMX1, ITPK,* and *PRDM14*) showing age-related methylation (Additional file 4: Figure S2) in 70 NSCLCs and 53 controls.

Feature selection for lung cancer classification and the performance evaluation of proposed models

The 123 samples were divided into a training set ($N = 82$) and a test set ($N = 41$), and the training set was used to build a classification model. Supervised machine learning algorithms, including support vector machine (SVM), random forest, decision tree, artificial neural network (ANN), logistic regression analysis, and K-nearest neighbor, were used to build models. An optimal subset of CpG features for use in building the classification models was selected from the training set with full β values of 485,577 CpGs. The performance of the models was evaluated on the test set using the ROC curve. Among the six algorithms, the logistic regression analysis showed the best classification performance: the sensitivity and specificity of one panel consisting of seven CpGs in *TFAP2A*, *TBX15*, *PRR15*, *HOXA11*, *PDGFRA*, *TOX2*, and *PHF11* genes (Fig. 1a) were 87.0 and 83.3% in the test set, respectively. The area under the receiver operating characteristic (ROC) curve was equal to 0.87 (95% confidence interval = 073–0.96, $p < 0.001$; Fig. 1b).

Methylation profiling was different between bronchial washing and surgically resected tumor tissue

To understand methylation profiling between bronchial washing and surgically resected tumor tissue, we compared the number and p values of CpGs showing statistical significance ($p < 1.0E–07$) in 123 bronchial washings and 897 TCGA primary lung tissues (821 primary tumor tissues and 76 normal tissues). All 24 CpGs showing statistical significance in bronchial washings were found to be significantly methylated in the TCGA cohort irrespective of histologic subtypes. The number of statistically significant CpGs was much higher in the TCGA cohort than that in bronchial washings (Fig. 2a). The degree of statistical

significance was also lower in bronchial washings compared to that in the TCGA cohort. p values of a CpG showing the strongest significance were 2.2E–16 and 2.1E–08 in the TCGA cohort and bronchial washings, respectively. Over 4000 CpGs were significantly ($p < 1.0E–07$) hypermethylated in TCGA tumor tissues compared to normal tissues. Figure 2b–e shows an example of four CpGs in *ITGA8*, *DLK1*, *HTR1B*, and *RSPO2* genes significantly hypermethylated in the TCGA cohort only. A Gene Ontology (GO) analysis showed that highly methylated genes in the TCGA cohort only were largely involved in the following: (i) positive regulation of transcription from RNA polymerase II promoter, (ii) homophilic cell adhesion via plasma membrane adhesion molecules, (iii) cell-cell signaling, and (iv) G-protein coupled receptor signaling pathway, coupled to cyclic nucleotide second messenger.

Smoking cessation is associated with reduction of methylated CpGs in nonmalignant bronchial epithelial cells

To understand the impact of smoking cessation on DNA methylation in bronchial washing, we first analyzed the association between levels of DNA methylation and three smoking-related variables: age at which smoking began, pack-years of cigarette smoking, and smoking status. The age at which smoking began was not associated with DNA methylation in bronchial washing (data not shown). However, aberrant methylation of nine CpGs in *RUNX3*, *MIR196A1*, *HOXA11*, *OTP*, *GATA4*, *PTPRU*, *SLC15A3*, *ZIC1*, and *TFAP2B* of 24 genes were found to be significantly associated with pack-years of smoking in controls (Additional file 5: Table S3). In addition, methylation patterns of these nine CpGs were different according to smoking status (Fig. 3). Methylation levels (β values) of seven of these nine CpGs were not associated with duration after smoking cessation in NSCLC or control group

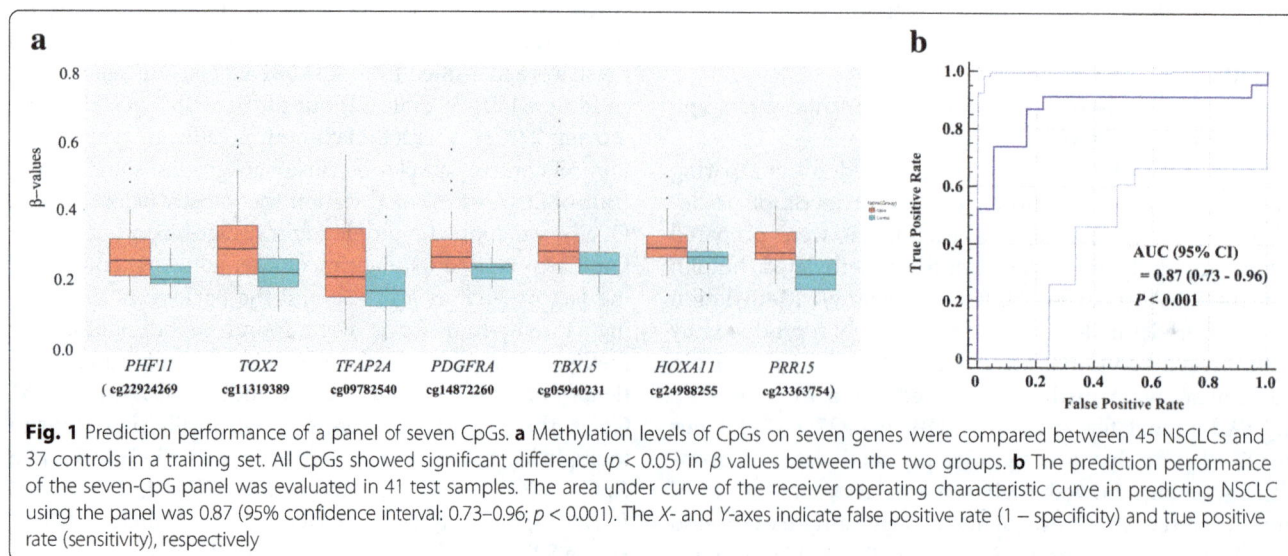

Fig. 1 Prediction performance of a panel of seven CpGs. **a** Methylation levels of CpGs on seven genes were compared between 45 NSCLCs and 37 controls in a training set. All CpGs showed significant difference ($p < 0.05$) in β values between the two groups. **b** The prediction performance of the seven-CpG panel was evaluated in 41 test samples. The area under curve of the receiver operating characteristic curve in predicting NSCLC using the panel was 0.87 (95% confidence interval: 0.73–0.96; $p < 0.001$). The *X*- and *Y*-axes indicate false positive rate (1 − specificity) and true positive rate (sensitivity), respectively

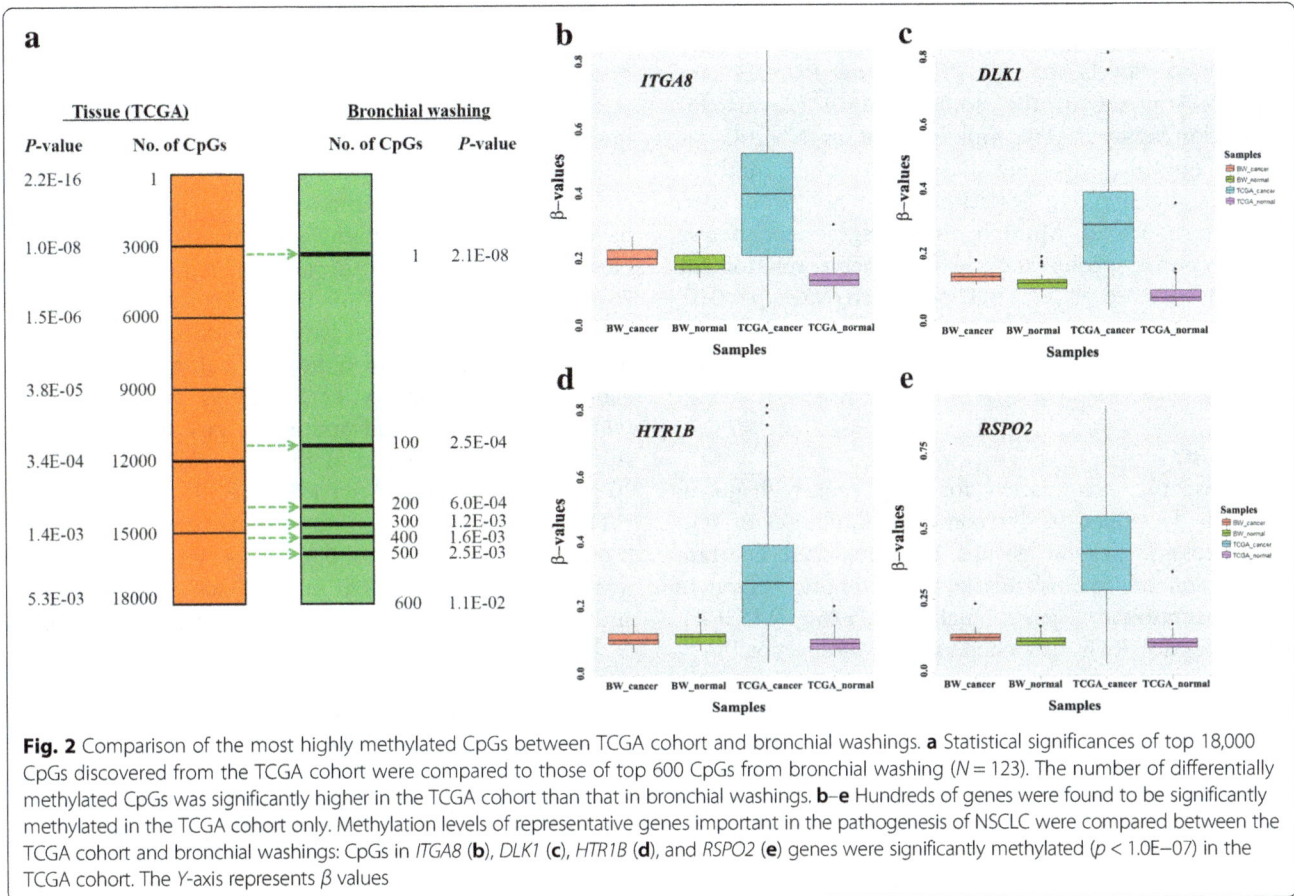

Fig. 2 Comparison of the most highly methylated CpGs between TCGA cohort and bronchial washings. **a** Statistical significances of top 18,000 CpGs discovered from the TCGA cohort were compared to those of top 600 CpGs from bronchial washing ($N = 123$). The number of differentially methylated CpGs was significantly higher in the TCGA cohort than that in bronchial washings. **b–e** Hundreds of genes were found to be significantly methylated in the TCGA cohort only. Methylation levels of representative genes important in the pathogenesis of NSCLC were compared between the TCGA cohort and bronchial washings: CpGs in *ITGA8* (**b**), *DLK1* (**c**), *HTR1B* (**d**), and *RSPO2* (**e**) genes were significantly methylated ($p < 1.0E{-}07$) in the TCGA cohort. The *Y*-axis represents β values

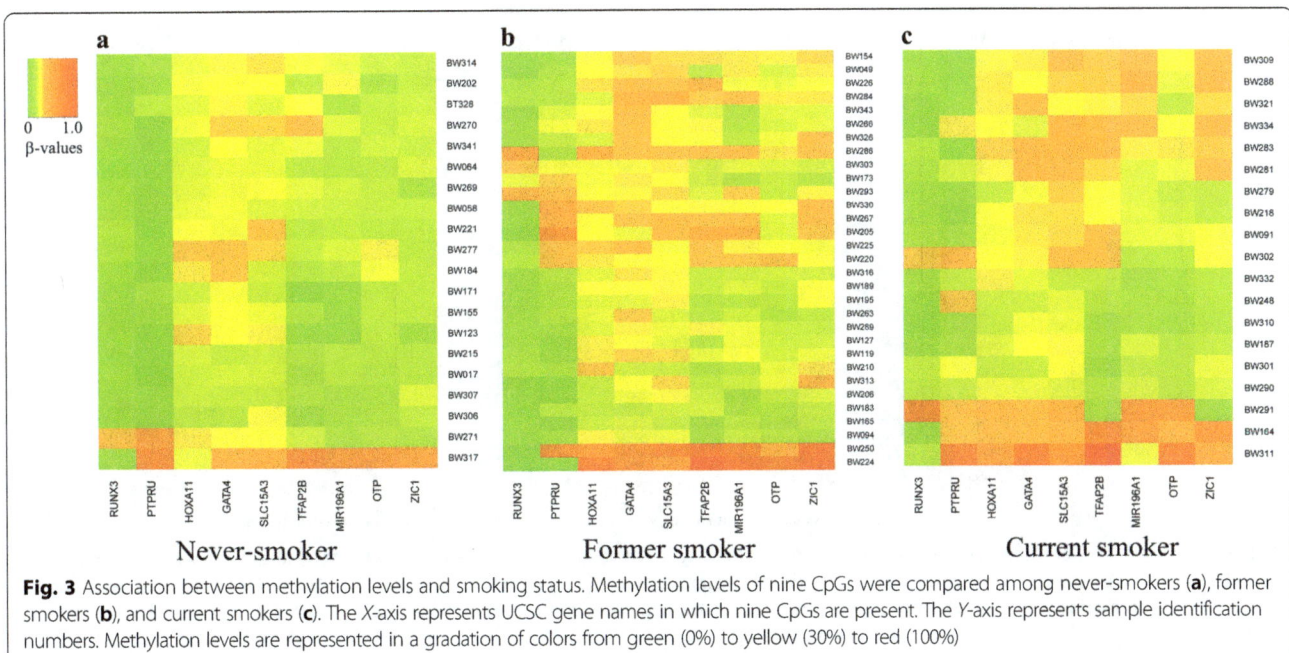

Fig. 3 Association between methylation levels and smoking status. Methylation levels of nine CpGs were compared among never-smokers (**a**), former smokers (**b**), and current smokers (**c**). The *X*-axis represents UCSC gene names in which nine CpGs are present. The *Y*-axis represents sample identification numbers. Methylation levels are represented in a gradation of colors from green (0%) to yellow (30%) to red (100%)

(data not shown). However, an inverse association was found between duration of smoking cessation and methylation levels of two CpGs in *RUNX3* and *MIR196A1* genes in the control group (Spearman's correlation analysis; Fig. 4a), but not in NSCLC patients (Fig. 4b), suggesting that a decrease in methylation level by smoking cessation might not occur after cancer has formed. Multiple linear regression analysis in the control group showed an inverse relationship of methylation levels of CpG loci on *RUNX3* ($p = 0.02$) and *MIR196A1* genes ($p = 0.006$) with duration of smoking cessation, after adjusting for pack-years of smoking (Table 1).

Discussion

Bronchoscopic examination for lung cancer diagnosis has been developed to overcome the limitation of sputum cytology. Several groups have reported aberrant methylation of CpG islands at the promoter region of tumor suppressor genes including *p16*, *RASSF1A*, *RARB2*, and *APC* in bronchial aspirate or sputum [3–9].

However, aberrant methylation does not indicate that methylation is tumor-specific since aberrant methylation can occur in bronchial epithelial cells due to aging. Age-related methylation has been reported for several genes, including *ER*, *N33*, *MYOD*, thrombospondin-4, and *IGF2* [18–22]. Epigenome-wide analysis has also shown changes in DNA methylation with age. Florath et al. [23] have analyzed DNA methylation using 450K array in blood DNA of 965 participants aged between 50 and 75 years and identified 65 novel CpG sites associated with aging. Bell et al. [24] have also reported age-related methylation changes in a healthy aging population at genome-wide level. Six of 31 CpGs with significant methylation in the univariate analysis of the present study showed age-related methylation in 53 controls and 70 NSCLCs (Additional file 4: Figure S2).

The number of CpGs showing statistical significance (Bonferroni-corrected $p < 0.05$) was less in bronchial washings compared to that in the TCGA cohort [25, 26] and bronchial biopsy [27]. CpGs of well-known genes such as *RARβ2*, *CDH13*, and *p16* were not included in

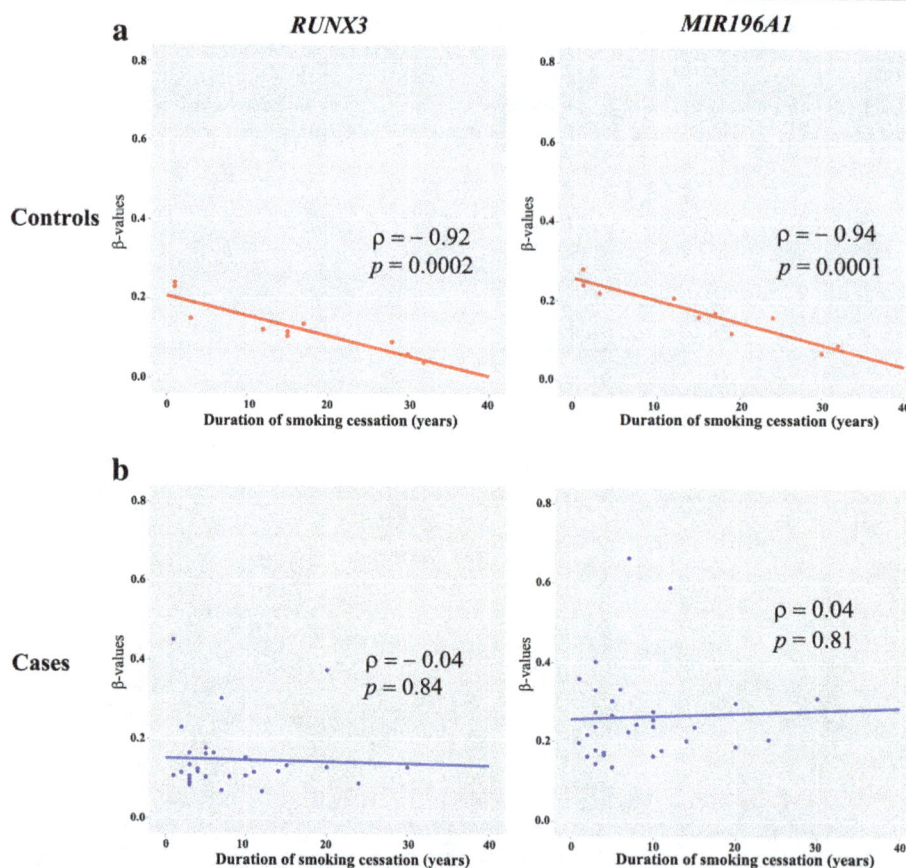

Fig. 4 Relationship between DNA methylation and duration of smoking cessation. A correlation between methylation levels and duration of smoking cessation was analyzed in NSCLC patients (**a**) and controls (**b**). Methylation levels of CpGs on two genes (*RUNX3* and *MIR196A1*) of nine genes associated with pack-years of smoking were inversely associated with duration of smoking cessation in the control group. *p* values are based on Spearman's correlation coefficient. The *X*- and *Y*-axes indicate duration of smoking cessation and *β* values, respectively

Table 1 Multivariate regression analysis (adjusted for pack-years of smoking) for the association between DNA methylation and smoking cessation in former smokers

Parameter	Cases ($N = 31$)		Controls ($N = 10$)	
	t value[a]	Pr > |t|	t value	Pr > |t|
(1) RUNX3	−0.32	0.75	−3.30	0.02
(2) MIR196A1	−0.30	0.76	−4.15	0.006

[a]The t value represents t-statistic

our final CpG list since they did not meet the Bonferroni significance threshold. The small number of CpGs with statistically significant results in bronchial washings compared to the TCGA cohort might be due to contamination of normal bronchial epithelial cells during bronchial washing. Another possibility is that invasive lung cancer cells might undergo more molecular changes than bronchial epithelial cells. In addition to 24 CpGs, hundreds of CpGs were found to be significantly hypermethylated in the TCGA cohort, supporting the concept of field cancerization [28]. Widespread cellular and molecular changes during transformation of a precancerous lesion into a cancerous lesion in airway epithelia exposed to carcinogens might also occur in lung tumor tissues. Abnormal methylation found in the TCGA cohort does not mean it has diagnostic value as it can be tumor related, inflammatory cell related, or stromal response related. However, 24 CpGs that were significantly methylated in our bronchial washing samples also showed significant methylation in the TCGA cohort, suggesting that abnormal methylation found in bronchial washing might reflect some methylation changes found in tumor tissue.

A positive relationship between aberrant methylation of genes and exposure to tobacco smoke has been reported by a few groups. For example, aberrant methylation of *p16* is associated with smoking duration in primary NSCLC [29]. It was induced by tobacco-specific carcinogen, 4-methylnitrosamino-1-(3-pyridyl)-1-butanone (NNK), in lung of Fischer 344 rats [30]. Aberrant methylation of *p16*, *RARβ2*, *CDH13*, and *RASSF1A* genes has also been found in specimens of bronchial epithelial cells from cancer-free heavy smokers [31]. Buro-Auriemma et al. [32] have also reported that cigarette smoking can alter methylation patterns in small airway epithelium. In this study, aberrant methylation of nine CpGs was found to be significantly associated with pack-years of smoking in bronchial washings of the control group. Among these genes, aberrant methylation of CpGs on *GATA4*, *EMX1*, and *RUNX3* genes is known to be associated with smoke exposure [33–36]. Wood smoke exposure is associated with lower percent predicted FEV1 of COPD patients in presence of aberrantly methylated *GATA4* [33]. Methylation levels of *EMX1* are associated with pack-years of smoking in gastric mucosa

of healthy individuals [34]. Positive relationship of *RUNX3* methylation to smoking has also been observed in DNA from blood leukocytes and placenta [35, 36].

Smoking cessation is a priority for preventing lung cancer. Epigenetic changes after smoking cessation have recently been identified by several groups. Several distinct CpG sites showing decreased methylation with increasing time after smoking cessation in peripheral blood lymphocytes of participants from KORA S3 survey [37] and the European Prospective Investigation into Cancer and Nutrition (EPIC) cohort [14, 15] have been reported, suggesting that a reduction of DNA methylation levels after smoking cessation may occur in a CpG site-specific manner. In this study, the impact of smoking cessation on aberrant methylation of CpG islands was analyzed in bronchial washings of former smokers. Of nine CpGs that were related to pack-years of smoking, two CpGs in *RUNX3* and *MIR196A1* genes showed an inverse relationship between the duration of smoking cessation and methylation levels of CpGs in the control group after adjusting for pack-years of smoking. Aberrant methylation of *MIR196A1* has not yet been reported in human cancer. However, *RUNX3* has been reported to be methylated in lung cancer [38, 39]. Runt-related transcription factor 3 (RUNX3) is known to function as a tumor suppressor. It also plays an important role in the regulation of cell proliferation, apoptosis, angiogenesis, cell adhesion, and invasion [40–42]. Reduction in DNA methylation levels after smoking cessation was not found in bronchial washings from lung cancer patients. Accordingly, smokers are encouraged to quit smoking prior to malignant transformation of bronchial epithelial cells.

Not many genes were found to be hypermethylated in bronchial washing in this study. This might be because only well-known genes found in lung cancer tissues were analyzed by candidate gene approach in bronchial washing fluids. Aberrant methylation of *DRD5*, *PHF11*, and *TPM1* genes discovered in this study has not been known in NSCLC up to date. CpG islands in *HOXA11* have been found to be hypermethylated in invasive NSCLC [43] and adenocarcinoma in situ (AIS) [44]. *PDGFRA* has been found to be significantly methylated in patients with NSCLC [25, 26]. *GDNF* and *TFAP2A* have been reported to be highly methylated in squamous cell carcinoma of the lung [45] and in adenocarcinoma [46], respectively. TOX high mobility group box family member 2 (*TOX2*) is not methylated in normal lung cancer cells. However, it is methylated in approximately 28% of lung cancer tissues [47].

This study was limited by several factors. First, this study was conducted in a small number of former smokers. The classification performance of a CpG panel from bronchial washing and the effect of smoking cessation on DNA methylation should be demonstrated in a large cohort in the future. Second, we did not measure the relative proportion of many other cell types (macrophages, lymphocytes, neutrophils) or total cell count in bronchial washing specimens. Therefore, it was unclear how much non-bronchial epithelial cell populations contributed to the analysis of methylation. Third, all cases were early-stage lung cancer and the size of some cancer tissues was small. Thus, we could not analyze methylation patterns of cancer tissues. Methylation patterns of tumor samples and bronchial washing samples should be compared in the same patient. Fourth, the potential impact of tumor heterogeneity and differences between methylation in invasive margin vs. tumor center need to be explored as explanations for the difference seen between bronchial washings and the TCGA cohort. Finally, the sensitivity and specificity of the CpG panel might be inflated because its prediction value was obtained from the same set of patients. Accordingly, an independent set of patients should be used in the future to determine their true values.

Conclusions

The present study suggests that methylation analysis in bronchial washing may be helpful for detecting NSCLC. Furthermore, smoking cessation in patients with benign lung diseases may result in decreased DNA methylation in a gene-specific manner.

Additional files

Additional file 1: Figure S1. Validation of 450K array. (A) A quality of 450K array was first checked by analyzing measured values for predefined subsets of methylation levels (0, 33, 66, and 100%). 2-D scatter plots were produced using plotColorBias2D in the Lumi package. The plotColorBias2D function separately plots methylated (green) and unmethylated (red) probe intensities in a 2-D scatter plot, and shows the interrogated CpG sites in red and green dots based on their color channels. (B) Methylation levels obtained by the 450K array were further validated using pyrosequencing. The sequencing output shows methylation levels at a cg27364741 locus at a promoter of OTX1 gene in cancer (top) and control sample (bottom). (C) Methylation levels at the cg27364741 locus were compared between β values from 450K array (Y-axis) and pyrosequencing (X-axis). Pyrosequencing was performed in 12 bronchial washing samples. Methylation levels at the cg27364741 locus were found to be higher in 450K array than in pyrosequencing. (TIF 25467 kb)

Additional file 2: Table S1. Clinicopathological characteristics (N = 123). (DOCX 17 kb)

Additional file 3: Table S2. Significantly methylated CpGs in bronchial washings of lung cancer. (DOCX 23 kb)

Additional file 4: Figure S2. Correlation coefficients for 6 CpGs showing positive correlation between patient's age and methylation. The relationship between patient's age and methylation levels. A correlation between methylation levels of EMX1 (A), ITPKA (B), EVX1 (C), HIST1H2BK (D), HOXA9 (F), and PRDM14 (FG) genes and patient's age was analyzed in 70 NSCLC patients and 53 controls separately. p values were based on Spearman's rank correlation coefficient. The X- and Y-axes indicate patient's age and β values, respectively. (TIF 2963 kb)

Additional file 5: Table S3. The correlation between pack-years of smoking and DNA methylation in 53 control groups. (DOCX 15 kb)

Abbreviations
AUC: Area under the curve; DNMT: DNA methyltransferase; GO: Gene Ontology; NSCLC: Non-small cell lung cancer; TCGA: The Cancer Genome Atlas; TNM: Tumor-node-metastasis

Acknowledgements
The authors wish to thank Eunkyung Kim and Jin-Hee Lee for data collection and management, and Hoon Suh for sample collection.

Funding
This work was supported by a grant (HI18C1098) from the Korea Health Technology R&D Project through the Korea Health Industry Development Institute (KHIDI), funded by the Ministry of Health & Welfare, Republic of Korea.

Authors' contributions
S-WU, YK, and D-HK participated in the design of the study, analyzed all data, and wrote the manuscript. Pathologic diagnosis was made by JH. Bronchoscopy was performed by S-WU, K-JL, and HK. YK, BBL, and DK conducted genome-wide methylation analysis and pyrosequencing. Surgical resection of lung cancer patients was performed by HKK and YMS. All authors read and approved the final manuscript.

Competing interests
The authors declare that they have no competing interests.

Author details
[1]Department of Internal Medicine, Samsung Medical Center, Sungkyunkwan University School of Medicine, Seoul 135-710, South Korea. [2]Department of Molecular Cell Biology, Samsung Biomedical Research Institute, Sungkyunkwan University School of Medicine, Suwon 440-746, South Korea. [3]Department of Thoracic and Cardiovascular Surgery, Samsung Medical Center, Sungkyunkwan University School of Medicine, Seoul 135-710, South Korea. [4]Department of Pathology, Samsung Medical Center, Sungkyunkwan University School of Medicine, Seoul 135-710, South Korea. [5]Samsung Medical Center, Research Institute for Future Medicine, #50 Ilwon-dong, Kangnam-gu, Professor Rm #5, Seoul 135-710, South Korea.

References
1. Siegel R, Naishadham D, Jemal A. Cancer statistics, 2012. CA Cancer J Clin. 2012;62:10–29.
2. Yamamoto K, Ohsumi A, Kojima F, Imanishi N, Matsuoka K, Ueda M, et al. Long-term survival after video-assisted thoracic surgery lobectomy for primary lung cancer. Ann Thorac Surg. 2010;89:353–9.
3. Ahrendt SA, Chow JT, Xu LH, Yang SC, Eisenberger CF, Esteller M, et al. Molecular detection of tumor cells in bronchoalveolar lavage fluid from patients with early stage lung cancer. J Natl Cancer Inst. 1999;91:332–9.
4. Kim H, Kwon YM, Kim JS, Lee H, Park JH, Shim YM, et al. Tumor-specific methylation in bronchial lavage for the early detection of non-small-cell lung cancer. J Clin Oncol. 2004;22:2363–70.
5. Kersting M, Friedl C, Kraus A, Behn M, Pankow W, Schuermann M. Differential frequencies of p16(INK4a) promoter hypermethylation, p53 mutation, and K-ras mutation in exfoliative material mark the development of lung cancer in symptomatic chronic smokers. J Clin Oncol. 2000;18:3221–9.
6. Grote HJ, Schmiemann V, Geddert H, Rohr UP, Kappes R, Gabbert HE, et al. Aberrant promoter methylation of p16(INK4a), RARB2 and SEMA3B in bronchial aspirates from patients with suspected lung cancer. Int J Cancer. 2005;116:720–5.
7. Nikolaidis G, Raji OY, Markopoulou S, Gosney JR, Bryan J, Warburton C, et al. DNA methylation biomarkers offer improved diagnostic efficiency in lung cancer. Cancer Res. 2012;72:5692–701.

8. Belinsky SA, Palmisano WA, Gilliland FD, Crooks LA, Divine KK, Winters SA, et al. Aberrant promoter methylation in bronchial epithelium and sputum from current and former smokers. Cancer Res. 2002;62:2370–7.

9. Millares L, Rosell A, Setó L, Sanz J, Andreo F, Monsó E. Variability in the measurement of the methylation status of lung cancer-related genes in bronchial secretions. Oncol Rep. 2014;32:1435–40.

10. Breitling LP, Yang R, Korn B, Burwinkel B, Brenner H. Tobacco-smoking-related differential DNA methylation: 27K discovery and replication. Am J Hum Genet. 2011;88:450–7.

11. Mortusewicz O, Schermelleh L, Walter J, Cardoso MC, Leonhardt H. Recruitment of DNA methyltransferase I to DNA repair sites. Proc Natl Acad Sci U S A. 2005;102:8905–9.

12. Di YP, Zhao J, Harper R. Cigarette smoke induces MUC5AC protein expression through the activation of Sp1. J Biol Chem. 2012;287:27948–58.

13. Lin RK, Hsieh YS, Lin P, Hsu HS, Chen CY, Tang YA, et al. The tobacco-specific carcinogen NNK induces DNA methyltransferase 1 accumulation and tumor suppressor gene hypermethylation in mice and lung cancer patients. J Clin Invest. 2010;120:521–32.

14. Ambatipudi S, Cuenin C, Hernandez-Vargas H, Ghantous A, Le Calvez-Kelm F, Kaaks R, et al. Tobacco smoking-associated genome-wide DNA methylation changes in the EPIC study. Epigenomics. 2016;8:599–618.

15. Guida F, Sandanger TM, Castagné R, Campanella G, Polidoro S, Palli D, et al. Dynamics of smoking-induced genome-wide methylation changes with time since smoking cessation. Hum Mol Genet. 2015;24:2349–59.

16. Edge SB, Byrd DR, Compton CC, Fritz AG, Greene FL, Troth A. American Joint Committee on Cancer. In: AJCC Cancer staging manual. 7th ed. New York: Springer; 2010. p. 253–70.

17. Pidsley R, Wong CCY, Volta M, Lunnon K, Mill J, Schalkwyk LC. A data-driven approach to preprocessing Illumina 450K methylation array data. BMC Genomics. 2013;14:293.

18. Issa JP, Ottaviano YL, Celano P, Hamilton SR, Davidson NE, Baylin SB. Methylation of the oestrogen receptor CpG island links ageing and neoplasia in human colon. Nat Genet. 1994;7:536–40.

19. Ahuja N, Li Q, Mohan AL, Baylin SB, Issa JP. Aging and DNA methylation in colorectal mucosa and cancer. Cancer Res. 1998;58:5489–94.

20. Greco SA, Chia J, Inglis KJ, Cozzi SJ, Ramsnes I, Buttenshaw RL, et al. Thrombospondin-4 is a putative tumour-suppressor gene in colorectal cancer that exhibits age-related methylation. BMC Cancer. 2010;10:494.

21. Issa JP, Vertino PM, Boehm CD, Newsham IF, Baylin SB. Switch from monoallelic to biallelic human IGF2 promoter methylation during aging and carcinogenesis. Proc Natl Acad Sci U S A. 1996;93:11757–62.

22. Li Q, Jedlicka A, Ahuja N, Gibbons MC, Baylin SB, Burger PC, et al. Concordant methylation of the ER and N33 genes in glioblastoma multiforme. Oncogene. 1998;16:3197–202.

23. Florath I, Butterbach K, Müller H, Bewerunge-Hudler M, Brenner H. Cross-sectional and longitudinal changes in DNA methylation with age: an epigenome-wide analysis revealing over 60 novel age-associated CpG sites. Hum Mol Genet. 2014;23:1186–201.

24. Bell JT, Tsai PC, Yang TP, Pidsley R, Nisbet J, Glass D, et al. Epigenome-wide scans identify differentially methylated regions for age and age-related phenotypes in a healthy ageing population. PLoS Genet. 2012;8:e1002629.

25. Cancer Genome Atlas Research Network. Comprehensive molecular profiling of lung adenocarcinoma. Nature. 2014;511:543–50.

26. Cancer Genome Atlas Research Network. Comprehensive genomic characterization of squamous cell lung cancers. Nature. 2012;489:519–25.

27. Um SW, Kim HK, Kim Y, Lee BB, Kim D, Han J, et al. Bronchial biopsy specimen as a surrogate for DNA methylation analysis in inoperable lung cancer. Clin Epigenetics. 2017;9:131.

28. Slaughter DP, Southwick HW, Smejkal W. Field cancerization in oral stratified squamous epithelium; clinical implications of multicentric origin. Cancer. 1953;6:963–8.

29. Kim DH, Nelson HH, Wiencke JK, Zheng S, Christiani DC, Wain JC, et al. p16INK4a and histology-specific methylation of CpG islands by exposure to tobacco smoke in non-small cell lung cancer. Cancer Res. 2001;61:3419–24.

30. Belinsky SA, Nikula KJ, Palmisano WA, Michels R, Saccomanno G, Gabrielson E, et al. Aberrant methylation of p16(INK4a) is an early event in lung cancer and a potential biomarker for early diagnosis. Proc Natl Acad Sci U S A. 1998;95:11891–6.

31. Zöchbauer-Müller S, Lam S, Toyooka S, Virmani AK, Toyooka KO, Seidl S, et al. Aberrant methylation of multiple genes in the upper aerodigestive tract epithelium of heavy smokers. Int J Cancer. 2003;107:612–6.

32. Buro-Auriemma LJ, Salit J, Hackett NR, Strulovici-Barel Y, Staudt MR, et al. Cigarette smoking induces small airway epithelial epigenetic changes with corresponding modulation of gene expression. Hum Mol Genet. 2013;22:4726–38.

33. Sood A, Petersen H, Blanchette CM, Meek P, Picchi MA, Belinsky SA, et al. Wood smoke exposure and gene promoter methylation are associated with increased risk for COPD in smokers. Am J Respir Crit Care Med. 2010;182:1098–104.

34. Shimazu T, Asada K, Charvat H, Kusano C, Otake Y, Kakugawa Y, et al. Association of gastric cancer risk factors with DNA methylation levels in gastric mucosa of healthy Japanese: a cross-sectional study. Carcinogenesis. 2015;36:1291–8.

35. Maccani JZ, Koestler DC, Houseman EA, Marsit CJ, Kelsey KT. Placental DNA methylation alterations associated with maternal tobacco smoking at the RUNX3 gene are also associated with gestational age. Epigenomics. 2013;5:619–30.

36. Zhu X, Li J, Deng S, Yu K, Liu X, Deng Q, et al. Genome-wide analysis of DNA methylation and cigarette smoking in a Chinese population. Environ Health Perspect. 2016;124:966–73.

37. Zeilinger S, Kühnel B, Klopp N, Baurecht H, Kleinschmidt A, Gieger C, et al. Tobacco smoking leads to extensive genome-wide changes in DNA methylation. PLoS One. 2013;8:e63812.

38. Yanada M, Yaoi T, Shimada J, Sakakura C, Nishimura M, Ito K, et al. Frequent hemizygous deletion at 1p36 and hypermethylation downregulate RUNX3 expression in human lung cancer cell lines. Oncol Rep. 2005;14:817–22.

39. Sato K, Tomizawa Y, Iijima H, Saito R, Ishizuka T, Nakajima T, et al. Epigenetic inactivation of the RUNX3 gene in lung cancer. Oncol Rep. 2006;15:129–35.

40. Subramaniam MM, Chan JY, Yeoh KG, Quek T, Ito K, Salto-Tellez M. Molecular pathology of RUNX3 in human carcinogenesis. Biochim Biophys Acta. 2009;1796:315–31.

41. Lund AH, van Lohuizen M. RUNX: a trilogy of cancer genes. Cancer Cell. 2002;1:213–5.

42. Chen LF. Tumor suppressor function of RUNX3 in breast cancer. J Cell Biochem. 2012;113:1470–7.

43. Hwang JA, Lee BB, Kim Y, Park SE, Heo K, Hong SH, et al. HOXA11 hypermethylation is associated with progression of non-small cell lung cancer. Oncotarget. 2013;4:2317–25.

44. Selamat SA, Galler JS, Joshi AD, Fyfe MN, Campan M, Siegmund KD, Kerr KM, Laird-Offringa IA, et al. DNA methylation changes in atypical adenomatous hyperplasia, adenocarcinoma in situ, and lung adenocarcinoma. PLoS One. 2011;6:e21443.

45. Anglim PP, Galler JS, Koss MN, Hagen JA, Turla S, Campan M, Weisenberger DJ, Laird PW, Siegmund KD, Laird-Offringa IA, et al. Identification of a panel of sensitive and specific DNA methylation markers for squamous cell lung cancer. Mol Cancer. 2008;7:62.

46. Rauch TA, Wang Z, Wu X, Kernstine KH, Riggs AD, Pfeifer GP. DNA methylation biomarkers for lung cancer. Tumour Biol. 2012;33:287–96.

47. Tessema M, Yingling CM, Grimes MJ, Thomas CL, Liu Y, Leng S, et al. Differential epigenetic regulation of TOX subfamily high mobility group box genes in lung and breast cancers. PLoS One. 2012;7:e34850.

12

Smoking induces coordinated DNA methylation and gene expression changes in adipose tissue with consequences for metabolic health

Pei-Chien Tsai[1,2,3]*, Craig A. Glastonbury[1,4], Melissa N. Eliot[5], Sailalitha Bollepalli[6], Idil Yet[1,7], Juan E. Castillo-Fernandez[1], Elena Carnero-Montoro[1,8], Thomas Hardiman[1,9], Tiphaine C. Martin[1,10,11], Alice Vickers[1,12], Massimo Mangino[1,13], Kirsten Ward[1], Kirsi H. Pietiläinen[14,15], Panos Deloukas[16,17], Tim D. Spector[1], Ana Viñuela[1,18,19,20], Eric B. Loucks[5], Miina Ollikainen[6], Karl T. Kelsey[5,21], Kerrin S. Small[1] and Jordana T. Bell[1]* (iD)

Abstract

Background: Tobacco smoking is a risk factor for multiple diseases, including cardiovascular disease and diabetes. Many smoking-associated signals have been detected in the blood methylome, but the extent to which these changes are widespread to metabolically relevant tissues, and impact gene expression or metabolic health, remains unclear.

Methods: We investigated smoking-associated DNA methylation and gene expression variation in adipose tissue biopsies from 542 healthy female twins. Replication, tissue specificity, and longitudinal stability of the smoking-associated effects were explored in additional adipose, blood, skin, and lung samples. We characterized the impact of adipose tissue smoking methylation and expression signals on metabolic disease risk phenotypes, including visceral fat.

Results: We identified 42 smoking-methylation and 42 smoking-expression signals, where five genes (*AHRR*, *CYP1A1*, *CYP1B1*, *CYTL1*, *F2RL3*) were both hypo-methylated and upregulated in current smokers. *CYP1A1* gene expression achieved 95% prediction performance of current smoking status. We validated and replicated a proportion of the signals in additional primary tissue samples, identifying tissue-shared effects. Smoking leaves systemic imprints on DNA methylation after smoking cessation, with stronger but shorter-lived effects on gene expression. Metabolic disease risk traits such as visceral fat and android-to-gynoid ratio showed association with methylation at smoking markers with functional impacts on expression, such as *CYP1A1*, and at tissue-shared smoking signals, such as *NOTCH1*. At smoking-signals, *BHLHE40* and *AHRR* DNA methylation and gene expression levels in current smokers were predictive of future gain in visceral fat upon smoking cessation.

Conclusions: Our results provide the first comprehensive characterization of coordinated DNA methylation and gene expression markers of smoking in adipose tissue. The findings relate to human metabolic health and give insights into understanding the widespread health consequence of smoking outside of the lung.

Keywords: Smoking, DNA methylation, Gene expression, RNA-sequencing, Adipose tissue

* Correspondence: pei-chien.tsai@kcl.ac.uk; jordana.bell@kcl.ac.uk
[1]Department of Twin Research and Genetic Epidemiology, King's College London, London SE1 7EH, UK
Full list of author information is available at the end of the article

Background

Tobacco smoking is a major environmental risk factor that predisposes an individual to chronic disease, cancer, and premature death [1, 2]. Smoking directly affects exposed regions of the lung [3], causes damage in organs throughout the body, and results in DNA mutations that have been linked to cancer [4]. The risk effects of smoking extend to multiple diseases, including cardiovascular and metabolic disease. Smoking cessation has also been linked to metabolic health complications and is associated with an increase in weight gain and in metabolic disease risk factors such as accumulation of visceral fat [5].

Persistent smoking has lasting effects on DNA methylation, and many epigenome-wide association studies (EWAS) have identified and replicated smoking-related differentially methylated signals across populations with the majority found in whole blood samples [6–20], buccal cells [21], and lung tissue [22, 23]. Most smoking methylation signals show lower levels of DNA methylation in current smokers compared to non-smokers, and variable dynamics upon cessation. Although some alterations persist over decades, smoking cessation can result in methylation levels reverting to those observed in non-smokers [13, 16, 18, 24]. However, most ex-smokers exhibit intermediate methylation levels between non-smokers and current smokers [13, 16, 18, 24]. Methylation levels correlate with the cumulative dose of smoking and are associated with time since smoking cessation [13, 16, 24, 25].

Smoking can also affect gene expression, as reported in the human airway epithelium [26, 27], lung tissue [28], alveolar macrophages [29], and lung cancer tissue [30].

However, few studies have examined DNA methylation and gene expression changes concurrently, and these studies were either conducted with low coverage genome assays (such as pyrosequencing [30] and HELP assay [8]) or targeted single genes of interest in small sample sizes [8, 30].

Here, we performed the first combined genome-wide analysis of smoking-related methylation and gene expression changes across tissues, focusing on adipose tissue. Exploring the molecular changes induced by smoking in a metabolically relevant tissue such as adipose tissue is of value to metabolic health research, because smoking is a risk factor for metabolic complications and smoking cessation has been linked to the accumulation of visceral fat. Here, we identify multiple genes that exhibit both methylation and expression changes within adipose tissue and across tissues, showing that smoking leaves a systemic imprint on DNA methylation and expression variation in the human body. Our data suggest that smoking leaves a stronger impact on gene expression, while DNA methylation smoking changes are more stable over time. By linking our findings to key human phenotypes related to metabolic health, we identify signals that could add understanding to some of the wide-ranging risk effects of smoking on metabolic diseases.

Results

Integrated DNA methylation and gene expression analyses in adipose tissue

Our study design is summarized in Fig. 1. Both DNA methylation and gene expression profiles were explored in adipose tissue biopsies from 542 subjects, comprising 54

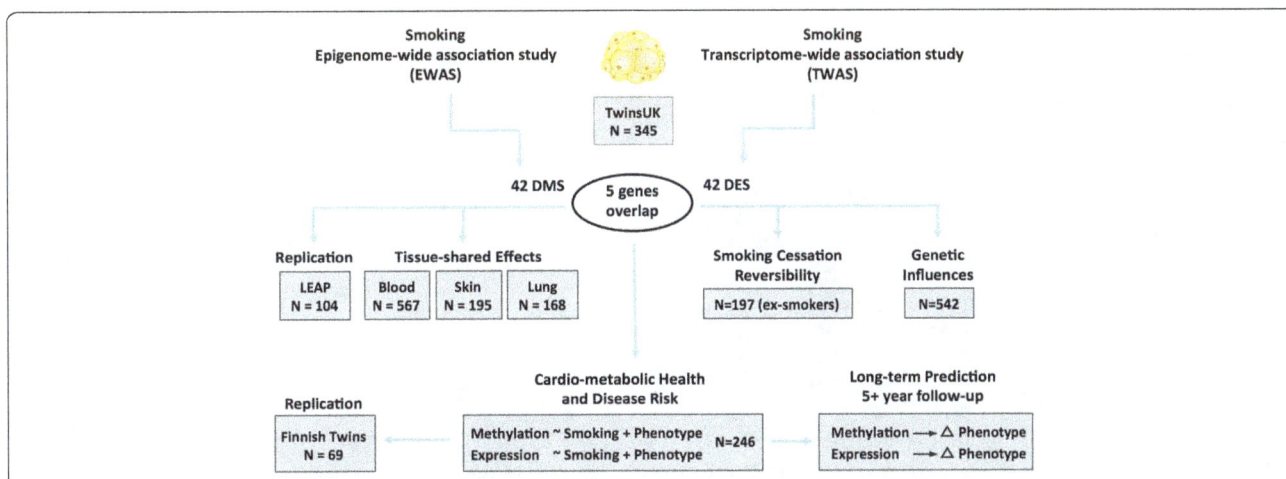

Fig. 1 Study design. Epigenome-wide and transcriptome-wide association studies were performed in 345 adipose tissue samples, identifying 42 smoking-DMS and 42 smoking-DES where five genes (14 CpG sites) overlapped. The 42 smoking-DMS were replicated in 104 independent subjects from the LEAP cohort, and the 14 smoking-DMS were further explored in blood, skin, and lung tissue for tissue-shared effects. DNA methylation and gene expression profiles at the 42 smoking-DMS and 42 smoking-DES were tested for smoking cessation reversibility in 197 ex-smokers. Heritability and QTL analyses testing genetic and environmental influences on methylation in the 542 adipose samples were also carried out. The final set of analyses focused on exploring the link between the 42 smoking-DMS and 42 smoking-DES with metabolic phenotypes. Phenotype associations with smoking-DMS were replicated in 69 Finnish twins. The last set of analyses explored the potential of methylation and gene expression levels at smoking-DMS and smoking-DES to predict future long-term changes in adiposity phenotypes in individuals who go on to quit smoking

current smokers, 197 ex-smokers, and 291 non-smokers. The 197 ex-smokers in our sample were excluded from analyses investigating methylation differences between current smokers and non-smokers, but were the focus of subsequent smoking cessation analyses. DNA methylation levels at 467,889 CpG sites from the Illumina Infinium HumanMethylation450 BeadChip were first compared between current smokers (mean BMI = 26.11 ± 4.66, mean age = 54.17 ± 8.31) and non-smokers (mean BMI = 26.95 ± 4.83, mean age = 59.18 ± 9.58). At a false discovery rate of 1% ($P < 8.37 \times 10^{-7}$), there were 42 smoking differentially methylated signals (smoking-DMS) or CpG sites, and these were located in 29 unique genomic regions comprising of 28 genes and 1 intergenic region (Fig. 2a). Smoking-DMS are located predominantly in the gene

body (47.6%), extended promoter region (38.1%), 3′UTR (4.7%), and intergenic region (9.5%), representing an enrichment of signals in the gene body relative to array composition. Using Roadmap annotations (adipose nuclei) [31], we observed that 16 smoking-DMS (38%) were located in enhancers and 9 (21%) were in or near active transcription start sites (TSS). Of these 25 enhancer or TSS signals, 9 were flanking bivalent enhancers ($n = 3$) or TSS ($n = 6$). As expected, methylation levels of current smokers were lower than those in non-smokers in the majority (90.5%) of the 42 signals (Table 1).

To assess the impact of potential confounders on these results, we performed two follow-up analyses. First, we considered the impact of adipose tissue cell-type composition heterogeneity by also analyzing these data within the

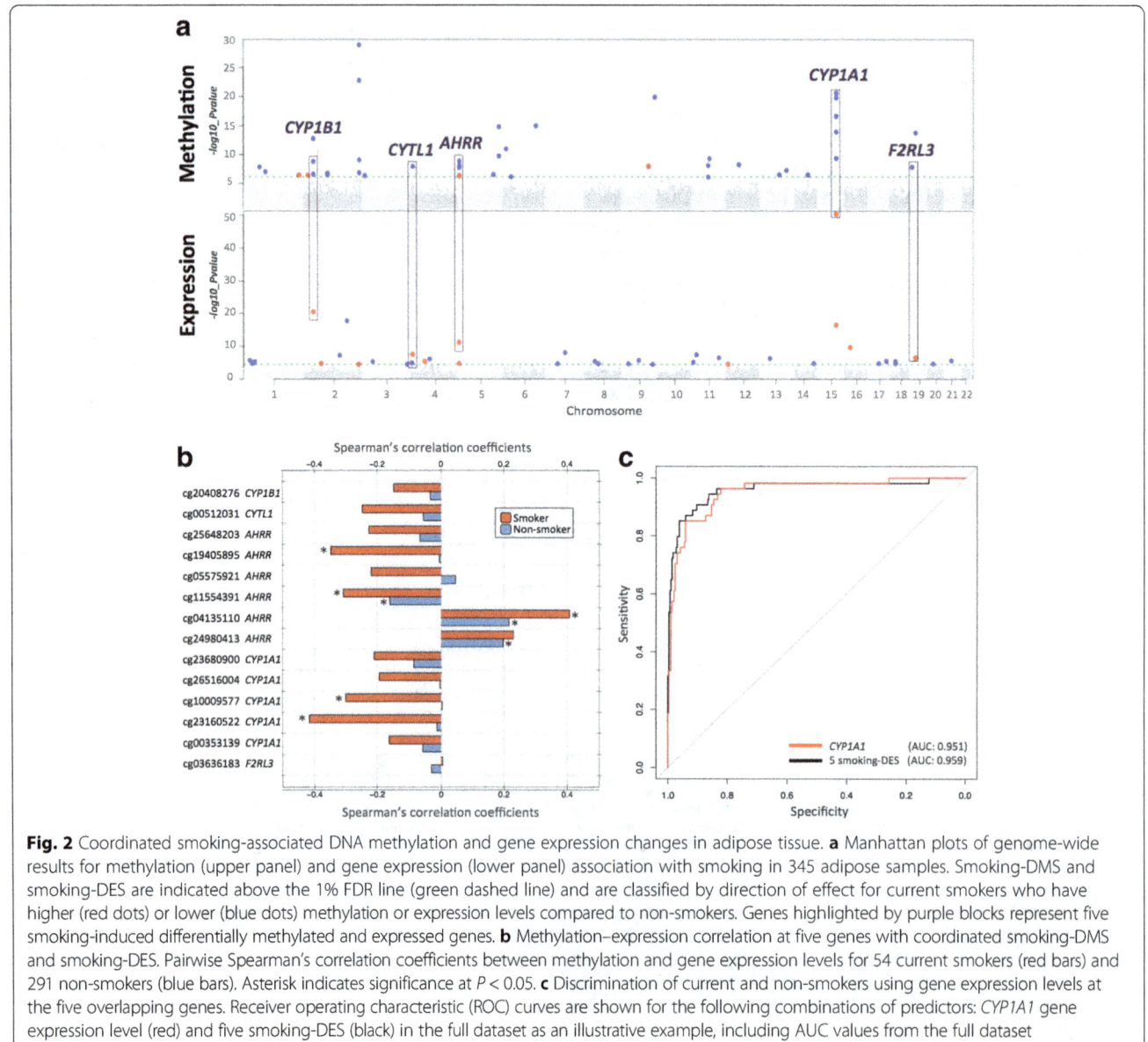

Fig. 2 Coordinated smoking-associated DNA methylation and gene expression changes in adipose tissue. **a** Manhattan plots of genome-wide results for methylation (upper panel) and gene expression (lower panel) association with smoking in 345 adipose samples. Smoking-DMS and smoking-DES are indicated above the 1% FDR line (green dashed line) and are classified by direction of effect for current smokers who have higher (red dots) or lower (blue dots) methylation or expression levels compared to non-smokers. Genes highlighted by purple blocks represent five smoking-induced differentially methylated and expressed genes. **b** Methylation–expression correlation at five genes with coordinated smoking-DMS and smoking-DES. Pairwise Spearman's correlation coefficients between methylation and gene expression levels for 54 current smokers (red bars) and 291 non-smokers (blue bars). Asterisk indicates significance at $P < 0.05$. **c** Discrimination of current and non-smokers using gene expression levels at the five overlapping genes. Receiver operating characteristic (ROC) curves are shown for the following combinations of predictors: CYP1A1 gene expression level (red) and five smoking-DES (black) in the full dataset as an illustrative example, including AUC values from the full dataset

Table 1 Smoking differentially methylated sites in adipose tissue (42 smoking-DMS)

IlmnID	CHR	Location	Gene name	Non-smoker β (mean ± SD)	Current smoker β (mean ± SD)	Coef.	S.E.	P value	cis-meQTL	S*
cg05951221	2	233284402	2q37.1	0.255 ± 0.054	0.172 ± 0.040	− 1.380	0.108	1.28×10^{-29}	rs2853386; 3.87×10^{-8}	
cg21566642	2	233284661	2q37.1	0.225 ± 0.040	0.167 ± 0.029	− 1.347	0.122	1.87×10^{-23}		
cg23680900	15	75017924	CYP1A1	0.202 ± 0.036	0.155 ± 0.030	− 1.198	0.118	2.96×10^{-21}		O
cg14120703	9	139416102	NOTCH1	0.748 ± 0.045	0.693 ± 0.044	− 1.172	0.118	1.44×10^{-20}		
cg26516004	15	75019376	CYP1A1	0.696 ± 0.047	0.628 ± 0.058	− 1.258	0.126	1.95×10^{-20}		Y
cg10009577	15	75018150	CYP1A1	0.068 ± 0.021	0.050 ± 0.016	− 0.810	0.090	2.48×10^{-17}		Y
cg01985595	6	136479501	PDE7B	0.961 ± 0.025	0.936 ± 0.032	− 1.015	0.119	1.09×10^{-15}		Y
cg22418620	5	172072885	NEURL1B	0.832 ± 0.049	0.765 ± 0.057	− 1.077	0.127	1.63×10^{-15}	rs57285944; 2.15×10^{-8}	Y
cg23160522	15	75015787	CYP1A1	0.622 ± 0.033	0.583 ± 0.044	− 0.991	0.122	1.33×10^{-14}		Y
cg03636183	19	17000585	F2RL3	0.506 ± 0.040	0.473 ± 0.038	− 0.826	0.103	1.80×10^{-14}		
cg07992500	2	37896583	CDC42EP3	0.771 ± 0.051	0.719 ± 0.052	− 1.087	0.141	1.88×10^{-13}	rs7595854; 1.32×10^{-7}	
cg12531611	6	11212619	NEDD9	0.909 ± 0.021	0.892 ± 0.024	− 0.855	0.120	1.12×10^{-11}		O
cg03646542	5	172076155	NEURL1B	0.689 ± 0.037	0.654 ± 0.035	− 0.880	0.133	1.87×10^{-10}	rs7715699; 1.72×10^{-10}	Y
cg00353139	15	75017914	CYP1A1	0.034 ± 0.013	0.022 ± 0.010	− 0.787	0.121	4.47×10^{-10}	rs11072498; 2.47×10^{-6}	Y
cg21124714	11	72983097	P2RY6	0.736 ± 0.037	0.707 ± 0.033	− 0.874	0.136	5.15×10^{-10}		Y
cg01940273	2	233284934	2q37.1	0.334 ± 0.045	0.302 ± 0.044	− 0.679	0.105	8.93×10^{-10}		
cg25648203	5	395444	AHRR	0.503 ± 0.044	0.459 ± 0.040	− 0.825	0.132	1.30×10^{-9}		
cg20408276	2	38300586	CYP1B1	0.548 ± 0.060	0.499 ± 0.059	− 0.781	0.125	1.61×10^{-9}		O
cg20131897	12	52305332	ACVRL1	0.694 ± 0.034	0.673 ± 0.028	−0.693	0.116	5.61×10^{-9}	rs1700159; 2.97×10^{-7}	Y
cg21611682	11	68138269	LRP5	0.370 ± 0.041	0.336 ± 0.035	−0.734	0.124	8.10×10^{-9}		
cg19405895	5	407315	AHRR	0.955 ± 0.014	0.942 ± 0.024	−0.768	0.128	8.38×10^{-9}		Y
cg05575921	5	373378	AHRR	0.713 ± 0.044	0.682 ± 0.039	− 0.611	0.104	1.07×10^{-8}	rs7731963; 3.97×10^{-8}	
cg13531977	9	112013420	EPB41L4B	0.807 ± 0.035	0.833 ± 0.029	0.831	0.140	1.14×10^{-8}		Y
cg00512031	4	5021976	CYTL1	0.880 ± 0.026	0.855 ± 0.028	−0.760	0.129	1.23×10^{-8}	chr4:5022470; 1.42×10^{-9}	Y
cg25189904	1	68299493	GNG12	0.100 ± 0.043	0.064 ± 0.030	−0.771	0.131	1.48×10^{-8}		
cg00378510	19	2291020	LINGO3	0.217 ± 0.059	0.181 ± 0.053	−0.781	0.134	1.53×10^{-8}	rs12609156; 6.83×10^{-18}	
cg11554391	5	321320	AHRR	0.065 ± 0.019	0.048 ± 0.014	−0.720	0.125	2.00×10^{-8}		
cg01802380	13	107865407	FAM155A	0.845 ± 0.030	0.825 ± 0.037	−0.737	0.133	5.69×10^{-8}	rs9520326; 1.52×10^{-12}	Y
cg14179389	1	92947961	GFI1	0.083 ± 0.030	0.063 ± 0.028	−0.665	0.122	1.07×10^{-7}		
cg06644428	2	233284112	2q37.1	0.036 ± 0.018	0.024 ± 0.010	− 0.704	0.130	1.61×10^{-7}		
cg12081267	2	98486185	TMEM131	0.878 ± 0.038	0.858 ± 0.035	− 0.650	0.122	1.97×10^{-7}		Y
cg02162897	2	38300537	CYP1B1	0.567 ± 0.060	0.520 ± 0.061	−0.674	0.127	2.89×10^{-7}		O
cg11555067	2	99081350	INPP4A	0.725 ± 0.047	0.700 ± 0.046	−0.717	0.138	3.18×10^{-7}	rs3754893; 2.27×10^{-7}	
cg04134818	5	148998446	FLJ41603	0.153 ± 0.026	0.133 ± 0.025	−0.690	0.132	3.26×10^{-7}	rs11950259; 7.83×10^{-6}	Y
cg03976650	13	77456505	KCTD12	0.667 ± 0.061	0.612 ± 0.067	−0.754	0.143	3.56×10^{-7}		Y
cg22851561	14	74214183	C14orf43	0.422 ± 0.041	0.390 ± 0.040	−0.634	0.121	3.92×10^{-7}		
cg10376100	1	236017278	LYST;MIR1537	0.923 ± 0.036	0.947 ± 0.030	0.615	0.117	4.03×10^{-7}		Y
cg04063216	2	14772482	FAM84A	0.071 ± 0.016	0.075 ± 0.019	0.441	0.085	4.39×10^{-7}		Y
cg16320419	3	5025570	BHLHE40	0.352 ± 0.052	0.315 ± 0.048	− 0.699	0.135	4.88×10^{-7}		
cg04135110	5	346695	AHRR	0.339 ± 0.061	0.384 ± 0.065	0.699	0.137	5.34×10^{-7}	rs2672748; 3.42×10^{-17}	
cg20109054	6	31804109	C6orf48;SNORD52	0.091 ± 0.026	0.072 ± 0.023	− 0.659	0.130	7.85×10^{-7}	rs3828922; 2.74×10^{-5}	
cg16721845	11	68518800	MTL5	0.018 ± 0.008	0.014 ± 0.007	− 0.530	0.106	8.37×10^{-7}		Y

IlmnID, Illumina probe ID; CHR, chromosome; Location, location of the CpG site (bp); β (mean ± SD), mean and standard deviation of the Illumina beta methylation levels in the non-smoker and current smoker group; Coef., regression coefficients from the linear mixed effect model, positive values denote hypermethylation in current smokers and negative values denote hypo-methylation in current smokers; cis-meQTL, top significant cis-meQTL for the CpG site; S*, adipose tissue-specific effect

Here, we compared our results to one of the biggest smoking-EWAS conducted in blood [20], probes not listed as their significant signals (on their Additional file 2: Table S2, FDR ≤ 0.05) were recorded as "Y" in this table; probes with significant effects in blood in the opposite direction are recorded as "O"

reference-free EWAS framework [32]. We observed that the 42 smoking-DMS remained significant at false discovery rate (FDR) of 1%, suggesting that cell composition within adipose tissue did not have a major impact on our findings (Additional file 1: Figure S1). Second, habitual smoking is strongly associated with alcohol consumption [33], and in our data, current smokers and ex-smokers have a higher alcohol intake compared to non-smokers (average alcohol intake = 5.96 (non-smokers), 10.03 (ex-smokers), and 11.67 (current smokers) grams per day, $P = 1.06 \times 10^{-5}$). Although our smoking analyses take into account alcohol consumption as a covariate, it is possible that the smoking-DMS still in part capture alcohol consumption. To test for the co-occurrence of differentially methylated signals for smoking and alcohol consumption, we performed an alcohol EWAS adjusting for smoking to compare the results with the 42 smoking-DMS. We observed no significant association between alcohol consumption and methylation at genome-wide significance after adjusting for smoking in adipose tissue, and only 7 smoking-DMS in *AHRR* (cg01802380, cg04134818, cg19405895), *CYP1B1* (cg19 405895, cg20408276), *FAM84A* (cg04063216), and *C6or f48* (cg20109054) surpassed nominal significance (*P* values between 0.05 and 0.005).

We next compared RNA-sequencing profiles from the same tissue biopsy between current smokers and non-smokers at the gene-based level using RPKM values across 17,399 genes. At an FDR of 1% ($P < 2.86 \times 10^{-5}$), there were 42 differentially expressed signals (smoking-DES) or genes (Fig. 2a), and 14 of these were up-regulated in current smokers (Table 2). The strongest smoking-related expression signal was in the *CYP1A1* gene—a lung cancer susceptibility gene, which was also one of the differentially methylated signals. Gene expression levels in *CYP1A1* were higher in current smokers compared to non-smokers (Figs. 2a and 3).

Comparison of the FDR 1% genome-wide significant smoking-DMS and smoking-DES showed overlapping signals at five genes comprising 14 CpG sites, and these included *AHRR, CYP1A1, CYP1B1, CYTL1,* and *F2RL3* (Fig. 2a). CpG sites within *AHRR, CYP1B1,* and *F2RL3* were located in the gene body, whereas CpG sites in or near *CYP1A1* and *CYTL1* were located 200 kb to 1500 kb away from the transcription start sites. All five genes were upregulated in current smokers, and in the majority of smoking-DMS (93%), current smokers showed lower methylation levels compared to non-smokers. These predominantly negative correlations between methylation and expression at these five genes suggested regulatory effects (Table 3, Fig. 2b). The methylation-expression correlations at some of these CpG sites were only observed in current smokers, and overall correlations were stronger in smokers compared to non-smokers.

Prediction of smoking status based on DNA methylation and gene expression

To assess the impact of smoking on DNA methylation and gene expression within the same analysis framework and at a comparable scale, we used methylation and expression changes at these five overlapping genes (14 CpG sites) to predict a subject's smoking status using a logistic regression model. We split the overall dataset into training and validation sets of equal size and report here the average area under curve (AUC) values from 1000 validation sets. The combination of 14 smoking-DMS levels and 5 smoking-DES levels resulted in reasonable discrimination of smoking status (AUC: 0.865). Compared to the prediction results based on 14 smoking-DMS levels alone (AUC: 0.888), smoking-DES levels are better predictors (all five genes, AUC: 0.951). This suggests that smoking leaves a greater impact on gene expression levels, compared to DNA methylation levels at these overlapping genes. A similar high predictive value can be achieved by using gene expression levels at just a single gene, *CYP1A1* (AUC: 0.952) (Fig. 2c). *CYP1A1* was the peak smoking differentially expressed gene, with differentially methylated signals in the promoter, and a negative correlation between methylation and expression (Fig. 3b).

Adipose-specific and tissue-shared smoking signals

To test if the effects of smoking are shared across tissues, we first compared our adipose findings to results from whole blood samples. To this end, we tested for association between smoking and whole blood genome-wide DNA methylation (in 569 individuals) and gene expression profiles (in 237 individuals), comparing current smokers with non-smokers. In blood, genome-wide significant results at FDR 1% for smoking DMS and DES overlapped at four genes (Additional file 2: Table S1). Altogether, comparison of FDR 1% significant smoking-DMS results across the adipose and whole blood datasets identified 14 CpG sites that were genome-wide differentially methylated in both blood and adipose tissue (Fig. 4a). The 14 tissue-shared CpG sites fell in eight genes, including *GNG12, GFI1, AHRR, NOTCH1, LRP5, C14orf43, LINGO3, F2RL3,* and in the 2q37.1 intergenic region (Table 4). All of these sites were previously reported as smoking differentially methylated sites in blood in previous studies [6–19] and include *AHRR*—the most robustly replicated smoking-methylation signal (Fig. 5a). DNA methylation changes in two genes (*AHRR* and *F2RL3*) that exhibit both expression and methylation smoking-associated effects in adipose tissue were also present in the blood (Figs. 4c and 5b).

We sought to explore the observed tissue-shared methylation effects at the 14 putative tissue-shared CpG sites in additional datasets including 195 skin tissue samples from healthy subjects [34] and 168 lung tissue

Table 2 Smoking differentially expressed genes in adipose tissue (42 smoking-DES)

ID	CHR	Name	Coef.	S.E.	P value	cis eQTLs
ENSG00000140465.7	15	CYP1A1	1.899	0.103	5.37×10^{-51}	rs35213055; 1.53×10^{-6}
ENSG00000138061.7	2	CYP1B1	1.373	0.131	2.83×10^{-21}	
ENSG00000144331.14	2	ZNF385B	-1.257	0.134	1.53×10^{-18}	rs9288034; 8.33×10^{-5}
ENSG00000179151.6	15	EDC3	1.167	0.129	3.10×10^{-17}	
ENSG00000063438.12	5	AHRR	1.059	0.149	6.03×10^{-12}	
ENSG00000175267.8	16	VWA3A	0.932	0.139	2.18×10^{-10}	
ENSG00000170381.7	7	SEMA3E	-0.821	0.137	8.35×10^{-9}	chr7:83264879;1.22×10^{-10}
ENSG00000170891.6	4	CYTL1	0.807	0.142	2.82×10^{-8}	
ENSG00000187486.5	11	KCNJ11	-0.859	0.148	3.27×10^{-8}	
ENSG00000168280.11	2	KIF5C	-0.813	0.145	4.74×10^{-8}	
ENSG00000006016.5	19	CRLF1	0.769	0.146	2.53×10^{-7}	chr19:18717389; 2.63×10^{-6}
ENSG00000127533.2	19	F2RL3	0.782	0.147	2.89×10^{-7}	
ENSG00000149294.11	11	NCAM1	-0.715	0.135	3.03×10^{-7}	rs17510563; 2.01×10^{-7}
ENSG00000120693.9	13	SMAD9	-0.733	0.140	4.76×10^{-7}	
ENSG00000169116.7	4	PARM1	-0.686	0.133	6.76×10^{-7}	
ENSG00000154330.6	9	PGM5	-0.716	0.147	1.72×10^{-6}	
ENSG00000162430.12	1	SEPN1	-0.663	0.137	1.82×10^{-6}	
ENSG00000154721.9	21	JAM2	-0.667	0.136	2.23×10^{-6}	
ENSG00000177303.4	17	CASKIN2	-0.669	0.140	2.90×10^{-6}	
ENSG00000157404.10	4	KIT	0.708	0.150	3.31×10^{-6}	
ENSG00000161544.4	17	CYGB	0.621	0.131	3.42×10^{-6}	
ENSG00000154065.9	18	ANKRD29	-0.684	0.144	3.49×10^{-6}	
ENSG00000176907.3	8	C8orf4	-0.714	0.151	3.56×10^{-6}	
ENSG00000168032.4	3	ENTPD3	-0.674	0.140	3.86×10^{-6}	rs34158576; 7.60×10^{-6}
ENSG00000162367.6	1	TAL1	-0.665	0.142	4.17×10^{-6}	
ENSG00000180785.8	11	OR51E1	-0.655	0.142	6.82×10^{-6}	rs11033126; 3.78×10^{-10}
ENSG00000164010.9	1	ERMAP	-0.690	0.154	9.50×10^{-6}	
ENSG00000068078.12	4	FGFR3	-0.643	0.143	9.68×10^{-6}	rs744658; 9.68×10^{-8}
ENSG00000246223.4	14	C14orf64	-0.633	0.142	1.44×10^{-5}	rs75700090; 2.00×10^{-5}
ENSG00000145506.9	5	NKD2	0.616	0.140	1.46×10^{-5}	
ENSG00000161649.7	17	CD300LG	-0.648	0.147	1.48×10^{-5}	
ENSG00000163873.5	1	GRIK3	-0.643	0.146	1.50×10^{-5}	
ENSG00000053747.9	18	LAMA3	-0.652	0.148	1.57×10^{-5}	
ENSG00000183733.6	2	FIGLA	0.406	0.093	1.57×10^{-5}	
ENSG00000164736.5	8	SOX17	-0.629	0.144	1.64×10^{-5}	
ENSG00000106078.12	7	COBL	-0.680	0.155	1.65×10^{-5}	
ENSG00000120156.14	9	TEK	-0.610	0.140	1.67×10^{-5}	
ENSG00000178726.5	20	THBD	-0.612	0.141	2.00×10^{-5}	
ENSG00000177675.4	12	CD163L1	0.635	0.148	2.40×10^{-5}	
ENSG00000136828.13	9	RALPGS1	-0.646	0.151	2.60×10^{-5}	
ENSG00000135914.4	2	HTR2B	0.613	0.144	2.82×10^{-5}	
ENSG00000090530.5	3	LEPREL1	-0.617	0.145	2.86×10^{-5}	rs6768989; 1.10×10^{-9}

ID, Ensemble ID; *CHR*, chromosome; *Coef.*, regression coefficients from the linear mixed effect model, positive values reflect higher expression in current smokers and negative values represent lower expression in current smokers; *eQTL*, expression quantitative trait locus

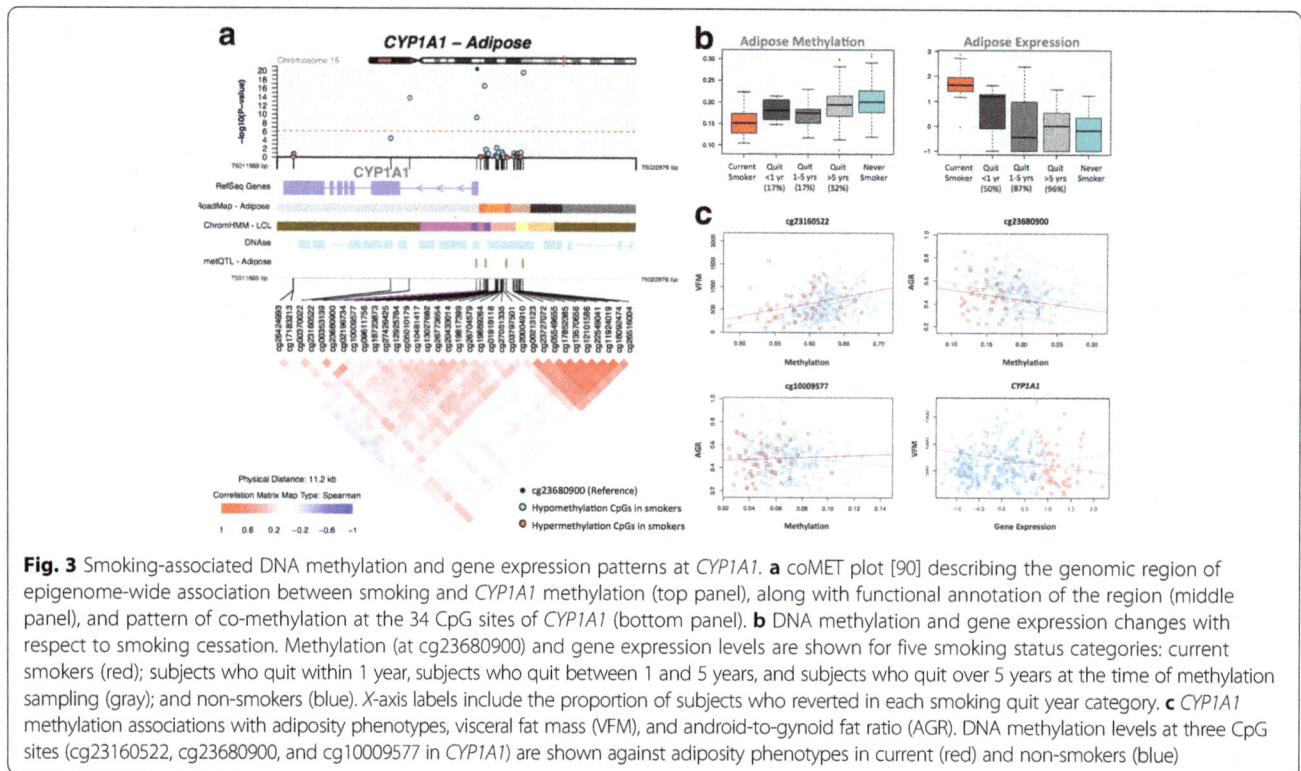

Fig. 3 Smoking-associated DNA methylation and gene expression patterns at *CYP1A1*. **a** coMET plot [90] describing the genomic region of epigenome-wide association between smoking and *CYP1A1* methylation (top panel), along with functional annotation of the region (middle panel), and pattern of co-methylation at the 34 CpG sites of *CYP1A1* (bottom panel). **b** DNA methylation and gene expression changes with respect to smoking cessation. Methylation (at cg23680900) and gene expression levels are shown for five smoking status categories: current smokers (red); subjects who quit within 1 year, subjects who quit between 1 and 5 years, and subjects who quit over 5 years at the time of methylation sampling (gray); and non-smokers (blue). *X*-axis labels include the proportion of subjects who reverted in each smoking quit year category. **c** *CYP1A1* methylation associations with adiposity phenotypes, visceral fat mass (VFM), and android-to-gynoid fat ratio (AGR). DNA methylation levels at three CpG sites (cg23160522, cg23680900, and cg10009577 in *CYP1A1*) are shown against adiposity phenotypes in current (red) and non-smokers (blue)

samples from subjects affected with lung cancer. Four of the 14 CpG sites validated in the skin in the intergenic region 2q37.1 (cg05951221, cg06644428, and cg21566642) and in *AHRR* (cg05575921). Furthermore, the majority ($n = 13$) of the 14 tissue-shared CpG sites had lower methylation levels in current smokers compared to non-smokers in both lung and skin methylation datasets, indicating a consistent direction of effect, which was not nominally significant (Table 4, Additional file 2: Table S2). In lung tissue from subjects affected with lung cancer, we validated 3 of the 14 CpG sites in the intergenic region 2q37.1 (cg21566642 and cg05951221) and in the *AHRR* gene (cg05575921) at a Bonferroni-corrected *P* value of 3.57×10^{-3} (Additional file 2: Table S2). The smoking-DMS effects observed across tissues were similar for CpG sites in the 2q37.1 region, while the smoking effect was much greater in blood at cg05575921 in *AHRR* (see Table 4, Fig. 4b).

In contrast to the methylation results, gene expression signals showed minimal evidence for tissue-shared impacts. Comparing our FDR 1% genome-wide smoking-DES across adipose and blood datasets showed that only *AHRR* was significantly upregulated in current smokers across both tissues (Fig. 5c). *AHRR* was the only signal that showed both differential methylation and expression changes across all of the datasets that we explored in this study, including blood, adipose, skin, and lung tissue.

A proportion of our smoking-DMS and most of our smoking-DES results appear to be adipose-specific. However, the sample size of the datasets used to explore tissue specificity in gene expression was much lower compared to that used for methylation; therefore, power to detect tissue-shared effects differs across the data types. Furthermore, we are limited by access to available multi-tissue datasets for follow-up, and further investigation of published findings reveals that some of our smoking adipose-specific signals have previously been detected in other tissues [20] For example, one of our peak results at *CYP1A1* showed methylation changes only in adipose tissue and not in the blood (Fig. 4), but has previously been reported as a smoking-methylation signal in blood [20], lung tissue [30, 35], cord blood [36], and placenta [37, 38]. Unlike the persistent tissue-shared effects identified in other smoking-DMS such as signals in *AHRR* and 2q37.1, we found that current smokers have lower *CYP1A1* methylation levels in adipose, skin, and lung tissue, but not in blood [20], placenta, and cord blood samples [36], overall suggesting that smoking may have contrasting effects, resulting in hyper- or hypo-methylation in different tissues (Fig. 4b). A similar contrast in direction of smoking methylation effects is observed at smoking-DMS in *NEDD9* and *CYP1B1* across adipose tissue and in blood (Table 1).

Table 3 Correlation between DNA methylation and gene expression

Gene name	IlmnID	CHR	Location	ID	r	P value
CYP1B1	cg20408276	2	38300586	ENSG00000138061.7	− 0.171	1.39×10^{-3}
CYTL1	cg00512031	4	5021976	ENSG00000170891.6	− 0.176	1.03×10^{-3}
AHRR	cg25648203	5	395444	ENSG00000063438.12	− 0.167	1.80×10^{-3}
AHRR	cg19405895	5	407315	ENSG00000063438.12	− 0.134	1.29×10^{-2}
AHRR	cg05575921	5	373378	ENSG00000063438.12	− 0.060	0.2633
AHRR	cg11554391	5	321320	ENSG00000063438.12	− 0.216	5.37×10^{-5}
AHRR	cg04135110	5	346695	ENSG00000063438.12	0.279	1.31×10^{-7}
AHRR	cg24980413	5	346987	ENSG00000063438.12	0.252	2.10×10^{-6}
CYP1A1	cg23680900	15	75017924	ENSG00000140465.7	− 0.329	3.94×10^{-10}
CYP1A1	cg26516004	15	75019376	ENSG00000140465.7	− 0.298	1.70×10^{-8}
CYP1A1	cg10009577	15	75018150	ENSG00000140465.7	-0.266	5.22×10^{-7}
CYP1A1	cg23160522	15	75015787	ENSG00000140465.7	− 0.299	1.48×10^{-8}
CYP1A1	cg00353139	15	75017914	ENSG00000140465.7	− 0.222	3.22×10^{-5}
F2RL3	cg03636183	19	17000585	ENSG00000127533.2	− 0.130	0.0159

IlmnID, Illumina probe ID; *CHR*, chromosome; *Location*, Illumina probe location (bp); *ID*, Ensemble ID; *r*, Spearman's correlation coefficients between methylation and gene expression data ($n = 345$)

Replication of adipose smoking methylation signals

We pursued replication of the adipose tissue smoking-DMS in an independent dataset of 104 participants from the LEAP cohort, within the New England Family Study (mean BMI 30.9 ± 7.03, mean age 47 ± 1.7, 48% male), described in detail elsewhere [39]. These individuals were not affected with common diseases and had available adipose biopsy methylation profiles for 46 current smokers and 58 non-smokers. We found that the smoking-methylation direction of association was consistent at all 42 adipose smoking-DMS (Additional file 2: Table S3), and 25 of these also surpassed nominal significance in the replication dataset ($P = 0.05$). At a more stringent threshold, the replication signal was significant at 13 sites, surpassing Bonferroni-adjusted P value for the replication analysis ($P = 1.19 \times 10^{-3}$).

Signatures of smoking cessation

We next assessed the effect of smoking cessation on the observed adipose DNA methylation and gene expression signals in ex-smokers from the discovery cohort. We considered reversal of smoking methylation or expression signals, that is, the longitudinal change in methylation to reach levels observed in non-smokers. We quantified the number of subjects who reverted to 25% of the change in methylation towards non-smokers, and estimated the proportion of subjects who reverted over time (in smoking-quit years), using the same approach in gene expression (see the "Methods" section).

We explored reversal patterns in adipose tissue at both the 42 smoking-DMS (Additional file 1: Figure S2) and 42 smoking-DES (Additional file 1: Figure S3) and focused on the five differentially methylated and expressed genes (14 CpG sites), where the average number of smoking-quit years was 24.8 (± 13.21) years among 197 ex-smokers. Overall, a rapid rate of reversal was observed in the first 10 years after smoking cessation, after which only subtle changes were detected in both methylation and gene expression. In the expression adipose data, ex-smokers showed a > 50% reversal rate 1 year after smoking cessation and reached > 85% reversal after 10 years (Additional file 1: Figure S3). In comparison, slower reversal was observed in the methylation dataset (Additional file 1: Figure S2). Among the 14 CpG sites, only three (two at *AHRR* and one at *CYP1A1*) showed a 50% reversal rate 1 year after cessation, while the remaining signals showed between 17 and 33% reversal (Figs. 3b and 5c, Additional file 1: Figure S3). Even after > 40 years of smoking cessation, a proportion of smoking-DMS ($n = 12$; 29%) showed less than 40% reversal (Additional file 1: Figure S3). This suggests that smoking leaves a longer lasting influence on DNA methylation levels than on gene expression levels after smoking cessation.

Controlling for genetic variation

Previous studies have shown heritable impacts on smoking behavior and nicotine addiction [40–43]. We explored the impact of genetic variation on the identified smoking methylation signals. Of the 42 smoking-DMS, 14 CpG sites had genome-wide significant meQTLs in *cis* in adipose tissue (Table 1). Of the 14 tissue-shared smoking-DMS, two signals in 2q37.1 and one in *LINGO3* had meQTLs in *cis* in adipose tissue, and three signals in *AHRR* and one in *F2RL3* had meQTLs in *cis* in blood samples.

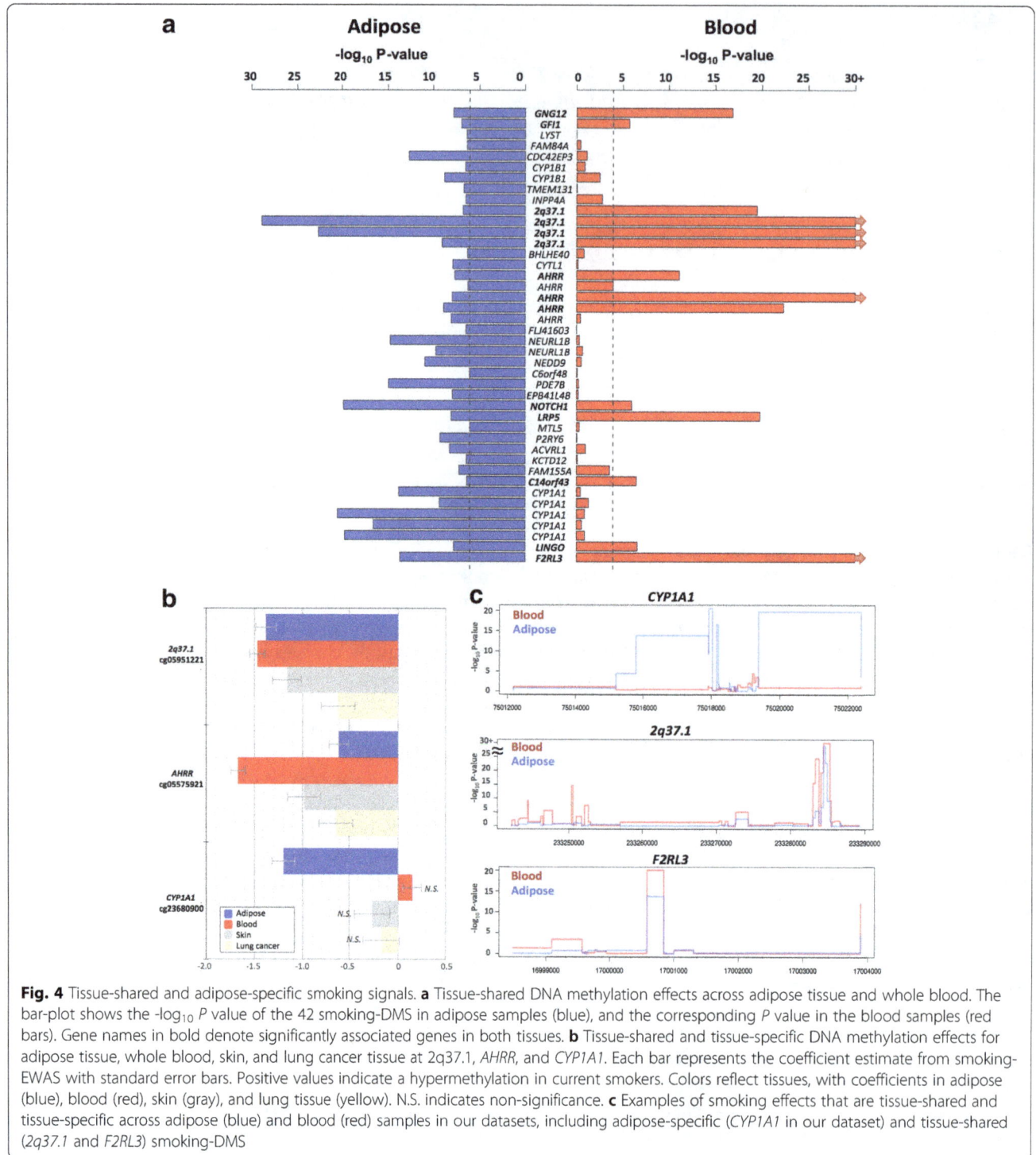

Fig. 4 Tissue-shared and adipose-specific smoking signals. **a** Tissue-shared DNA methylation effects across adipose tissue and whole blood. The bar-plot shows the -log$_{10}$ P value of the 42 smoking-DMS in adipose samples (blue), and the corresponding P value in the blood samples (red bars). Gene names in bold denote significantly associated genes in both tissues. **b** Tissue-shared and tissue-specific DNA methylation effects for adipose tissue, whole blood, skin, and lung cancer tissue at 2q37.1, *AHRR*, and *CYP1A1*. Each bar represents the coefficient estimate from smoking-EWAS with standard error bars. Positive values indicate a hypermethylation in current smokers. Colors reflect tissues, with coefficients in adipose (blue), blood (red), skin (gray), and lung tissue (yellow). N.S. indicates non-significance. **c** Examples of smoking effects that are tissue-shared and tissue-specific across adipose (blue) and blood (red) samples in our datasets, including adipose-specific (*CYP1A1* in our dataset) and tissue-shared (2q37.1 and *F2RL3*) smoking-DMS

Given our observed genetic influences on smoking-DMS, we asked if previously reported genetic variants associated with smoking behavior [42] or nicotine metabolism [43] could impact DNA methylation levels in adipose tissue. We first focused on common genetic variants that were previously associated with smoking phenotypes in the largest smoking genetic association study to date (*n* = 15,907) [42]. We observed that all genetic variants previously strongly linked to smoking behavior (14 SNPs) [42] had an impact on adipose DNA methylation levels in *cis* (Additional file 2: Table S4). We then explored a recently reported association between

Table 4 Tissue-shared smoking-induced differentially methylated sites in cancer-free subjects

IlmnID	CHR	Location	Gene name	Adipose tissue (n = 345)		Blood samples (n = 567)		Skin tissue (n = 195)	
				Coef.	P value	Coef.	P value	Coef.	P value
cg25189904	1	68299493	GNG12	− 0.771	1.48×10^{-8}	− 0.974	6.92×10^{-18}	− 0.434	1.58×10^{-2}
cg14179389	1	92947961	GFI1	− 0.665	1.07×10^{-7}	− 0.404	4.74×10^{-6}	− 0.408	1.89×10^{-2}
cg06644428	2	233284112	2q37.1	− 0.704	1.61×10^{-7}	− 0.864	1.76×10^{-19}	− 0.641	3.39×10^{-4}
cg05951221	2	233284402	2q37.1	− 1.38	1.28×10^{-29}	− 1.471	3.65×10^{-60}	− 1.161	6.13×10^{-13}
cg21566642	2	233284661	2q37.1	− 1.347	1.87×10^{-23}	− 1.491	9.67×10^{-61}	− 1.138	4.83×10^{-11}
cg01940273	2	233284934	2q37.1	− 0.679	8.93×10^{-10}	− 1.415	3.17×10^{-52}	− 0.302	3.09×10^{-2}
cg11554391	5	321320	AHRR	− 0.72	2.00×10^{-8}	− 0.694	8.10×10^{-12}	− 0.494	4.91×10^{-3}
cg05575921	5	373378	AHRR	− 0.611	1.07×10^{-8}	− 1.672	2.45×10^{-80}	− 0.982	7.24×10^{-8}
cg25648203	5	395444	AHRR	− 0.825	1.30×10^{-9}	− 0.937	3.50×10^{-22}	− 0.398	7.29×10^{-3}
cg14120703	9	139416102	NOTCH1	− 1.172	1.44×10^{-20}	− 0.352	1.84×10^{-6}	− 0.423	8.69×10^{-3}
cg21611682	11	68138269	LRP5	− 0.734	8.10×10^{-9}	− 0.874	4.23×10^{-20}	0.075	6.38×10^{-1}
cg22851561	14	74214183	C14orf43	− 0.634	3.92×10^{-7}	− 0.5	5.24×10^{-7}	− 0.326	7.07×10^{-2}
cg00378510	19	2291020	LINGO3	− 0.781	1.53×10^{-8}	− 1.478	3.59×10^{-62}	− 0.133	4.66×10^{-1}
cg03636183	19	17000585	F2RL3	− 0.826	1.80×10^{-14}	− 0.466	2.37×10^{-7}	− 0.372	1.45×10^{-2}

IlmnID, Illumina probe ID; *CHR*, chromosome; *Location*, Illumina probe location (bp); *Coef.*, regression coefficients from the linear mixed effect model, positive values denote hypermethylation in non-smokers and negative values denote hypermethylation in current smokers

a cluster of SNPs on chromosome 19 and nicotine metabolism, where the same genetic variants were also associated with blood DNA methylation levels in the same region as meQTLs [43]. We replicate the chromosome 19 meQTL findings in our adipose DNA methylation data at CpGs in genes *CYP2A7*, *ENGL2*, and *LTBP4* (Additional file 2: Table S5), suggesting that these are strong genetic impacts on DNA methylation that are shared across tissues. Taken together, these genetic-methylation association results provide additional support for the hypothesis that some of the observed genetic impacts on smoking behavior and nicotine metabolism may be mediated by DNA methylation.

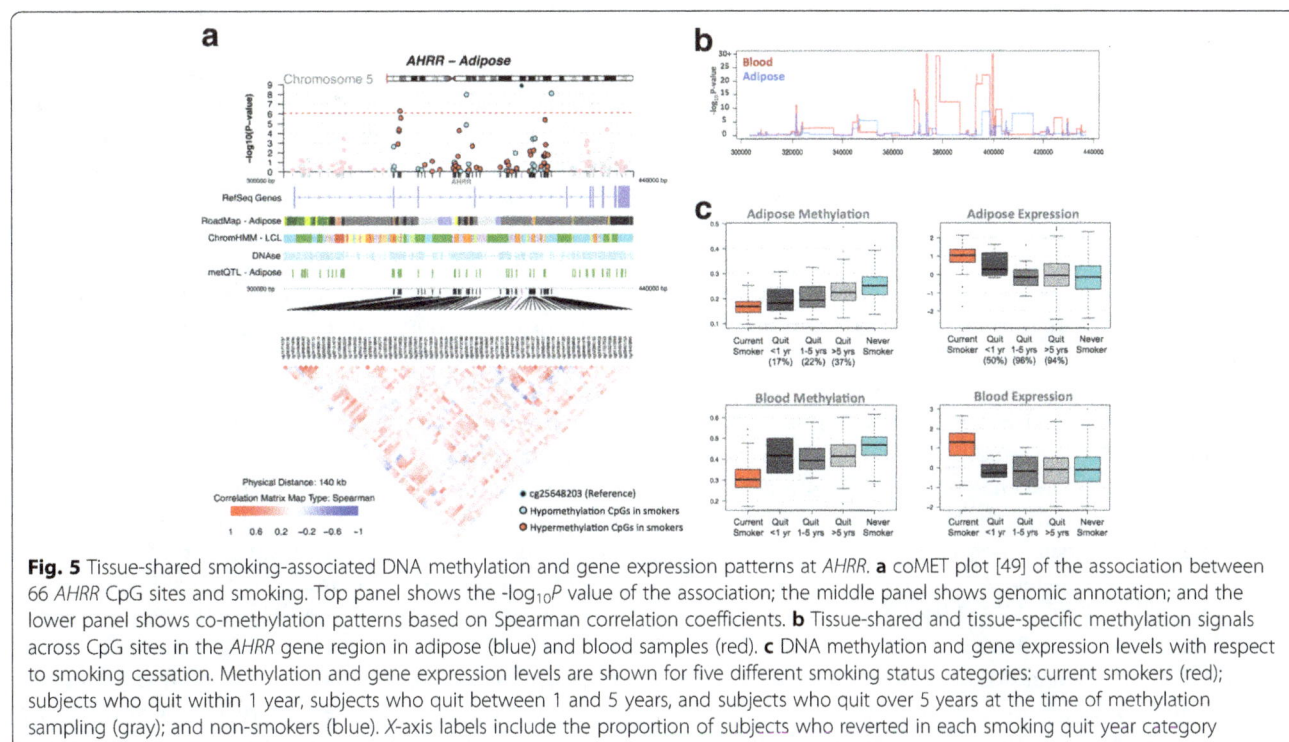

Fig. 5 Tissue-shared smoking-associated DNA methylation and gene expression patterns at *AHRR*. **a** coMET plot [49] of the association between 66 *AHRR* CpG sites and smoking. Top panel shows the -$\log_{10}P$ value of the association; the middle panel shows genomic annotation; and the lower panel shows co-methylation patterns based on Spearman correlation coefficients. **b** Tissue-shared and tissue-specific methylation signals across CpG sites in the *AHRR* gene region in adipose (blue) and blood samples (red). **c** DNA methylation and gene expression levels with respect to smoking cessation. Methylation and gene expression levels are shown for five different smoking status categories: current smokers (red); subjects who quit within 1 year, subjects who quit between 1 and 5 years, and subjects who quit over 5 years at the time of methylation sampling (gray); and non-smokers (blue). X-axis labels include the proportion of subjects who reverted in each smoking quit year category

Impacts on metabolic health and disease risk

Given the wide-ranging effects of smoking on human disease, we explored the links between the identified adipose methylation and expression smoking signals and phenotypes that are major risk factors for metabolic disease. Three metabolic disease risk phenotypes—total fat mass (TFM), visceral fat mass (VFM), and android-to-gynoid fat ratio (AGR)—were profiled using dual X-ray absorptiometry in 288 subjects with adipose methylation and expression profiles. We assessed the association of the 42 smoking-DMS and 42 smoking-DES with these adiposity phenotypes using a twofold approach.

First, we tested for association between adipose methylation levels at the 42 smoking-DMS and the three phenotypes, adjusting for covariates including age, BMI, and smoking. We observed that smoking-DMS in *CYP1A1* and *NOTCH1* were significantly associated with measures of metabolic disease risk. First, methylation levels at three CpG sites in *CYP1A1* were significantly associated with VFM and AGR, either as main effects (cg23160522 and VFM, beta = 1.35×10^{-3}, SE = 3.03×10^{-3}, $P = 4.35 \times 10^{-7}$; cg23680900 and AGR, beta = -1.59, SE = 0.44, $P = 6.58 \times 10^{-6}$) or taking into account interactions (cg10009577 and AGR, $P = 5.50 \times 10^{-4}$), where current smokers and non-smokers have different patterns of association between DNA methylation at *CYP1A1* cg10009577 and AGR (Fig. 3c). Probe cg10009577 is located in the *CYP1A1* promoter, suggesting gene regulatory impacts on *CYP1A1* expression levels. Correspondingly, we observed a nominally significant association between *CYP1A1* gene expression and VFM (Fig. 3c), where current smokers and non-smokers have different patterns of association ($P = 0.042$). A significant negative association between DNA methylation levels and AGR was also observed with cg14120703 in *NOTCH1* (beta = -1.80, SE = 0.43, $P = 1.07 \times 10^{-7}$). We pursued replication of these associations in an independent sample of 69 younger Finnish twins with adipose tissue Illumina 450K methylation profiles. We replicated the overall negative association between *CYP1A1* cg10009577 and AGR (discovery sample beta = -0.95, SE = 0.31; replication sample beta = -0.58, SE = 0.25, $P = 0.02$) and observed a similar direction of interaction effects, which did not reach nominal significance in the replication sample (Additional file 2: Table S5).

We performed similar analyses with the 42 smoking-DES and observed main effects at *F2RL3* on the three phenotypes (VFM beta = -1.5×10^{-3}, SE = 3.78×10^{-4}, $P = 7.8 \times 10^{-4}$; AGR beta = 2.3, SE = 0.56, $P = 4.5 \times 10^{-5}$; TFM beta = 1.6×10^{-3}, SE = 3.9×10^{-4}, $P = 5.8 \times 10^{-5}$), and *OR51E1* on VFM (beta = -1.5×10^{-3}, SE = 3.78×10^{-4}, $P = 7.8 \times 10^{-4}$) and AGR (beta = -2.85, SE = 0.51, $P = 3.1 \times 10^{-8}$). We did not observe significant evidence for interaction effects in the gene expression results.

In the second set of phenotypic analyses, we explored the role of the 42 smoking-DMS and 42 smoking-DES on weight gain after smoking cessation. Recent studies have reported not only a gain in weight on smoking cessation, but also an increase in visceral fat [5]. We considered adiposity phenotypes in 246 of the individuals in our study at two time points, where time point 1 was the initial adipose DNA methylation profiling and phenotype measurement, and time point 2 was a phenotype measurement on average 5 years later. We found that current smokers who go on to quit smoking over this 5-year interval show a gain in adiposity across all phenotypes (Fig. 6a), and this effect is also observed in individuals who quit within up to 4 years at time point 1. However, our data suggests that this gain in adiposity is not long lasting, because we do not observe this effect in the group of ex-smokers who had quit for > 5 years at time point 1. In comparison, there were no major phenotype changes within constant smokers (current smokers at both time points) or never smokers (non-smokers at both time points) across the two time points.

We tested if the 42 smoking-DMS and 42 DES in adipose tissue could predict future changes in adiposity upon smoking cessation, focusing on visceral fat accumulation as the major risk factor for the development of adiposity-related metabolic diseases. Based on the phenotype results (Fig. 6a), we compared two groups of individuals: first, the combined group ($n = 18$) of current smokers at the time of methylation profiling (time point 1) who subsequently quit smoking ($n = 5$), and individuals who had quit within 1–4 years at time point 1 ($n = 13$); and second, the combined group ($n = 228$) of ex-smokers who had quit for > 5 years at time point 1 ($n = 92$), as well as constant smokers ($n = 12$) and never smokers ($n = 124$) across the two time points. We assessed the impact of methylation or expression at the 42 smoking-DMS (Additional file 1: Figure S4) and 42 smoking-DES (Additional file 1: Figure S5) on future changes in visceral fat, selecting results that showed significantly different patterns of association in the two groups of 18 and 228 subjects.

After Bonferroni correction for multiple testing, we found one DMS and one DES significantly associated with future changes in visceral fat, where a strong association effect was only observed in the group 18 subjects. This group consists of current smokers who go on to quit smoking ($n = 5$) and recent ex-smokers who remain ex-smokers ($n = 13$), and where all subjects exhibit a gain in adiposity over time. The first signal was observed in cg16320419 in *BHLHE40* (methylation by group interaction term $P = 9.3 \times 10^{-4}$), where methylation levels in current smokers or recent ex-smokers explain 35.5% of the variation in future gain in visceral fat

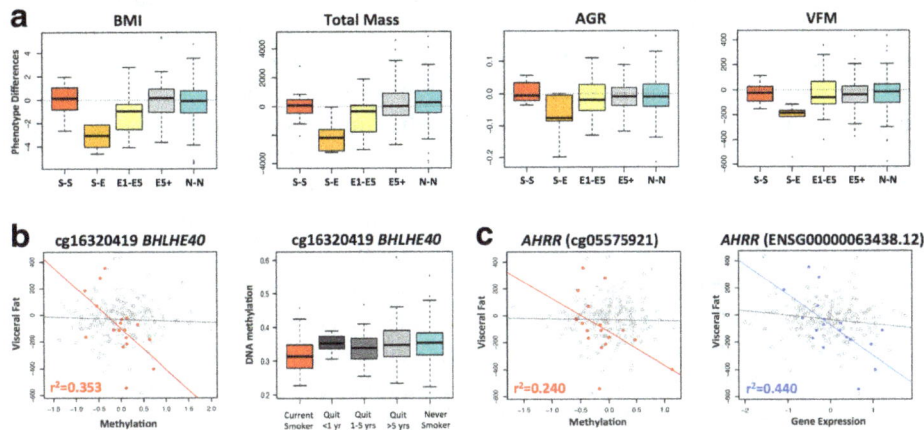

Fig. 6 Smoking-DMS and smoking-DES relate to future changes in visceral fat mass on smoking cessation. **a** Adiposity phenotype changes over a 5-year time period between time point 1 (2007–2008) and time point 2 (2012–2013). Adiposity phenotypes include BMI, total fat mass (TFM), android-to-gynoid fat ratio (AGR), and visceral fat mass (VFM). Phenotype changes are shown for five categories of subjects: current smokers at the two time points (S-S, $n = 12$), current smokers at time point 1 who quit smoking by time point 2 (S-E, $n = 5$), ex-smokers (who quit smoking within 1–5 year) at time point 1 who remain ex-smokers at time point 2 (E1-E5, $n = 13$), ex-smokers who quit > 5 years at time point 1 who remain ex-smokers at time point 2 (E5+, $n = 92$), and non-smokers at both time points (N-N, $n = 124$). **b** Left panel shows the association between DNA methylation levels at cg16320419 in *BHLHE40* and future changes in visceral fat mass in 18 subjects in categories S-E and E1-E5 (red points), compared to all remaining subjects (gray points). Right panel shows methylation cessation patterns at cg16320419 in *BHLHE40*. **c** Association between DNA methylation (left panel, red points) and gene expression (right panel, blue points) in *AHRR* with future changes in visceral fat mass in 18 subjects in categories S-E and E1-E5, compared to all remaining subjects (gray points)

(Fig. 6b). The second signal was observed in *AHRR* (gene expression by group interaction term $P = 4.7 \times 10^{-5}$), where gene expression levels in current smokers or recent ex-smokers explain 44% of the variation in future gain in visceral fat (Fig. 6c). The results were similar after correcting for smoking years and years since smoking cessation.

Discussion

Tobacco smoking is a major disease risk factor. Our study is the first to identify smoking-associated DNA methylation and gene expression changes in adipose tissue in humans. Approximately 30% of the identified smoking-methylation signals showed significant coordinated changes in gene expression levels in five genes, giving insights into the cascade of molecular events that are triggered in response to smoking, toxin exposure, and nicotine metabolism. At least a third of smoking-methylation signals (in nine genomic regions) were shared across tissues, showing that smoking leaves tissue-shared signatures. Given that our target tissue was adipose, we considered the impact of the identified smoking methylation and expression signals on metabolic disease risk. Significant associations were observed between visceral fat and android-to-gynoid fat ratio and several smoking-methylation and expression markers. Furthermore, methylation and expression levels at *BHLHE40* and *AHRR* in current smokers or recent ex-smokers were predictive of future gain in visceral fat observed after smoking cessation. Our findings provide a first comprehensive assessment of methylation and expression changes related to

smoking in adipose tissue, with insights for metabolic health and disease risk.

Coordinated smoking methylation and expression changes overlapped at five genes (*AHRR*, *CYP1A1*, *CYP1B1*, *CYTL1*, and *F2RL3*), which include well-known and strongly replicated smoking-methylation signals, such as *AHRR* and *F2RL3*. Some of these genes have previously been linked to human phenotypes. For example, GWAS associations have been reported with multiple diseases and traits, such as drinking behavior (*CYTL1*) [44], cystic fibrosis severity (*AHRR*) [45], caffeine consumption (*CYP1A1*) [46], and diastolic blood pressure (*CYP1A1*) [47], and methylation levels at *AHRR* have been linked to multiple phenotypes including lung function [48] and BMI [49]. At the five overlapping genes, methylation levels were predominantly negatively correlated with expression levels. CpG sites in *AHRR*, *CYP1B1*, and *F2RL3* were located on the gene body, whereas those in *CYTL1* and *CYP1A1* were in the promoter. Our results are consistent with the expectation that promoter-based CpG sites negatively associate with gene expression [50–52]. Studies have reported both positive and negative correlations between methylation and expression for CpG sites in the gene body [53–56]. DNA methylation sites in the gene body that are negatively associated with expression levels may be located in alternative promoters that regulate the expression of particular isoforms.

CYP1A1, or cytochrome P4501A1, is a lung cancer susceptibility gene. Although in our data, *CYP1A1* smoking signals appear adipose-specific, independent studies have reported links to smoking in multiple tissues. *CYP1A1* smoking-associated methylation signals are present in the lung in the fetus [57] and in adults [30, 35]. In adults, effects are observed in normal lung tissue from lung cancer patients at both the *CYP1A1* promoter [35] and enhancer [30], which is also differentially methylated between normal tissue and lung tumor tissue [30]. A recent large-scale meta-analysis of smoking methylation signals in blood also reported a moderate effect at *CYP1A1* [20]. Maternal tobacco use was also associated with alterations in promoter methylation of placental *CYP1A1*, and these changes were correlated with *CYP1A1* gene expression and fetal growth restriction [58]. Furthermore, *CYP1A1* gene expression is downregulated by *AHRR*. *CYP1A1* is inducible by agonists of the aryl hydrocarbon receptor (AhR), which include environmental pollutants and components of cigarette smoke. Following activation of AhR by an agonist in the cytoplasm, the AhR-ligand complex translocates to the nucleus, where it dimerizes with the aryl hydrocarbon receptor nuclear translocator (ARNT) [59]. This heterodimer binds to the xenobiotic response element (XRE) site of *CYP1A1* in the upstream enhancer region, which activates transcription. *CYP1A1* metabolizes drug molecules and environmental pollutants, including polycyclic aromatic hydrocarbons, dioxin, and benzo(α)pyrene, into highly reactive intermediates. These derivatives can bind to DNA and form adducts, which may contribute to carcinogenesis [60]. AhR, in a complex with xenobiotic compounds and ARNT, induces *CYP1A1* expression, which subsequently detoxifies toxic components of cigarette smoke. *AHRR* suppresses the effects of *AhR* through binding to ARNT. Hypo-methylation of *AHRR* and increased *AHRR* expression may therefore reduce cellular responses to smoking, potentially through *CYP1A1* [61]. However, our findings of increased gene expression levels at both *AHRR* and *CYP1A1* in current smokers suggest that smoking-induced *AHRR* changes do not impact the *CYP1A1* response to smoking in adipose tissue. The smoking effects at *CYP1A1* in our study appear to be adipose-specific; therefore, these observations do not extend to blood, skin, or lung samples.

In addition to *CYP1A1*, other smoking signals that we identify in this study have also been previously linked to lung cancer. *CYP1B1* differentially methylated effects have been reported for smoking, for lung cancer, and for age at cancer diagnosis in non-small cell lung carcinoma (NSCLC) samples [62]. Several of our smoking signals were previously reported to be differentially methylated in lung adenocarcinoma tumor and matched non-tumor tissue [63]. These included two of our top smoking-DMS, *CYTL1* and *ACVRL1*, and seven of our top smoking-DES, *CYTL1*, *JAM2*, *CYGB*, *TAL1*, *GRIK3*, *SOX17*, and *TEK*.

In line with previous studies, we observe that genetic variation can impact the smoking-DMS, with potential implications for genotype influences on the rates of toxin elimination and nicotine metabolism in the human body. Importantly, we observe that all of the major smoking genetic variants detected in the largest smoking GWAS to date appear to influence DNA methylation levels in *cis*. These findings strongly suggest that DNA methylation may mediate some of the effects of genetic influences on smoking behavior, toxin elimination, or nicotine metabolism. We also replicate results from a genome-wide association study of nicotine metabolite ratio, identifying a 4.2-Mb region on chromosome 19q13 where GWAS SNPs were also associated with DNA methylation levels [43]. Taken together, these findings suggests some of the observed genetic impacts on smoking behavior and nicotine metabolism may be mediated by DNA methylation and that such effects are robust and shared across tissues.

Our analyses specifically in ex-smokers show variability in the extent of signal reversal over time, which is consistent with previous findings. We observe an overall trend towards at least partial reversal at most of the identified smoking-associated signals. Importantly, our study is the first to show that this trend is also observed in gene expression levels. Our findings suggest that smoking has a longer lasting influence on the methylome compared to the transcriptome, where the majority of reversal effects occur within the first year after smoking cessation.

The smoking-methylation signals were assessed for association with adiposity phenotypes that constitute major metabolic disease risk. Significant associations were observed between visceral fat mass and android-to-gynoid fat ratio with methylation levels at smoking markers with functional impacts on gene expression, such as *CYP1A1* with replication, and in signals that were shared across tissues, such as *NOTCH1*. Associations were also detected with smoking-DES. These results may help improve our understanding of how smoking impacts metabolic health, and to explore this further, we considered smoking effects on future changes in metabolic phenotypes on smoking cessation. Visceral fat has a strong association with obesity-related metabolic diseases, such as type 2 diabetes and cardiovascular disease [64, 65] and is a major metabolic disease risk factor. At smoking markers *BHLHE40* and *AHRR*, DNA methylation and gene expression levels in current smokers were predictive of future gain in visceral fat observed after smoking cessation. Although the sample size of current smokers who go on to quit smoking in our data is modest, these findings provide an interesting insight into potential molecular mechanisms mediating environmental effects on metabolic disease risk and require replication in larger samples.

A limitation to our study is partial correction for the influence of expected covariates. These include, first, alcohol consumption, which co-occurs with smoking. In our co-occurrence analyses, none of the alcohol-associated CpG sites reached genome-wide significance after adjusting for smoking. In a previous alcohol EWAS in blood, Liu et al. [66] also found that the effect size of the majority alcohol-DMS was not affected by smoking status suggesting that despite their co-occurrence, smoking and alcohol impact DNA methylation in different aspects. A related question is optimal correction for cell composition in adipose tissue. Since we only had access to subcutaneous adipose tissue biopsies, rather than isolated cell subtypes, we corrected for cell composition by using the analytical approach within the reference-free EWAS [32] framework and found that the majority of results remained largely unchanged. However, it is possible that this does not fully capture the effect of a heterogeneous population of cells as a confounder. Some of the smoking-DMS such as *BHLHE40*, which was also found to be predictive of future gain in visceral fat, may reflect cell-specific methylation profiles. *BHLHE40* was previously reported to be hypo-methylated in activated NK cells (but not in naive NKs, T, and B cells) [67] and a similar trend was observed for *AHRR* [67]. One interpretation of these findings is that some smoking signals are cell subtype specific [68, 69], potentially reflecting a selective enhancement of activated cells, because smoking can also induce changes in blood count [70]. In adipose tissue, this particular effect may be represented as an infiltration of activated NK cells, and this infiltration may increase with obesity, diabetes, and smoking. On the other hand, the relative abundance of NK DNA compared with adipose DNA in adipose tissue is minimal; therefore, these effects should be minimal. Future studies are needed to assess the impact of these potential confounding effects using for example histological and immunological staining of adipose tissue.

Conclusion

Our results show that smoking can impact DNA methylation and gene expression levels in adipose tissue. To our knowledge, this is the first study that performed genome-wide analyses of smoking in adipose tissue DNA methylation and gene expression profiles. The key results are that, first, smoking leaves a signature on both the methylome and transcriptome with overlapping signals; second, smoking methylation signals tend to be tissue-shared effects; third, smoking has a longer lasting influence on DNA methylation levels than on gene expression after smoking cessation; and forth, specific smoking methylation and expression signals are associated with metabolic disease risk phenotypes, as well as future weight gain after smoking cessation.

Methods

Study population and sample collection

The primary sample of subjects is twins from the TwinsUK cohort who were recruited as part of the MuTHER (Multiple Tissue Human Expression Resource) study [71]. All subjects are Caucasian females and ascertained to be free from severe disease when the samples were collected. The sample consisted of 542 female twins, comprising 54 current smokers, 197 ex-smokers, and 291 non-smokers. The 542 twins included 84 MZ twin pairs, 112 DZ twin pairs, and 150 unrelated individuals (Additional file 2: Table S6). Adipose tissue biopsies were obtained from all subjects between August 2007 and May 2009. Details of biopsy procedures and sample descriptions are described previously [72]. Briefly, subcutaneous adipose tissue biopsies were dissected from near the umbilicus of the abdominal region; the fat layer was separated from skin layers and stored immediately in liquid nitrogen. Both DNA and RNA were extracted from the same adipose tissue biopsy, as previously described [72, 73]. Ethical approval was granted by the National Research Ethics Service London-Westminster, the St Thomas' Hospital Research Ethics Committee (EC04/015 and 07/H0802/84). All research participants have signed an informed consent prior to taking part in any research activities.

To explore tissue-shared effects, peripheral blood samples from 789 and 362 subjects from TwinsUK were also explored for genome-wide methylation and expression profiling, respectively. The blood samples for methylation measurement were taken from 1992 to 2012, and the samples for gene expression measurement were taken from 2007 to 2009. From the 542 subjects with available adipose tissue samples, 200 and 222 subjects donated blood samples for methylation and expression profiling, respectively. Blood samples and adipose tissues were collected during the subject's visit to the clinic.

The majority of data analysis focused on methylation and expression level differences between current smokers and non-smokers. The sample subsets of current smokers and non-smokers comprised 345 subjects in adipose methylation and expression samples, 567 subjects in blood methylation samples, and 237 in blood expression samples.

Replication and validation analyses

The 42 smoking-DMS that we identified in the TwinsUK cohort were further explored in five independent datasets: (1) 104 subjects from the LEAP cohort were used for adipose smoking-DMS replication (dataset 1); (2) 69 subjects from the Finnish Twins were used for replication of methylation associations with metabolic phenotypes (dataset 2); and (3) 195 subjects (skin, dataset 3), (4) 168 subjects (lung, dataset 4), and (5) 567 subjects (blood, dataset 5) were used to explore tissue-shared effects at the 42 smoking-DMS. Details of dataset 5 were described in the previous section.

Dataset 1: LEAP cohort adipose tissue (USA)

To replicate the 42 adipose tissue smoking-DMS, we studied 104 participants from the New England Family Study, the LEAP cohort (mean BMI 30.9 ± 7.03, mean age 47 ± 1.7, 48% male; see Additional file 2: Table S6), described in detail elsewhere [39]. The individuals are of mixed ancestry (63.5% white) and were not affected with disease. There were 46 current smokers and 58 non-smokers. Subcutaneous adipose tissue samples in these participants were collected from the upper outer quadrant of the buttock, followed by DNA extraction, and Infinium HumanMethylation450 BeadChip array profiling as previously described [37]. Replication analyses were performed using a linear regression model adjusting for age, gender, BMI, and batch effect.

Dataset 2: Finnish twin adipose tissue

To replicate the methylation associations with metabolic health traits, we studied 69 Finnish twins (mean age 31.1 ± 4.43 years, mean BMI 27.5 ± 4.72, 44.9% male; see Additional file 2: Table S6), who were recruited as a part of the Finnish twin cohort. Adipose tissue sample collection and DNA extraction in this sample have been previously described in detail [74, 75]. The sample included 34 full MZ twin pairs and 21 current smokers. DNA methylation profiling was measured by Infinium HumanMethylation450 BeadChip array and TFM and AGR were determined by dual energy X-ray absorptiometry (DEXA). Replication analyses were performed using a linear mixed effect regression model adjusting for age, gender, BMI, family, batch effect, and alcohol intake. Sample characteristics of the replication cohorts are shown in Additional file 2: Table S6.

To examine the tissue specificity of the 42 smoking-DMS, we included two additional datasets (dataset 3 and dataset 4) for validation of tissue-shared smoking effects.

Dataset 3: TwinsUK skin tissue

The first validation dataset for identifying tissue-shared effects included 195 skin tissue samples from twins (mean age 59.1 ± 9.71 years, mean BMI 26.7 ± 4.71; see Additional file 2: Table S6) from the TwinsUK cohort. This analysis included 37 current smokers and 158 non-smokers cancer-free female subjects only, and some subjects also provided adipose samples in the current study. The TwinsUK skin samples and the evaluation of DNA methylation in the samples are described elsewhere [34]. We performed the analysis using a linear mixed effects model adjusting for age, BMI, alcohol consumption, batch effect, family structure, and zygosity. Sample characteristics are shown in Additional file 2: Table S6.

Dataset 4: Lung cancer tissue

The second validation dataset for identifying tissue-shared smoking effects included 168 lung cancer female subjects (mean age 65.1 ± 10.66 years; see Additional file 2: Table S6) from a multicenter cohort of 450 subjects with non-small cell lung cancer (GEO dataset: GSE39279) [76]. In the validation analysis, we selected only female subjects who had smoking records (129 current smokers and 39 non-smokers) and used a linear regression model to test for the effect of smoking on methylation, adjusting for age, cancer stage [1 to 4], and cancer type (adenocarcinoma or squamous). DNA methylation levels were obtained using the Infinium HumanMethylation450 BeadChip, and BMIQ normalization was performed prior to analysis.

Phenotype collection

During a subject's clinical visit, basic demographic information was collected, with on-site measurements such as height and weight, DEXA measurements, and biopsy collection. Self-reported smoking status is obtained through longitudinal questionnaires. Data included answers to the following questions: "Do you currently smoke (more than 3 days per week)?" (yes/no), "How long has it been since you gave up smoking (in years/months)?", "How long have you smoked for in total (in years/months)?", "On average how many cigarettes do you smoke a day (cigarette numbers)?", "How many cigarette you smoke in the past 100 days (cigarette numbers)?". Longitudinal data were available for each subject, and we excluded subjects who did not have consistent longitudinal smoking records. Smoking status was defined in three categories: current smokers, ex-smokers, and non-smokers. Current smokers were defined as subjects who consistently smoked cigarettes (and have not stopped at any point) according to their longitudinal records up to the clinical visit when the adipose tissue biopsy was obtained. Ex-smokers were individuals who have successfully (and consistently) reported to have quit smoking cigarettes for at least 3 months prior to the adipose tissue biopsy. Non-smokers were individuals who never smoked according to the longitudinal questionnaire records. Other phenotypes such as age, body mass index (BMI), and alcohol consumption were also collected during the clinical visit. The alcohol consumption data were obtained by questionnaires, and subjects were asked about the quantity (mL) and beverage types (beer, cider, lager, wine, spirits) drank per week. We then summarized the total alcohol intake as units per week and then converted to grams/day (one unit of alcohol in the UK is defined as 7.9 g [77]). Adiposity phenotypes, such as total fat mass (TFM), visceral fat mass (VFM), and android-to-gynoid ratio (AGR) were measured by DEXA scan.

Some participants have regular clinical research visits, approximately every 2 years. To study the weight gain after smoking cessation, we used phenotype information for VFM collected at two time points: the first time point is the date nearest to the adipose tissue collection date, and the second time point is the most recent clinical research visit of the subject where VFM data were collected. The time between longitudinal clinical research visits used in this study ranged between 3 and 7 years with a mean of 5.1 ± 0.70.

Genome-wide DNA methylation profiles

The Infinium HumanMethylation450 BeadChip (Illumina Inc., San Diego, CA) was used to measure DNA methylation in both adipose and blood samples. Details of experimental approaches have been previously described [72, 78]. At each probe, the methylation levels are characterized as a finite bounded quantitative trait ranging between 0 and 1, and represented as beta values. To overcome biases caused by the two Illumina probe types and two-color channels [79], we performed the beta mixture quantile dilation (BMIQ) method [80] and background correction for each sample. DNA methylation probes that mapped incorrectly or to multiple locations in the reference sequence were removed. Probes with more than 1% of subjects with detection P value > 0.05 were also removed. All the probes have non-missing values in blood samples and less than 1% missing subjects in adipose samples. Probes located on chromosomes X and Y were removed from the analysis. To check for sample swaps, we compared 65 single nucleotide polymorphism (SNP) markers that featured as control probes on the array to genotypes for each subject and removed subjects with incomparable genotypes. Because methylation levels on the majority of probes do not follow the normal distribution, which might violate the regression assumption for downstream analysis, we normalized the methylation levels to $N(0,1)$ prior to analysis. For all the other methylation datasets (USA adipose, Finnish adipose, lung cancer tissues, TwinsUK skin samples, and TwinsUK blood samples), we performed exactly the same quality control steps for data cleaning and normalization prior to the analysis.

RNA-sequencing data

The twin adipose RNA-seq data and quality control have been previously described [81, 82]. Briefly, sequenced paired-end reads (49 bp) were mapped to the human genome (GRCh37) by Burrows-Wheeler aligner (BWA) software v0.5.9 [83], then genes were annotated as defined by protein coding in GENCODE v10 [84]. Samples were excluded if they failed during library preparation or sequencing. Samples were only considered to have good quality if more than 10 million reads were sequenced and mapped to exons. Gene expression levels were

quantified per gene, estimated as RPKM values (reads per kilobase of transcript per million mapped reads) and rank normal transformed prior to analysis. The genotype of each subject was used for identity checks in case of sample swaps. After removing genes located on chromosomes X and Y, and non-coding transcripts, 17,399 genes were included in the gene expression analysis for adipose tissues and blood samples.

Genotype data

Genotypes were available for all subjects in study. Genotyping of the larger TwinsUK dataset was performed using HumanHap300, HumanHap610Q, HumanHap1M Duo, and HumanHap1.2M Duo 1M arrays. Imputation was done in two datasets separately and subsequently merged with GTOOL. Genotype data were pre-phased using IMPUTE2 without a reference panel, then using the resulting haplotypes to perform fast imputation from 1000 Genome phase1 dataset [85, 86]. We used 1000 Genomes Phase I (interim) as reference set, based on a sequence data freeze from 23 Nov 2010; the phased haplotypes were released Jun 2011. After imputation, SNPs were filtered at a MAF $> 5\%$. Genotypes were used for identification of meQTLs and eQTLs in the 542 adipose samples.

Statistical analysis
Differential methylation and expression analyses

Principal component analysis (PCA) was used to identify potential batch effects and covariates to be included in the statistical model for both methylation and gene expression adipose data. To identify the adipose methylation differences between current smokers and non-smokers, a linear mixed effect regression model (LMER) was applied adjusting for batch effects (plate, position on the plate, bisulfite conversion levels, and bisulfite conversion efficiency), age, BMI, alcohol consumption, family and zygosity structure. In the blood, the methylation differences between current smokers and non-smokers were tested adjusting for batch effects (plate and position on the plate), age, BMI, alcohol consumption, and seven predicted cell count estimates (plasma blast, CD8pCd28nCD45Ran, CD8 naïve, CD4T, NK, monocytes, and granulocytes), family and zygosity structure. Blood cell counts were calculated using the Horvath online calculator [87]. A linear mixed effect regression model was applied as the data contained MZ and DZ twins. Family structure and zygosity were included as random effect terms, while all the other covariates were included as fixed effect terms. Similarly, in the RNA-seq data analysis, the adipose and blood expression differences between current smokers and non-smokers were examined using LMER adjusting for age, BMI, alcohol consumption (grams/day), GC mean, primer index, clinic visit date, family structure, and zygosity. Family structure, zygosity, primer index, and clinic visit date were taken as random effect, and all the other covariates were included as fixed terms. For each CpG site or gene, a full model that regressed all of the covariates was compared to a null model that excluded smoking status. The models were compared using the ANOVA F statistic. A genome-wide significance level was set at 1% false discovery rate for all analyses.

In order to account for mixtures of cell types in adipose tissue, we performed a EWAS using the reference-free approach proposed by Houseman et al. [32]. The method is similar to surrogate variable analysis (SVA) and independent surrogate variable analysis (ISVA), which is used to adjust for technical errors (e.g., batch effect) and confounders. In addition, the reference-free approach also includes a bootstrap step to account for the correlation in the structure of standard errors. Using this approach, we can estimate direct epigenetic effects that account for cell compositions and use bootstrap-based P values to assess their significance. Due to the limitation that the reference-free approach can currently only be applied to datasets of unrelated individuals, we used 251 unrelated individuals from the original 542 twins and compared the top results between two EWASs.

To identify tissue-shared smoking differentially methylated signals across adipose and whole blood datasets, we compared the genome-wide FDR 1% signals across adipose and whole blood DNA methylation analyses. In whole blood samples, we tested for association between smoking status and DNA methylation levels at 452,874 CpG sites in 86 current and 481 non-smokers in blood. We compared the FDR 1% adipose DMS to 2782 CpG sites that were associated with smoking in blood at FDR 1% ($P = 1.14 \times 10^{-5}$). To further explore tissue specificity in other tissues, we explored the 14 tissue-shared smoking-DMS identified in both adipose and blood samples. We used previously published datasets of 196 cancer-free female subjects with skin tissue biopsies [34] and a lung cancer DNA methylation dataset [76], applying a Bonferroni-adjusted P value of 3.6×10^{-4} as the significance threshold.

Receiver operative curve (ROC) analysis
We tested several models for predicting smoking status based on the different combinations of the adipose smoking-DMS and smoking-DES. The sensitivity and specificity of these prediction models were calculated using receiver operative curve (ROC). The ROC analysis was performed in R using the "pROC" package [88] with the "lme" function for logistic regression, where outcomes are categorized as current smokers and non-smokers. We then used the "predict" function to predict the expected probabilities under different combinations of predicting factors (methylation levels of 14 CpG sites and expression

levels at five genes), and the "roc" function to predict the sensitivity and specificity and draw the area under the curve. We selected 27 current smokers and 145 non-smokers as a training set to construct a logistic model for smoking status classification, and then used the remaining set of 173 subjects (27 current smokers) as a validation set, in which we obtained the AUC values. We repeated this procedure 1000 times and report the average AUC values across 1000 validation sets.

Smoking cessation analyses
We quantified "reversal" time by estimating the time (in smoking-quit years) required for ex-smokers to revert to 25% of the change in methylation towards non-smokers. We first calculate the difference between methylation levels in current smokers and those in non-smokers and use 25% change of that difference as a "reversal" threshold. For example, at cg05575921 in *AHRR*, the median level of methylation residual is − 0.234 in current smokers and 0.037 in non-smokers, resulting in a 0.271 methylation change. Therefore, ex-smokers who reached methylation levels of − 0.031 were classified as subjects who "reversed". We quantified the proportion of subjects who reversed within different quit years. For example, at cg05575921, 6 ex-smokers quit in less than 1 year, but only one had methylation reverting to 25% of the methylation change towards non-smokers; therefore, the reversal rate was 16.7%. We quantified reversal at the gene expression level using the same approach.

Methylation QTL (meQTL) analyses
Genome-wide meQTL analyses were performed testing for the association between common genetic variants and DNA methylation at CpG sites in the two adipose tissue samples. We only considered SNPs that were significantly associated with DNA methylation in *cis* to be meQTLs. If multiple SNPs were identified for a single CpG site, we reported only the most significant SNP per CpG site ($P = 5 \times 10^{-5}$, as described in Grundberg et al. [72]). In total, methylation levels of 102,461 CpG sites were associated with genetic factors in *cis*, and 25,531 sites in *trans*.

We tested for adipose tissue meQTLs first by fitting a LME model regressed all the identified covariates, then performed a linear regression of the residuals on the SNPs using the MatrixeQTL R package [89]. Results from meQTL analyses are presented at a P value of 10^{-5} for the smoking-DMS, the smoking-DES, and at the smoking GWAS genetic variants. For meQTL analyses replicating the results from Loukola et al. [43], we applied a different threshold. Loukola et al. [43] conducted a genome-wide association study of nicotine metabolite ratio, identifying many strongly associated SNPs in a 4.2-Mb region on chromosome 19q13. Among the 158

CpG sites within that region, 16 CpG sites showed statistically significant association with 173 SNPs. We compared our meQTL findings to those from Loukola et al. [43] at a modified Bonferroni significance threshold of 1.81×10^{-5} ($= 0.05/(16 \times 173)$) and identified SNPs that influence methylation levels at 5 CpG sites (in *CYP2A7*, *ENGL2*, and *LTBP4* genes) (Additional file 2: Table S5).

Correlations between methylation and gene expression levels

We compared the 542 subjects' adipose methylation and gene expression levels at the five overlapping genes identified in the two genome-wide association analyses. Both the methylation and expression data were first adjusted for covariates, and Spearman's correlation test was then performed on the residuals.

Metabolic disease risk phenotype analyses

We studied the impacts of smoking methylation signals on obesity and metabolic phenotypes. We explored 288 adipose subjects (42 current smokers and 246 non-smokers, mean BMI = 26.70 ± 4.62) who had available DEXA profiles at or within up to 1 year of the adipose tissue biopsy. We compared the association between DNA methylation and the adiposity phenotypes, such as visceral fat mass (VFM), total fat mass (TFM), and android-to-gynoid fat ratio (AGR). Analyses were carried out at the 42 smoking-DMS using a linear regression model adjusting for BMI, age, and smoking status. A significance level was set at a Bonferroni-adjusted threshold of $P = 5.7 \times 10^{-4}$. We used a similar approach to test for phenotype associations with the 42 smoking-DES.

To further investigate the effect of 42 smoking-DMS and 42 smoking-DES on weight gain after smoking cessation, the adiposity phenotype differences were obtained at two time points in a reduced sample size of 248 subjects. Depending on a subjects' smoking behavior at the two time points, we categorized subjects into five categories: current smokers at the two time points (constant smokers, S-S, $n = 12$), current smokers at time point 1 who quit smoking by time point 2 (S-E, $n = 5$), ex-smokers (who quit smoking within 1–5 years) at time point 1 who remain ex-smokers at time point 2 (E1-E5, $n = 13$), ex-smokers who quit > 5 years at time point 1 who remain ex-smokers at time point 2 (E5+, $n = 92$), and non-smokers at both time points (never smokers, N-N, $n = 124$). We then calculated the phenotype differences (phenotype at time point 2 minus phenotypes at time point 1) for each subject and correlated this differences to their adipose methylation (42 smoking-DMS) and gene expression levels (42 smoking-DES).

We used the R statistical software (https://www.r-project.org/) for all analyses and figures, and the regional plots were generated using the coMET package [90].

Abbreviations
AGR: Android-to-gynoid fat ratio; AhR: Aryl hydrocarbon receptor; AUC: Area under curve; BMI: Body mass index; BWA: Burrows-Wheeler aligner; DES: Differentially expressed signals; DEXA: Dual energy X-ray absorptiometry; DMS: Differentially methylated signals; EWAS: Epigenome-wide association study; FDR: False discovery rate; LME model: Linear mixed effect model; MAF: Minor allele frequency; meQTL: Methylation quantitative trait locus; NSCLC: Non-small cell lung carcinoma; PCA: Principal component analysis; RNA-seq: RNA-sequencing; ROC: Receiver operative curve; SE: Standard error; SNP: Single nucleotide polymorphism; SVA: Surrogate variable analysis; TFM: Total fat mass; TSS: Transcription start site; TWAS: Transcriptome-wide association study; VFM: Visceral fat mass

Funding
This work was supported by the Economic and Social Research Council [grant number ES/N000404/1 to J.T.B], Medical Research Council [Project grant number MR/L01999X/1 to K.S.S; grant number MR/N013700/1 and King's College London member of the MRC Doctoral Training Partnership in Biomedical Sciences (A.Vic.)], and the Academy of Finland [grant number 297908 to M.O.]. The TwinsUK study was funded by the Wellcome Trust; European Community's Seventh Framework Programme (FP7/2007–2013); National Institute for Health Research (NIHR)-funded BioResource, Clinical Research Facility and Biomedical Research Centre based at Guy's and St Thomas' NHS Foundation Trust in partnership with King's College London. SNP genotyping was performed by The Wellcome Trust Sanger Institute and National Eye Institute via NIH/CIDR. The Finnish twin study was funded by the Academy of Finland [grant numbers 266286, 272376, 314383], Helsinki University Central Hospital, The University of Helsinki Research Funds, Novo Nordisk Foundation, Ane and Signe Gyllenberg Foundation, Finnish Diabetes Research Foundation, Finnish Foundation for Cardiovascular Research. The funding bodies did not impact the design of the study, analysis and interpretation of data, and writing of the manuscript.

Authors' contributions
JTB designed the study and outlined the main conceptual ideas. JTB, KSS, KK, MO, EL, TDS, and KHP supervised the work in each contributing research group. TDS, PD, KSS, and JTB generated the primary datasets. P-CT leads the data analysis. CAG, MNE, SB, IY, JEC-F, TH, TCM, AV, MM, KW, and AV contributed to the data analysis. JTB and P-CT wrote the article, and all authors provided critical feedback and helped shape the research, analysis, and manuscript. All authors read and approved the final manuscript.

Author details
[1]Department of Twin Research and Genetic Epidemiology, King's College London, London SE1 7EH, UK. [2]Department of Biomedical Sciences, Chang Gung University, Taoyuan, Taiwan. [3]Division of Allergy, Asthma, and Rheumatology, Department of Pediatrics, Chang Gung Memorial Hospital, Linkou, Taiwan. [4]Big Data Institute at the Li Ka Shing Centre for Health Information and Discovery, University of Oxford, Oxford OX3 7LF, UK. [5]Department of Epidemiology, Brown University School of Public Health, Providence, RI 02912, USA. [6]Institute for Molecular Medicine Finland (FIMM) and Department of Public Health, University of Helsinki, Helsinki, Finland. [7]Department of Bioinformatics, Institute of Health Sciences, Hacettepe University, 06100 Ankara, Turkey. [8]Pfizer - University of Granada - Andalusian Government Center for Genomics and Oncological Research (GENYO), Granada, Spain. [9]Division of Cancer Studies, King's College London, London SE1 9RT, UK. [10]Department of Oncological Sciences, Icahn School of Medicine at Mount Sinai, New York City, NY 10029, USA. [11]The Tisch Cancer

Institute, Icahn School of Medicine at Mount Sinai, New York City, NY 10029, USA. [12]Centre for Stem Cells and Regenerative Medicine, King's College London, Floor 28, Tower Wing, Guy's Hospital, Great Maze Pond, London SE1 9RT, UK. [13]NIHR Biomedical Research Centre at Guy's and St Thomas' Foundation Trust, London SE1 9RT, UK. [14]Research Programs Unit, Diabetes and Obesity, Obesity Research Unit, University of Helsinki, Helsinki, Finland. [15]Endocrinology, Abdominal Center, Helsinki University Hospital, Helsinki, Finland. [16]William Harvey Research Institute, Barts and The London School of Medicine and Dentistry, Queen Mary University of London, London EC1M 6BQ, UK. [17]Princess Al-Jawhara Al-Brahim Centre of Excellence in Research of Hereditary Disorders (PACER-HD), King Abdulaziz University, Jeddah, Saudi Arabia. [18]Department of Genetic Medicine and Development, University of Geneva Medical School, 1211 Geneva, Switzerland. [19]Institute for Genetics and Genomics in Geneva (iGE3), University of Geneva, 1211 Geneva, Switzerland. [20]Swiss Institute of Bioinformatics, 1211 Geneva, Switzerland. [21]Department of Laboratory Medicine & Pathology, Brown University, Providence, RI 02912, USA.

References

1. Thun MJ, DeLancey JO, Center MM, Jemal A, Ward EM. The global burden of cancer: priorities for prevention. Carcinogenesis. 2010;31(1):100–10.
2. Ezzati M, Lopez AD. Estimates of global mortality attributable to smoking in 2000. Lancet. 2003;362(9387):847–52.
3. United States. Public Health Service. Office of the Surgeon General. How tobacco smoke causes disease : the biology and behavioral basis for smoking-attributable disease : a report of the Surgeon General. Rockville, MD Washington, DC: U.S. Dept. of Health and Human Services, Public Health Service For sale by the Supt. of Docs., U.S. G.P.O.; 2010. xv, 704 p p.
4. Pfeifer GP, Denissenko MF, Olivier M, Tretyakova N, Hecht SS, Hainaut P. Tobacco smoke carcinogens, DNA damage and p53 mutations in smoking-associated cancers. Oncogene. 2002;21(48):7435–51.
5. Matsushita Y, Nakagawa T, Yamamoto S, Takahashi Y, Noda M, Mizoue T. Associations of smoking cessation with visceral fat area and prevalence of metabolic syndrome in men: the Hitachi health study. Obesity (Silver Spring). 2011;19(3):647–51.
6. Besingi W, Johansson A. Smoke-related DNA methylation changes in the etiology of human disease. Hum Mol Genet. 2014;23(9):2290–7.
7. Breitling LP, Yang R, Korn B, Burwinkel B, Brenner H. Tobacco-smoking-related differential DNA methylation: 27K discovery and replication. Am J Hum Genet. 2011;88(4):450–7.
8. Buro-Auriemma LJ, Salit J, Hackett NR, Walters MS, Strulovici-Barel Y, Staudt MR, et al. Cigarette smoking induces small airway epithelial epigenetic changes with corresponding modulation of gene expression. Hum Mol Genet. 2013;22(23):4726–38.
9. Elliott HR, Tillin T, McArdle WL, Ho K, Duggirala A, Frayling TM, et al. Differences in smoking associated DNA methylation patterns in South Asians and Europeans. Clin Epigenetics. 2014;6(1):4.
10. Monick MM, Beach SR, Plume J, Sears R, Gerrard M, Brody GH, et al. Coordinated changes in AHRR methylation in lymphoblasts and pulmonary macrophages from smokers, American journal of medical genetics part BNeuropsychiatr Genet 2012;159B(2):141 151.
11. Dogan MV, Shields B, Cutrona C, Gao L, Gibbons FX, Simons R, et al. The effect of smoking on DNA methylation of peripheral blood mononuclear cells from African American women. BMC Genomics. 2014;15:151.
12. Philibert RA, Beach SR, Lei MK, Brody GH. Changes in DNA methylation at the aryl hydrocarbon receptor repressor may be a new biomarker for smoking. Clin Epigenetics. 2013;5(1):19.
13. Shenker NS, Ueland PM, Polidoro S, van Veldhoven K, Ricceri F, Brown R, et al. DNA methylation as a long-term biomarker of exposure to tobacco smoke. Epidemiology. 2013;24(5):712–6.
14. Sun YV, Smith AK, Conneely KN, Chang Q, Li W, Lazarus A, et al. Epigenomic association analysis identifies smoking-related DNA methylation sites in African Americans. Hum Genet. 2013;132(9):1027–37.
15. Wan ES, Qiu W, Baccarelli A, Carey VJ, Bacherman H, Rennard SI, et al. Cigarette smoking behaviors and time since quitting are associated with differential DNA methylation across the human genome. Hum Mol Genet. 2012;21(13):3073–82.

16. Zeilinger S, Kuhnel B, Klopp N, Baurecht H, Kleinschmidt A, Gieger C, et al. Tobacco smoking leads to extensive genome-wide changes in DNA methylation. PLoS One. 2013;8(5):e63812.
17. Zhang H, Herman AI, Kranzler HR, Anton RF, Zhao H, Zheng W, et al. Array-based profiling of DNA methylation changes associated with alcohol dependence. Alcohol Clin Exp Res. 2013;37 Suppl 1:E108–15.
18. Guida F, Sandanger TM, Castagne R, Campanella G, Polidoro S, Palli D, et al. Dynamics of smoking-induced genome-wide methylation changes with time since smoking cessation. Hum Mol Genet. 2015;24(8):2349–59.
19. Harlid S, Xu Z, Panduri V, Sandler DP, Taylor JA. CpG sites associated with cigarette smoking: analysis of epigenome-wide data from the sister study. Environ Health Perspect. 2014;122(7):673–8.
20. Joehanes R, Just AC, Marioni RE, Pilling LC, Reynolds LM, Mandaviya PR, et al. Epigenetic signatures of cigarette smoking. Circ Cardiovasc Genet. 2016; 9(5):436–47.
21. Teschendorff AE, Yang Z, Wong A, Pipinikas CP, Jiao Y, Jones A, et al. Correlation of smoking-associated DNA methylation changes in buccal cells with DNA methylation changes in epithelial cancer. JAMA Oncol. 2015;1(4): 476–85.
22. Freeman JR, Chu S, Hsu T, Huang YT. Epigenome-wide association study of smoking and DNA methylation in non-small cell lung neoplasms. Oncotarget. 2016;7(43):69579–91.
23. Stueve TR, Li WQ, Shi J, Marconett CN, Zhang T, Yang C, et al. Epigenome-wide analysis of DNA methylation in lung tissue shows concordance with blood studies and identifies tobacco smoke-inducible enhancers. Hum Mol Genet. 2017;26(15):3014–27.
24. Zhang Y, Yang R, Burwinkel B, Breitling LP, Brenner H. F2RL3 methylation as a biomarker of current and lifetime smoking exposures. Environ Health Perspect. 2014;122(2):131–7.
25. Wilson R, Wahl S, Pfeiffer L, Ward-Caviness CK, Kunze S, Kretschmer A, et al. The dynamics of smoking-related disturbed methylation: a two time-point study of methylation change in smokers, non-smokers and former smokers. BMC Genomics. 2017;18(1):805.
26. Schembri F, Sridhar S, Perdomo C, Gustafson AM, Zhang X, Ergun A, et al. MicroRNAs as modulators of smoking-induced gene expression changes in human airway epithelium. Proc Natl Acad Sci U S A. 2009;106(7):2319–24.
27. Woenckhaus M, Klein-Hitpass L, Grepmeier U, Merk J, Pfeifer M, Wild P, et al. Smoking and cancer-related gene expression in bronchial epithelium and non-small-cell lung cancers. J Pathol. 2006;210(2):192–204.
28. McLemore TL, Adelberg S, Liu MC, McMahon NA, Yu SJ, Hubbard WC, et al. Expression of CYP1A1 gene in patients with lung cancer: evidence for cigarette smoke-induced gene expression in normal lung tissue and for altered gene regulation in primary pulmonary carcinomas. J Natl Cancer Inst. 1990;82(16):1333–9.
29. Ito K, Lim S, Caramori G, Chung KF, Barnes PJ, Adcock IM. Cigarette smoking reduces histone deacetylase 2 expression, enhances cytokine expression, and inhibits glucocorticoid actions in alveolar macrophages. FASEB J. 2001; 15(6):1110–2.
30. Tekpli X, Zienolddiny S, Skaug V, Stangeland L, Haugen A, Mollerup S. DNA methylation of the CYP1A1 enhancer is associated with smoking-induced genetic alterations in human lung. Int J Cancer. 2012;131(7):1509–16.
31. Roadmap Epigenomics C, Kundaje A, Meuleman W, Ernst J, Bilenky M, Yen A, et al. Integrative analysis of 111 reference human epigenomes. Nature. 2015;518(7539):317–30.
32. Houseman EA, Molitor J, Marsit CJ. Reference-free cell mixture adjustments in analysis of DNA methylation data. Bioinformatics. 2014;30(10):1431–9.
33. Weitzman ER, Chen YY. The co-occurrence of smoking and drinking among young adults in college: national survey results from the United States. Drug Alcohol Depend. 2005;80(3):377–86.
34. Roos L, Sandling JK, Bell CG, Glass D, Mangino M, Spector TD, et al. Higher nevus count exhibits a distinct DNA methylation signature in healthy human skin: implications for melanoma. J Invest Dermatol. 2017;137(4):910–20.
35. Anttila S, Hakkola J, Tuominen P, Elovaara E, Husgafvel-Pursiainen K, Karjalainen A, et al. Methylation of cytochrome P4501A1 promoter in the lung is associated with tobacco smoking. Cancer Res. 2003;63(24):8623–8.
36. Kupers LK, Xu X, Jankipersadsing SA, Vaez A, la Bastide-van Gemert S, Scholtens S, et al. DNA methylation mediates the effect of maternal smoking during pregnancy on birthweight of the offspring. Int J Epidemiol. 2015;44(4):1224–37.

37. Fa S, Larsen TV, Bilde K, Daugaard TF, Ernst EH, Lykke-Hartmann K, et al. Changes in first trimester fetal CYP1A1 and AHRR DNA methylation and mRNA expression in response to exposure to maternal cigarette smoking. Environ Toxicol Pharmacol. 2018;57:19–27.

38. Janssen BG, Gyselaers W, Byun HM, Roels HA, Cuypers A, Baccarelli AA, et al. Placental mitochondrial DNA and CYP1A1 gene methylation as molecular signatures for tobacco smoke exposure in pregnant women and the relevance for birth weight. J Transl Med. 2017;15(1):5.

39. Loucks EB, Huang YT, Agha G, Chu S, Eaton CB, Gilman SE, et al. Epigenetic mediators between childhood socioeconomic disadvantage and mid-life body mass index: the New England family study. Psychosom Med. 2016; 78(9):1053–65.

40. Vink JM, Willemsen G, Boomsma DI. Heritability of smoking initiation and nicotine dependence. Behav Genet. 2005;35(4):397–406.

41. Vink JM, Smit AB, de Geus EJ, Sullivan P, Willemsen G, Hottenga JJ, et al. Genome-wide association study of smoking initiation and current smoking. Am J Hum Genet. 2009;84(3):367–79.

42. Tobacco, Genetics C. Genome-wide meta-analyses identify multiple loci associated with smoking behavior. Nat Genet. 2010;42(5):441–7.

43. Loukola A, Buchwald J, Gupta R, Palviainen T, Hallfors J, Tikkanen E, et al. A genome-wide association study of a biomarker of nicotine metabolism. PLoS Genet. 2015;11(9):e1005498.

44. Chen XD, Xiong DH, Yang TL, Pei YF, Guo YF, Li J, et al. ANKRD7 and CYTL1 are novel risk genes for alcohol drinking behavior. Chin Med J. 2012;125(6): 1127–34.

45. Wright FA, Strug LJ, Doshi VK, Commander CW, Blackman SM, Sun L, et al. Genome-wide association and linkage identify modifier loci of lung disease severity in cystic fibrosis at 11p13 and 20q13.2. Nat Genet. 2011;43(6):539–46.

46. Amin N, Byrne E, Johnson J, Chenevix-Trench G, Walter S, Nolte IM, et al. Genome-wide association analysis of coffee drinking suggests association with CYP1A1/CYP1A2 and NRCAM. Mol Psychiatry. 2012;17(11):1116–29.

47. Ehret GB, Caulfield MJ. Genes for blood pressure: an opportunity to understand hypertension. Eur Heart J. 2013;34(13):951–61.

48. Kodal JB, Kobylecki CJ, Vedel-Krogh S, Nordestgaard BG, Bojesen SE. AHRR hypomethylation, lung function, lung function decline and respiratory symptoms. Eur Respir J. 2018;51:1701512.

49. Demerath EW, Guan W, Grove ML, Aslibekyan S, Mendelson M, Zhou YH, et al. Epigenome-wide association study (EWAS) of BMI, BMI change and waist circumference in African American adults identifies multiple replicated loci. Hum Mol Genet. 2015;24(15):4464–79.

50. Ball MP, Li JB, Gao Y, Lee JH, LeProust EM, Park IH, et al. Targeted and genome-scale strategies reveal gene-body methylation signatures in human cells. Nat Biotechnol. 2009;27(4):361–8.

51. Eckhardt F, Lewin J, Cortese R, Rakyan VK, Attwood J, Burger M, et al. DNA methylation profiling of human chromosomes 6, 20 and 22. Nat Genet. 2006;38(12):1378–85.

52. Lister R, Pelizzola M, Dowen RH, Hawkins RD, Hon G, Tonti-Filippini J, et al. Human DNA methylomes at base resolution show widespread epigenomic differences. Nature. 2009;462(7271):315–22.

53. Zemach A, McDaniel IE, Silva P, Zilberman D. Genome-wide evolutionary analysis of eukaryotic DNA methylation. Science. 2010;328(5980):916–9.

54. Zilberman D, Gehring M, Tran RK, Ballinger T, Henikoff S. Genome-wide analysis of Arabidopsis thaliana DNA methylation uncovers an interdependence between methylation and transcription. Nat Genet. 2007; 39(1):61–9.

55. Jjingo D, Conley AB, Yi SV, Lunyak VV, Jordan IK. On the presence and role of human gene-body DNA methylation. Oncotarget. 2012;3(4):462–74.

56. Gutierrez-Arcelus M, Lappalainen T, Montgomery SB, Buil A, Ongen H, Yurovsky A, et al. Passive and active DNA methylation and the interplay with genetic variation in gene regulation. eLife. 2013;2:e00523.

57. Chhabra D, Sharma S, Kho AT, Gaedigk R, Vyhlidal CA, Leeder JS, et al. Fetal lung and placental methylation is associated with in utero nicotine exposure. Epigenetics. 2014;9(11):1473–84.

58. Suter M, Ma J, Harris A, Patterson L, Brown KA, Shope C, et al. Maternal tobacco use modestly alters correlated epigenome-wide placental DNA methylation and gene expression. Epigenetics. 2011;6(11):1284 94.

59. Beischlag TV, Luis Morales J, Hollingshead BD, Perdew GH. The aryl hydrocarbon receptor complex and the control of gene expression. Crit Rev Eukaryot Gene Expr. 2008;18(3):207–50.

60. Khlifi R, Messaoud O, Rebai A, Hamza-Chaffai A. Polymorphisms in the human cytochrome P450 and arylamine N-acetyltransferase: susceptibility to head and neck cancers. Biomed Res Int. 2013;2013:582768.

61. Novakovic B, Ryan J, Pereira N, Boughton B, Craig JM, Saffery R. Postnatal stability, tissue, and time specific effects of AHRR methylation change in response to maternal smoking in pregnancy. Epigenetics. 2014;9(3):377–86.

62. Kang HJ, Kim EJ, Kim BG, You CH, Lee SY, Kim DI, et al. Quantitative analysis of cancer-associated gene methylation connected to risk factors in Korean colorectal cancer patients. J Prev Med Public Health. 2012;45(4):251–8.

63. Selamat SA, Chung BS, Girard L, Zhang W, Zhang Y, Campan M, et al. Genome-scale analysis of DNA methylation in lung adenocarcinoma and integration with mRNA expression. Genome Res. 2012;22(7):1197–211.

64. Wajchenberg BL. Subcutaneous and visceral adipose tissue: their relation to the metabolic syndrome. Endocr Rev. 2000;21(6):697–738.

65. Fontana L, Eagon JC, Trujillo ME, Scherer PE, Klein S. Visceral fat adipokine secretion is associated with systemic inflammation in obese humans. Diabetes. 2007;56(4):1010–3.

66. Liu C, Marioni RE, Hedman AK, Pfeiffer L, Tsai PC, Reynolds LM, et al. A DNA methylation biomarker of alcohol consumption. Mol Psychiatry. 2018;23(2): 422–33.

67. Wiencke JK, Butler R, Hsuang G, Eliot M, Kim S, Sepulveda MA, et al. The DNA methylation profile of activated human natural killer cells. Epigenetics. 2016;11(5):363–80.

68. Bauer M, Linsel G, Fink B, Offenberg K, Hahn AM, Sack U, et al. A varying T cell subtype explains apparent tobacco smoking induced single CpG hypomethylation in whole blood. Clin Epigenetics. 2015;7:81.

69. Su D, Wang X, Campbell MR, Porter DK, Pittman GS, Bennett BD, et al. Distinct epigenetic effects of tobacco smoking in whole blood and among leukocyte subtypes. PLoS One. 2016;11(12):e0166486.

70. Higuchi T, Omata F, Tsuchihashi K, Higashioka K, Koyamada R, Okada S. Current cigarette smoking is a reversible cause of elevated white blood cell count: cross-sectional and longitudinal studies. Prev Med Rep. 2016;4:417–22.

71. Moayyeri A, Hammond CJ, Valdes AM, Spector TD. Cohort profile: TwinsUK and healthy ageing twin study. Int J Epidemiol. 2013;42(1):76–85.

72. Grundberg E, Meduri E, Sandling JK, Hedman AK, Keildson S, Buil A, et al. Global analysis of DNA methylation variation in adipose tissue from twins reveals links to disease-associated variants in distal regulatory elements. Am J Hum Genet. 2013;93(5):876–90.

73. Grundberg E, Small KS, Hedman AK, Nica AC, Buil A, Keildson S, et al. Mapping cis- and trans-regulatory effects across multiple tissues in twins. Nat Genet. 2012;44(10):1084–9.

74. Kaprio J. Twin studies in Finland 2006. Twin Res Human Genet. 2006;9(6): 772–7.

75. Pietilainen KH, Ismail K, Jarvinen E, Heinonen S, Tummers M, Bollepalli S, et al. DNA methylation and gene expression patterns in adipose tissue differ significantly within young adult monozygotic BMI-discordant twin pairs. Int J Obes. 2016;40(4):654–61.

76. Sandoval J, Mendez-Gonzalez J, Nadal E, Chen G, Carmona FJ, Sayols S, et al. A prognostic DNA methylation signature for stage I non-small-cell lung cancer. J Clin Oncol. 2013;31(32):4140–7.

77. Brennan A, Meng Y, Holmes J, Hill-McManus D, Meier PS. Potential benefits of minimum unit pricing for alcohol versus a ban on below cost selling in England 2014: modelling study. BMJ. 2014;349:g5452.

78. Tsaprouni LG, Yang TP, Bell J, Dick KJ, Kanoni S, Nisbet J, et al. Cigarette smoking reduces DNA methylation levels at multiple genomic loci but the effect is partially reversible upon cessation. Epigenetics. 2014;9(10):1382–96.

79. Dedeurwaerder S, Defrance M, Bizet M, Calonne E, Bontempi G, Fuks F. A comprehensive overview of Infinium HumanMethylation450 data processing. Brief Bioinform. 2014;15(6):929–41.

80. Teschendorff AE, Marabita F, Lechner M, Bartlett T, Tegner J, Gomez-Cabrero D, et al. A beta-mixture quantile normalization method for correcting probe design bias in Illumina Infinium 450 k DNA methylation data. Bioinformatics. 2013;29(2):189–96.

81. Brown AA, Buil A, Vinuela A, Lappalainen T, Zheng HF, Richards JB, et al. Genetic interactions affecting human gene expression identified by variance association mapping. eLife. 2014;3:e01381.

82. Buil A, Brown AA, Lappalainen T, Vinuela A, Davies MN, Zheng HF, et al. Gene-gene and gene-environment interactions detected by transcriptome sequence analysis in twins. Nat Genet. 2015;47(1):88–91.

83. Li H, Durbin R. Fast and accurate short read alignment with Burrows-Wheeler transform. Bioinformatics. 2009;25(14):1754–60.

84. Harrow J, Frankish A, Gonzalez JM, Tapanari E, Diekhans M, Kokocinski F, et al. GENCODE: the reference human genome annotation for The ENCODE Project. Genome Res. 2012;22(9):1760–74.

85. Howie B, Marchini J, Stephens M. Genotype imputation with thousands of genomes. G3. 2011;1(6):457–70.

86. Howie B, Fuchsberger C, Stephens M, Marchini J, Abecasis GR. Fast and accurate genotype imputation in genome-wide association studies through pre-phasing. Nat Genet. 2012;44(8):955–9.

87. Horvath S. DNA methylation age of human tissues and cell types. Genome Biol. 2013;14(10):R115.

88. Robin X, Turck N, Hainard A, Tiberti N, Lisacek F, Sanchez JC, et al. pROC: an open-source package for R and S+ to analyze and compare ROC curves. BMC Bioinformatics. 2011;12:77.

89. Shabalin AA. Matrix eQTL: ultra fast eQTL analysis via large matrix operations. Bioinformatics. 2012;28(10):1353–8.

90. Martin TC, Yet I, Tsai PC, Bell JT. coMET: visualisation of regional epigenome-wide association scan results and DNA co-methylation patterns. BMC Bioinformatics. 2015;16:131.

13

Paternal sepsis induces alterations of the sperm methylome and dampens offspring immune responses—an animal study

Katharina Bomans, Judith Schenz, Sandra Tamulyte, Dominik Schaack, Markus Alexander Weigand and Florian Uhle*

Abstract

Background: Sepsis represents the utmost severe consequence of infection, involving a dysregulated and self-damaging immune response of the host. While different environmental exposures like chronic stress or malnutrition have been well described to reprogram the germline and subsequently offspring attributes, the intergenerational impact of sepsis as a tremendous immunological stressor has not been examined yet.

Methods: Polymicrobial sepsis in 12-week-old male C57BL/6 mice was induced by cecal ligation and puncture (CLP), followed by a mating of the male survivors (or appropriate sham control animals) 6 weeks later with healthy females. Alveolar macrophages of offspring animals were isolated and stimulated with either LPS or Zymosan, and supernatant levels of TNF-α were quantified by ELISA. Furthermore, systemic cytokine response to intraperitoneally injected LPS was assessed after 24 h. Also, morphology, motility, and global DNA methylation of the sepsis survivors' sperm was examined.

Results: Comparative reduced reduction bisulfite sequencing (RRBS) of sperm revealed changes of DNA methylation ($n = 381$), most pronounced in the intergenic genome as well as within introns of developmentally relevant genes. Offspring of sepsis fathers exhibited a slight decrease in body weight, with a more pronounced weight difference in male animals (CLP vs. sham). Male descendants of sepsis fathers, but not female descendants, exhibited lower plasma concentrations of IL-6, TNF-alpha, and IL-10 24 h after injection of LPS. In line, only alveolar macrophages of male descendants of sepsis fathers produced less TNF-alpha upon Zymosan stimulation compared to sham descendants, while LPS responses kept unchanged.

Conclusion: We can prove that male—but surprisingly not female—descendants of post-sepsis fathers show a dampened systemic as well as pulmonary immune response. Based on this observation of an immune hypo-responsivity, we propose that male descendants of sepsis fathers are at risk to develop fungal and bacterial infections and might benefit from therapeutic immune modulation.

Keywords: Intergenerational inheritance, Epigenetic, Germline, Methylation

* Correspondence: florian.uhle@med.uni-heidelberg.de
Department of Anesthesiology, Heidelberg University Hospital, Im Neuenheimer Feld 110, 69120 Heidelberg, Germany

Background

Globally, more than 30 million people are estimated to suffer from sepsis each year [1]. Recently redefined as organ dysfunction resulting from an exaggerated systemic immune response to an underlying bacterial, fungal, or viral infection, the syndrome sepsis belongs to the ongoing challenges of modern intensive care medicine [2]. Steady improvements of treatment bundles resulted in a gradual decline in mortality over the past years, remaining anyhow on an unacceptable high level of 20–50% [3]. Sepsis not only does affect elderly persons but also can strike all ages, including patients before or within the onset of their sexual activity [4–6]. During the immune response in the early stage of sepsis, a systemic activation of immune cells leads to an uncontrolled release of cytokines, chemokines, and other mediators, e.g., reactive oxygen species [7]. The consequence is an avalanche-like forward amplifying response, impacting in its severity not only cells of the immune system but also, e.g., endothelial cells, cardiomyocytes, or skeletal muscle cells [8–10]. Furthermore, changes in progenitor cells like hematopoietic stem cells (HSC) of the bone marrow have been hypothesized to occur during inflammation [11], with recent proof of this concept during chronic inflammation in diabetes [12] as well as in the acute inflammatory condition of sepsis [13, 14]. Epigenetic mechanisms have been proposed to mediate the changes and are also found in monocytes of patients with sepsis [15]. Besides the bone marrow, also the germline contains multipotent cells, developing in males into sperm cells. While the negative impact of inflammation on the overall male fertility has been well characterized [16, 17], it is unclear if individual sperm cells or even their progenitors might also be affected on a more subtle epigenetic level, enabling the carrying forward of information onto the next generation.

Today, evidence for the non-genetic "inclusive inheritance" of a variety of environmental exposures by epigenetic and behavioral transmission to following generations is steadily growing [18, 19]. Most available evidence exists for parental exposure to different diets and emotional stress [20], with no information about the situation after severe infections or sepsis. To approach this point, we performed an animal study utilizing a clinically relevant model of polymicrobial abdominal sepsis to evaluate the transmissibility of an immunological phenotype after paternal sepsis.

Results

Sepsis impairs sperm function and alters the DNA methylome

After CLP, nearly half of the paternal animals died within 5 days (9/20 animals), while no animal of the sham group died (Fig. 1b). The pronounced loss of body weight and higher clinical scores of CLP animals indicate the infection-associated severity of induced abdominal sepsis (Fig. 1c, d). To evaluate impact of sepsis on the paternal germline, we initially assessed sperm morphology and function. We found an increased number of sperm cells in animals after CLP (Fig. 2a), but these tended to be immobile (Fig. 2b) or to show a defect appearance (e.g., double tails or heads) (Fig. 2c).

Our phenotypical sperm results drove us to dig deeper and to examine the sperm methylome for sepsis-induced changes. We used an independent animal cohort with comparable mortality as the mating cohort (Additional file 1: Figure S1). Six weeks after CLP, respectively after sham procedure, we isolated sperm DNA and subjected it to methylation analysis via RRBS. We can identify 381 differentially methylated cytosines (dmCs; both hypo- and hypermethylated) distributed over all chromosomes (methylation change $\geq 25\%$, q value ≤ 0.01) (Fig. 3a). The majority of dmCs was located in intergenic regions (57%) followed by introns (24%), exons (13%), and promoters (6%) (Fig. 3b). Using these 381 dmCs, the animals distinctively clustered according to their paternal exposure (Fig. 3c, d; Additional file 2: Figure S2). For dmCs located within promoter regions, exons or introns, the corresponding genes were extracted and resulting lists were separately analyzed for overrepresentation of biological functions. The results provide evidence for alterations within genes involved in metabolic, biosynthetic, and developmental processes, e.g., "regulation of endothelial cell development" ($p = 4 \times 10^{-3}$), "cellular carbohydrate biosynthetic process" ($p = 1.3 \times 10^{-4}$), and "cell differentiation" ($p = 6.22 \times 10^{-6}$) (Fig. 3e–g).

Paternal sepsis increases postnatal mortality and influences development

Descendants of CLP fathers showed a significantly lower survival compared to control animals (76/98: 77.6% vs. 95/110: 86.4%; $p = 0.0454$) (Fig. 1e, Additional file 3: Table S1). The difference became evident early within the first week after birth, and with the exception of one animal (which was euthanized due to teeth malposition), no delayed deaths occurred.

Also, the number of litters, litter size, and sex distribution did not differ between the groups (Fig. 1f, g). Female and male descendants of CLP fathers both exhibited a subtle lower gain of body weight compared to descendants of control animals (Fig. 1h, i). On day 57 after weaning, the mean difference in body weight was significantly present in both genders, but more pronounced in males (25.7 vs. 27.1 g, $p = 0.001$) than in females (19.9 vs. 20.5 g, $p = 0.0072$) (Fig. 1j).

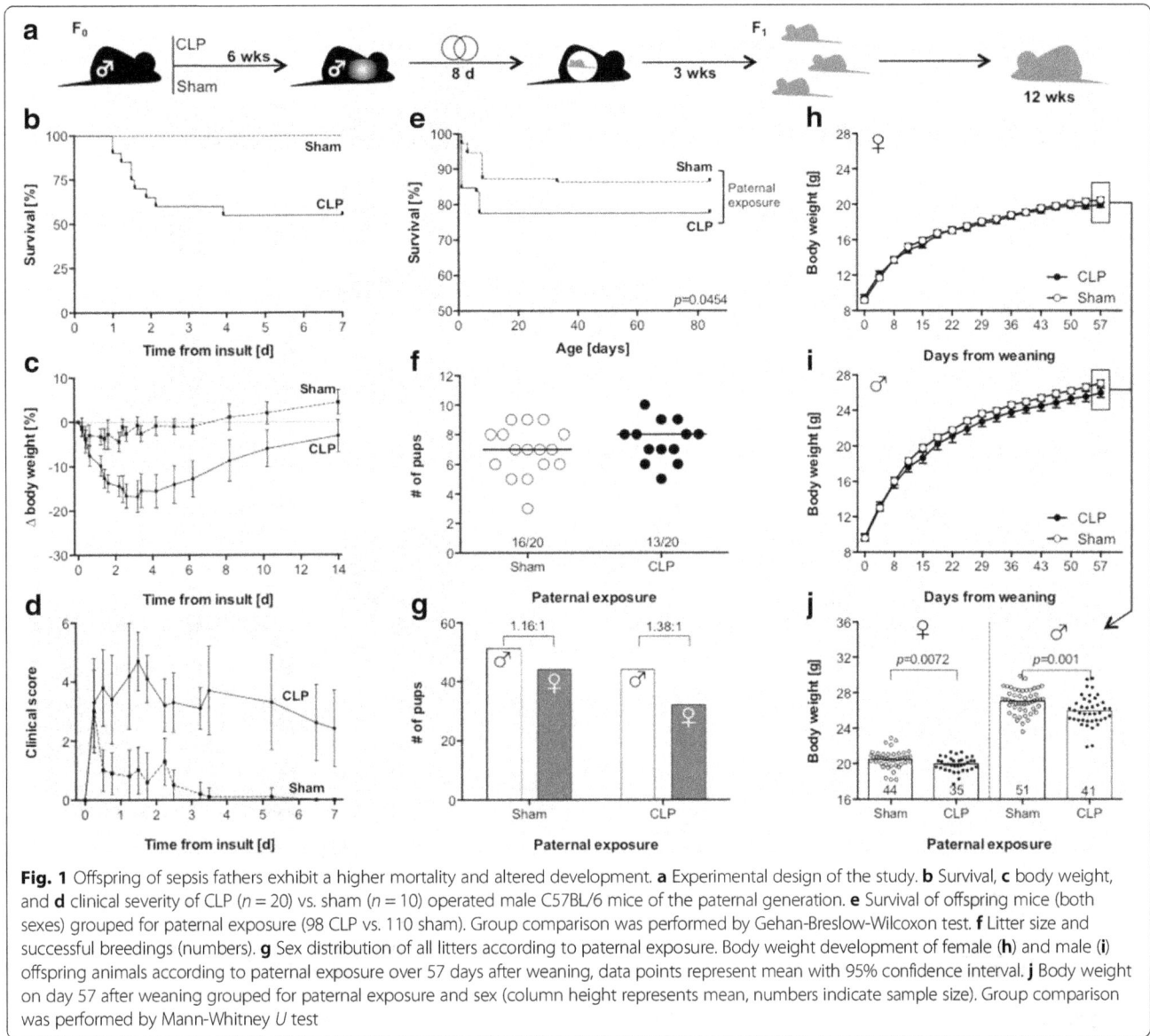

Fig. 1 Offspring of sepsis fathers exhibit a higher mortality and altered development. **a** Experimental design of the study. **b** Survival, **c** body weight, and **d** clinical severity of CLP ($n = 20$) vs. sham ($n = 10$) operated male C57BL/6 mice of the paternal generation. **e** Survival of offspring mice (both sexes) grouped for paternal exposure (98 CLP vs. 110 sham). Group comparison was performed by Gehan-Breslow-Wilcoxon test. **f** Litter size and successful breedings (numbers). **g** Sex distribution of all litters according to paternal exposure. Body weight development of female (**h**) and male (**i**) offspring animals according to paternal exposure over 57 days after weaning, data points represent mean with 95% confidence interval. **j** Body weight on day 57 after weaning grouped for paternal exposure and sex (column height represents mean, numbers indicate sample size). Group comparison was performed by Mann-Whitney U test

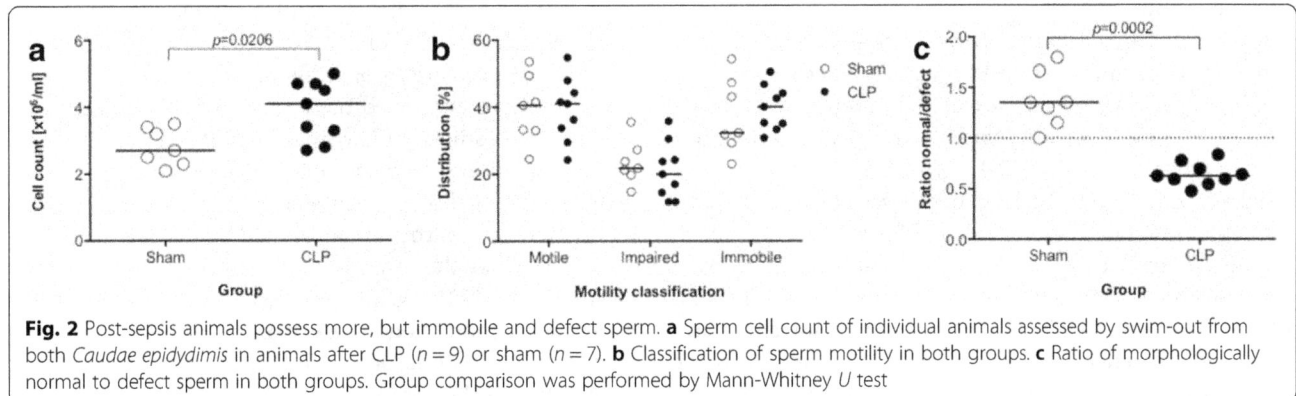

Fig. 2 Post-sepsis animals possess more, but immobile and defect sperm. **a** Sperm cell count of individual animals assessed by swim-out from both *Caudae epidydimis* in animals after CLP ($n = 9$) or sham ($n = 7$). **b** Classification of sperm motility in both groups. **c** Ratio of morphologically normal to defect sperm in both groups. Group comparison was performed by Mann-Whitney U test

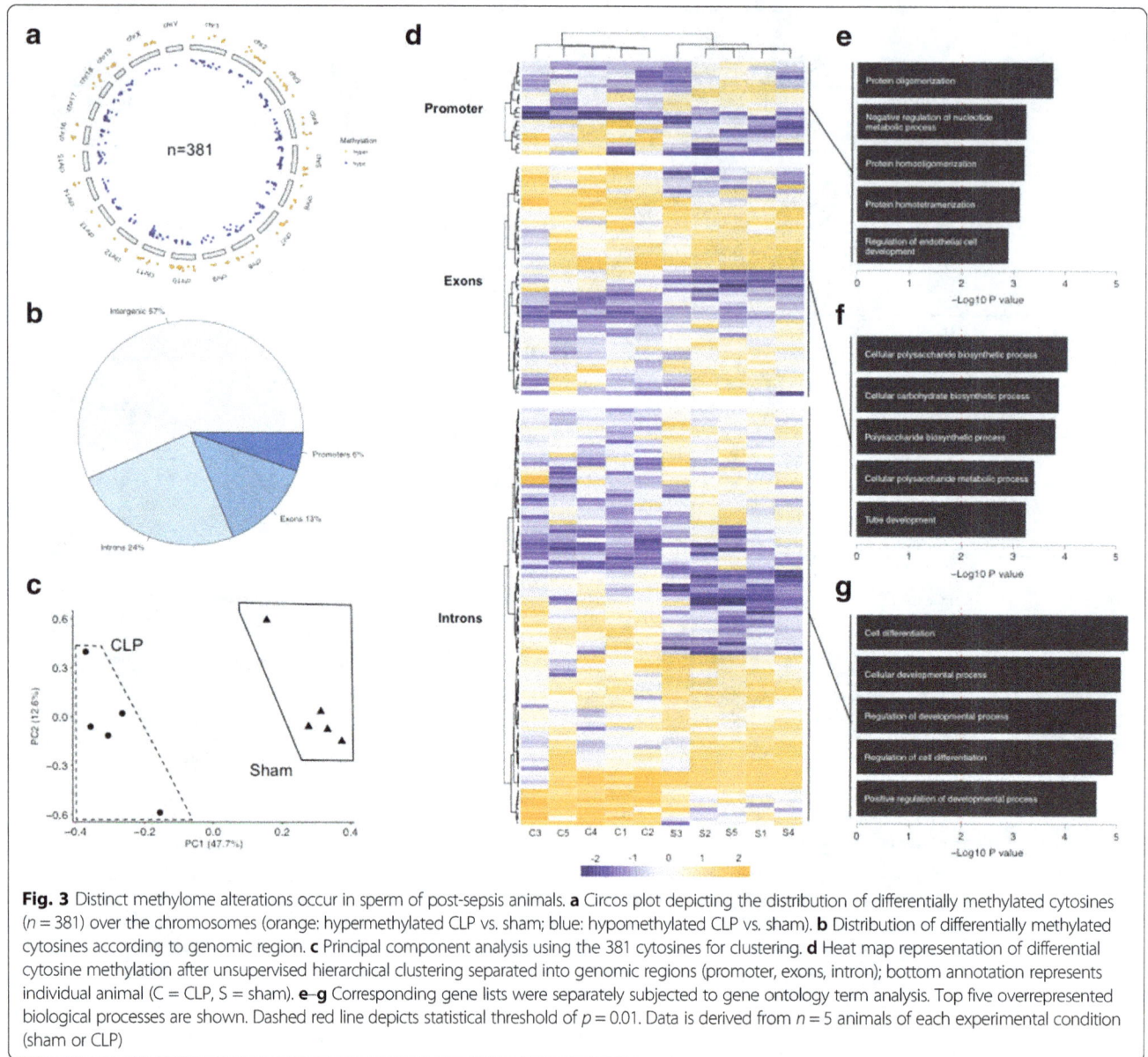

Fig. 3 Distinct methylome alterations occur in sperm of post-sepsis animals. **a** Circos plot depicting the distribution of differentially methylated cytosines (*n* = 381) over the chromosomes (orange: hypermethylated CLP vs. sham; blue: hypomethylated CLP vs. sham). **b** Distribution of differentially methylated cytosines according to genomic region. **c** Principal component analysis using the 381 cytosines for clustering. **d** Heat map representation of differential cytosine methylation after unsupervised hierarchical clustering separated into genomic regions (promoter, exons, intron); bottom annotation represents individual animal (C = CLP, S = sham). **e–g** Corresponding gene lists were separately subjected to gene ontology term analysis. Top five overrepresented biological processes are shown. Dashed red line depicts statistical threshold of *p* = 0.01. Data is derived from *n* = 5 animals of each experimental condition (sham or CLP)

Immunological responses are disturbed exclusively in male offspring

We evaluated the systemic cytokine response of the animals after stimulation with the *Toll-like receptor*-4 (TLR4) agonist LPS. Males exhibited differences depending on paternal exposure, with lower pro-inflammatory IL-6 (median 151.3 vs. 738.4 pg/ml; *p* = 0.0047), TNF-α (median 26.8 vs. 51.1 pg/ml; *p* = 0.0407), and anti-inflammatory IL-10 (median 27.4 vs. 61.0 pg/ml; *p* = 0.0062) levels in the blood (Fig. 4a–d). MCP-1 levels did not differ between the paternal exposure groups. With the exception of IL-10, females did not show any response differences in respect to paternal exposure or analyzed cytokine, but generally reduced cytokine levels

(Fig. 4e–h). Weight changes after LPS injection resembled these results with a trend towards a pronounced weight loss of male CLP offspring as soon as 24 h after injection of LPS (Additional file 4: Figure S3).

Furthermore, we tested the response of isolated alveolar macrophages stimulated with either LPS or the Dectin-1 agonist zymosan. Alveolar macrophages from male CLP offspring showed a reduced TNF-α response to zymosan compared to controls (median 4182 vs. 6357 pg/ml, *p* = 0.0083), while the response to LPS was not affected (median 1510 vs. 1719 pg/ml) (Fig. 5a). In contrast, the same experiment conducted in alveolar macrophages isolated from female offspring showed no difference in response, irrespective of the stimulus (Fig. 5b).

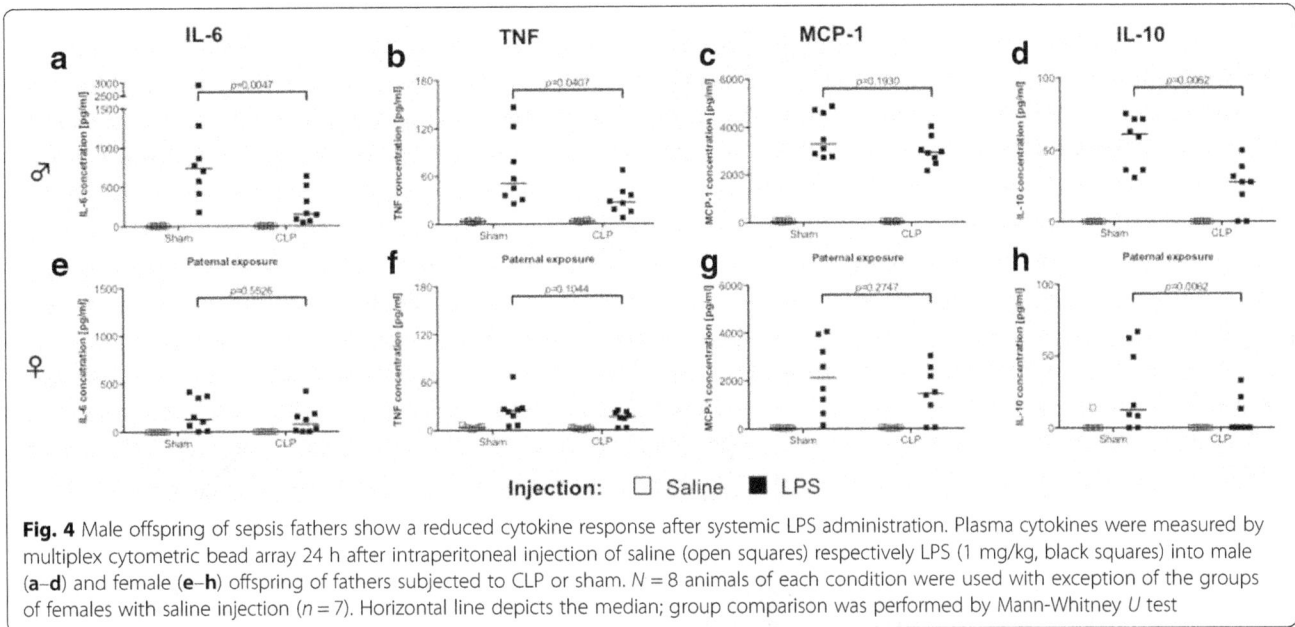

Fig. 4 Male offspring of sepsis fathers show a reduced cytokine response after systemic LPS administration. Plasma cytokines were measured by multiplex cytometric bead array 24 h after intraperitoneal injection of saline (open squares) respectively LPS (1 mg/kg, black squares) into male (**a–d**) and female (**e–h**) offspring of fathers subjected to CLP or sham. $N = 8$ animals of each condition were used with exception of the groups of females with saline injection ($n = 7$). Horizontal line depicts the median; group comparison was performed by Mann-Whitney U test

Discussion

Using a polymicrobial animal model of abdominal sepsis, our results are the first to our knowledge providing evidence for an intergenerational transmission of immunological changes from fathers to their male, but apparently not female, offspring. We further propose the sperm methylome as a potential carrier of information between the generations, as we can show differentially hypo- and hypermethylation of cytosine residues spread over the genome. The mechanisms of epigenetic inheritance through the male germline are still under debate, especially considering the replacement of histones to protamine during spermatozoa development and the global erasure of DNA methylation after fertilization [20]. Nevertheless, several studies involving paternal (mal-)nutritional exposures as, e.g., high-fat, low-protein, or low-folate [21–23] or the exposure to environmental toxicants [24, 25] clearly indicate a crucial role of changes in the sperm methylome. As a mechanistic rationale, Guibert and colleagues provided evidence that certain methylated cytosines "escape" the TET-mediated wave of demethylation during the development of primordial germ cells [26, 27]. Besides, DNA methylation of disease-associated loci in sperms changes with age, and the association of impaired DNA methylation with male infertility has been proven in several studies so far [28, 29]. Interestingly, we can recapitulate this concept in our animal model of sepsis with more immobile sperm and the occurrence of morphologically aberrant sperm cells even 6 weeks after the insult. In contrast, survivors of sepsis exhibited more sperm cells,

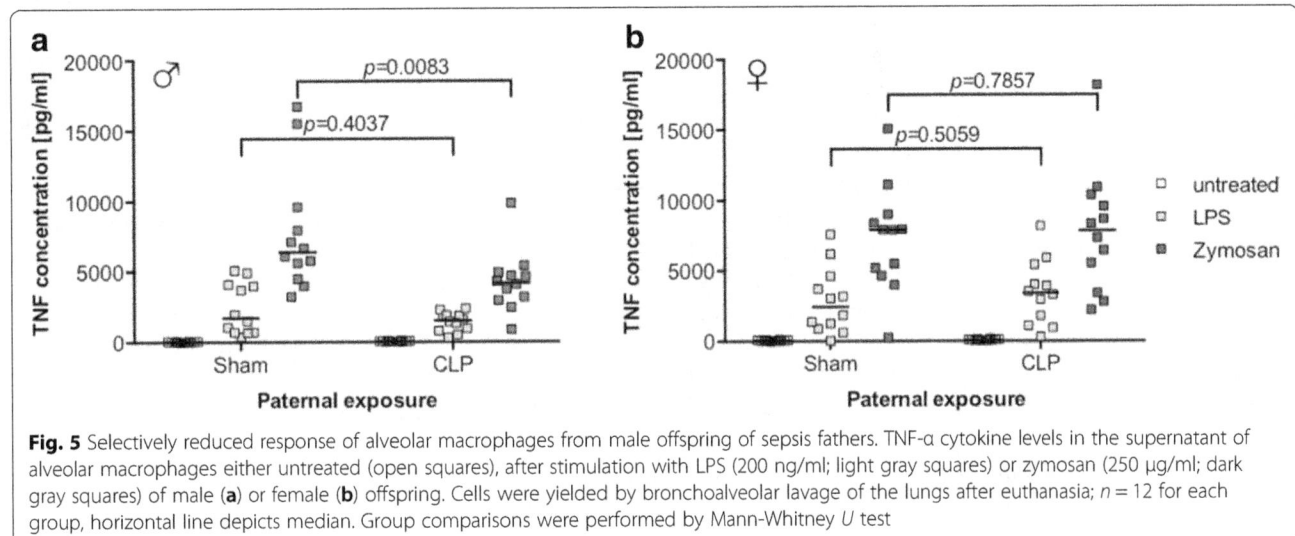

Fig. 5 Selectively reduced response of alveolar macrophages from male offspring of sepsis fathers. TNF-α cytokine levels in the supernatant of alveolar macrophages either untreated (open squares), after stimulation with LPS (200 ng/ml; light gray squares) or zymosan (250 μg/ml; dark gray squares) of male (**a**) or female (**b**) offspring. Cells were yielded by bronchoalveolar lavage of the lungs after euthanasia; $n = 12$ for each group, horizontal line depicts median. Group comparisons were performed by Mann-Whitney U test

hinting towards a compensatory mechanism. This finding is in line with results of Kajihara et al., which used bacterial LPS to induce testicular dysfunction in mice and found this phenomenon to happen transiently after 1 week due to apoptotic cell death followed by a prolonged overcompensation of sperm production up to 5 weeks [30]. Despite the observed epigenetic and morphological alterations, the overall reproductive performance of the male survivors in our study was not impaired. Considering the time since septic insult in respect to duration of murine spermiogenesis [31], we can exclude that the sperm cells present at mating have been exposed themselves to the systemic inflammation or its mediators, hinting towards a long-lasting impact of inflammation on the spermatogonia precursors.

Leaping forward, the impact of these alterations were obvious in the early postnatal stage, with a higher loss of animals occurring in sepsis offspring than control offspring. This result might be driven by a maternal rejection of or aggression behavior against the pups, maybe as a consequence of poor offspring health. The differential weight gain of surviving pups after weaning points towards a developmental genetic trait carried forward from the fathers. In line with this, the methylation changes in intronic and promoter regions of genes associated with developmental processes have been found overrepresented, besides alterations of cytosine methylation within promoters and exons of genes involved in metabolism. Strong evidence for the intergenerational impact of subtle alterations of the sperm methylome on offspring's metabolic function has been provided recently [32]. This study used in utero undernourishment as metabolic stressor and found metabolic alterations in the descendants. Comparably, during the acute phase of abdominal sepsis, the mice transiently lost substantial weight due to a sickness behavior-associated lower food intake aggravated by the high metabolic demand of the activated immune system, closely mimicking the clinical condition. Besides the abovementioned, several studies report inter- and transgenerational heredity of parental under- and overnutrition as a genetic trait for offspring's metabolism and body weight, making it a potential contributing factor also in our study [22, 33–36]. Alternatively, other studies involving animals and human subjects prove the transgenerational inheritance of experienced environmental stress (e.g., noise) [37–39]. With sepsis resembling an enormous stressful condition involving the excessive activation of, e.g., the neuroendocrine hypothalamic–pituitary–adrenal axis [35, 40], these might also adaptively lower the offspring's stress response threshold, thereby again increasing basal energy consumption and lowering body weight. Also, emerging evidence shows the importance of different cellular metabolic pathways as fundamental determinants of immune cell function in sepsis and other conditions [41, 42].

We report here a loss of immunological responsivity of male descendants of sepsis fathers upon intraperitoneal LPS injection, indicated by reduced plasma cytokines. We can neither rule out functional or numerical alterations in immune cell populations in the peritoneal cavity nor in the circulation as underlying reason for the observed phenotype. However, considering the fact that alveolar macrophages from our male mice showed comparably reduced, but yet stimuli dependent, responses might underline the conceptual framework of germline transmission and cellular reprogramming, happening already in the development of embryonic tissues of immunological relevance (e.g., the bone marrow or fetal liver). The lungs of adult mice are populated by macrophages originating from different tissue sources, with Mac2 expressing macrophages from fetal liver being the dominating and self-renewing population within the alveoli and therefore in our experimental design [43]. Alternatively, recent work from Roquilly et al. was able to prove that the lung microenvironment after infection induces anergy of dendritic cells by a regulatory T cell dependent and TGF-β-mediated mechanism [44]. How the specific reduction of the response to zymosan, a fungal cell wall component, but not bacterial LPS, is mediated remains elusive. Taken together, our current results hint towards a predisposing phenotype for invasive fungal infections, especially at the lung barrier.

Our findings might be interpreted in two ways: either the observed F_1 phenotype is a "protective burden" of host tolerance to evade excessive inflammation as experienced by the fathers or it represents a compensatory maladaptive state, rendering male descendants more susceptible to microbial encounters. An example for the latter has been shown in an experimental model of paternal chronic colitis, in which offspring exhibited an increased susceptibility and disease severity [45].

Considering the phenotype of lower body weight shared from both genders, it seems to be obvious that our immunological findings must result from a synergistic interaction of the transmitted epimutations and the well-known gender dimorphism of immune responses [46]. Also, other groups showed sex-specific intergenerational phenotypes: Sanchez-Garido and colleagues proved a pronounced impact of paternal obesity on male offspring, explained by hormonal synergism [47]. In contrast, Ng et al. found paternal high-fat diet to exclusively reprogram female offspring's pancreatic beta cells [48]. Nevertheless, especially in respect to the observed weight phenotype, we cannot rule out that when applying other immunological challenges (e.g., infection or autoimmune models), female offspring might uncover changes in responsivity and vulnerability as well.

As a mechanistical framework, we propose that paternal sepsis alters spermatogonia progenitors, which propagate their acquired epigenetic changes through meiosis into the mature sperm methylome. This information is then carried over into the zygote. Earlier studies in zebrafish prove that the sperm methylome is in fact inherited and even dominates over the maternal methylome during early embryonic development [49, 50], potentially assisted by the layer of histones [51]. With changes of the methylome present in the early embryo, the stage is set for the further propagation into all developing tissues, including the seeding immune cells. Further studies need to unravel how the identified changes are maintained through embryogenesis and how it penetrates and modulates offspring's post-natal development and immune function. Furthermore, research involving patients in the reproductive age after sepsis is necessary to prove the translation of this concept to the post-clinical setting in regard to fertility and molecular alterations of sperm cells. From a methodical point, we just measured the tip of the iceberg, as RRBS only covers 5–10% of the genome's cytosine content and a tremendous amount of information might be still hidden, extractable by single-base-resolution sequencing methods.

In summary, we can provide evidence for sepsis-induced epigenetic changes of the sperm methylome as a hub of non-sequence coded intergenerational information transfer, shaping offsprings' development and immune competence.

Conclusion

While the incidence of sepsis is steadily rising, modern high-performance medicine increases the number of surviving patients. Our results of epigenetically transmitted, intergenerational immunological changes in the offspring of sepsis sires open a whole new perspective, driving the necessity to undertake further research measures to understand the post-sepsis challenges.

Methods

Study approval

All animal procedures were conducted in accordance with the German Protection of Animals Act law and were approved by the regional council Karlsruhe (reference number G-132/15).

CLP sepsis model

Male C57BL/6 mice aged 10–12 weeks were obtained from Janvier Laboratories (Le Genest Saint Isle, France). Mice were housed in a 12-h light/dark cycle at 22 °C. Food and water were provided ad libidum. Animals were allowed to acclimatize for 7 days before any experimental procedure. Polymicrobial sepsis was induced using the cecal ligation and puncture (CLP) model [52]. In total, 20 mice were anesthetized with 100 mg/kg

ketamine (Ketanest®S, Pfizer Pharma, Berlin, Germany) and 20 mg/kg xylazine (Xylavet, CP-Pharma, Burgdorf, Germany) intraperitoneally. After a midline laparotomy and mobilization of the cecum, 5 mm was ligated and punctured once with a 23-G needle (BD Microlance™ 3, BD Medical, Heidelberg, Germany). The ligated cecum was pressed gently to extrude fecal contents. Afterwards, the cecum was relocated, the mice were supplemented with 400 μl 0.9% NaCl (B. Braun, Melsungen, Germany), given directly into the abdominal region, and the abdomen was closed with a double suture. For control, 10 animals underwent a laparotomy surgery only applying the same anesthesia regime. After surgery, pain relieve in both groups was achieved by treatment with 0.05 mg/kg bodyweight buprenorphine (Temgesic, RB Pharmaceuticals, Slough, UK) every 8 h for 2 days. For the isolation and analysis of sperm, a separate cohort of animals, both CLP as well as sham, was operated.

Sperm isolation and analysis

Mature sperm cells were isolated from the Cauda epididymis of 9 CLP and 7 sham mice into Donners medium (135 mM NaCl (Sigma-Aldrich, Steinheim, Germany), 5 mM KCl (Merck, Darmstadt, Germany), 1 mM $MgSO_4$ (Sigma-Aldrich, Steinheim, Germany), 2 mM $CaCl_2$ (Sigma-Aldrich, Steinheim, Germany), 30 mM HEPES pH 7.4 (Roth, Karlsruhe, Germany); freshly supplemented with 0.53% sodium lactate (Caelo, Hilden, Germany), 1 mM sodium pyruvate (Life Technologies, Darmstadt, Germany), 20 mg/mL BSA (Roth, Karlsruhe, Germany) and 25 mM $NaHCO_3$ (Roth, Karlsruhe, Germany)) at 37 °C and 5% CO_2 for 40 min via swim-up assay. To avoid contamination with somatic cells, only the top fractions were used for further examinations.

Sperm motility, morphology, and total cell numbers from CLP and sham mice were assessed according to WHO guidelines [53]. Total cell numbers were counted using a hemocytometer. For both, sperm motility and morphology, 200 cells of each isolation were analyzed (in replicate) using a Keyence Biozero microscope (Keyence, Neu-Isenburg, Germany). Sperm motility was scaled into three categories: progressive motility (PR), non-progressive motility (NP), and immotile (IM). Cell-VU® Prestained Morphology Slides (Millenium Sciences, NY, USA) were used according to the manufacturer's protocol for proper visualization. Sperm cells morphology was judged as normal or defect.

Details on DNA extraction, sequencing, and bioinformatics are given in Additional file 3: Document S1.

Breeding scheme and characterization of litters

For breeding, all CLP survivors and sham mice were used. Each male was mated with two infection-naive C57BL/6 females (aged 12 weeks) 6 weeks after induction of sepsis (Fig. 1a). To exclude paternal effects on maternal care and subsequently offspring survival as well as development, males were separated after 8 days resembling two full estrous cycles [23].

After birth, litter size was determined and survival of pups assessed over 12 weeks while held under standard housing conditions within the same facility. Pregnancy occurred in 13 of 20 CLP breeding pairs and 16 of 20 sham breeding groups. Maternal weaning and offspring sex determination occurred on day 23 postnatally. For the investigation of weight development, offspring were weighted two times per week for a total of 57 days after weaning.

TNF-α levels of alveolar macrophages in offspring

Alveolar macrophages were isolated via bronchoalveolar lavage (BAL) in 12-week-old animals. Offspring from CLP survivors and control sires ($n = 12$ for each sex and parental exposure) were euthanized by bleeding under ketanest/xylazin anesthesia, and BAL was performed by flushing the lung with 1 ml ice-cold phosphate-buffered saline (PBS) (Life Technologies, Umkirch, Germany) for 10 times through an incision of the trachea. Cells were counted, and 1×10^6 cells were seeded in a 96-well plate (Sarstedt, Nuembrecht, Germany) with Aim V Media (Life Technologies, Darmstadt, Germany). Stimulation was done with 200 ng/ml ultrapure LPS or 250 µg/ml depleted Zymosan (both Invivogen, Toulouse, France). No stimulating agent was added to controls. After incubation for 24 h (37 °C with 5% CO_2), supernatant was collected and TNF-α levels were determined using Mouse TNF-alpha DuoSet ELISA (R&D Systems, Minneapolis, USA) according to the manufacturer's instruction. In case of low BAL cell yield, lower cell numbers were used for stimulation and response was normalized accordingly.

In vivo stimulation and cytokine analysis of offspring

Offspring from CLP survivors and sham sires (aged 32 weeks) were injected with LPS (1 mg/kg). For each group, eight animals were used except for saline-treated female groups ($n = 7$) After 24 h, mice were euthanized and the blood was collected by cardiac puncture. Mice were weighted before injection as well as before euthanasia.

For flow cytometry-based multiplex cytokine analysis, the CBA Mouse Inflammation Kit (BD Biosciences, Heidelberg, Germany) was used according to the manufacturer's protocol. Detection was performed with a BD FACSVerse flow cytometer and data analyzed by FCAP Array 3.0 software (BD Biosciences, Heidelberg, Germany).

Statistics

All statistical analysis and visualizations were done in GraphPad Prism (V6.0 for Mac, GraphPad Software, La Jolla, USA). Comparisons between two groups were performed depending on the sample size and distribution either by non-parametric Mann-Whitney U test (two-tailed; for non-normal distribution and $n \leq 30$) or unpaired t test (two-tailed; normally distributed data or $n > 30$). Survival time analysis was done by applying the Gehan-Breslow-Wilcoxon test to take into account the occurrence of early events over the observation time. Statistical significance was assumed with a p value of less than 0.05 for all analysis.

Abbreviations
CLP: Cecal ligation and puncture; dmCs: Differentially methylated cytosines; DNA: Deoxyribonucleic acid; HSC: Hematopoietic stem cells; IL-6/-10: Interleukin-6/-10; LPS: Lipopolysaccharide; MCP-1: Monocyte chemoattractant protein 1; RRBS: Reduced reduction bisulfite sequencing; TGF-β: Transforming growth factor β; TLR4: Toll-like receptor 4; TNF-α: Tumor necrosis factor α

Acknowledgements
The authors thank Ute Krauser, Birgit Prior, and Sabine Stegmaier for outstanding technical support.

Authors' contributions
KB and FU planned and performed the animal experiments. KB, JS, ST, and DS conducted the analysis. KB, DS, MAW, and FU performed the data interpretation and statistics. FU and MAW wrote the manuscript. All authors critically revised and drafted the manuscript. All authors read and approved the final manuscript.

Competing interests
The authors declare that they have no competing interests.

References
1. Fleischmann C, Scherag A, Adhikari NKJ, Hartog CS, Tsaganos T, Schlattmann P, et al. Assessment of global incidence and mortality of hospital-treated sepsis. Current estimates and limitations. Am J Respir Crit Care Med. 2016;193:259–72.
2. Singer M, Deutschman CS, Seymour CW, Shankar-Hari M, Annane D, Bauer M, et al. The third international consensus definitions for sepsis and septic shock (Sepsis-3). JAMA. 2016;315:801–10.
3. Kaukonen K-M, Bailey M, Suzuki S, Pilcher D, Bellomo R. Mortality related to severe Sepsis and septic shock among critically ill patients in Australia and New Zealand, 2000-2012. JAMA. 2014;311:1308–9.
4. Martin GS, Mannino DM, Moss M. The effect of age on the development and outcome of adult sepsis. Crit Care Med. 2006;34:15–21.
5. Gaieski DF, Edwards JM, Kallan MJ, Carr BG. Benchmarking the incidence and mortality of severe sepsis in the United States. Crit Care Med. 2013;41:1167–74.

6. Hartman ME, Linde-Zwirble WT, Angus DC, Watson RS. Trends in the epidemiology of pediatric severe sepsis*. Pediatr Crit Care Med. 2013;14:686–93.

7. Uhle F, Chousterman BG, Grützmann R, Brenner T, Weber GF. Pathogenic, immunologic, and clinical aspects of sepsis - update 2016. Expert Rev Anti-Infect Ther. 2016;14:917–27.

8. Matkovich S, Khiami Al B, Efimov IR, Evans S, Vader J, Jain A, et al. Widespread down-regulation of cardiac mitochondrial and sarcomeric genes in patients with Sepsis. Crit Care Med. 2017;45(3):407–14. https://doi.org/10.1097/CCM.0000000000002207.

9. Rocheteau P, Chatre L, Briand D, Mebarki M, Jouvion G, Bardon J, et al. Sepsis induces long-term metabolic and mitochondrial muscle stem cell dysfunction amenable by mesenchymal stem cell therapy. Nat Commun. 2015;6:10145.

10. Schouten M, Wiersinga WJ, Levi M, van der Poll T. Inflammation, endothelium, and coagulation in sepsis. J Leukoc Biol Society for Leukocyte Biology. 2008;83:536–45.

11. Carson WF, Cavassani KA, Dou Y, Kunkel SL. Epigenetic regulation of immune cell functions during post-septic immunosuppression. Epigenetics. 2011;6:273–83.

12. Gallagher KA, Joshi A, Carson WF, Schaller M, Allen R, Mukerjee S, et al. Epigenetic changes in bone marrow progenitor cells influence the inflammatory phenotype and alter wound healing in type 2 diabetes. Diabetes. 2015;64:1420–30.

13. Zhang H, Rodriguez S, Wang L, Wang S, Serezani H, Kapur R, et al. Sepsis induces hematopoietic stem cell exhaustion and myelosuppression through distinct contributions of TRIF and MYD88. Stem Cell Reports. 2016;6:940–56.

14. Faivre V, Lukaszewicz AC, Payen D. Downregulation of blood monocyte HLA-DR in ICU patients is also present in bone marrow cells. PLoS One. 2016;11:e0164489.

15. Weiterer S, Uhle F, Lichtenstern C, Siegler BH, Bhuju S, Jarek M, et al. Sepsis induces specific changes in histone modification patterns in human monocytes. Mariño-Ramírez L, editor. PLoS ONE. Public Libr Sci; 2015;10:e0121748.

16. Azenabor A, Ekun AO, Akinloye O. Impact of inflammation on male reproductive tract. J Reprod Infertil. 2015;16:123–9.

17. Rusz A, Pilatz A, Wagenlehner F, Linn T, Diemer T, Schuppe HC, et al. Influence of urogenital infections and inflammation on semen quality and male fertility. World J Urol. 2012;30:23–30.

18. Danchin É, Charmantier A, Champagne FA, Mesoudi A, Pujol B, Blanchet S. Beyond DNA: integrating inclusive inheritance into an extended theory of evolution. Nat Rev Genet. 2011;12:475–86.

19. Miska EA, Ferguson-Smith AC. Transgenerational inheritance: models and mechanisms of non-DNA sequence-based inheritance. Science. 2016;354:59–63.

20. Heard E, Martienssen RA. Transgenerational epigenetic inheritance: myths and mechanisms. Cell. 2014;157:95–109.

21. de Castro Barbosa T, Ingerslev LR, Alm PS, Versteyhe S, Massart J, Rasmussen M, et al. High-fat diet reprograms the epigenome of rat spermatozoa and transgenerationally affects metabolism of the offspring. Molecular Metabolism. 2016;5:184–97.

22. Carone BR, Fauquier L, Habib N, Shea JM, Hart CE, Li R, et al. Paternally induced transgenerational environmental reprogramming of metabolic gene expression in mammals. Cell. 2010;143:1084–96.

23. Lambrot R, Xu C, Saint-Phar S, Chountalos G, Cohen T, Paquet M, et al. Low paternal dietary folate alters the mouse sperm epigenome and is associated with negative pregnancy outcomes. Nat Commun. 2013;4:2889.

24. Skinner MK, Ben Maamar M, Sadler-Riggleman I, Beck D, Nilsson E, McBirney M, et al. Alterations in sperm DNA methylation, non-coding RNA and histone retention associate with DDT-induced epigenetic transgenerational inheritance of disease. Epigenetics Chromatin. 2018;11:8.

25. Beck D, Sadler-Riggleman I, Skinner MK. Generational comparisons (F1 versus F3) of vinclozolin induced epigenetic transgenerational inheritance of sperm differential DNA methylation regions (epimutations) using MeDIP-Seq. Environ Epigenet. 2017;3:dvx016.

26. Guibert S, Forné T, Weber M. Global profiling of DNA methylation erasure in mouse primordial germ cells. Genome Res. 2012;22:633–41.

27. Hackett JA, Sengupta R, Zylicz JJ, Murakami K, Lee C, Down TA, et al. Germline DNA demethylation dynamics and imprint erasure through 5-hydroxymethylcytosine. Science. 2013;339:448–52.

28. Jenkins TG, Aston KI, Pflueger C, Cairns BR, Carrell DT. Age-associated sperm DNA methylation alterations: possible implications in offspring disease susceptibility. PLoS Genet. 2014;10:e1004458.

29. Santi D, De Vincentis S, Magnani E, Spaggiari G. Impairment of sperm DNA methylation in male infertility: a meta-analytic study. Andrology. 2017;5:695–703.

30. Kajihara T, Okagaki R, Ishihara O. LPS-induced transient testicular dysfunction accompanied by apoptosis of testicular germ cells in mice. Med Mol Morphol. 2006;39:203–8.

31. Oakberg EF. A description of spermiogenesis in the mouse and its use in analysis of the cycle of the seminiferous epithelium and germ cell renewal. Am J Anat Wiley Subscription Services, Inc, A Wiley Company. 1956;99:391–413.

32. Radford EJ, Ito M, Shi H, Corish JA, Yamazawa K, Isganaitis E, et al. In utero effects. In utero undernourishment perturbs the adult sperm methylome and intergenerational metabolism. Science. 2014;345:1255903.

33. Huypens P, Sass S, Wu M, Dyckhoff D, Tschöp M, Theis F, et al. Epigenetic germline inheritance of diet-induced obesity and insulin resistance. Nat Genet. 2016;48:497–9.

34. Fullston T, Ohlsson Teague EMC, Palmer NO, DeBlasio MJ, Mitchell M, Corbett M, et al. Paternal obesity initiates metabolic disturbances in two generations of mice with incomplete penetrance to the F2 generation and alters the transcriptional profile of testis and sperm microRNA content. FASEB J. 2013;27:4226–43.

35. Cropley JE, Eaton SA, Aiken A, Young PE, Giannoulatou E, Ho JWK, et al. Male-lineage transmission of an acquired metabolic phenotype induced by grand-paternal obesity. Molecular Metabolism. 2016;5:699–708.

36. Grandjean V, Fourré S, De Abreu DAF, Derieppe M-A, Remy J-J, Rassoulzadegan M. RNA-mediated paternal heredity of diet-induced obesity and metabolic disorders. Sci Rep. 2015;5:18193.

37. Rodgers AB, Morgan CP, Bronson SL, Revello S, Bale TL. Paternal stress exposure alters sperm microRNA content and reprograms offspring HPA stress axis regulation. J Neurosci. 2013;33:9003–12.

38. Crews D, Gillette R, Scarpino SV, Manikkam M, Savenkova MI, Skinner MK. Epigenetic transgenerational inheritance of altered stress responses. Proc Natl Acad Sci U S A. 2012;109:9143–8.

39. Morgan CP, Bale TL. Early prenatal stress epigenetically programs dysmasculinization in second-generation offspring via the paternal lineage. J Neurosci. 2011;31:11748–55.

40. Lesur O, Roussy J-F, Chagnon F, Gallo-Payet N, Dumaine R, Sarret P, et al. Proven infection-related sepsis induces a differential stress response early after ICU admission. Crit Care. BioMed Central; 2010;14:R131.

41. Ganeshan K, Chawla A. Metabolic regulation of immune responses. Annu Rev Immunol Annual Reviews. 2014;32:609–34.

42. Cheng S-C, Scicluna BP, Arts RJW, Gresnigt MS, Lachmandas E, Giamarellos-Bourboulis EJ, et al. Broad defects in the energy metabolism of leukocytes underlie immunoparalysis in sepsis. Nat Immunol. 2016;17:406–13.

43. Tan SYS, Krasnow MA. Developmental origin of lung macrophage diversity. Development. 2016;143:1318–27.

44. Roquilly A, McWilliam HEG, Jacqueline C, Tian Z, Cinotti R, Rimbert M, et al. Local modulation of antigen-presenting cell development after resolution of pneumonia induces long-term susceptibility to secondary infections. Immunity. 2017;47:135.

45. Tschurtschenthaler M, Kachroo P, Heinsen F-A, Adolph TE, Rühlemann MC, Klughammer J, et al. Paternal chronic colitis causes epigenetic inheritance of susceptibility to colitis. Sci Rep. 2016;6:31640.

46. Klein SL, Flanagan KL. Sex differences in immune responses. Nature Publishing Group Nature Publishing Group. 2016;16:626–38.

47. Sanchez-Garrido MA, Ruiz-Pino F, Velasco I, Barroso A, Fernandois D, Heras V, et al. Intergenerational influence of paternal obesity on metabolic and reproductive health parameters of the offspring: male-preferential impact and involvement of Kiss1-mediated pathways. Endocrinology. 2018;159:1005–18.

48. Ng S-F, Lin RCY, Laybutt DR, Barrès R, Owens JA, Morris MJ. Chronic high-fat diet in fathers programs β-cell dysfunction in female rat offspring. Nature. Nature Publishing Group; 2010;467:963–966.

49. Jiang L, Zhang J, Wang J-J, Wang L, Zhang L, Li G, et al. Sperm, but not oocyte, DNA methylome is inherited by zebrafish early embryos. Cell. 2013; 153:773–84.

50. Potok ME, Nix DA, Parnell TJ, Cairns BR. Reprogramming the maternal zebrafish genome after fertilization to match the paternal methylation pattern. Cell. 2013;153:759–72.

51. Murphy PJ, Wu SF, James CR, Wike CL, Cairns BR. Placeholder nucleosomes underlie germline-to-embryo DNA methylation reprogramming. Cell. 2018; 172:993–1006. e13

52. Rittirsch D, Huber-Lang MS, Flierl MA, Ward PA. Immunodesign of experimental sepsis by cecal ligation and puncture. Nat Protoc. 2008;4:31–6.

53. World Health Organization. WHO Laboratory manual for the examination and processing of human semen. 5th edition. World Health Organization; 2010.

rs10732516 polymorphism at the *IGF2/H19* locus associates with genotype-specific effects on placental DNA methylation and birth weight of newborns conceived by assisted reproductive technology

Heidi Marjonen[1], Pauliina Auvinen[1], Hanna Kahila[2], Olga Tšuiko[3,4], Sulev Kõks[5,6], Airi Tiirats[7,8], Triin Viltrop[3], Timo Tuuri[2], Viveca Söderström-Anttila[2,9], Anne-Maria Suikkari[9], Andres Salumets[2,3,4,7], Aila Tiitinen[2] and Nina Kaminen-Ahola[1*] [iD]

Abstract

Background: Assisted reproductive technology (ART) has been associated with low birth weight of fresh embryo transfer (FRESH) derived and increased birth weight of frozen embryo transfer (FET)-derived newborns. Owing to that, we focused on imprinted insulin-like growth factor 2 (*IGF2*)/*H19* locus known to be important for normal growth. This locus is regulated by *H19* imprinting control region (ICR) with seven binding sites for the methylation-sensitive zinc finger regulatory protein (CTCF). A polymorphism rs10732516 G/A in the sixth binding site for CTCF, associates with a genotype-specific trend to the DNA methylation. Due to this association, 62 couples with singleton pregnancies derived from FRESH (44 IVF/18 ICSI), 24 couples from FET (15 IVF/9 ICSI), and 157 couples with spontaneously conceived pregnancies as controls were recruited in Finland and Estonia for genotype-specific examination. DNA methylation levels at the *H19* ICR, *H19* DMR, and long interspersed nuclear elements in placental tissue were explored by MassARRAY EpiTYPER ($n = 122$). Allele-specific changes in the methylation level of *H19* ICR in placental tissue ($n = 26$) and white blood cells (WBC, $n = 8$) were examined by bisulfite sequencing. Newborns' ($n = 243$) anthropometrics was analyzed by using international growth standards.

Results: A consistent trend of genotype-specific decreased methylation level was observed in paternal allele of rs10732516 paternal A/maternal G genotype, but not in paternal G/maternal A genotype, at *H19* ICR in ART placentas. This hypomethylation was not detected in WBCs. Also genotype-specific differences in FRESH-derived newborns' birth weight and head circumference were observed ($P = 0.04$, $P = 0.004$, respectively): FRESH-derived newborns with G/G genotype were heavier ($P = 0.04$) and had larger head circumference ($P = 0.002$) compared to newborns with A/A genotype. Also, the placental weight and birth weight of controls, FRESH- and FET-derived newborns differed significantly in rs10732516 A/A genotype ($P = 0.024$, $P = 0.006$, respectively): the placentas and newborns of FET-derived pregnancies were heavier compared to FRESH-derived pregnancies ($P = 0.02$, $P = 0.004$, respectively).

(Continued on next page)

---

* Correspondence: nina.kaminen@helsinki.fi
[1]Department of Medical and Clinical Genetics, Medicum, University of Helsinki, Helsinki, Finland
Full list of author information is available at the end of the article

(Continued from previous page)

Conclusions: The observed DNA methylation changes together with the phenotypic findings suggest that rs10732516 polymorphism associates with the effects of ART in a parent-of-origin manner. Therefore, this polymorphism should be considered when the effects of environmental factors on embryonic development are studied.

Keywords: Assisted reproductive technology, IVF, Fresh embryo transfer, Frozen embryo transfer, Imprinting, IGF2/H19, rs10732516, DNA methylation, Placenta, Birth weight,

Background

Although the results of assisted reproductive technology (ART) in Western countries are impressive and the children born are generally healthy, they have been associated with increased risk of adverse perinatal outcome [1]. Especially, an increased risk of low birth weight and preterm birth have been observed in in vitro fertilized (IVF) singleton pregnancies compared to natural conception [2–4]. Furthermore, there has been a suspicion of a higher frequency of imprinting disorders, such as Angelman, Beckwith-Wiedemann, and Silver-Russell syndromes [5, 6]. On the other hand, increased birth weight has been associated with newborns derived from frozen embryo transfer (FET) [7–9]. The reason for the differences in perinatal outcome is unclear, but it could be explained by parental characteristics, subfertility, or gonadotrophin stimulation of the ovaries [10–12]. Furthermore, some adverse effect of laboratory procedures involving use of culture media, prolonged culturing of the embryos and freezing/thawing methods has not been excluded [10].

The procedures of IVF and intracytoplasmic sperm injection (ICSI) are performed in the beginning of embryonic development, which is a period of epigenetic reprogramming. During this dynamic period of cell divisions, the epigenetic marks are erased and then established again [13]. The adequate methylation profiles are needed for normal embryonic development, and indeed, it has been recently shown that many developmentally important transcription factors display preference for sequences containing DNA methylation [14]. Altered levels of DNA methylation have been observed not only in different human tissues derived from IVF/ICSI pregnancies [15–17] but also in mouse [18, 19], suggesting that IVF protocol, even without infertility can alter the epigenome. Although the results are inconsistent, theoretically IVF could affect the epigenetic reprogramming of early embryo and consequently influence the perinatal outcome.

Owing to the low birth weight associated with IVF and increased birth weight of newborns derived from FET, we focused on the imprinted insulin-like growth factor 2 (IGF2)/H19 locus on chromosome 11p15.5. These two genes are expressed in parent-of-origin manner; IGF2, a major driver of growth, is expressed from paternal allele

[20] and non-coding, negative growth controller H19 from maternal allele [21]. Allele-specific gene expression is needed for normal placental and embryonic growth. The locus is regulated by allele-specific DNA methylation at the H19 imprinting control region (H19 ICR) locating between the genes, as well as H19 promoter region (H19 DMR) and three differentially methylated regions (DMR0, DMR1, and DMR2) at the IGF2 (Fig. 1). H19 ICR contains seven binding sites for a methylation-sensitive, zinc-finger protein CCCTC-binding factor (CTCF). These binding factors organize chromatin contacts and have a critical role in the establishment and maintenance of imprinting [22]. According to mouse studies, unmethylated H19 ICR sequence on the maternal allele enables binding of the CTCF protein, which is required to prevent enhancers from acting on maternal IGF2, thus, repressing its expression [23].

Imprinting disorders have shown the importance of the adequate H19 ICR methylation: hypomethylation results in downregulation of IGF2 and biallelic expression of H19, leading to a growth restriction disorder, Silver-Russell syndrome. By contrast, hypermethylation of H19 ICR leads to overexpression of IGF2, downregulation of H19, and consequently fetal over-growth known as Beckwith-Wiedemann syndrome [24, 25]. Hypomethylation of the sixth CTCF binding site (CTCF6) at the H19 ICR has been previously associated with placental cells [15], buccal epithelium cells [16], and cord blood mononuclear cells [17] in human pregnancies conceived by IVF or ICSI. Also, increased inter- and intra-individual variation in allele-specific DNA methylation and decreased IGF2 and H19 expression have been observed in placental tissue of in vitro conceived children [26].

In our recent study, we observed a single nucleotide polymorphism rs10732516 G/A in CTCF6, which associated with the distinct DNA methylation profiles of H19 ICR in human placenta [27]. Moreover, when the samples were divided in four groups according to the genotype (rs10732516 G/G, paternal G/maternal A, paternal A/maternal G, and A/A), we observed decreased methylation level in alcohol-exposed placentas of paternal A/maternal G genotype, but not in paternal G/maternal A genotype. Surprisingly, alcohol exposure associated with decreased head circumference in all genotypes except A/A, in which increased head circumference was observed

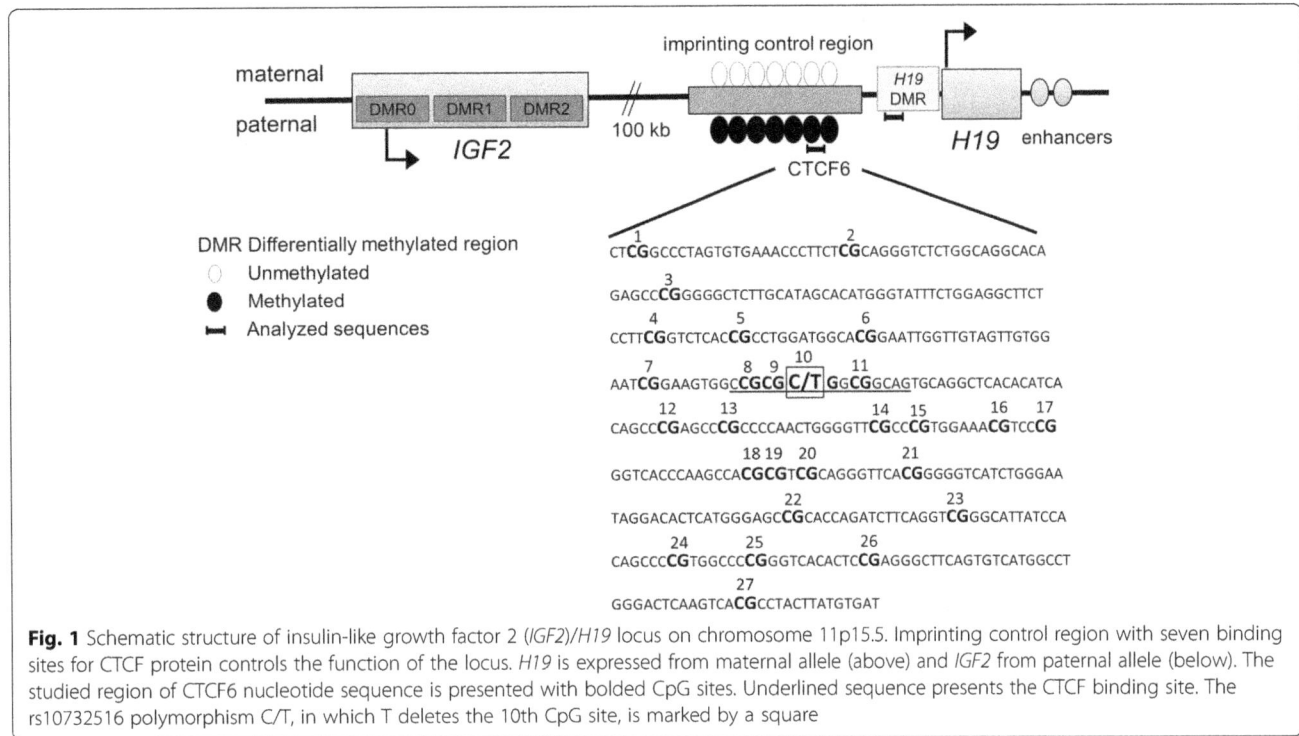

Fig. 1 Schematic structure of insulin-like growth factor 2 (*IGF2*)/*H19* locus on chromosome 11p15.5. Imprinting control region with seven binding sites for CTCF protein controls the function of the locus. *H19* is expressed from maternal allele (above) and *IGF2* from paternal allele (below). The studied region of CTCF6 nucleotide sequence is presented with bolded CpG sites. Underlined sequence presents the CTCF binding site. The rs10732516 polymorphism C/T, in which T deletes the 10th CpG site, is marked by a square

[27]. Interestingly, previous studies have shown parent-of-origin associations between birth weight and polymorphisms rs4929984 and rs2071094, which both are in linkage to rs10732516 [28, 29].

Although prenatal alcohol exposure and IVF are very different environmental factors, they both have been associated with growth-restricted phenotype of newborns. To examine if there is similar genotype-specific decreased DNA methylation level at the *IGF2/H19* locus caused by ART, we collected placental tissue from fresh embryo transfer (FRESH) and frozen embryo transfer (FET)-derived pregnancies of Finnish and Estonian couples (Table 1; Additional file 1: Table S1). We compared them to placentas of spontaneous, naturally conceived pregnancies. We explored the methylation levels of *H19* ICR and *H19* DMR in placenta. Owing to the previously detected ART-associated changes in global DNA methylation levels [30], also long interspersed nuclear elements (LINE-1) were examined. In addition to placenta, we collected umbilical cord blood to explore if we could see similar changes in DNA methylation in both extra embryonic placental cells and embryonic blood cells of the newborns. Potential genotype-specific effects of ART on the newborns' phenotype were studied by using international growth standards [31].

Results

Participants characteristics
Significant differences between mothers in studied groups (controls, FRESH- and FET-derived pregnancies) were observed in age ($P < 0.0001$, two-way ANOVA) and parity ($P = 0.003$, two-way ANOVA), but not in maternal BMI (Table 1). Finnish and Estonian mothers differed significantly in age ($P = 0.005$, two-way ANOVA) and parity ($P = 0.04$, two-way ANOVA); however, the interaction effect was not significant ($P = 0.8$, $P = 1$, respectively). There was a significant difference in gestational age between the study groups ($P = 0.002$, two-way ANOVA), as well as between the Finnish and Estonian study populations ($P = 0.01$, two-way ANOVA), although the interaction effect was not significant ($P = 0.7$). Furthermore, ART had no effect on the 5 min Apgar score which is used to evaluate the vitality of the newborn at birth.

Birth weight, birth length, and head circumference were examined for FRESH and FET derived as well as control newborns using international growth standards [31]. The placental weights differed significantly between the controls, FRESH- and FET-derived newborns ($P = 0.04$, two-way ANOVA) (Table 1, Fig. 2a). Although there was a significant difference in the placental weights between Finnish and Estonian newborns ($P < 0.001$, two-way ANOVA), the interaction effect was not significant ($P = 0.4$) and the data was combined. Placentas of FET-derived pregnancies were heavier compared to FRESH-derived placentas and control placentas ($P < 0.001$, $P = 0.01$, respectively, Bonferroni post hoc). Also FRESH-derived placentas were lighter compared to controls ($P = 0.01$, Bonferroni post hoc) (Fig. 2a). According to the international growth standards, the standard deviations (SDs)

Table 1 General characteristics of the controls, fresh embryo transfer (FRESH) and frozen embryo transfer (FET)-derived newborns, and their mothers included in the study. The SD of measures based on international growth references adjusted for gestational age at birth and gender. The mean values ± SD are presented and the significant difference between studied groups for total amount of samples is calculated by Two-Way ANOVA (P value)

	Country	Control (n = 157)	Fresh embryo transfer (FRESH) (n = 62)	Frozen embryo transfer (FET) (n = 24)	P value
Newborns					
Birth weight (g)	Total	3700 ± 436	3525 ± 548	3805 ± 601	0.02
	FI	3667.7 ± 412.2 (n = 100)	3443.4 ± 502.8 (n = 29)	3846.3 ± 451.4 (n = 18)	
	EE	3758.9 ± 473.9 (n = 57)	3595.8 ± 582.4 (n = 33)	3679.8 ± 970 (n = 6)	
Birth weight SD	Total	0.21 ± 0.8	0.1 ± 1	0.6 ± 1	NS
	FI	0.1 ± 0.9 (n = 100)	−0.1 ± 0.9 (n = 29)	0.6 ± 0.9 (n = 18)	
	EE	0.4 ± 0.6 (n = 57)	0.4 ± 1 (n = 33)	0.6 ± 0.9 (n = 6)	
Length (cm)	Total	51.0 ± 1.9	50.3 ± 2.3	51.1 ± 2.3	0.04
	FI	51 ± 2 (n = 100)	50 ± 2 (n = 29)	51 ± 2 (n = 18)	
	EE	51 ± 2 (n = 57)	51 ± 2 (n = 33)	51 ± 4 (n = 6)	
Length SD	Total	−0.1 ± 0.8	−0.1 ± 0.8	0.1 ± 0.8	NS
	FI	−0.2 ± 0.9 (n = 100)	−0.3 ± 0.8 (n = 29)	−0.0 ± 0.9 (n = 18)	
	EE	0.2 ± 0.8 (n = 57)	0.1 ± 0.7 (n = 33)	0.6 ± 0.5 (n = 6)	
Head circumference (cm)	Total	35.5 ± 1.3 (n = 155)	35.2 ± 1.7	35.4 ± 1.9	NS
	FI	35.5 ± 1 (n = 100)	34.7 ± 2 (n = 29)	35.6 ± 2 (n = 18)	
	EE	35.5 ± 1 (n = 55)	35.5 ± 2 (n = 33)	34.9 ± 2 (n = 6)	
Head circumference SD	Total	0.3 ± 0.8 (n = 155)	0.3 ± 1.1	0.4 ± 1.3	NS
	FI	0.3 ± 0.9 (n = 100)	−0.1 ± 1 (n = 29)	0.4 ± 1.4 (n = 18)	
	EE	0.4 ± 0.8 (n = 55)	0.7 ± 1 (n = 33)	0.4 ± 0.7 (n = 6)	
Placenta (g)	Total	565 ± 141	514 ± 118 (n = 61)	642 ± 187	0.04
	FI	626.5 ± 126.4 (n = 100)	578.4 ± 105.3 (n = 29)	687.4 ± 176 (n = 18)	
	EE	456.7 ± 90.5 (n = 57)	454.8 ± 97.9 (n = 32)	504.5 ± 159.6 (n = 6)	
Gestational age (weeks)	Total	40.3 ± 1.2	39.6 ± 1.4	39.8 ± 1.7	0.002
	FI	40.4 ± 1 (n = 100)	39.9 ± 1.3 (n = 29)	40 ± 1 (n = 18)	
	EE	40 ± 1.4 (n = 57)	39.3 ± 1.4 (n = 33)	39.3 ± 3 (n = 6)	
Males	Total	53%	55%	58%	NS
	FI	52%	41%	67%	
	EE	54%	67%	33%	
Females	Total	47%	45%	42%	NS
	FI	48%	59%	33%	
	EE	46%	33%	67%	
Apgar score (5 min)	Total	9 ± 1 (n = 156)	9 ± 1	9 ± 1	NS
	FI	9 ± 1 (n = 100)	9 ± 0.5 (n = 29)	9 ± 0.5 (n = 18)	
	EE	9 ± 1 (n = 56)	9 ± 0.7 (n = 33)	9 ± 0.8 (n = 6)	
Mothers					
Age (years)	Total	31 ± 5	34 ± 5	35 ± 4	< 0.001
	FI	32 ± 5 (n = 100)	35 ± 4 (n = 29)	36 ± 3 (n = 18)	
	EE	29 ± 6 (n = 57)	33 ± 5 (n = 33)	33 ± 5 (n = 6)	

Table 1 General characteristics of the controls, fresh embryo transfer (FRESH) and frozen embryo transfer (FET)-derived newborns, and their mothers included in the study. The SD of measures based on international growth references adjusted for gestational age at birth and gender. The mean values ± SD are presented and the significant difference between studied groups for total amount of samples is calculated by Two-Way ANOVA (P value) *(Continued)*

	Country	Control (n = 157)	Fresh embryo transfer (FRESH) (n = 62)	Frozen embryo transfer (FET) (n = 24)	P value
Parity	Total	0.7 ± 0.9	0.3 ± 0.5	0.4 ± 0.6	0.003
	FI	0.6 ± 0.7 (n = 100)	0.2 ± 0.5 (n = 29)	0.3 ± 0.5 (n = 18)	
	EE	0.8 ± 1 (n = 57)	0.4 ± 0.6 (n = 33)	0.7 ± 0.8 (n = 6)	
BMI	Total	23.1 ± 4 (n = 155)	23.0 ± 4	24.2 ± 4	NS
	FI	22.8 ± 3.5 (n = 99)	22.9 ± 3.4 (n = 29)	23.8 ± 3.4 (n = 18)	
	EE	23.7 ± 5 (n = 56)	23.2 ± 5 (n = 33)	25.5 ± 4.3 (n = 6)	

FI Finland, *EE* Estonia, *NS* not significant

of birth weight (Fig. 2b) or head circumference did not differ significantly between the Finnish and Estonian newborns or between the studied groups. Birth length differed significantly between Finnish and Estonian newborns ($P = 0.001$, two-way ANOVA), although the interaction effect was not significant ($P = 0.9$) and no difference could be observed between the study groups ($P = 0.2$). We did not observe significant differences between sexes, when all samples were compared.

DNA methylation profiles at *H19* ICR, *H19* DMR, and LINE-1
To explore the potential association between ART and placental DNA methylation changes, we compared the methylation levels of *H19* imprinting control region (ICR) and *H19* differentially methylated region (DMR) by EpiTYPER (Sequenom). We did not observe differences between ART and control placentas (Additional file 2:

Table S1). We also determined the effects of ART on global methylation level in placenta by examining methylation in LINE-1 by EpiTYPER. However, we did not observe any significant alterations in global methylation level either (Additional file 2: Table S1).

Genotype-specific DNA methylation at *H19* ICR and *H19* DMR by EpiTYPER
Owing to the genotype-specific DNA methylation profiles of CTCF6 at *H19* ICR [27], we divided our samples into four groups according to the genotype: rs10732516 G/G, paternal G/maternal A (patG/matA), paternal A/maternal G (patA/matG), and A/A. The allele frequencies of this polymorphism are almost equal in Finnish population (G = 0.47, A = 0.53) [32], and there were no differences in the prevalence of rs10732516 genotypes

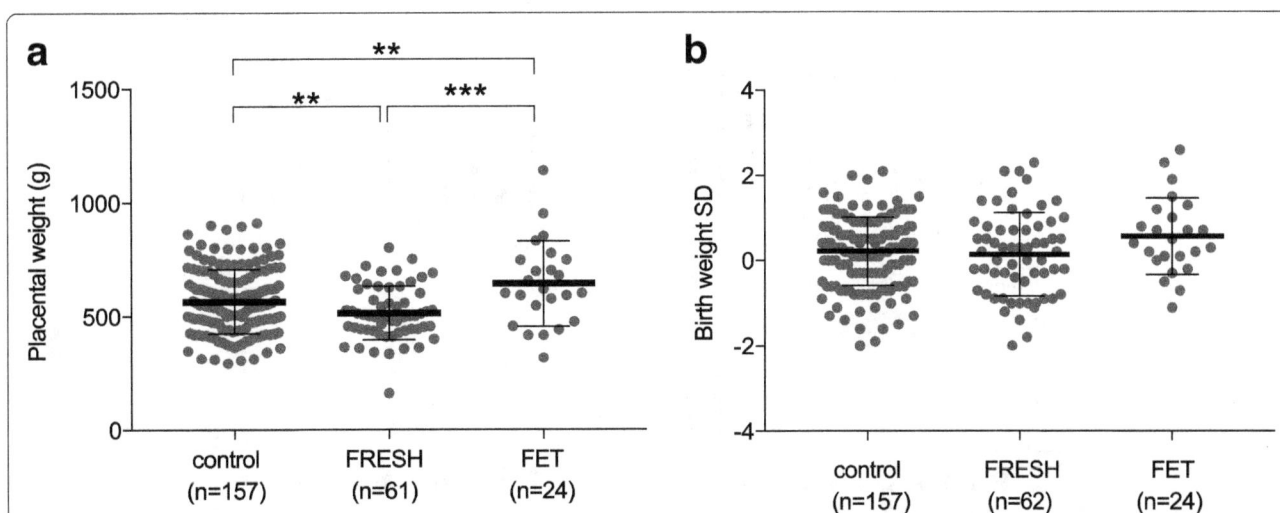

Fig. 2 Placental weights and birth weights (SD) of control, fresh embryo transfer (FRESH) and frozen embryo transfer (FET) derived newborns. **a** The placental weights differ significantly between the groups ($P = 0.04$, Two-Way ANOVA). FET-derived placentas are heavier compared to FRESH ($P = 0.001$, Bonferroni pos hoc) and FRES-derived lighter compared to controls ($P = 0.01$, Bonferroni post hoc). **b** There are no significant differences in birth weights between the groups. Bonferroni post hoc test for Two-Way ANOVA. Bonferroni post hoc test for two-way ANOVA: *$P < 0.05$, **$P < 0.01$, ***$P \leq 0.001$

between controls and ART-derived samples in this study ($X^2(3) = 5.52$, $P = 0.138$, chi-square test).

We compared first the genotype-specific methylation levels of placental CTCF6 at *H19* ICR and *H19* DMR by EpiTYPER to explore potential effects of ART. We did not see any genotype-specific differences between control and ART samples at *H19* ICR (Additional file 2: Table S1). At the *H19* DMR, we observed increased methylation level in CpG_3 and CpG_16 units in A/A genotype of ART samples (nominal *P* values: $P = 0.03$ and $P = 0.05$, respectively, Student's *t* test), but changes were not significant after Bonferroni multiple testing correction.

Genotype-specific DNA methylation at *H19* ICR by bisulfite sequencing

We also compared genotype-specific methylation levels of CTCF6 at *H19* ICR between control and ART placentas by traditional bisulfite sequencing. To discern maternal and paternal alleles, we used only heterozygous samples (patG/matA and patA/matG). We observed a bias in PCR

product: hypomethylated maternal allele of patA/matG genotype was amplified more efficiently compared to hypermethylated paternal allele. Owing to that, we counted the average methylation percentages separately for both alleles and then calculated the total methylation level for each CpG sites (CpG_1-27). We observed similar, but much more prominent common genotype-specific methylation profiles in placenta as we detected by EpiTYPER (Additional file 2: Table S1 and S2).

When comparing genotype-specific DNA methylation within heterozygotes (patG/matA and patA/matG) controls to ART samples, we observed decreased methylation level at sites CpG_1-3, CpG_5, CpG_14, and CpG_24 patA/matG genotype in the ART placentas (nominal *P* values 0.008, 0.02, 0.001, 0.013, 0.013, and 0.029, respectively, Mann-Whitney) (Fig. 3d). Instead of hypomethylation, we observed increased methylation level at site CpG_26 in patG/matA genotype (nominal *P* value = 0.041, Mann-Whitney). However, changes in methylation level were not significant after multiple testing correction. We did not see similar trend of decreased methylation

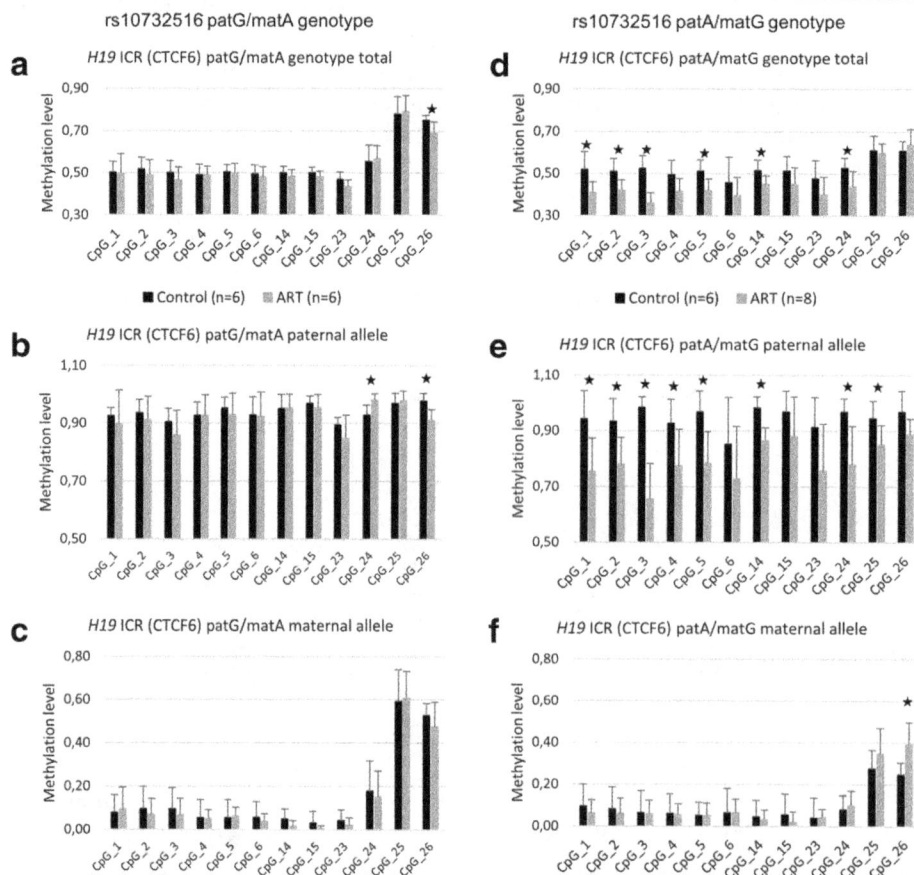

Fig. 3 Genotype- and allele-specific DNA methylation levels at *H19* ICR (CTCF6) in control and ART placentas measured by traditional bisulfite sequencing. Methylation levels of selected CpG sites in the **a** patG/matA genotype, **b** paternal allele of patG/matA genotype, **c** maternal allele of patG/matA genotype, **d** patA/matG genotype, **e** paternal allele of patA/matG genotype, and **f** maternal allele of patA/matG genotype. Error bars denote the SD. The numbers of samples are in brackets. A star (★) illustrates nominal *P* value < 0.05, Mann–Whitney

in the patA/matG genotype by EpiTYPER method (Additional file 2: Table S1 and S2), which could be explained by the amplification bias in PCR.

Allele-specific DNA methylation at *H19* ICR

We next assessed the allele-specific methylation levels of CTCF6 at *H19* ICR in heterozygous genotypes (patG/matA and patA/matG) in placenta by bisulfite sequencing. When comparing the methylation levels of paternal and maternal alleles separately in control and ART samples, we observed consistently decreased methylation level in paternal allele of patA/matG genotype at sites CpG_1-5, CpG_14, CpG_24, and CpG_25 in ART placentas (nominal *P* values 0.013, 0.013, 0.001, 0.029, 0.013, 0.003, 0.005, and 0.029, respectively, Mann-Whitney) (Fig. 3e, Additional file 2: Table S2). Conversely, increased methylation level was observed at site CpG_26 in the maternal allele of patA/matG genotype (nominal *P* value = 0.005, Mann Whitney) (Fig. 3f), and both increased and decreased methylation at sites CpG_24 and CpG_26, respectively, in the paternal allele of patG/matA genotype (nominal *P* value = 0.026 and 0.015, respectively, Mann-Whitney) (Fig. 3b). However, changes in methylation levels were not significant after multiple testing correction.

To see if similar decreased methylation level in patA/matG genotype can be seen also in the blood, we examined white blood cells (WBCs) of newborns' umbilical cord blood from the same ART-derived pregnancies. However, we did not observe similar decreased methylation level in the paternal allele of patA/matG genotype in ART-derived WBCs as we saw in placental tissue (Fig. 4, Additional file 2: Table S3). Conversely, a subtle but consistent increased methylation level in ART-derived WBCs was detected. The methylation level of CpG_4 site in the paternal allele of ART samples was clearly increased (*P* = 0.03, Mann-Whitney), but the difference is not significant after multiple testing correction.

Genotype-specific phenotypes of newborns

Finally, we assessed genotype-specific phenotypes of newborns by using international growth standards. Genotype-specific examination revealed differences in FRESH-derived newborns' birth weight and head circumference (*P* = 0.04 and *P* = 0.004, respectively, one-way ANOVA). FRESH-derived newborns with G/G genotype were heavier (*P* = 0.04, Bonferroni post hoc) and had larger head circumference (*P* = 0.002, Bonferroni post hoc) compared to newborns with A/A genotype (Fig. 5a, b). We did not observe significant differences in birth length. Genotype-specific differences were not compared in the FET-derived newborns since the sample size was too low in the heterozygous genotypes. We also saw that the placental weight and birth weight differed significantly between controls, FRESH-derived and FET-derived newborns in the A/A genotype (*P* = 0.024 and *P* = 0.006, one-way ANOVA) (Fig. 5a, c). Both the placentas and newborns of FET-derived pregnancies were heavier than FRESH-derived pregnancies (*P* = 0.02 and *P* = 0.004, respectively, Bonferroni post hoc). We did not see similar differences between the groups in the G/G genotype.

Discussion

Owing to the decreased birth weight and decreased methylation level at the *H19* ICR associated previously with IVF treatments, we focused on the imprinted *IGF2/H19* locus, which is crucial for normal placental and embryonic growth. In our previous study, a polymorphism rs10732516 at this locus associated with a genotype-specific trend in placental DNA methylation and head circumference of prenatally alcohol-exposed newborns [27]. Due to the growth-restricted phenotype in both prenatal alcohol exposure and IVF, we explored if these rather different environmental factors could associate with similar changes. We observed consistently decreased DNA methylation at the sixth binding site (CTCF6) of *H19* ICR in ART-derived placentas, which is consistent with previous ART study

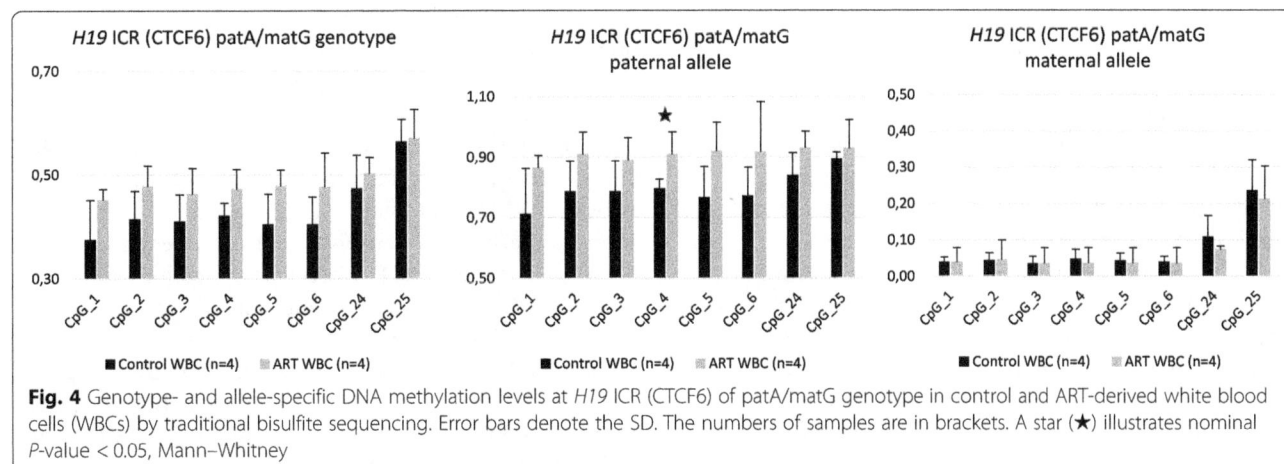

Fig. 4 Genotype- and allele-specific DNA methylation levels at *H19* ICR (CTCF6) of patA/matG genotype in control and ART-derived white blood cells (WBCs) by traditional bisulfite sequencing. Error bars denote the SD. The numbers of samples are in brackets. A star (★) illustrates nominal *P*-value < 0.05, Mann–Whitney

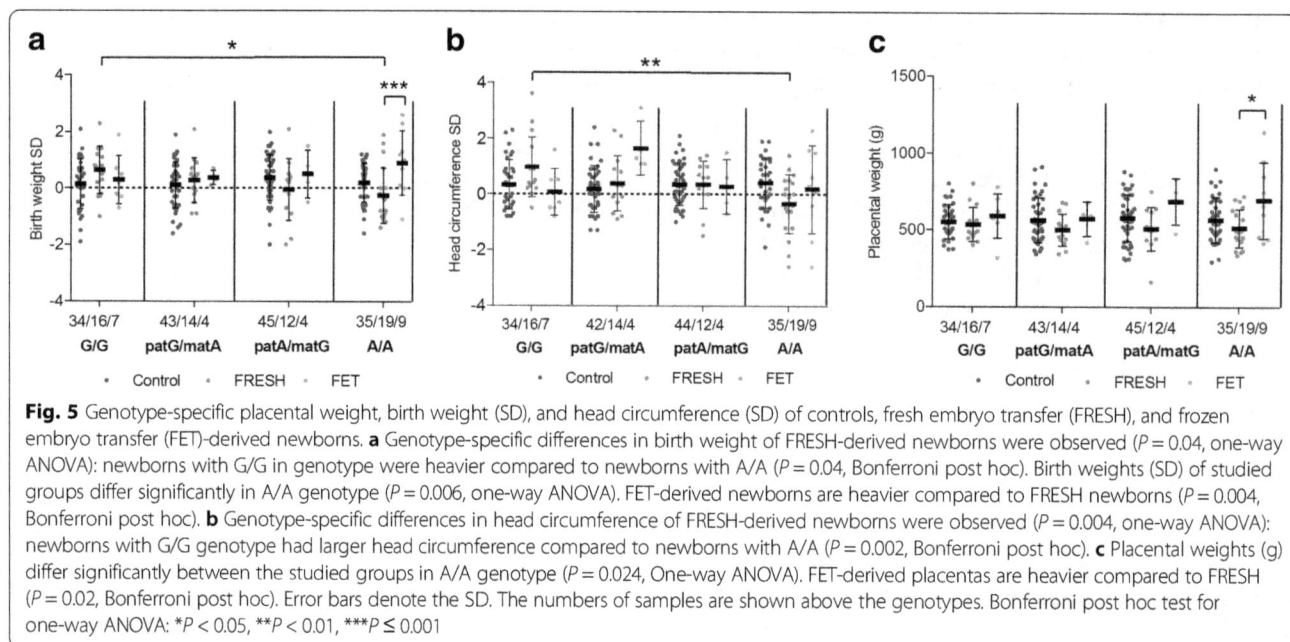

Fig. 5 Genotype-specific placental weight, birth weight (SD), and head circumference (SD) of controls, fresh embryo transfer (FRESH), and frozen embryo transfer (FET)-derived newborns. **a** Genotype-specific differences in birth weight of FRESH-derived newborns were observed ($P = 0.04$, one-way ANOVA): newborns with G/G in genotype were heavier compared to newborns with A/A ($P = 0.04$, Bonferroni post hoc). Birth weights (SD) of studied groups differ significantly in A/A genotype ($P = 0.006$, one-way ANOVA). FET-derived newborns are heavier compared to FRESH newborns ($P = 0.004$, Bonferroni post hoc). **b** Genotype-specific differences in head circumference of FRESH-derived newborns were observed ($P = 0.004$, one-way ANOVA): newborns with G/G genotype had larger head circumference compared to newborns with A/A ($P = 0.002$, Bonferroni post hoc). **c** Placental weights (g) differ significantly between the studied groups in A/A genotype ($P = 0.024$, One-way ANOVA). FET-derived placentas are heavier compared to FRESH ($P = 0.02$, Bonferroni post hoc). Error bars denote the SD. The numbers of samples are shown above the genotypes. Bonferroni post hoc test for one-way ANOVA: $*P < 0.05$, $**P < 0.01$, $***P \leq 0.001$

[15]. Interestingly, the decreased methylation level was detected only in the paternal allele in rs10732516 patA/matG genotype of two studied heterozygous genotypes, and alteration was even more profound than in the alcohol-exposed placentas in our previous study. This suggests that the effect of ART on DNA methylation in placenta is genotype-specific.

We did not observe similar changes in the methylation level of paternal allele in WBCs from cord blood of ART-derived newborns. This could be explained by the more advanced differentiation stage of the extraembryonic trophoblast cells compared to inner cell mass, the location of the cells in the blastocyst, or the better DNA methylation repairing and maintaining mechanisms of the embryonic cells. However, our result is consistent with the earlier study, where decreased methylation in this same region was detected only in mononuclear cells, not in WBCs [17]. This suggests that these genotype-specific changes in methylation have not occurred in blood cells in the early embryonic development or they are not fixed in all cell types.

We are aware of some limitations in this study. Traditional bisulfite sequencing is useful only for allele-specific examination of heterozygous genotypes, and thus, the methylation information about homozygous genotypes is lacking. Furthermore, we did not observe similar trend of decreased methylation by EpiTYPER, indicating that as a PCR-based method, it is not a convenient method to detect relatively small but consistent allele specific methylation changes in this specific imprinted region. Also, based on these results, it is not possible to see if decreased methylation at the *H19* ICR is caused by ART or infertility.

The number of FET samples was too low to explore the phenotypic effects on each genotype, but the genotype-specific variation in the birth weight and head circumference of FRESH-derived newborns suggest that the polymorphism could associate with the growth. Genotype-specific examination also revealed that in the rs10732516 A/A genotype, the placental weight and birth weight (SD) of controls, FRESH- and FET-derived newborns, differed from each other. Interestingly, we did not see the same in the G/G genotype. Both the placentas and newborns of FET-derived pregnancies were the heaviest in the A/A genotype. This is consistent with the increased head circumference of prenatally alcohol-exposed children [27] as well as the strongest growth phenotype of infantile hemangiomas [33], which both associate with this specific genotype.

Conclusion

Both genotype-specific methylation profiles and phenotypic findings suggest that rs10732516 polymorphism associates with the effects of ART in a parent-of-origin manner. The polymorphism locates on the binding sequence of CTCF protein, and allele A deletes a CpG binding site for a methyl group. Whether the A allele affects slightly the binding efficiency of CTCF protein and consequently makes A/A genotype particularly sensitive to environmental factors, it needs to be clarified in functional studies. More studies are also needed to find out if changes in this locus have occurred already in the very beginning of the embryonic development, in the period of epigenetic reprogramming, and the causality of the alterations: could the genotype-specific changes in DNA methylation affect the gene expression and thus the phenotype of developing embryo. Owing to the genotype-specific methylation changes at the *H19* ICR in ART-derived placentas and previous associations between ART and imprinting disorders, it would be interesting to find out if the prevalence of imprinting disorders associates with the rs10732516 G/A polymorphism.

Methods

Study design and sample collection

Couples applied to fertilization treatment in the Reproductive Medicine Unit of Helsinki University Central Hospital, Finland or Fertility Clinic of the Family Federation of Finland or Tartu University Hospital were recruited to this study. IVF or ICSI have been used in the treatments. The conception has been done using fresh embryo transfer (FRESH) or frozen embryo transfer (FET). Placental and cord blood samples from 47 Finnish cases (29 FRESH: 23 IVF/6 ICSI and 18 FET: 12 IVF/6 ICSI) are collected during years 2013–2017 and 39 Estonian cases (33 FRESH: 21 IVF/12 ICSI and 6 FET: 3 IVF/3 ICSI) 2016–2017. Spontaneously conceived 100 Finnish controls have been collected during years 2013–2015 in Helsinki University Central Hospital, Finland [27], and 57 Estonian controls in Tartu University Hospital. All the samples were Caucasian origin, from Finnish and Estonian newborns. Sample information and variation between Finnish and Estonian samples are shown in Table 1 and Additional file 1: Table S1.

The placental biopsies (1 cm³) and umbilical cord blood samples were collected immediately after delivery. The placental biopsies were collected from the fetal side of placenta within a radius of 2–3 cm from the umbilical cord, rinsed in cold 1× PBS and stored in RNAlater® (Thermo Fisher Scientific, Vilnius, Lithuania) at − 80 °C. White blood cells (WBCs) were extracted as soon as possible, at latest 16 h after birth (Additional file 3: Protocol S1).

Birth weight (g), birth length (cm), and head circumference (cm) were examined for both Finnish and Estonian newborns using international growth standards, the Fentom Preterm Growth Chart by PediTools (http://peditools.org/), in which the gestational age at birth and sex are considered when calculating the SD (*z*-score) of birth measures [31]. This chart has also been used previously for full-term deliveries [34, 35]. Measures deviating more than ± 2 SDs are commonly considered abnormal.

Methylation analysis

EpiTYPER

Placental genomic DNA was extracted by commercial QIAamp Fast DNA Tissue Kit (Finnish samples, Qiagen, Valencia, CA, USA) or PureLink Genomic DNA Kit (Estonian samples, Invitrogen, Life Technologies, USA). The extractions were done from one to four pieces (on average from three pieces) of placental tissue. The total DNA methylation levels of *H19* ICR (CTCF6), *H19*

DMR, and LINE-1 regions in placental samples were measured by MassARRAY EpiTYPER (SEQUENOM Inc.) based on matrix-assisted laser desorption/ionization time-of-flight (MALDI-TOF) mass spectrometry. First, DNA (1000 ng) was bisulfite converted (EZ-96 DNA Methylation™ kit, Zymo Research, Irvine, CA, USA) and PCR was performed in three independent 10 µl reactions using HotStar PCR kit (Qiagen, Valencia, CA, USA) according to manufacturer's instructions. Primers for the regions of interest were obtained from previous publications [36, 37] (Additional file 3: Table S2). The EpiTYPER measurements were done for pooled PCR reactions. Altogether, 60 controls and 62 ART-derived (48 FRESH: 33 IVF/15 ICSI and 14 FET: 8 IVF/6 ICSI) Finnish and Estonian placental samples were analyzed by EpiTYPER.

Bisulfite sequencing

To find out the allele-specific methylation profiles and to confirm the EpiTYPER results as well as genotypes, the CTCF6 at *H19* ICR of heterozygous ART-derived placental samples with patG/matA genotype (4 FRESH: 4 IVF, and 2 FET: 1 IVF/1 ICSI) and patA/matG genotype (7 FRESH: 4 IVF/3 ICSI, and 1 FET: IVF), and eight WBC samples with patA/matG genotype (4 controls and 4 ART-derived samples: 3 FRESH: 1 IVF/2 ICSI, and 1 FET: IVF) were subjected to bisulfite sequencing. All the samples were from Finnish newborns. The control placental samples had been published previously [27]. Due to heterozygosity and imprinting, the paternal and maternal alleles could be distinguished. Two separate bisulfite conversions were performed for 500 ng of genomic DNA (EZ DNA Methylation™ kit, Zymo Research, Irvine, CA, USA) and pooled afterwards. To avoid possible PCR bias, three independent 20 µl PCR reactions (HotStar PCR kit, Qiagen, Valencia, CA, USA) were performed per sample. Primers were obtained from previous publication and allowed to detect the polymorphism in units CpG_17,18,19,20 [38] (Additional file 2: Table S3). PCR reactions were gel isolated, and the three reactions of each sample were pooled and purified using NucleoSpin Gel and PCR Clean-up Kit (Macherey-Nagel, Düren, Germany). The purified PCR fragments were ligated into pGEM®-T Easy Vector (Promega, Madison, WI, USA) and cloned by standard protocol. The recombinant-DNA clones were purified using NucleoSpin® Plasmid EasyPure kit (Macherey-Nagel, Düren, Germany) according to manufacturer's instructions. Fifty to eighty clones of each individual were sequenced. The sequences were analyzed by BIQ Analyzer [39] excluding the clones with lower than 90% conversion rate from the dataset.

Genotype analysis

Placental samples were genotyped by Sanger sequencing. According to our sequencing analyses, the heterozygous samples were able to distinguish from each other due to uneven amplification and hence different signal levels of the alleles. The peak of rs10732516 A in sequence of patA/matG genotype was lower compared to patG/matA genotype. One 20 μl PCR reaction was performed for each sample using commercial HotStar PCR kit (Qiagen Valencia, CA, USA) with 100–300 ng of template DNA. Primers were designed by using NCBI/Primer Blast (Additional file 3: Table S2). PCR products were purified with SAP treatment (FastAP Thermosensitive Alkaline Phosphatase (1 U/μL), Thermo Scientific, Waltham, MA, USA) according to manufacturer's instructions. The genotypes of samples that were analyzed by EpiTYPER could be confirmed by detecting genotype-specific fragmentation and distinct methylation levels in unit CpG_10 of *H19* ICR. The methylation level in patG/matA was ∼ 0.80, in G/G ∼ 0.30, in patA/matG ∼ 0.02, and in A/A there was no value.

Statistical analysis

Statistical analyses were conducted using either SPSS software for Windows version 22.0 (NY, USA) or Graph-Pad Prism 7 software (GraphPad Software, Inc., La Jolla, CA, USA). All data are expressed as the mean with ±SD for a normal distribution of variables. Samples were divided into four groups according to the genotype and the chi-square test was used to compare the prevalence of the rs1072516 in the control and ART samples. The non-parametric Mann–Whitney test was used to compare the methylation level of CpG sites analyzed by bisulfite sequencing. Student's t test was used to compare CpG units analyzed by EpiTYPER. In the methylation analysis, the nominal P value was considered significant when < 0.05 and Bonferroni correction was used for multiple testing correction. Two-way ANOVA, followed by Bonferroni post hoc test when significant, was used to identify the differences among the study groups as well as to eliminate the interaction effect if significant differences between the Finnish and Estonian newborns were observed.

Additional files

Additional file 1: Table S1. Information of ART samples. (PDF 165 kb)

Additional file 2: Table S1. DNA methylation levels of *H19* ICR (CTCF6), *H19* DMR and LINE-1 in control and ART-derived placentas by EpiTYPER method. Methylation average values with SDs (±) of CpG units are presented. Gray boxes present significant methylation level difference at CpG sites in *H19* DMR between ART and control samples within A/A genotype (nominal p-value < 0.05, Student's t-test). Table S2. Total, rs10732516 genotype-specific (patG/matA and patA/matG) and allele-specific (paternal and maternal) DNA methylation levels at *H19* ICR (CTCF6) in control and ART-derived placentas by traditional bisulfite sequencing. Gray boxes present significant methylation level difference at CpG sites between control and ART samples within genotypes and alleles (nominal p-value < 0.05, Mann-Whitney). Total methylation levels:

total means of both genotypes and both alleles are included. Genotype-specific methylation levels: total means of both alleles are included. Allele-specific methylation levels: maternal and paternal alleles are presented separately. Table S3. rs10732516 patA/matG genotype- and allele-specific DNA methylation levels at *H19* ICR1 (CTCF6) in controls and ART-derived newborns' white blood cells (WBCs) in cord blood by traditional bisulfite sequencing. Genotype-specific methylation levels: total means of both alleles are included. Allele-specific methylation levels: maternal and paternal alleles are presented separately. (PDF 145 kb)

Additional file 3: Protocol S1. Extraction of total white blood cells (WBC) from EDTA-tube. Table S2. Primers (A) and PCR reactions (B). (PDF 306 kb)

Abbreviations

ART: Assisted reproductive technology; CTCF: Zinc-finger protein CCCTC-binding factor; CTCF6: The sixth binding site for CTCF; DMR: Differentially methylated region; FET: Frozen embryo transfer; FRESH: Fresh embryo transfer; ICR: Imprinting control region; ICSI: Intracytoplasmic sperm injection; IGF2: Insulin-like growth factor 2; IVF: In vitro fertilization; LINE-1: Long interspersed nuclear elements; WBC: White blood cell

Acknowledgements

We thank all participants in Finland and Estonia for their invaluable contributions to the study and research nurses Teija Karkkulainen and Riikka Hiltunen.

Funding

The study was funded by Faculty of Medicine, University of Helsinki, and Helsinki University Hospital, Estonian Ministry of Education and Research (IUT34-16), Enterprise Estonia (EU48695), Horizon 2020 innovation program (WIDENLIFE, 692065), European Union's FP7 Marie Curie Industry-Academia Partnerships and Pathways funding (IAPP, SARM, EU324509), and MSCA-RISE-2015 project MOMENDO (691058).

Authors' contributions

HM, HK, OT, SK, AT, TV, TT, VSA, AMS, AS, AT, and NKA collected the samples and the clinical data. HM and NKA designed the study and the statistical analysis of the data. HM, PA, and NKA performed laboratory experiments. HM, PA, and NKA wrote the manuscript. All authors have read, commented, and approved the final manuscript.

Competing interests

The authors declare that they have no competing interests.

Author details

[1]Department of Medical and Clinical Genetics, Medicum, University of Helsinki, Helsinki, Finland. [2]Department of Obstetrics and Gynecology, University of Helsinki and Helsinki University Hospital, Helsinki, Finland. [3]Department of Biomedicine, Institute of Biomedicine and Translational Medicine, University of Tartu, Tartu, Estonia. [4]Competence Centre on Health Technologies, Tartu, Estonia. [5]Department of Pathophysiology, Institute of Biomedicine and Translational Medicine, University of Tartu, Tartu, Estonia. [6]Department of Reproductive Biology, Estonian University of Life Sciences, Tartu, Estonia. [7]Department of Obstetrics and Gynaecology, Institute of Clinical Medicine, University of Tartu, Tartu, Estonia. [8]Department of

Paediatric ICU, Tartu University Hospital, Tartu, Estonia. [9]The Family Federation of Finland, Fertility Clinic, Helsinki, Finland.

References

1. Qin JB, Sheng XQ, Wu D, Gao SY, You YP, Yang TB, Wang H. Worldwide prevalence of adverse pregnancy outcomes among singleton pregnancies after in vitro fertilization/intracytoplasmic sperm injection: a systematic review and meta-analysis. Arch Gynecol Obstet. 2017;295:285–301.

2. Jackson RA, Gibson KA, Wu YW, Croughan MS. Perinatal outcomes in singletons following in vitro fertilization: a meta-analysis. Obstet Gynecol. 2004;103:551–63.

3. Pandey S, Shetty A, Hamilton M, Bhattacharya S, Maheshwari A. Obstetric and perinatal outcomes in singleton pregnancies resulting from IVF/ICSI: a systematic review and meta-analysis. Hum Reprod Update. 2012;18:485–503.

4. Malchau SS, Loft A, Henningsen AK, Nyboe Andersen A, Pinborg A. Perinatal outcomes in 6,338 singletons born after intrauterine insemination in Denmark, 2007 to 2012: the influence of ovarian stimulation. Fertil Steril. 2014;102:1110–6.

5. Maher ER, Brueton LA, Bowdin SC, Luharia A, Cooper W, Cole TR, Macdonald F, Sampson JR, Barratt CL, Reik W, et al. Beckwith-Wiedemann syndrome and assisted reproduction technology (ART). J Med Genet. 2003;40:62–4.

6. Lazaraviciute G, Kauser M, Bhattacharya S, Haggarty P, Bhattacharya S. A systematic review and meta-analysis of DNA methylation levels and imprinting disorders in children conceived by IVF/ICSI compared with children conceived spontaneously. Hum Reprod Update. 2014;20:840–52.

7. Pelkonen S, Koivunen R, Gissler M, Nuojua-Huttunen S, Suikkari AM, Hyden-Granskog C, Martikainen H, Tiitinen A, Hartikainen AL. Perinatal outcome of children born after frozen and fresh embryo transfer: the Finnish cohort study 1995–2006. Hum Reprod. 2010;25:914–23.

8. Wennerholm UB, Henningsen AK, Romundstad LB, Bergh C, Pinborg A, Skjaerven R, Forman J, Gissler M, Nygren KG, Tiitinen A. Perinatal outcomes of children born after frozen-thawed embryo transfer: a Nordic cohort study from the CoNARTaS group. Hum Reprod. 2013;28:2545–53.

9. Maheshwari A, Pandey S, Amalraj Raja E, Shetty A, Hamilton M, Bhattacharya S. Is frozen embryo transfer better for mothers and babies? Can cumulative meta-analysis provide a definitive answer? Hum Reprod Update. 2018;24:35–58.

10. Pinborg A, Loft A, Romundstad LB, Wennerholm UB, Söderström-Anttila V, Bergh C, Aittomäki K. Epigenetics and assisted reproductive technologies. Acta Obstet Gynecol Scand. 2016;95:10–5.

11. Sunkara SK, La Marca A, Seed PT, Khalaf Y. Increased risk of preterm birth and low birthweight with very high number of oocytes following IVF: an analysis of 65 868 singleton live birth outcomes. Hum Reprod. 2015;30:1473–80.

12. Kamath MS, Kirubakaran R, Mascarenhas M, Sunkara SK. Perinatal outcomes after stimulated versus natural cycle IVF: a systematic review and meta-analysis. Reprod BioMed Online. 2018;36:94–101.

13. Reik W, Dean W, Walter J. Epigenetic reprogramming in mammalian development. Science. 2010;293:1089–93.

14. Yin Y, Morgunova E, Jolma A, Kaasinen E, Sahu B, Khund-Sayeed S, Das PK, Kivioja T, Dave K, Zhong F, et al. Impact of cytosine methylation on DNA binding specificities of human transcription factors. Science. 2017;356:eaaj2239.

15. Nelissen EC, Dumoulin JC, Daunay A, Evers JL, Tost J, van Montfoort AP. Placentas from pregnancies conceived by IVF/ICSI have a reduced DNA methylation level at the H19 and MEST differentially methylated regions. Hum Reprod. 2013;28:1117–26.

16. Loke YJ, Galati JC, Saffery R, Craig JM. Association of in vitro fertilization with global and IGF2/H19 methylation variation in newborn twins. J Dev Orig Health Dis. 2015;6:115–24.

17. Castillo-Fernandez JE, Loke YJ, Bass-Stringer S, Gao F, Xia Y, Wu H, Lu H, Liu Y, Wang J, Spector TD, et al. DNA methylation changes at infertility genes in newborn twins conceived by in vitro fertilisation. Genome Med. 2017;9:1–15.

18. Mann MR, Lee SS, Doherty AS, Verona RI, Nolen LD, Schultz RM, Bartolomei MS. Selective loss of imprinting in the placenta following preimplantation development in culture. Development. 2004;131:3727–35.

19. Market-Velker BA, Fernandes AD, Mann MR. Side-by-side comparison of five commercial media systems in a mouse model: suboptimal in vitro culture interferes with imprint maintenance. Biol Reprod. 2010;83:938–50.

20. DeChiara TM, Robertson EJ, Efstratiadis A. Parental imprinting of the mouse insulin-like growth factor II gene. Cell. 1991;64:849–59.

21. Gabory A, Ripoche MA, Le Digarcher A, Watrin F, Ziyyat A, Forne T, Jammes H, Ainscough JF, Surani MA, Journot L, et al. H19 acts as a trans regulator of the imprinted gene network controlling growth in mice. Development. 2009;136:3413–21.

22. Phillips JE, Corces VG. CTCF: master weaver of the genome. Cell. 2009; 137:1194–211.

23. Hark AT, Schoenherr CJ, Katz DJ, Ingram RS, Levorse JM, Tilghman SM. CTCF mediates methylation-sensitive enhancer-blocking activity at the H19/Igf2 locus. Nature. 2000;405:486–9.

24. Soejima H, Higashimoto K. Epigenetic and genetic alterations of the imprinting disorder Beckwith–Wiedemann syndrome and related disorders. J Hum Genet. 2013;58:402–9.

25. Gicquel C, Rossignol S, Cabrol S, Houang M, Steunou V, Barbu V, et al. Epimutation of the telomeric imprinting center region on chromosome 11p15 in Silver-Russell syndrome. Nat Genet. 2005;37:1003–7.

26. Turan N, Katari S, Gerson LF, Chalian R, Foster MW, Gaughan JP, Coutifaris C, Sapienza C. Inter- and intra-individual variation in allele-specific DNA methylation and gene expression in children conceived using assisted reproductive technology. PLoS Genet. 2010;6:e1001033.

27. Marjonen H, Kahila H, Kaminen-Ahola N. rs10732516 polymorphism at the IGF2/H19 locus associates with a genotype-specific trend in placental DNA methylation and head circumference of prenatally alcohol-exposed newborns. Hum Reprod Open. 2017;(3):hox014.

28. Adkins RM, Somes G, Morrison JC, Hill JB, Watson EM, Magann EF, Krushkal J. Association of birth weight with polymorphisms in the IGF2, H19, and IGF2R genes. Pediatr Res. 2010;68:429–34.

29. Petry CJ, Seear RV, Wingate DL, Acerini CL, Ong KK, Hughes IA, Dunger DB. Maternally transmitted foetal H19 variants and associations with birth weight. Hum Genet. 2011;130:663–70.

30. Ghosh J, Coutifaris C, Sapienza C, Mainigi M. Global DNA methylation levels are altered by modifiable clinical manipulations in assisted reproductive technologies. Clin Epigenetics. 2017;6:14.

31. Fenton TR, Nasser R, Eliasziw M, Kim JH, Bilan D, Sauve R. Validating the weight gain of preterm infants between the reference growth curve of the fetus and the term infant. BMC Pediatr. 2013;13:92.

32. Auton A, Brooks LD, Durbin RM, Garrison EP, Kang HM, Korbel JO, Marchini JL, McCarthy S, McVean GA, et al. Genomes Project C: a global reference for human genetic variation. Nature. 2015;526:68–74.

33. Schultz B, Yao X, Deng Y, Waner M, Spock C, Tom L, Persing J, Narayan D. A common polymorphism within the IGF2 imprinting control region is associated with parent of origin specific effects in infantile hemangiomas. PLoS One. 2015;10:e0113168.

34. Gilbert-Diamond D, Emond JA, Baker ER, Korrick SA, Karagas MR. Relation between in utero arsenic exposure and birth outcomes in a cohort of mothers and their newborns from New Hampshire. Environ Health Perspect. 2016;124:1299–307.

35. Vanker A, Barnett W, Workman L, Nduru PM, Sly PD, Gie RP, Zar HJ. Early-life exposure to indoor air pollution or tobacco smoke and lower respiratory tract illness and wheezing in African infants: a longitudinal birth cohort study. Lancet Planet Health. 2017;1:e328–36.

36. Ollikainen M, Smith KR, Joo EJ, Ng HK, Andronikos R, Novakovic B, Abdul Aziz NK, Carlin JB, Morley R, Saffery R, et al. DNA methylation analysis of multiple tissues from newborn twins reveals both genetic and intrauterine components to variation in the human neonatal epigenome. Hum Mol Genet. 2010;19:4176–88.

37. Wang L, Wang F, Guan J, Le J, Wu L, Zou J, Zhao H, Pei L, Zheng X, Zhang T. Relation between hypomethylation of long interspersed nucleotide elements and risk of neural tube defects. Am J Clin Nutr. 2010;91:1359–67.

38. Coolen MW, Statham AL, Gardiner-Garden M, Clark SJ. Genomic profiling of CpG methylation and allelic specificity using quantitative high-throughput mass spectrometry: critical evaluation and improvements. Nucleic Acids Res. 2007;35:e119.

39. Bock C, Reither S, Mikeska T, Paulsen M, Walter J, Lengauer T. BiQ analyzer: visualization and quality control for DNA methylation data from bisulphite sequencing. Bioinformatics. 2005;21:4067–8.

15

PLD3 epigenetic changes in the hippocampus of Alzheimer's disease

Idoia Blanco-Luquin[1], Miren Altuna[1,2], Javier Sánchez-Ruiz de Gordoa[1,2], Amaya Urdánoz-Casado[1], Miren Roldán[1], María Cámara[2], Victoria Zelaya[3], María Elena Erro[1,2], Carmen Echavarri[1,4] and Maite Mendioroz[1,2]*

Abstract

Background: Whole-exome sequencing has revealed a rare missense variant in *PLD3* gene (rs145999145) to be associated with late onset Alzheimer's disease (AD). Nevertheless, the association remains controversial and little is known about the role of *PLD3* in AD. Interestingly, *PLD3* encodes a phospholipase that may be involved in amyloid precursor protein (APP) processing. Our aim was to gain insight into the epigenetic mechanisms regulating *PLD3* gene expression in the human hippocampus affected by AD.

Results: We assessed *PLD3* mRNA expression by qPCR and protein levels by Western blot in frozen hippocampal samples from a cohort of neuropathologically confirmed pure AD cases and controls. Next, we profiled DNA methylation at cytosine-phosphate-guanine dinucleotide (CpG) site resolution by pyrosequencing and further validated results by bisulfite cloning sequencing in two promoter regions of the *PLD3* gene. A 1.67-fold decrease in *PLD3* mRNA levels (*p* value < 0.001) was observed in the hippocampus of AD cases compared to controls, and a slight decrease was also found by Western blot at protein level. Moreover, *PLD3* mRNA levels inversely correlated with the average area of β-amyloid burden (tau-b = − 0,331; *p* value < 0.01) in the hippocampus. A differentially methylated region was identified within the alternative promoter of *PLD3* gene showing higher DNA methylation levels in the AD hippocampus compared to controls (21.7 ± 4.7% vs. 18.3 ± 4.8%; *p* value < 0.05).

Conclusions: *PLD3* gene is downregulated in the human hippocampus in AD cases compared to controls. Altered epigenetic mechanisms, such as differential DNA methylation within an alternative promoter of *PLD3* gene, may be involved in the pathological processes of AD. Moreover, *PLD3* mRNA expression inversely correlates with hippocampal β-amyloid burden, which adds evidence to the hypothesis that PLD3 protein may contribute to AD development by modifying APP processing.

Keywords: PLD3, Alzheimer's disease, Epigenetics, DNA methylation, Gene and protein expression, Hippocampus, APP, Lysosome

Background

Alzheimer's disease (AD) is a genetically complex process where ε4 allele of the *APOE* gene (APOE4) is by far the best-established genetic susceptibility risk factor. In addition, genome-wide association studies have revealed a considerable number of small-effect common variants in genes related to AD [1–3]. However, those variants do not explain the full heritability of this disease. More recently, novel sequencing technologies are enabling the identification of other rare genetic variants that could potentially contribute to the development of sporadic AD. Notable recent discoveries in this area include rare disease variants in *TREM2, UNC5C, AKAP9, TM2D3, ADAM10,* and *PLD3* genes [2, 4, 5].

PLD3 (phospholipase D family, member 3) (*OMIM* * 615698) gene is located at chromosome 19q13.2 and encodes a lysosomal protein that belongs to the phospholipase D (PLD) superfamily, which catalyzes the hydrolysis of membrane phospholipids. However, PLD3 catalytic function has not yet been demonstrated [6, 7]. *PLD3* gene is highly expressed in the brain of healthy

* Correspondence: maitemendilab@gmail.com
[1]Neuroepigenetics Laboratory-Navarrabiomed, Complejo Hospitalario de Navarra, Universidad Pública de Navarra (UPNA), IdiSNA (Navarra Institute for Health Research), C/ Irunlarrea, 3, 31008 Pamplona, Navarra, Spain
[2]Department of Neurology, Complejo Hospitalario de Navarra- IdiSNA (Navarra Institute for Health Research), C/ Irunlarrea, 3, 31008 Pamplona, Navarra, Spain
Full list of author information is available at the end of the article

controls, particularly in several brain regions vulnerable to AD pathology, such as frontal, temporal, and occipital cortices and hippocampus, but reduced in neurons from AD brains [3, 8]. Nevertheless, little is known on the regulation, the function, and the involvement of *PLD3* in AD pathogenesis.

Interestingly, controversial association exists about this gene conferring increased risk for the development of AD. Cruchaga et al. performed whole-exome sequencing on AD patients and identified a rare missense variant (rs145999145) in exon 7 of the *PLD3* gene which resulted in a val232-to-met (V232M) substitution [8]. Their results revealed that carriers of the *PLD3* coding variant had a twofold increased risk for late onset AD. Moreover, they showed that PLD3 influences amyloid precursor protein (APP) processing, acting as a negative regulator, since PLD3 overexpression in cultured neuroblastoma cells correlated with lower intracellular APP, extracellular Aβ42, and Aβ40 levels and that PLD3 protein could be co-immunoprecipitated with APP. In that regard, Satoh et al. showed an accumulation of PLD3 on neuritic plaques in AD brains and suggested a key role for PLD3 in the pathological processes of AD [9].

Other authors confirmed that *PLD3* gene variant V232M was associated with AD risk and significantly lower cognitive function [10] providing a systematic view of the involvement of *PLD3* in AD at genetic, mRNA, and protein level expression. However, additional studies were not able to define an essential role of *PLD3* rare variants in AD [11], neither to support an important contribution of *PLD3* rare variants in the etiology of AD, given the high variability of the frequency of *PLD3* Val232Met variant across populations [12]. Indeed, follow-up studies have questioned the role of *PLD3* rare variants in AD, obtaining negative replication data [13–15] and suggesting a more complex role of *PLD3* in the etiology of the disease.

Keeping in mind the results mentioned above, we wanted to gain insight into the epigenetic mechanisms regulating *PLD3* expression in order to add evidence to the potential contribution of *PLD3* to AD. Further knowledge on these mechanisms may provide opportunities for new AD therapeutic strategies. Here, we profiled *PLD3* gene expression and methylation in the human hippocampus, one of the most vulnerable brain regions to AD. To that end, we selected a cohort of neuropathologically defined "pure" AD cases and controls to measure hippocampal *PLD3* expression by quantitative PCR and Western blot. Next, we explored the correlation of *PLD3* expression with AD neuropathological changes. Finally, DNA methylation levels at two distinct promoter regions of the *PLD3* gene were assessed by pyrosequencing and bisulfite cloning sequencing.

Methods

Human hippocampal samples and neuropathological examination

Brain hippocampal samples from 30 AD patients and 12 controls were provided by Navarrabiomed Brain Bank. After death, half brain specimens from donors were cryopreserved at − 80 °C. Neuropathological examination was completed following the usual recommendations [16] and according to the updated National Institute on Aging-Alzheimer's Association guidelines [17]. Assessment of β-amyloid deposition was carried out by immunohistochemical staining of paraffin-embedded sections (3–5 μm thick) with a mouse monoclonal (S6F/3D) anti β-amyloid antibody (Leica Biosystems Newcastle Ltd., Newcastle upon Tyne, UK). Evaluation of neurofibrillary pathology was performed with a mouse monoclonal antibody anti-human PHF-TAU, clone AT-8, (Tau AT8) (Innogenetics, Gent, Belgium), which identifies hyperphosphorylated tau (p-tau) [18]. The reaction product was visualized using an automated slide immunostainer (Leica Bond Max) with Bond Polymer Refine Detection (Leica Biosystems, Newcastle Ltd.).

To avoid spurious findings related to multiprotein deposits, "pure" AD cases with deposits of only p-tau and β-amyloid were eligible for the study and controls were free of any pathological protein aggregate. This approach maximizes chances of finding true associations with AD, even though reducing the final sample size. A summary of characteristics of subjects included in this study is shown in Additional file 1: Table S1. AD subjects were older than controls (82.3 ± 11.3 versus 50.7 ± 21.5; p value < 0.01), and no differences were found regarding gender (p value $= 0.087$). The postmortem interval (PMI) were not significantly different between groups (8.2 ± 4.4 h in the control group versus 7.9 ± 7.1 h in the AD group; p value $= 0.91$).

PLD3 mRNA expression analysis by RT-qPCR

Total RNA was isolated from hippocampal homogenates using RNeasy Lipid Tissue Mini kit (QIAGEN, Redwood City, CA, USA), following the manufacturer's instructions. Genomic DNA was removed with recombinant DNase (TURBO DNA-free™ Kit, Ambion, Inc., Austin, TX, USA). RNA integrity was checked by 1.25% agarose gel electrophoresis under denaturing conditions. Concentration and purity of RNA were both evaluated with NanoDrop spectrophotometer. Only RNA samples showing a minimum quality index (260 nm/280 nm absorbance ratios between 1.8 and 2.2 and 260 nm/230 nm absorbance ratios higher than 1.8) were included in the study. Complementary DNA (cDNA) was reverse transcribed from 1500 ng total RNA with SuperScript® III First-Strand Synthesis Reverse Transcriptase (Invitrogen, Carlsbad, CA, USA) after priming with oligo-d (T) and random primers. RT-qPCR reactions were performed in triplicate with Power SYBR Green PCR Master Mix (Invitrogen, Carlsbad, CA, USA) in a QuantStudio 12K Flex Real-Time PCR System (Applied Biosystems, Foster City, CA, USA) and repeated twice within independent cDNA sets. Sequences of primer pair were designed using Real Time PCR tool (IDT, Coralville, IA, USA) and are listed in Additional file 1: Table S2. Relative expression level of *PLD3* mRNA in a particular sample was calculated as previously described [19] and *ACTB* gene was used as the reference gene to normalize expression values.

PLD3 protein expression analysis by Western blot

Human hippocampus tissue from patients and control samples was lysed with 100 µL lysis buffer containing urea, thiourea, and DTT. After centrifugation at 35.000 rpm for 1 h at 15 °C, extracted proteins were quantified following the Bradford-Protein Assay (Bio-Rad, Hercules, CA, USA) by using a spectrophotometer.

Next, 5 µg of protein per sample were resolved in 4–20% Criterion TGX stain-free gels (Bio-Rad) and electrophoretically transferred onto nitrocellulose membranes using a Trans-blot Turbo transfer system (25 V, 7 min) (Bio-Rad). Equal loading of the gel was assessed by stain-free digitalization and by Ponceau staining. Membranes were probed with rabbit anti-human PLD3 primary antibody (Sigma-Aldrich; 1:250) in 5% nonfat milk and incubated with peroxidase-conjugated anti-rabbit secondary antibody (Cell Signaling; 1:2000). Immunoblots were then visualized by exposure to an enhanced chemiluminescence Clarity Western ECL Substrate (Bio-Rad) using a ChemidocMP Imaging System (Bio-Rad). Expression levels of PLD3 were standardized by the corresponding band intensity of GAPDH (Calbiochem; 1:10000).

Quantitative assessment of β-amyloid and p-tau deposits in hippocampal samples

In order to quantitatively assess the β-amyloid and p-tau burden for further statistical analysis, we applied a method to quantify protein deposits, as described in detail elsewhere [20]. In brief, hippocampal sections were examined after performing immunostaining with anti β-amyloid and anti p-tau antibodies. Focal deposit of β-amyloid, including neuritic, immature, and compact plaques [21], was analyzed with the ImageJ software. Moreover, β-amyloid plaque count, referred to as amyloid plaque score (APS), was measured. Finally, p-tau deposit was also analyzed with ImageJ software in order to obtain an average quantitative measure of the global p-tau deposit for each section.

PLD3 methylation measurement by pyrosequencing

Genomic DNA was isolated from frozen hippocampal tissue by phenol-chloroform method [22]. Next, 500 ng of genomic DNA was bisulfite converted using the EpiTect Bisulfite Kit (Qiagen, Redwood City, CA, USA) according to the manufacturer's protocol. Primers to amplify and sequence two promoter regions of *PLD3* were designed with PyroMark Assay Design version 2.0.1.15 (Qiagen) (Additional file 1: Table S2), and PCR reactions were carried out on a VeritiTM Thermal Cycler (Applied Biosystems, Foster City, CA, USA). Next, 20 µl of biotinylated PCR product was immobilized using streptavidin-coated sepharose beads (GE Healthcare Life Sciences, Piscataway, NJ, USA) and 0.3 µM sequencing primer was annealed to purified DNA strands. Pyrosequencing was performed using the PyroMark Gold Q96 reagents (Qiagen) on a PyroMark™ Q96 ID System (Qiagen). For each particular cytosine-phosphate-guanine dinucleotide (CpG), methylation levels were expressed as percentage of methylated cytosines over the sum of total cytosines. Unmethylated and methylated DNA samples (EpiTect PCR Control DNA Set, Qiagen) were used as controls for the pyrosequencing reaction.

PLD3 methylation validations by bisulfite cloning sequencing

Bisulfite-converted genomic DNA was used to validate pyrosequencing results. Primer pair sequences were designed by MethPrimer [23] and are listed in Additional file 1: Table S2. PCR products were cloned using the TopoTA Cloning System (Invitrogen, Carlsbad, CA, USA), and a minimum of 10–12 independent clones were sequenced for each examined subject and region. Methylation graphs were obtained with QUMA software [24].

Statistical data analysis

Statistical analysis was performed with SPSS 21.0 (IBM, Inc., USA). Before performing differential analysis, we checked that all continuous variables showed a normal distribution, as per one-sample Kolgomorov-Smirnov test and the normal quantil-quantil (QQ) plots. Data represents the mean ± standard deviation (SD). Significance level was set at p value < 0.05. Statistical significance for *PLD3* mRNA levels and pyrosequecing intergroup differences was assessed by T test. One-way analysis of variance (ANOVA) followed by Games-Howell *post hoc* analysis was used to analyze differences in the expression levels of *PLD3* mRNA between Braak and Braak stage groups. A logistic regression model (ENTER method) was fit to assess the independent association of *PLD3* mRNA levels with AD status, using gender and age as covariates. Kendall's tau-b correlation coefficient was used to determine correlation between AD-related pathology and *PLD3* mRNA expression levels. Difference between two bisulfite cloning sequencing groups was evaluated with Mann-Whitney U test. GraphPad Prism version 6.00 for Windows (GraphPad Software, La Jolla, CA, USA) was used to draw graphs except for methylation figures that were obtained by QUMA software.

Results

PLD3 expression is downregulated in Alzheimer's disease hippocampus

As the first step in this study, we measured PLD3 mRNA expression levels by real-time quantitative PCR (RT-qPCR) in the hippocampus of AD patients compared to controls. Five samples did not pass the RNA quality threshold (see the "Methods" section) and so were not included in the experiments. Eventually, 26 AD cases were compared to 11 controls. As shown in Fig. 1a, PLD3 mRNA levels were significantly decreased by 1.67-fold in the hippocampus of AD cases compared to controls [p value < 0.001]. Next, a disease-staging analysis was performed to investigate changes of PLD3 mRNA levels depending on the AD severity measured by Braak & Braak staging [21] . We found that PLD3 mRNA levels were significantly reduced across Braak & Braak stages [p value < 0.005; Fig. 1b]. Games-Howell post hoc analysis revealed that PLD3 mRNA expression was significantly different between control and Braak stages III–IV [p value < 0.05] and between control and Braak stages V–VI [p value < 0.05] (Fig. 1).

Then, to identify adjusted estimates of the association of PLD3 mRNA levels with AD status (control = 0; AD = 1), a logistic regression model was designed. Age and gender were included into the model to adjust for potentially confounding variables. As shown in Table 1, PLD3 mRNA expression levels remained as an independent predictor of AD status after adjusting for age and gender [p value < 0.05] (Table 1).

In order to examine whether the decrease in PLD3 mRNA levels in the AD hippocampus extended to the protein level, a Western blot analysis was performed. Protein extracts from frozen hippocampal samples that were included in the qPCR experiment were obtained, and a polyclonal antibody against a recombinant protein epitope signature tag (PrEST) of PLD3 was used. GAPDH protein detection was used as housekeeping. In line with the PLD3 mRNA expression results, we observed that PLD3 protein expression tends to be decreased in samples from hippocampus of AD patients as compared to controls (Fig. 1c).

Correlation of PLD3 mRNA expression levels with p-tau and amyloid deposits

Next, we aimed to correlate PLD3 mRNA levels with AD-related neuropathological changes in hippocampal

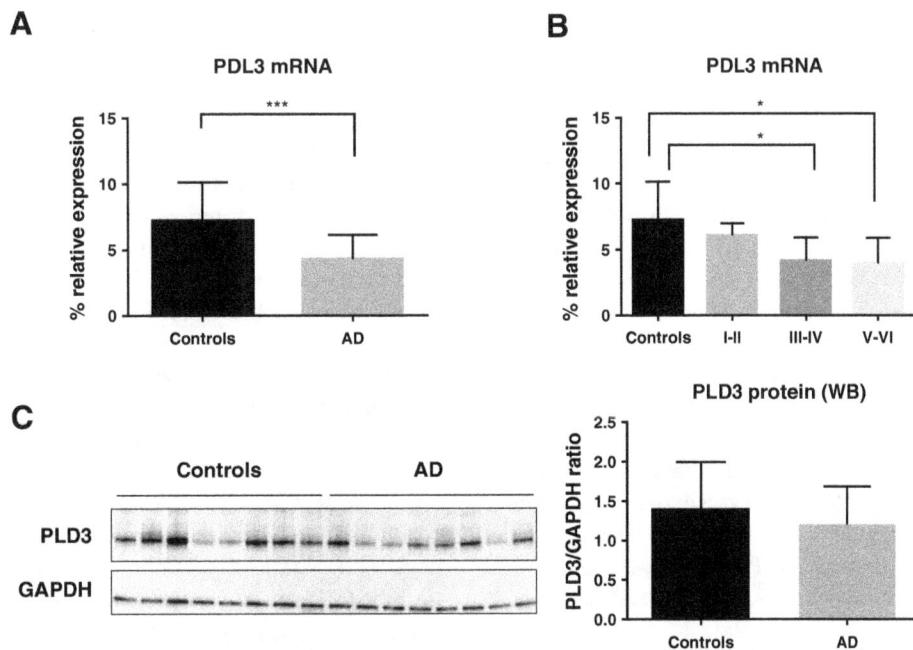

Fig. 1 PLD3 expression is decreased in human hippocampus in Alzheimer's disease (AD). **a** The graph shows a significant 1.67-fold decrease in PLD3 mRNA levels in AD hippocampal samples compared to control hippocampal samples. **b** PLD3 mRNA expression decreased across AD stages, as shown when PLD3 mRNA expression levels are sorted by Braak and Braak stages. Bars represent percentage of PLD3 mRNA expression relative to ACTB housekeeping gene expression. Vertical lines represent the standard error of the mean. *p value < 0.05; ***p value < 0.001. **c** Western blot analysis of PLD3 shows a mild protein expression decrease in AD. Human hippocampus samples from controls or AD patients were loaded as labeled on top of lanes. GADPH expression is shown as reference control. The bar chart represents the quantitative measurement of the PLD3 protein relative to GAPDH protein expression

Table 1 Adjusted logistic regression model to predict AD status

Variable	B	Wald	p value	OR
PLD3 mRNA levels	− 0.544	4.212	0.040*	0.581
Gender (female)	0.613	0.286	0.593	1.847
Age < 65 years old	2.774	5.981	0.014*	16.02
Constant	− 1.494	0.254	0.614	0.224

Alzheimer status (control = 0; AD = 1) was considered as the dependent variable and PLD3 mRNA expression levels, gender, and age were included as covariates
B regression coefficient, OR odds ratio
*p value < 0.05

sections. In brief, β-amyloid and hyperphosphorylated tau (p-tau) burden were measured and averaged for each subject by a semi-automated quantitative method by using the ImageJ software (see the "Methods" section). The amyloid plaque score (APS) was also recorded. As β-amyloid and p-tau data were not normally distributed, the non-parametric Kendall's tau-b correlation coefficient was used. We found that the average area of β-amyloid burden in the hippocampus was inversely correlated with PLD3 mRNA levels [tau-b = − 0,331; p value < 0.01], and accordingly, an inverse association was found between APS and PLD3 mRNA levels [tau-b = − 0,319; p value < 0.01]. Regarding p-tau deposits, a statistically significant correlation was found for an inverse correlation [tau-b = − 0,306; p value < 0.01].

DNA methylation in PLD3 is increased in hippocampus of AD cases compared to controls

DNA methylation levels of regulatory regions in the genome modulate the expression of related or nearby genes. Thus, we tested whether DNA methylation levels in PLD3 gene were also altered in the AD hippocampus. PLD3 gene is located in the long arm of chromosome 19 (19q13.2) and has two distinct CpG island-containing promoter regions as shown by the UCSC Genome Browser website [25] (Fig. 2a). The principal promoter, which is placed at the 5′ end of the gene, contains a 553 bp CpG island (chr19:40854181-40854733; GRCh37/hg19) while an alternative promoter overlapping exon 2 contains a smaller 207 bp CpG island (chr19:40871 618-40871824; GRCh37/hg19). Pyrosequencing primers were designed to amplify and sequence specific CpGs within both promoters regions (P_prom CpG1 and CpG2 for the principal promoter and A_prom CpG1 and CpG2 for the alternative promoter) (Fig. 2a).

We observed that the principal promoter of PLD3 was mostly demethylated [mean ± SD, 1.8 ± 2.9%], as it corresponds to the constitutive promoter of an actively expressed gene. Average DNA methylation levels were slightly higher in AD cases compared to controls only for P_prom CpG2 [2.6 ± 3.13% vs. 0 ± 0%; p value < 0.001]. The alternative promoter showed intermediate levels of

DNA methylation [20.5 ± 4.91%]. A_prom CpG1 showed a statistical trend to be highly methylated in AD cases compared to controls [23 ± 7.8% vs. 18.4 ± 6.2%; p value = 0.09] and a statistically significant difference in DNA methylation levels was observed for A_prom CpG2 in AD cases compared to controls [21.5 ± 5.8% vs. 15.3 ± 3.8%; p value < 0.01].

Next, we sought to replicate pyrosequencing results by extending the initial cohort with additional AD and control hippocampal samples for which DNA was available. These samples came from Navarrabiomed Brain Bank and were used to increase the sample size for the methylation experiments. Eventually, 36 AD patients and 18 controls were analyzed by pyrosequencing. In the principal promoter, average DNA methylation levels showed a trend to be higher in AD cases compared to controls at P_prom CpG2 [2.3 ± 2% vs. 1 ± 2.4% p value = 0.094]. In the alternative promoter, no differences were found for A_prom CpG1 between AD cases and controls [p value > 0.05]. However, we observed a statistically significant difference in DNA methylation levels for A_prom CpG2 between AD cases and controls [21.7 ± 4.7% vs. 18.3 ± 4.8%; p value < 0.05], pointing to a differentially methylated region located within the alternative promoter of PLD3 in the AD hippocampus (Fig. 2b). In order to test whether A_prom CpG2 methylation was an independent predictor of AD status (control = 0; AD = 1), a binary logistic regression model was performed. After adjusting for age and gender, A_prom CpG2 methylation levels remain as an independent predictor of AD (Additional file 1: Table S3).

We validated the pyrosequencing results and extended the methylation local mapping by using bisulfite cloning sequencing in two independent amplicons overlapping both PLD3 promoter regions. DNA methylation percentage was measured at CpG site resolution and further averaged across all the CpG sites for each amplicon. In line with the previous pyrosequencing results, we found that average DNA methylation levels of the amplicon at PLD3 principal promoter were very low and showed no differences between AD patients and controls (Fig. 2c). On the contrary, average DNA methylation levels of the amplicon at PLD3 alternative promoter were increased in AD patients compared to controls [19.1 ± 7.8% vs. 6 ± 4%; p value < 0.05] (Fig. 2c).

Since DNA methylation is one of the major mechanisms to regulate gene expression, we analyzed the correlation between PLD3 mRNA expression and PLD3 DNA methylation in our sample set. No significant correlation was found between expression and DNA methylation measured by pyrosequencing [A_prom CpG1 r = − 0.264, p value = 0.114; A_prom CpG2 r = − 0.275, p value = 0.110]. However, a significant inverse correlation was observed between expression and DNA methylation

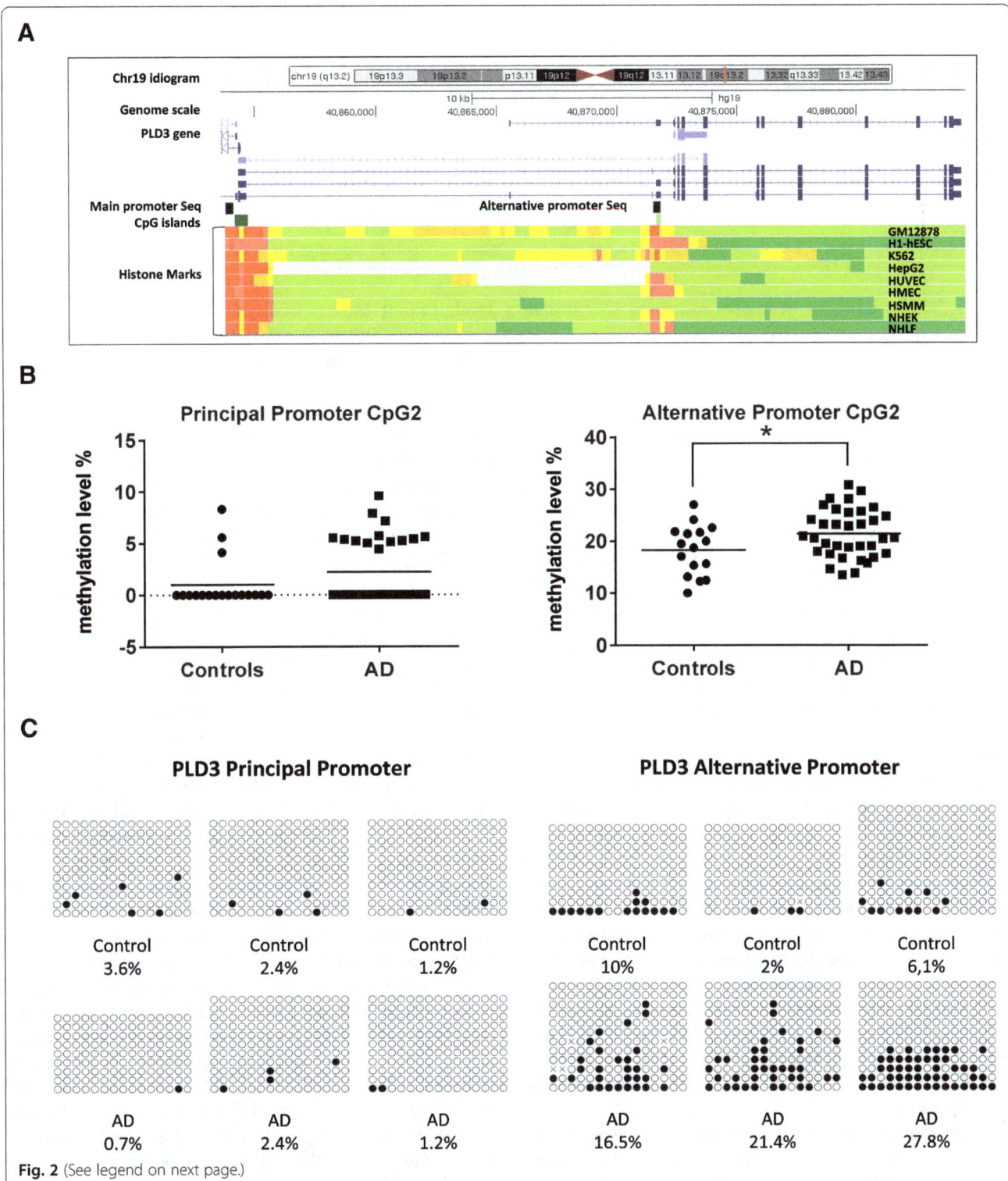

Fig. 2 (See legend on next page.)

(See figure on previous page.)
Fig. 2 *PLD3* DNA methylation levels in human hippocampal samples. **a** The graph shows genomic position of the amplicons (black boxes) validated by bisulfite cloning sequencing which contain the cytosines assayed by pyrosequencing (CpG1 and CpG2) within the promoter regions (principal and alternative) of the *PLD3* gene. *PLD3* is located on the long arm of chromosome 19 (chr19:40,854,332-40,884,390 -GRchr19/hg19 coordinates). CpG islands are represented by isolated green boxes. At the bottom of the graph, predicted functional elements are shown for each of nine human cell lines explored by chromatine imunoprecipitation (ChIP) combined with massively parallel DNA sequencing. Boxes represent promoter regions (red), enhancers (yellow), transcriptional transition and elongation (dark green), and weak transcribed regions (light green). The track was obtained from the *Chromatin State Segmentation by HMM from ENCODE/Broad* track shown at the UCSC Genome Browser. **b** Dot-plot charts representing methylation levels for principal and alternative promoter of *PLD3* by pyrosequencing. Horizontal lines represent median methylation values for each group.*p value < 0.05. **c** Representative examples of bisulfite cloning sequencing validation for the two independent amplicons (principal and alternative promoter regions). Black and white circles denote methylated and unmethylated cytosines respectively. Each column symbolizes a unique CpG site in the examined amplicon, and each line represents an individual DNA clone

in the *PLD3* alternative promoter measured by bisulfite cloning sequencing [$r = -0.683$; p value < 0.05].

Discussion

We report *PLD3* gene to be downregulated at both transcript and protein level in the human hippocampus affected by AD. In addition, we show that the decrease in *PLD3* mRNA expression inversely correlates with β-amyloid burden in the hippocampus. An important finding of this study is that an alternative promoter of *PLD3* gene is differentially methylated in the hippocampus of AD patients compared to controls suggesting that epigenetic disturbances in *PLD3* may occur in the pathological process of AD.

Our results showing a reduction in *PLD3* expression in the AD hippocampus add to previous evidence supporting the idea that *PLD3* gene is downregulated in brain areas affected by AD processes [8, 9]. Cruchaga et al. [8] used data from genome-wide transcriptomics in laser-captured neurons from 33 AD cases and 16 controls (GEO dataset GSE5281) [26] to reveal that *PLD3* gene expression was significantly lower in AD cases compared to controls. In addition, Satoh et al. found a marginal reduction in *PLD3* mRNA levels in the frontal cortex of 7 AD cases compared to 14 non-AD subjects, including other neurodegenerative disorders such as amyotrophic lateral sclerosis and Parkinson disease [9]. In agreement with the previous results, we observed a statistically significant decrease in *PLD3* mRNA expression in the hippocampus, a vulnerable region to AD pathology, and also show that *PLD3* is reduced across Braak & Braak stages indicating that *PLD3* is somehow related to the progressive neurodegenerative processes of AD.

A number of different mechanisms could explain the decrease in *PLD3* gene expression in the AD hippocampus, including the progressive loss of neuronal populations, changes in cellular composition with increasing astrogliosis in late stages of AD, or cell-type-specific decrease in *PLD3* gene expression. A limitation of the present study is that it has been designed on a tissue-specific basis, and therefore, changes in gene expression at cell-specific level, including neuron-specific

level, cannot be assessed. In fact, the ratio of cellular components in the human hippocampus may change across different stages of AD. In this case, and if the expression of *PLD3* were cell type specific, the gene expression changes observed globally in the hippocampus could be attributed to the loss of a given cell population and not reflect actual *PLD3* expression changes. However, the fact of having found epigenetic modifications in the same sample set would support the existence of a true alteration in the regulation of *PLD3* gene expression. To know whether the difference in *PLD3* gene expression is driven by a decreased expression in neurons or by changes in the ratio of cell populations in the brain of AD patients, other technologies, such as the emerging single-cell techniques, should be used.

The reduction in *PLD3* expression is in line with the classical β-amyloid cascade hypothesis of AD, since PLD3 protein seems to act as a negative regulator of APP processing [8]. It has been shown that knockdown of *PLD3* expression in cells results in higher levels of extracellular Aβ42 and Aβ40 levels, and conversely, overexpression of *PLD3* is associated with reduced extracellular Aβ42 and Aβ40 levels [8]. Furthermore, PLD3 protein is accumulated in neuritic plaques in human AD brains [9]. Indeed, it has been demonstrated that PLD3 protein can be co-immunoprecipitated with APP in cultured cells [8]. Even more, *PLD3* protein has been recently characterized as a novel endosome-to-Golgi retrieval gene that regulates the endosomal protein sorting, whose loss of function results in increased processing of APP [27]. Accordingly, we have found an inverse correlation between *PLD3* mRNA expression levels and the burden of hippocampal β-amyloid assessed by two measurements, averaged deposit of β-amyloid and amyloid plaque score (APS). All these data supports the notion that PLD3 protein could display a protective effect against AD pathology through its role in APP trafficking, as other authors have previously suggested [27].

Interestingly, PLD3 protein is co-expressed with other lysosomal proteins [9], including progranulin, which regulates lysosomal functioning and is also accumulated in neuritic plaques [9, 28]. Moreover, PLD3 protein is required to preserve the structure of lysosomes in vivo and, therefore, impairment of the endosomal-lysosomal systems has been proposed as an alternative mechanism by which PLD3 could contribute to the development of AD [29]. Most interestingly, another genetic variant in *PLD3*, p.Leu308Pro, was recently found to cause autosomal dominant spinocerebellar ataxia [30], a neurodegenerative condition where lysosomal disturbances are thought to be crucial [31, 32]. As an additional alternative explanation, PLD3 might also influence AD pathological processes by altering adult neurogenesis since *PLD3* gene expression seems to be turned on at late stages of neurogenesis [33].

Finally, we describe an altered pattern of DNA methylation within an alternative promoter of the *PLD3* gene in the human hippocampus affected by AD. To our knowledge, no previous reports on altered DNA methylation in *PLD3* gene have been published and very little is known about regulation of *PLD3* gene expression. The alternative promoter of *PLD3* is placed ~17,500 bp downstream the principal promoter overlapping exon 2. It contains a small CpG island and is conserved across several cell types (Fig. 2a). In our study, it was found to be differentially methylated showing higher DNA methylation levels in AD patients than in controls. Since DNA methylation of CpG islands is one of the major epigenetic mechanisms that influence gene expression, our results indicate that altered DNA methylation at this particular regulatory region might contribute to downregulate *PLD3* expression in AD.

In this regard, we also show a significant correlation between *PLD3* mRNA expression and DNA methylation in our dataset when measured by bisulfite cloning sequencing, while the pyrosequencing results did not show correlation with expression. It is intriguing why the significant correlation is found only for the bisulfite cloning sequencing results. First of all, although not significant, an inverse correlation appears in the statistical analysis for the pyrosequencing results. However, it is only a statistical trend. One possible explanation would be that DNA methylation levels measured by bisulfite cloning sequencing average the methylation levels of an extended genomic region (15 CpGs), and therefore, this result may be more close to the real functional effect of methylation on gene expression than the result of individual CpGs.

Epigenetic disturbances are increasingly being described for a number of genes related to AD, including genes harboring rare variants that contribute to developing AD [34–40]. In this sense, our work provides new knowledge about the epigenetic alterations involved in gene transcription regulation in key brain regions for the development of AD. Additionally, our results support the involvement of *PLD3* in the pathology of AD.

Conclusions

To sum up, this study confirms that *PLD3* gene is downregulated in the hippocampus of AD patients. Moreover, *PLD3* expression inversely correlates with β-amyloid burden, which adds evidence to the hypothesis that PLD3 protein may contribute to AD development through modifying APP processing. Having identified a differentially methylated region in an alternative promoter of *PLD3*, our study suggests that epigenetic disturbances in *PLD3* gene may be involved in the pathological processes of AD.

Abbreviations

AD: Alzheimer's disease; ANOVA: Analysis of variance; APOE4: ε4 allele of the *APOE* gene; APP: Amyloid precursor protein; APS: Amyloid plaque score; cDNA: Complementary DNA; CpG: Cytosine-phosphate-guanine dinucleotide; GEO: Gene Expression Omnibus; *PLD3*: Phospholipase D family, member 3; PrEST: Protein epitope signature tag; p-tau: Hyperphosphorylated tau; QQ: Quantil-quantil plots; RT-qPCR: Real-time quantitative PCR; Tau AT8: Mouse monoclonal antibody anti-human PHF-TAU, clone AT-8; UCSC: University of California, Santa Cruz; V232M: Val232-to-met substitution

Acknowledgements

We want to kindly thank Teresa Tuñón M.D., Ph.D (Department of Pathology, Complejo Hospitalario de Navarra, technical support), Federico García-Bragado M.D., Ph.D (Department of Pathology, Complejo Hospitalario de Navarra, technical support), Iván Méndez M.D., (Department of Internal Medicine, Hospital García Orcoyen, technical editing), and Isabel Gil M.D. (Navarrabiomed BrainBank, technical support) for their help. Finally, we are very grateful to the patients and relatives that generously donor the brain tissue to the Navarrabiomed Brain Bank.

Funding

This work was supported by the Spanish Government through grants from the Institute of Health Carlos III (FIS PI13/02730 & PI17/02218), jointly funded by the European Regional Development Fund (ERDF), European Union, "A way of shaping Europe"; the Regional Basque Government through a grant from The Basque Foundation for Health Innovation and Research (BIOEF) (BIO12/ALZ/007), a grant from Fundación Caja-Navarra; and the Trans-Pyrenean Biomedical Research Network (REFBIO). In addition, AUC received a grant "Doctorados industriales 2018-2020" founded by the Government of Navarra and MM received a grant "Programa de intensificación" funded by Fundación Bancaria "la Caixa" and Fundación Caja-Navarra.

Authors' contributions

IBL contributed to the acquisition of the data, analysis and interpretation of the data, and drafting/revising of the manuscript for content. MR contributed to the acquisition of the data and drafting/revising of the manuscript for content. JSR contributed to the analysis and interpretation of the data (p-tau and amyloid deposits), sorting of the patients into different stages, and acquisition of the image data. AU contributed to the analysis of the data, figure drawing, and drafting/revising of the manuscript for content. MR contributed to the running of the experiments and was involved in the interpretation of the data. MC contributed to the acquisition of the data and drafting/revising of the manuscript for content. MVZ participated in the revision of the subject diagnosis and classification of patients and contributed to the drafting/revising the manuscript for content. MEE contributed to the analysis of the results and drafting/revising of the manuscript for content. CE contributed to the acquisition of the data, diagnosis of the subjects, and drafting/revising of the manuscript for content. MM contributed to the drafting/revising of the manuscript for content, study concept and design, analysis and interpretation of the data, acquisition of the data, statistical analysis, study supervision, and obtaining the funding. All authors read and approved the final manuscript.

Author details

[1]Neuroepigenetics Laboratory-Navarrabiomed, Complejo Hospitalario de Navarra, Universidad Pública de Navarra (UPNA), IdiSNA (Navarra Institute for Health Research), C/ Irunlarrea, 3, 31008 Pamplona, Navarra, Spain. [2]Department of Neurology, Complejo Hospitalario de Navarra- IdiSNA (Navarra Institute for Health Research), C/ Irunlarrea, 3, 31008 Pamplona, Navarra, Spain. [3]Department of Pathology, Complejo Hospitalario de Navarra-IdiSNA (Navarra Institute for Health Research), 31008 Pamplona, Navarra, Spain. [4]Hospital Psicogeriátrico Josefina Arregui, 31800 Alsasua, Navarra, Spain.

References

1. Bettens K, Sleegers K, Van Broeckhoven C. Genetic insights in Alzheimer's disease. Lancet Neurol. 2013;12(1):92–104. https://doi.org/10.1016/S1474-4422(12)70259-4.
2. Zhu JB, Tan CC, Tan L, Yu JT. State of play in Alzheimer's disease genetics. J Alzheimers Dis. 2017;58(3):631–59. https://doi.org/10.3233/JAD-170062.
3. Humphries C, Kohli MA. Rare variants and transcriptomics in Alzheimer disease. Curr Genet Med Rep. 2014;2(2):75–84. https://doi.org/10.1007/s40142-014-0035-9.
4. Giri M, Zhang M, Lü Y. Genes associated with Alzheimer's disease: an overview and current status. Clin Interv Aging. 2016;11:665–81. https://doi.org/10.2147/CIA.S105769.
5. Guimas Almeida C, Sadat Mirfakhar F, Perdigão C, Burrinha T. Impact of late-onset Alzheimer's genetic risk factors on beta-amyloid endocytic production. Cell Mol Life Sci. 2018; https://doi.org/10.1007/s00018-018-2825-9.
6. Munck A, Böhm C, Seibel NM, Hashemol Hosseini Z, Hampe W. Hu-K4 is a ubiquitously expressed type 2 transmembrane protein associated with the endoplasmic reticulum. FEBS J. 2005;272(7):1718–26. https://doi.org/10.1111/j.1742-4658.2005.04601.x.
7. Gonzalez AC, Schweizer M, Jagdmann S, Bernreuther C, Reinheckel T, Saftig P, et al. Unconventional trafficking of mammalian phospholipase D3 to lysosomes. Cell Rep. 2018;22(4):1040–53. https://doi.org/10.1016/j.celrep.2017.12.100.
8. Cruchaga C, Karch CM, Jin SC, Benitez BA, Cai Y, Guerreiro R, et al. Rare coding variants in the phospholipase D3 gene confer risk for Alzheimer's disease. Nature. 2014;505(7484):550–4. https://doi.org/10.1038/nature12825.
9. Satoh J, Kino Y, Yamamoto Y, Kawana N, Ishida T, Saito Y, et al. PLD3 is accumulated on neuritic plaques in Alzheimer's disease brains. Alzheimers Res Ther. 2014;6(9):70. https://doi.org/10.1186/s13195-014-0070-5.
10. Engelman CD, Darst BF, Bilgel M, Vasiljevic E, Koscik RL, Jedynak BM, et al. The effect of rare variants in TREM2 and PLD3 on longitudinal cognitive function in the Wisconsin Registry for Alzheimer's Prevention. Neurobiol Aging. 2018;66:177.e1–5. https://doi.org/10.1016/j.neurobiolaging.2017.12.025.
11. Zhang DF, Fan Y, Wang D, Bi R, Zhang C, Fang Y, et al. PLD3 in Alzheimer's disease: a modest effect as revealed by updated association and expression analyses. Mol Neurobiol. 2016;53(6):4034–45. https://doi.org/10.1007/s12035-015-9353-5.
12. van der Lee SJ, Holstege H, Wong TH, Jakobsdottir J, Bis JC, Chouraki V, et al. PLD3 variants in population studies. Nature. 2015;520(7545):E2–3. https://doi.org/10.1038/nature14038.
13. Cacace R, Van den Bossche T, Engelborghs S, Geerts N, Laureys A, Dillen L, et al. Rare variants in PLD3 do not affect risk for early-onset Alzheimer disease in a European Consortium Cohort. Hum Mutat. 2015;36(12):1226–35. https://doi.org/10.1002/humu.22908.
14. Lambert JC, Grenier-Boley B, Bellenguez C, Pasquier F, Campion D, Dartigues JF, et al. PLD3 and sporadic Alzheimer's disease risk. Nature. 2015;520(7545):E1. https://doi.org/10.1038/nature14036.
15. Heilmann S, Drichel D, Clarimon J, Fernández V, Lacour A, Wagner H, et al. PLD3 in non-familial Alzheimer's disease. Nature. 2015;520(7545):E3–5. https://doi.org/10.1038/nature14039.
16. Bell JE, Alafuzoff I, Al-Sarraj S, Arzberger T, Bogdanovic N, Budka H, et al. Management of a twenty-first century brain bank: experience in the BrainNet Europe consortium. Acta Neuropathol. 2008;115(5):497–507. https://doi.org/10.1007/s00401-008-0360-8.
17. Montine TJ, Phelps CH, Beach TG, Bigio EH, Cairns NJ, Dickson DW, et al. National Institute on Aging-Alzheimer's Association guidelines for the neuropathologic assessment of Alzheimer's disease: a practical approach. Acta Neuropathol. 2012;123(1):1–11. https://doi.org/10.1007/s00401-011-0910-3.
18. Braak H, Alafuzoff I, Arzberger T, Kretzschmar H, Del Tredici K. Staging of Alzheimer disease-associated neurofibrillary pathology using paraffin sections and immunocytochemistry. Acta Neuropathol. 2006;112(4):389–404. https://doi.org/10.1007/s00401-006-0127-z.
19. Livak KJ, Schmittgen TD. Analysis of relative gene expression data using real-time quantitative PCR and the 2(-Delta Delta C(T)) Method. Methods (San Diego, Calif). 2001;25(4):402–8. https://doi.org/10.1006/meth.2001.1262.
20. Celarain N, Sánchez-Ruiz de Gordoa J, Zelaya MV, Roldán M, Larumbe R, Pulido L, et al. TREM2 upregulation correlates with 5-hydroxymethycytosine enrichment in Alzheimer's disease hippocampus. Clin Epigenetics. 2016;8:37. https://doi.org/10.1186/s13148-016-0202-9.
21. Braak H, Braak E. Neuropathological stageing of Alzheimer-related changes. Acta Neuropathol. 1991;82(4):239–59.
22. Miller SA, Dykes DD, Polesky HF. A simple salting out procedure for extracting DNA from human nucleated cells. Nucleic Acids Res. 1988;16(3):1215.
23. Li LC, Dahiya R. MethPrimer: designing primers for methylation PCRs. Bioinformatics. 2002;18(11):1427–31.
24. Kumaki Y, Oda M, Okano M. QUMA: quantification tool for methylation analysis. Nucleic Acids Res. 2008;36(Web Server issue):W170–5. https://doi.org/10.1093/nar/gkn294.
25. Kent WJ, Sugnet CW, Furey TS, Roskin KM, Pringle TH, Zahler AM, et al. The human genome browser at UCSC. Genome research. 2002;12(6):996–1006. https://doi.org/10.1101/gr.229102. Article published online before print in May 2002
26. Liang WS, Reiman EM, Valla J, Dunckley T, Beach TG, Grover A, et al. Alzheimer's disease is associated with reduced expression of energy metabolism genes in posterior cingulate neurons. Proc Natl Acad Sci U S A. 2008;105(11):4441–6. https://doi.org/10.1073/pnas.0709259105.
27. Mukadam AS, Breusegem SY, Seaman MNJ. Analysis of novel endosome-to-Golgi retrieval genes reveals a role for PLD3 in regulating endosomal protein sorting and amyloid precursor protein processing. Cell Mol Life Sci. 2018; https://doi.org/10.1007/s00018-018-2752-9.
28. Tanaka Y, Suzuki G, Matsuwaki T, Hosokawa M, Serrano G, Beach TG, et al. Progranulin regulates lysosomal function and biogenesis through acidification of lysosomes. Hum Mol Genet. 2017;26(5):969–88. https://doi.org/10.1093/hmg/ddx011.
29. Fazzari P, Horre K, Arranz AM, Frigerio CS, Saito T, Saido TC, et al. PLD3 gene and processing of APP. Nature. 2017;541(7638):E1–2. https://doi.org/10.1038/nature21030.
30. Nibbeling EAR, Duarri A, Verschuuren-Bemelmans CC, Fokkens MR, Karjalainen JM, Smeets CJLM, et al. Exome sequencing and network analysis identifies shared mechanisms underlying spinocerebellar ataxia. Brain. 2017;140(11):2860–78. https://doi.org/10.1093/brain/awx251.
31. Unno T, Wakamori M, Koike M, Uchiyama Y, Ishikawa K, Kubota H, et al. Development of Purkinje cell degeneration in a knockin mouse model

reveals lysosomal involvement in the pathogenesis of SCA6. Proc Natl Acad Sci U S A. 2012;109(43):17693–8. https://doi.org/10.1073/pnas.1212786109.

32. Alves S, Cormier-Dequaire F, Marinello M, Marais T, Muriel MP, Beaumatin F, et al. The autophagy/lysosome pathway is impaired in SCA7 patients and SCA7 knock-in mice. Acta Neuropathol. 2014;128(5):705–22. https://doi.org/10.1007/s00401-014-1289-8.

33. Pedersen KM, Finsen B, Celis JE, Jensen NA. Expression of a novel murine phospholipase D homolog coincides with late neuronal development in the forebrain. J Biol Chem. 1998;273(47):31494–504.

34. Bakulski KM, Dolinoy DC, Sartor MA, Paulson HL, Konen JR, Lieberman AP, et al. Genome-wide DNA methylation differences between late-onset Alzheimer's disease and cognitively normal controls in human frontal cortex. J Alzheimers Dis. 2012;29(3):571–88. https://doi.org/10.3233/jad-2012-111223.

35. Sanchez-Mut JV, Aso E, Heyn H, Matsuda T, Bock C, Ferrer I, et al. Promoter hypermethylation of the phosphatase DUSP22 mediates PKA-dependent TAU phosphorylation and CREB activation in Alzheimer's disease. Hippocampus. 2014;24(4):363–8. https://doi.org/10.1002/hipo.22245.

36. Lunnon K, Smith R, Hannon E, De Jager PL, Srivastava G, Volta M, et al. Methylomic profiling implicates cortical deregulation of ANK1 in Alzheimer's disease. Nat Neurosci. 2014;17(9):1164–70. https://doi.org/10.1038/nn.3782.

37. De Jager PL, Srivastava G, Lunnon K, Burgess J, Schalkwyk LC, Yu L, et al. Alzheimer's disease: early alterations in brain DNA methylation at ANK1, BIN1, RHBDF2 and other loci. Nat Neurosci. 2014;17(9):1156–63. https://doi.org/10.1038/nn.3786.

38. Yu L, Chibnik LB, Srivastava GP, Pochet N, Yang J, Xu J, et al. Association of Brain DNA methylation in SORL1, ABCA7, HLA-DRB5, SLC24A4, and BIN1 with pathological diagnosis of Alzheimer disease. JAMA Neurol. 2015;72(1): 15–24. https://doi.org/10.1001/jamaneurol.2014.3049.

39. Watson CT, Roussos P, Garg P, Ho DJ, Azam N, Katsel PL, et al. Genome-wide DNA methylation profiling in the superior temporal gyrus reveals epigenetic signatures associated with Alzheimer's disease. Genome Med. 2016;8(1):5. https://doi.org/10.1186/s13073-015-0258-8.

40. Celarain N, Sanchez-Ruiz de Gordoa J, Zelaya MV, Roldan M, Larumbe R, Pulido L, et al. TREM2 upregulation correlates with 5-hydroxymethycytosine enrichment in Alzheimer's disease hippocampus. Clinical Epigenetics. 2016; 8:37. https://doi.org/10.1186/s13148-016-0202-9.

16

Type 2 diabetes and cardiometabolic risk may be associated with increase in DNA methylation of *FKBP5*

Robin Ortiz[1], Joshua J. Joseph[2], Richard Lee[3], Gary S. Wand[4] and Sherita Hill Golden[4*] ⓘ

Abstract

Background: Subclinical hypercortisolism and hypothalamic-pituitary-adrenal (HPA) axis dysfunction are associated with type 2 diabetes (T2DM), cardiovascular disease, and metabolic dysfunction. Intronic methylation of *FKBP5* has been implicated as a potential indicator of chronic cortisol exposure. Our overall objective in this study was to determine the association of chronic cortisol exposure, measured via percent methylation of *FKBP5* at intron 2, with percent glycosylated hemoglobin (HbA1c), low-density lipoprotein cholesterol (LDL-cholesterol), waist circumference (WC), and body mass index (BMI), in a clinic-based sample of 43 individuals with T2DM.

Results: Greater percent methylation of the *FKBP5* intron 2 at one CpG-dinucleotide region was significantly associated with higher HbA1c ($\beta = 0.535$, $p = 0.003$) and LDL cholesterol ($\beta = 0.344$, $p = 0.037$) and a second CpG-dinucleotide region was significantly associated with higher BMI and WC ($\beta = 0.516$, $p = 0.001$; $\beta = 0.403$, $p = 0.006$, respectively).

Conclusions: *FKBP5* methylation may be a marker of higher metabolic risk in T2DM, possibly secondary to higher exposure to cortisol. Further work should aim to assess the longitudinal association of *FKBP5* with cardiovascular disease and glycemic outcomes in T2DM as a first step in understanding potential preventive and treatment-related interventions targeting the HPA axis.

Keywords: FKBP5, Methylation, Epigenetics, Cortisol, Diabetes, Cardiovascular disease, Obesity, Body mass index (BMI), Waist circumference, Hemoglobin A1c

Background

Subclinical hypercortisolism and hypothalamic-pituitary-adrenal (HPA) axis dysfunction are associated with type 2 diabetes (T2DM), cardiovascular disease, and metabolic dysfunction [1–3]. While recent research has shown alterations of the cortisol diurnal profile in those with T2DM, further research in this area has been hindered by lack of a chronic total cortisol (glucocorticoid) exposure measure. Recently, epigenetic modification of HPA axis-targeted genes has been identified as a potential measure of chronic exposure to cortisol and HPA axis dysfunction [4, 5]. Understanding the role of HPA dysfunction, assessed via epigenetic modifications, in metabolic disorders, T2DM, and cardiovascular disease,

may lead to a unifying pathophysiology, thus setting the stage for preventive and therapeutic interventions targeting the HPA axis. It has been proposed that identifying a target, such as a specific modulator or receptor, could allow for restoration of HPA axis function to a homeostatic physiological state thereby reversing subclinical hypercortisolism and its associated comorbidities including metabolic syndrome, T2DM, and cardiovascular disease [6].

The FK506-binding protein 51 kDa (*FKBP5*) gene is a modulator, or co-chaperone, of the glucocorticoid receptor by limiting translocation of the receptor complex to the nucleus [7]. An observation that changes in *FKBP5* methylation at intron 2, specifically, were associated with shaping the human brain and function was one of the first demonstrations of the epigenetic interaction between genetics and environment [8]. *FKBP5* has been linked to metabolic dysfunction including regulation of body weight after bariatric surgery and insulin resistance

---
* Correspondence: Sahill@jhmi.edu
[4]Division of Endocrinology, Diabetes and Metabolism, Department of Medicine, Johns Hopkins University School of Medicine, 1830 E. Monument Street Suite 333, Baltimore, MD 21287, USA
Full list of author information is available at the end of the article

in non-diabetic individuals [9, 10]. Epigenetic modification via loss of intronic methylation of *FKBP5* has been associated with Cushing's syndrome and can serve as an indicator of chronic exposure to cortisol [11]. Cushing's can often manifest with cardiovascular and metabolic dysfunction including truncal obesity, hypertension, and glucose intolerance. *FKBP5* methylation has also been associated with neuropsychiatric disease [8, 12]. However, *FKBP5* methylation has not been studied in individuals with T2DM, or in the context of specific measures of metabolic and cardiovascular disease. Given its importance in the function of the HPA axis via regulation of the glucocorticoid receptor, if *FKBP5* is shown to be associated with metabolic syndrome, T2DM, and cardiovascular disease, it may serve as a promising target for interventions aimed at restoring HPA axis function.

Our overall objective in this study was to determine the association of chronic cortisol exposure, measured via percent methylation of *FKBP5* at, specifically, intron 2, as was studied by Klengel, et al. [8], with markers of metabolic and cardiovascular disease in those with T2DM. Specifically, the association of percent methylation of *FKBP5* with percent glycosylated hemoglobin (HbA1c), low-density lipoprotein cholesterol (LDL cholesterol), body mass index (BMI), and waist circumference (WC), which is a surrogate for central obesity and an independent risk factor for cardiovascular disease [13]. We further explored the association between methylation of *FKBP5* and (1) cardiovascular disease risk modifier, exercise, and (2) the presence of cardiovascular disease, assessed by the need for coronary artery disease intervention.

Methods

Aims

The aim of this study was to primarily assess methylation of *FKBP5* at intron 2 with markers of metabolic and cardiovascular disease in those with T2DM including HbA1c, LDL cholesterol, BMI, and WC. A secondary aim was to assess the potential relationship between *FKBP5* and exercise as well as a history of cardiovascular procedures in the study cohort.

Study participants

MinD, a study assessing the crude prevalence of minor depressive disorder (MinD) in a clinic-based population of 128 consented adults with T2DM, participant data was used for this analysis. Because the primary aim of the MinD study focused on data assessing minor depression prevalence and comorbidity with associated cardiovascular and metabolic measures in subjects with T2DM, control subjects without diabetes were not included in the original design. Further, participants taking antipsychotic medication or glucocorticoids were excluded as both medications may be associated with major mood disorders. The detailed

methods of study design were previously described elsewhere and are described here briefly [14]. Individuals with physician-confirmed T2DM who were 18 years of age or older were recruited between 2011 and 2013 from the Diabetes Center clinics at Johns Hopkins Hospital during routine visits. Patients who were willing to participate in the study provided written informed consent. This study was approved by the Johns Hopkins University School of Medicine Institutional Review Board.

Exposures and outcomes samples

Baseline information was obtained during clinic visits using standardized questionnaires including demographics, race, level of education, and annual income. Calibrated devices were used by certified technicians and nurses to measure participants' weight, WC (average of two measurements around the umbilicus), and height. BMI was calculated as weight (kilograms)/height^2 (m^2). Resting seated blood pressure (BP) was measured twice at 5-min intervals using an appropriately sized cuff with standard Hawksley random-zero instruments, and measurements were averaged for analysis. Hypertension was defined as systolic BP of 140 mmHg or greater, diastolic BP of 90 mmHg or greater, or use of antihypertensive therapy. HbA1c and lipid panels (including low-density lipoprotein, triglycerides, and high-density lipoprotein) were also collected and analyzed by Johns Hopkins Clinical Core Laboratory with LDL cholesterol calculated from total cholesterol.

A secondary aim of the MinD data collection was to assess the relationship of *FKBP5* with measures of cardiometabolic risk in diabetes. Therefore, a subset of patients consented to provide blood samples to be used for future research purposes. Only subjects who did not consent to blood collection of DNA for research purposes were excluded. DNA was extracted from the blood and stored at − 20 °C, until epigenetic analyses were conducted.

Bisulfite pyrosequencing for DNA methylation (DNAm) quantification

Two sets of bisulfite polymerase chain reaction (PCR) primers were designed to target each of two regions in the second intron of the human *FKBP5* gene. The two regions flanked a glucocorticoid response element (GRE) [15] and contained consecutive cytosine-guanine dinucleotides (CpGs) implicated in previous studies [8, 11]. The coordinates of the nine CpGs on chromosome 6 are Chr6: 35,606,441–35,606,662 (CpG1-4) and Chr6: 35,609,542–35,609,666 (CpG5-9), according to the UCSC Genome Browser build GRCh37.hg19 assembly [16]. Two rounds of a nested PCR amplification were performed. In the first PCR, 3.5 μL bisulfate converted DNA was used. In the second PCR, 2 μL template from the PCR was used. One of the nested bisulfite primers was biotinylated and HPLC-purified, allowing it to bind to sepharose beads and become single-stranded, in preparation for bisulfite pyrosequencing. The single-stranded amplicons were annealed to pyrosequencing primers and subjected to primer extension and nucleotide incorporation using the PyroMark Q96 MD pyrosequencer (Qiagen). The pyrosequencer QCpG program determined percent DNA methylation (DNAm) at all of the CpG dinucleotides downstream of the annealed primer at > 90% precision.

Statistical analysis

Subject demographics were analyzed using descriptive statistics. Outliers in methylation assays were identified if the value was greater than three standard deviations away from the mean suggesting sub- or supra-physiologic levels and likely erroneous. Multivariable linear regression was performed to examine the association of percent DNAm of *FKBP5* (dependent variable) with HbA1c, LDL cholesterol, BMI, and WC (independent variables). Age, sex, and race were included as covariates in all regression analyses, based on previous cortisol analyses [1, 17]. Beta regression coefficients with a p value < 0.05 were considered statistically significant. Given this was established as a hypothesis-generating study, no adjustments were made for multiple comparisons as such tests were considered too conservative for correlated hypotheses as we propose here. For all independent variables with significant beta regression coefficients, basic correlation R values were used to assess effect size using Cohen's effect size such that $r = 0.1$ was considered of small effect size, $r = 0.3$ was considered of medium effect size, and $r = 0.5$ was considered of large effect size [18]. Based on preliminary results, a secondary analysis was completed including a multivariate regression with the number of cardiovascular procedures as a dependent variable and another with the number of days of physical activity greater than 30 min as an independent variable. All statistical analyses were performed using IBM SPSS Statistics Version 23.

Results

A total of 65 subjects had given consent for blood samples for epigenetic analysis. After excluding individuals with missing data on HbA1c ($n = 5$), LDL cholesterol ($n = 11$), BMI ($n = 1$), and WC ($n = 11$), 43 participants were included in the analysis (Additional file 1: Figure S1). The participants were 48.8% female, 60.5% non-Hispanic black with a mean age of 61.9 years (SD ±9.0 years); other demographics are described in Table 1. Given that all participants had diabetes and were on anti-hypertensive medication, 81.4% of subjects with WC ≥ 94 cm in men or ≥ 80 cm in women, therefore, met the National Cholesterol Education Program Adult Treatment Panel III (NCEP:ATPIII) criteria for metabolic syndrome [19].

We analyzed by pyrosequencing nine CpG-dinucleotides in intron 2 of *FKBP5* that were implicated in metabolic

Table 1 Participant demographic characteristics ($n = 43$)

Characteristic	Percentage or mean (standard deviation)
Sex (%)	
Female	48.8% ($n = 21$)
Race (%)	
Non-Hispanic White	37.2% ($n = 16$)
Non-Hispanic Black	60.5% ($n = 26$)
Asian	2.3% ($n = 1$)
Age (years)	61.9 ± 9.0
WC (cm)	109.7 ± 21.6
WC ≥ 94 cm (men) or 80 cm (women) (%)	81.5% ($n = 35$)
BMI (kg/m²)	34.1 ± 8.3
Antihypertensive medication use (%)	100% ($n = 43$)
HbA1c (%)	8.3 ± 1.6
LDL cholesterol (mg/dL)	89 ± 40
Cardiovascular procedure (%)*	
Catheterization	11.6% ($n = 5$)
Percutaneous coronary intervention (PCI)	4.7% ($n = 2$)
Coronary artery bypass surgery (CABG)	7.0% ($n = 3$)
PCI and CABG	4.7% ($n = 2$)

*Collectively this represents the total number of individuals included in the FKBP5 analysis model with a history of cardiovascular procedures ($n = 12$)

disorders in previous studies and flanked an experimentally validated GRE [8, 11]. We observed a significant association between intronic *FKBP5* DNAm in subjects with T2DM and multiple cardiometabolic outcomes in two different CpG-dinucleotides in intron 2 (Fig. 1). Greater percent DNAm of the *FKBP5* intron 2 CpG9-dinucleotide (CpG9) (coordinates chr6: 35,609,542) was significantly associated with higher HbA1c ($\beta = 0.535$, $p = 0.003$, Fig. 1a) and LDL cholesterol ($\beta = 0.344$, $p = 0.037$, Fig. 1b). Greater percent DNAm of the *FKBP5* intron 2 CpG7-dinucleotide (CpG7) (coordinates chr6: 35,609,628) was significantly associated with higher BMI and WC ($\beta = 0.516$, $p = 0.001$, Fig. 1c, and $\beta = 0.403$, $p = 0.006$, Fig. 1d, respectively). The associations with HbA1c, BMI, and WC were all of medium to large effect sizes (Table 2). These findings remained stable regardless of using the complete case sample ($n = 43$) or all available cases despite missing data (Additional file 2: Table S1, Additional file 3: Figure S2). Results for non-significant associations are shown in Additional file 2: Table S2.

In a secondary analysis, it was observed that having a history of more invasive cardiovascular procedures was associated with greater percent DNAm at CpG9 when adjusting for LDL cholesterol ($\beta = 0.344$, $p = 0.033$) (Table 3). Greater percent DNAm at CpG7 was inversely associated with more days a week completing more than 30 min of physical activity even when controlling for WC ($\beta = -0.390$, $p = 0.011$) (Table 3).

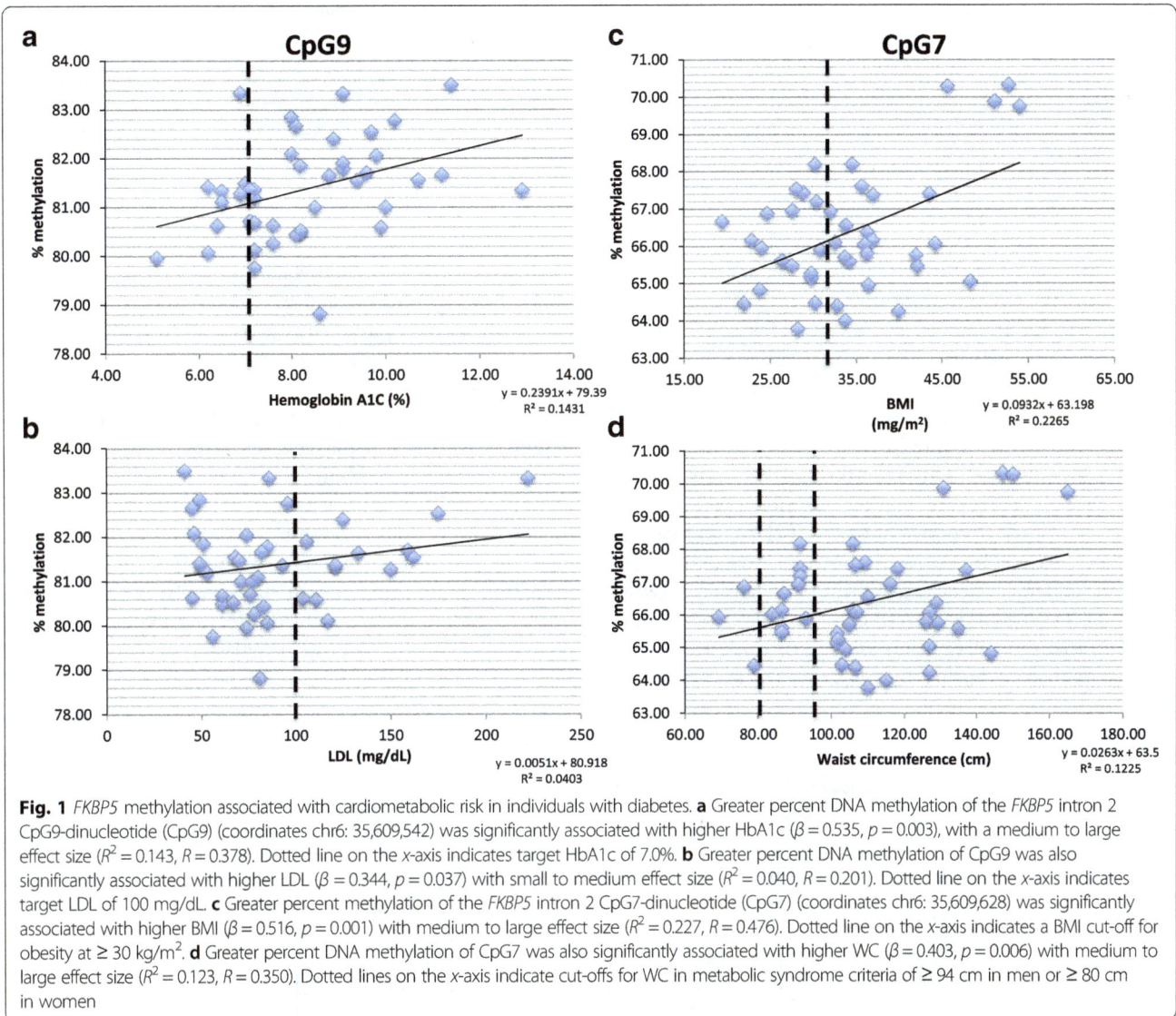

Fig. 1 *FKBP5* methylation associated with cardiometabolic risk in individuals with diabetes. **a** Greater percent DNA methylation of the *FKBP5* intron 2 CpG9-dinucleotide (CpG9) (coordinates chr6: 35,609,542) was significantly associated with higher HbA1c ($\beta = 0.535$, $p = 0.003$), with a medium to large effect size ($R^2 = 0.143$, $R = 0.378$). Dotted line on the *x*-axis indicates target HbA1c of 7.0%. **b** Greater percent DNA methylation of CpG9 was also significantly associated with higher LDL ($\beta = 0.344$, $p = 0.037$) with small to medium effect size ($R^2 = 0.040$, $R = 0.201$). Dotted line on the *x*-axis indicates target LDL of 100 mg/dL. **c** Greater percent methylation of the *FKBP5* intron 2 CpG7-dinucleotide (CpG7) (coordinates chr6: 35,609,628) was significantly associated with higher BMI ($\beta = 0.516$, $p = 0.001$) with medium to large effect size ($R^2 = 0.227$, $R = 0.476$). Dotted line on the *x*-axis indicates a BMI cut-off for obesity at ≥ 30 kg/m^2. **d** Greater percent DNA methylation of CpG7 was also significantly associated with higher WC ($\beta = 0.403$, $p = 0.006$) with medium to large effect size ($R^2 = 0.123$, $R = 0.350$). Dotted lines on the *x*-axis indicate cut-offs for WC in metabolic syndrome criteria of ≥ 94 cm in men or ≥ 80 cm in women

Discussion

In our study of individuals with T2DM, we observed that one pyrosequenced CpG-dinucleotide in intron 2 of the *FKBP5* gene (CpG9) was significantly associated with higher HbA1c and LDL, and another CpG-dinucleotide (CpG7) site with BMI and WC, though results should be interpreted in the context of a small sample size of 43 subjects. In the study population, mean HbA1c was above 7% (8.3%), mean BMI was categorized as obese (> 30 kg/m^2), there was a presence of hyperlipidemia (LDL cholesterol

Table 2 *FKBP5* methylation associated with cardiometabolic risk in individuals with diabetes

Independent variables	Model including the covariates age, sex, and race		Effect size	
	β	p	R	Effect size
Percent methylation of CpG9				
HbA1c	0.535	0.003**	0.378	Medium-large
LDL	0.344	0.037*	0.201	Small to medium
Percent methylation of CpG7				
BMI	0.516	0.001**	0.476	Large
WC	0.403	0.006**	0.350	Medium-large

The analysis included 43 subjects. Percent methylation of CpG9 and CpG7 were the dependent variables in the model
*$p < 0.05$; **$p < 0.01$

Table 3 *FKBP5* methylation associated with cardiovascular procedures and days of physical activity in individuals with diabetes

Dependent variable	Independent variable	Model including the covariates age, sex, and race	Model including additional covariate[a]
Number of cardiovascular procedures	Percent methylation of CpG9	$\beta = 0.247$, $p = 0.112$	LDL; $\beta = 0.344$, $p = 0.033*$
Percent methylation of CpG7	Number of days of physical activity	$\beta = -0.492$, $p = 0.001**$	WC; $\beta = -0.390$, $p = 0.011*$

[a]This model includes covariates of age, sex, and race in addition to the covariate listed below
*$p < 0.05$; **$p < 0.01$

greater than 100 mg/dL) in 30% of subjects, and a majority of subjects (81.4%) were above target WC and thus met criteria for metabolic syndrome. This suggests that the associations between DNAm of *FKBP5* and the outcome measures for cardiovascular and metabolic dysfunction observed in our study population including HbA1c, LDL cholesterol, BMI, and WC, are clinically meaningful as risk for disease. The relationship between *FKBP5* methylation, a surrogate marker for presumed chronic cortisol exposure, glycemic control in T2DM, and cardiovascular disease (CVD) risk, is notably indicated by the medium to large effect size of the association between intron 2% DNAm with HbA1c and WC, and the medium effect size of the relationship with LDL cholesterol. Our secondary analysis further suggests that the association of *FKBP5* with CVD as methylation of *FKBP5* is also associated with cardiovascular interventions including catheterization, percutaneous intervention (PCI), and coronary artery bypass grafting (CABG), and inversely associated with exercise.

There is a higher incidence of CVD in individuals with diabetes due to both macrovascular pathology and associated comorbid metabolic disorders, including hyperlipidemia [20, 21]. However, current treatments continue to target individual disease processes. Though our findings are correlative and cannot be used to determine causality, they support our hypothesis of a potential unifying pathophysiology of underlying hypercortisolism related to activation of glucocorticoid receptor signaling (Fig. 2), which may implicate the glucocorticoid pathway

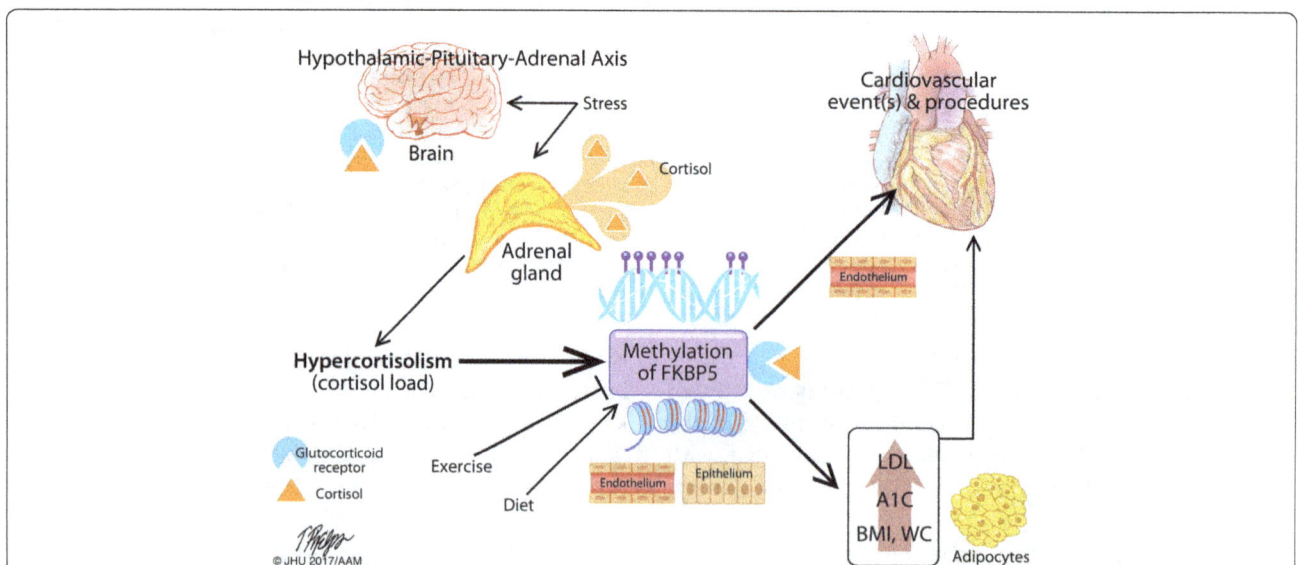

Fig. 2 The hypothesized relationship of *FKBP5* DNA methylation and cardiometabolic risk. Our findings demonstrate evidence that *FKBP5*, and therefore likely the hypothalamic-pituitary-adrenal axis, play a role in metabolic and cardiovascular disease risk and outcome. *FKBP5*, and the glucocorticoid receptor, is expressed in the brain, intestinal endothelial, and epithelial tissues. *FKBP5* expression in the brain (hypothalamus and hippocampus) as well as these other tissues has been associated previously with the influences of stress and cortisol load, exercise, and diet. Prior demonstration has also shown the function of *FKBP5* to play a role in adipogenesis and in endothelial changes in myocardial infarction. Taken together, these associations are hypothesized to link to risk and outcomes in cardiometabolic disease through methylation of *FKBP5*, and therefore, potentially expression or sensitivity of the glucocorticoid receptor. The methylation of *FKBP5* is associated with increased clinical risk factors for disease including hyperlipidemia (elevated LDL), chronic hyperglycemia (elevated HbA1c), and obesity (high BMI and WC) in individuals with diabetes. Further, methylation of *FKBP5* may be associated with cardiovascular procedures and inversely associated with exercise independent of LDL and obesity. Though many clinical trials have established the classical model of pathophysiologic associations with diabetes and hyperglycemia, hyperlipidemia, obesity, and cardiometabolic disease, the findings illustrated here demonstrate that there may be a role for the hypothalamic-pituitary-adrenal axis and glucocorticoid pathway dysfunction in the underlying pathophysiology of cardiometabolic disease risk and outcomes

as a new potential target for preventive and therapeutic interventions.

Our study corroborates current literature demonstrating the significance of *FKBP5* in associations with metabolic dysfunction and dysglycemia. For example, a polymorphism, rs1360780, has been associated with insulin resistance in children and adolescents with obesity and also with lower weight loss up to 26 months after bariatric surgery in adults [10, 22]. Studies have also demonstrated that *FKBP5* protein expression is responsive to certain environmental stimuli. For example, animal studies have shown that higher levels of *FKBP5* expression in the hypothalamus are related to increases in body weight and, further, hypothalamic, hippocampal, and intestinal colon epithelial expression of *FKBP5* may be responsive to dietary intake and environmental stress [23–25]. In humans, adipose tissue *FKBP5* expression and insulin resistance increase with dexamethasone exposure [9].

The observations in our secondary analysis that higher *FKBP5* methylation is inversely associated with current exercise activity and positively associated with a history of cardiovascular procedures are also supported by the literature. It has been demonstrated that *FKBP5* may play a role in vascular endothelial function in exercise in obese individuals as well as on endothelial platelet aggregation in individuals with acute myocardial infarction [26–28]. This dysfunction may be the underpinnings of the associations between cortisol and coronary artery calcifications, mortality after cardiac surgery (CABG), and all-cause CVD mortality [29–31]. Similarly, elevated hair cortisol levels as a measure of chronic cortisol exposure predict myocardial infarction and heart failure severity [32, 33].

Epigenetics is the concept that the genome may be modifiable through environmental exposures. One method of epigenetic modification is methylation of CpG-dinucleotide sites of DNA. One study demonstrated that a decrease in methylation of an intron 2 site of *FKBP5* is present in Cushing's syndrome [11]. Only one study to our knowledge, an animal study, exists assessing methylation and expression of *FKBP5* as a result of chronic steroid exposure, which showed persistent loss of methylation correlating with increased steroid exposure [4]. These studies suggest hypomethylation in association with chronic glucocorticoid exposure and our study identified hypermethylation associated with risk factors for CVD in T2DM. However, we note that two of the *FKBP5* intronic CpGs analyzed by Klengel et al. also showed increase in DNAm associated with the trauma exposure [8]. While gain of methylation events are usually associated with gene silencing, there are notable examples, such as at imprinted loci, where increase in DNAm inhibit binding of insulator proteins such as CTCF that govern complex enhancer-promoter interactions and gene activation [34]. If lower *FKBP5* expression is the outcome of hypermethylation in this group, it could indicate that these subjects are more responsive at the tissue level to cortisol since lower *FKBP5* protein expression allows more cortisol signaling. The increased responsiveness in adipose and other tissues could be the reason for the correlation [9, 24, 25, 28]. In this scenario, methylation is not a marker of cortisol exposure but of cortisol sensitivity. Additional in vitro experiments are needed to identify methylation-dependent binding of disease-specific factors whose presence in intron 2 may increase expression of *FKBP5* and its relationship with chronicity of cortisol exposure. Though further studies are needed to elucidate these gene loci-specific environment interactions, taken together with the findings in the current literature, our study may suggest that chronic exposure to glucocorticoids in obesity and T2DM may be in part responsible for associated cardiovascular and metabolic dysfunction through *FKBP5* expression.

Our study has many strengths. First, our sample includes a clinically generalizable sample of patients with T2DM and clinical outcome measures relevant to the assessment of disease in this population, especially HbA1c as a marker of glucose control, LDL cholesterol as a marker of increased risk of CVD, and BMI and WC as markers of a diagnosis of metabolic syndrome. Second, our study is one of the first studies to explore the epigenetics of *FKBP5* in humans with T2DM, in relation to metabolic and CVD risk and clinical characteristics including exercise and cardiac procedures. Finally, there is strength in the specificity of selecting a region of interest within the *FKBP5* gene, intron 2. This offers a specific target for future studies and potentially future interventions.

Our study does have some potential limitations. First, this is a small sample size and only includes individuals with T2DM seen in a tertiary care practice without a control group, which limits generalizability. The small sample size also limits the ability to adjust for multiple confounders and permits risk of overfitting the data in analyses. Given the small sample size and that the *FKBP5* analysis was hypothesis generating as a secondary aim of the MinD study, it may have been underpowered to accurately assess the effect sizes listed in Table 2. Also, control subjects without T2DM were not included in the original design. Future studies should include larger samples with control subjects in order to more stringently establish, and then validate, methylation as a potential biomarker for chronic glucocorticoid exposure. Second, our study is correlative and does not offer insight into causative association between glucocorticoid receptor function and disease outcomes. Third, we do not have longitudinal cortisol measures to assess the association with percent methylation as a surrogate for chronic hyper- or hypocortisolism nor did we measure peripheral *FKBP5* protein expression and, therefore, cannot assess whether the increase in DNA methylation we observe is associated with *FKBP5* or cortisol levels. Therefore, we propose that future studies of greater sample size, including a matched control group, assess both chronic, longitudinal assessment of cortisol load, such as hair cortisol levels, and RNA expression of *FKBP5* protein. We also assessed peripheral blood samples for *FKBP5* methylation and not adipocytes, epithelial, or endothelial cells. Finally, in our statistical analyses, our associations were interpreted without corrections for multiple comparisons, as typical multiple corrections assume that the tests are independent and are too conservative for correlated hypotheses as we have tested here.

Conclusion

In conclusion, we examined *FKBP5* methylation among individuals with T2DM and found that *FKBP5* DNAm was associated with higher levels of HbA1c, LDL cholesterol, BMI, and WC, which are all risk factors for CVD. We also found that increased percent *FKBP5* methylation was associated with greater number of cardiac procedures, supporting our initial finding of the relationship between *FKBP5* and adverse cardiovascular risk factors. Thus, *FKBP5* DNAm may be a marker of higher cardiovascular risk in T2DM, possibly secondary to higher exposure to cortisol. There is a critical need for further characterization of the longitudinal association of *FKBP5* with CVD in T2DM as a first step in understanding potential causation, and future directions for preventive and treatment interventions targeting the HPA axis.

Abbreviations
BMI: Body mass index (kg/m^2); BP: Blood pressure; CABG: Coronary artery bypass graft; Chr: Chromosome; CpG: Cytosine guanine dinucleotide; CVD: Cardiovascular disease; DNA: Deoxyribonucleic acid; DNAm: DNA methylation; *FKBP5*: FK506-binding protein 51 kDa gene; GRE: Glucocorticoid response element; HbA1c: Glycosylated hemoglobin (%); HPA: Hypothalamic-pituitary-adrenal; HPLC: High-performance liquid chromatography; LDL: Low-density lipoprotein cholesterol (mg/dL); MinD: Minor depressive disorder; PCR: Polymerase chain reaction; T2DM: Type 2 diabetes mellitus; TG: Triglycerides; WC: Waist circumference (cm)

Acknowledgements
The authors would like to acknowledge Timothy Phelps, Professor and Medical Illustrator, Graduate Program of Art as Applied to Medicine, Johns Hopkins in Baltimore, Maryland, for his help in the design of Fig. 2 in our manuscript.

Funding
The project described was supported by Award Number Grant UL1TR001070 from the National Center For Advancing Translational Sciences. The content is solely the responsibility of the authors and does not necessarily represent the official views of the National Center For Advancing Translational Sciences or the National Institutes of Health.
This study was supported by the National Institute of Diabetes, Digestive, and Kidney Diseases (R03 DK088997 awarded to SHG) and the National Institute of Alcohol Abuse and Alcoholism (U01 AA020890 awarded to GSW).

Authors' contributions
RO contributed to study design, data analysis, manuscript writing, and manuscript revising. JJ was involved in project design, data gathering, data analysis, and manuscript revising. RL was responsible for laboratory analyses, data analysis, and manuscript revising. GW contributed to the original study design, laboratory analyses, data analysis, and manuscript revising. SG obtained funding and contributed to the original study design, project design, data gathering, data analysis, and manuscript revising. All authors read and approved the final manuscript.

Competing interests
The authors declare that they have no competing interests.

Author details
[1]Departments of Internal Medicine & Pediatrics, Johns Hopkins University School of Medicine, 600 North Wolfe Street, Harvey Bldg. Rm 805, Baltimore, MD 21287, USA. [2]Division of Endocrinology, Diabetes, and Metabolism, Department of Medicine, The Ohio State University Wexner Medical Center, 566 McCampbell Hall, 1581 Dodd Drive, Columbus, OH 43210, USA. [3]Department of Psychiatry and Behavioral Sciences, Johns Hopkins University School of Medicine, 720 Rutland Ave. Ross Bldg. 1068, Baltimore, MD 21205, USA. [4]Division of Endocrinology, Diabetes and Metabolism, Department of Medicine, Johns Hopkins University School of Medicine, 1830 E. Monument Street Suite 333, Baltimore, MD 21287, USA.

References
1. Joseph JJ, Wang X, Spanakis E, Seeman T, Wand G, Needham B, Golden SH. Diurnal salivary cortisol, glycemia and insulin resistance: the multi-ethnic study of atherosclerosis. Psychoneuroendocrinology. 2015;62:327–35.
2. Nederhof E, van Oort FV, Bouma EM, Laceulle OM, Oldehinkel AJ, Ormel J. Predicting mental disorders from hypothalamic-pituitary-adrenal axis functioning: a 3-year follow-up in the TRAILS study. Psychol Med. 2015; 45:2403–12.
3. Joseph JJ, Golden SH. Cortisol dysregulation: the bidirectional link between stress, depression, and type 2 diabetes mellitus. Ann N Y Acad Sci. 2017; 1391:20–34.
4. Lee RS, Tamashiro KL, Yang X, Purcell RH, Harvey A, Willour VL, Huo Y, Rongione M, Wand GS, Potash JB. Chronic corticosterone exposure increases expression and decreases deoxyribonucleic acid methylation of Fkbp5 in mice. Endocrinology. 2010;151:4332–43.

5. Lee RS, Tamashiro KL, Yang X, Purcell RH, Huo Y, Rongione M, Potash JB, Wand GS. A measure of glucocorticoid load provided by DNA methylation of Fkbp5 in mice. Psychopharmacology. 2011;218:303–12.

6. Gragnoli C. Hypothesis of the neuroendocrine cortisol pathway gene role in the comorbidity of depression, type 2 diabetes, and metabolic syndrome. Appl Clin Genet. 2014;7:43–53.

7. Cattaneo A, Riva MA. Stress-induced mechanisms in mental illness: a role for glucocorticoid signalling. J Steroid Biochem Mol Biol. 2016;160:169–74.

8. Klengel T, Mehta D, Anacker C, Rex-Haffner M, Pruessner JC, Pariante CM, Pace TW, Mercer KB, Mayberg HS, Bradley B, et al. Allele-specific FKBP5 DNA demethylation mediates gene-childhood trauma interactions. Nat Neurosci. 2013;16:33–41.

9. Pereira MJ, Palming J, Svensson MK, Rizell M, Dalenback J, Hammar M, Fall T, Sidibeh CO, Svensson PA, Eriksson JW. FKBP5 expression in human adipose tissue increases following dexamethasone exposure and is associated with insulin resistance. Metabolism. 2014;63:1198–208.

10. Hartmann IB, Fries GR, Bucker J, Scotton E, von Diemen L, Kauer-Sant'Anna M. The FKBP5 polymorphism rs1360780 is associated with lower weight loss after bariatric surgery: 26 months of follow-up. Surg Obes Relat Dis. 2016;12:1554–60.

11. Resmini E, Santos A, Aulinas A, Webb SM, Vives-Gilabert Y, Cox O, Wand G, Lee RS. Reduced DNA methylation of FKBP5 in Cushing's syndrome. Endocrine. 2016;54:768–77.

12. Argentieri MA, Nagarajan S, Seddighzadeh B, Baccarelli AA, Shields AE. Epigenetic pathways in human disease: the impact of DNA methylation on stress-related pathogenesis and current challenges in biomarker development. EBioMedicine. 2017;18:327–50.

13. Klein S, Allison DB, Heymsfield SB, Kelley DE, Leibel RL, Nonas C, Kahn R, Association for Weight Management and Obesity Prevention, NAASO, et al. Waist circumference and cardiometabolic risk: a consensus statement from shaping America's health: Association for Weight Management and Obesity Prevention; NAASO, the Obesity Society; the American Society for Nutrition; and the American Diabetes Association. Diabetes Care. 2007;30:1647–52.

14. Golden SH, Shah N, Naqibuddin M, Payne JL, Hill-Briggs F, Wand GS, Wang NY, Langan S, Lyketsos C. The prevalence and specificity of depression diagnosis in a clinic-based population of adults with type 2 diabetes mellitus. Psychosomatics. 2017;58:28–37.

15. Klengel T, Binder EB. FKBP5 allele-specific epigenetic modification in gene by environment interaction. Neuropsychopharmacology. 2015;40:244–6.

16. Aken BL, Achuthan P, Akanni W, Amode MR, Bernsdorff F, Bhai J, Billis K, Carvalho-Silva D, Cummins C, Clapham P, et al. Ensembl 2017. Nucleic Acids Res. 2017;45:D635–42.

17. Hajat A, Diez-Roux A, Franklin TG, Seeman T, Shrager S, Ranjit N, Castro C, Watson K, Sanchez B, Kirschbaum C. Socioeconomic and race/ethnic differences in daily salivary cortisol profiles: the multi-ethnic study of atherosclerosis. Psychoneuroendocrinology. 2010;35:932–43.

18. Cohen J. A power primer. Psychol Bull. 1992;112:155–9.

19. Kassi E, Pervanidou P, Kaltsas G, Chrousos G. Metabolic syndrome: definitions and controversies. BMC Med. 2011;9:48.

20. Tehrani DM, Zhao Y, Blaha MJ, Mora S, Mackey RH, Michos ED, Budoff MJ, Cromwell W, Otvos JD, Rosenblit PD, Wong ND. Discordance of low-density lipoprotein and high-density lipoprotein cholesterol particle versus cholesterol concentration for the prediction of cardiovascular disease in patients with metabolic syndrome and diabetes mellitus (from the multi-ethnic study of atherosclerosis [MESA]). Am J Cardiol. 2016;117:1921–7.

21. Katz R, Budoff MJ, O'Brien KD, Wong ND, Nasir K. The metabolic syndrome and diabetes mellitus as predictors of thoracic aortic calcification as detected by non-contrast computed tomography in the multi-ethnic study of atherosclerosis. Diabet Med. 2016;33:912–9.

22. Fichna M, Krzysko-Pieczka I, Zurawek M, Skowronska B, Januszkiewicz-Lewandowska D, Fichna P. FKBP5 polymorphism is associated with insulin resistance in children and adolescents with obesity. Obes Res Clin Pract. 2016;12(1):62–70.

23. Balsevich G, Uribe A, Wagner KV, Hartmann J, Santarelli S, Labermaier C, Schmidt MV. Interplay between diet-induced obesity and chronic stress in mice: potential role of FKBP51. J Endocrinol. 2014;222:15–26.

24. Zhang L, Qiu B, Wang T, Wang J, Liu M, Xu Y, Wang C, Deng R, Williams K, Yang Z, et al. Loss of FKBP5 impedes adipocyte differentiation under both normoxia and hypoxic stress. Biochem Biophys Res Commun. 2017;485:761–7.

25. Chen Q, Swist E, Beckstead J, Green J, Matias F, Roberts J, Qiao C, Raju J, Brooks SP, Scoggan KA. Dietary fructooligosaccharides and wheat bran elicit specific and dose-dependent gene expression profiles in the proximal colon epithelia of healthy Fischer 344 rats. J Nutr. 2011;141:790–7.

26. Laughlin MH, Padilla J, Jenkins NT, Thorne PK, Martin JS, Rector RS, Akter S, Davis JW. Exercise training causes differential changes in gene expression in diaphragm arteries and 2A arterioles of obese rats. J Appl Physiol (1985). 2015;119:604–16.

27. Eicher JD, Wakabayashi Y, Vitseva O, Esa N, Yang Y, Zhu J, Freedman JE, McManus DD, Johnson AD. Characterization of the platelet transcriptome by RNA sequencing in patients with acute myocardial infarction. Platelets. 2016;27:230–9.

28. Zhao J, An Q, Goldberg J, Quyyumi AA, Vaccarino V. Promoter methylation of glucocorticoid receptor gene is associated with subclinical atherosclerosis: a monozygotic twin study. Atherosclerosis. 2015;242:71–6.

29. Kumari M, Shipley M, Stafford M, Kivimaki M. Association of diurnal patterns in salivary cortisol with all-cause and cardiovascular mortality: findings from the Whitehall II study. J Clin Endocrinol Metab. 2011;96:1478–85.

30. Ronaldson A, Kidd T, Poole L, Leigh E, Jahangiri M, Steptoe A. Diurnal cortisol rhythm is associated with adverse cardiac events and mortality in coronary artery bypass patients. J Clin Endocrinol Metab. 2015;100:3676–82.

31. Vogelzangs N, Beekman AT, Milaneschi Y, Bandinelli S, Ferrucci L, Penninx BW. Urinary cortisol and six-year risk of all-cause and cardiovascular mortality. J Clin Endocrinol Metab. 2010;95:4959–64.

32. Pereg D, Chan J, Russell E, Berlin T, Mosseri M, Seabrook JA, Koren G, Van Uum S. Cortisol and testosterone in hair as biological markers of systolic heart failure. Psychoneuroendocrinology. 2013;38:2875–82.

33. Pereg D, Gow R, Mosseri M, Lishner M, Rieder M, Van Uum S, Koren G. Hair cortisol and the risk for acute myocardial infarction in adult men. Stress. 2011;14:73–81.

34. Bell AC, Felsenfeld G. Methylation of a CTCF-dependent boundary controls imprinted expression of the Igf2 gene. Nature. 2000;405:482–5.

17

T cell epigenetic remodeling and accelerated epigenetic aging are linked to long-term immune alterations in childhood cancer survivors

Sara Daniel[1], Vibe Nylander[2], Lars R. Ingerslev[2], Ling Zhong[3], Odile Fabre[2], Briana Clifford[1], Karen Johnston[4], Richard J. Cohn[4], Romain Barres[1,2]*[†] and David Simar[1,2]*[†] (iD)

Abstract

Background: Cancer treatments have substantially improved childhood cancer survival but are accompanied by long-term complications, notably chronic inflammatory diseases. We hypothesize that cancer treatments could lead to long-term epigenetic changes in immune cells, resulting in increased prevalence of inflammatory diseases in cancer survivors.

Results: To test this hypothesis, we established the epigenetic and transcriptomic profiles of immune cells from 44 childhood cancer survivors (CCS, > 16 years old) on full remission (> 5 years) who had received chemotherapy alone or in combination with total body irradiation (TBI) and hematopoietic stem cell transplant (HSCT). We found that more than 10 years post-treatment, CCS treated with TBI/HSCT showed an altered DNA methylation signature in T cell, particularly at genes controlling immune and inflammatory processes and oxidative stress. DNA methylation remodeling in T cell was partially associated with chronic expression changes of nearby genes, increased frequency of type 1 cytokine-producing T cell, elevated systemic levels of these cytokines, and over-activation of related signaling pathways. Survivors exposed to TBI/HSCT were further characterized by an Epigenetic-Aging-Signature of T cell consistent with accelerated epigenetic aging. To investigate the potential contribution of irradiation to these changes, we established two cell culture models. We identified that radiation partially recapitulated the immune changes observed in survivors through a bystander effect that could be mediated by circulating factors.

Conclusion: Cancer treatments, in particular TBI/HSCT, are associated with long-term immune disturbances. We propose that epigenetic remodeling of immune cells following cancer therapy augments inflammatory- and age-related diseases, including metabolic complications, in childhood cancer survivors.

Keywords: Epigenetic aging, DNA methylation, inflammation, cancer survivors, T cell

Background

Improvement in the cure rate of childhood cancer, and in particular acute lymphoblastic leukemia, has led to a significant increase in the number of long-term survivors [1]. However, more than 95% of childhood cancer survivors (CCS) develop chronic health conditions by the age of 45 [2]. The most frequently reported complications include cardiac, endocrine, or neurological conditions [3], chronic diseases that all share an inflammatory component. While a combination of cancer treatment, lifestyle and environmental factors could contribute to the development of these chronic conditions [4, 5], we and others have identified total body irradiation (TBI) and hematopoietic stem cells transplant (HSCT) as major risk factors for the development of metabolic, cardiovascular, and other health conditions in childhood cancer survivors [6, 7]. When compared to chemotherapy alone,

---

* Correspondence: barres@sund.ku.dk; d.simar@unsw.edu.au
[†]Romain Barres and David Simar contributed equally to this work.
[1]Mechanisms of Disease and Translational Research, School of Medical Sciences, UNSW Sydney, Wallace Wurth Building East Room 420, Sydney, NSW 2052, Australia
Full list of author information is available at the end of the article

exposure to radiation resulted in a higher cumulative incidence of several chronic health conditions 20 years post-diagnosis, with TBI being the mode of radiation causing the highest incidence of severe conditions [3]. We further reported in a cohort of 248 CCS that the prevalence of metabolic complications was more than doubled at a median of 12.7 years after remission [7]. More recently, we have established in a mouse model that irradiation in the absence of HSCT led to altered muscle and adipose lineage commitment and metabolic dysfunction later in life [8].

Immune disturbances contribute to cardiovascular, neurological, and metabolic conditions, notably in early development of these diseases [9, 10]. Radiation-induced immune response, including macrophage activation, neutrophil, and lymphocyte recruitment, leads to the production of pro-inflammatory mediators to support anti-tumor activity and clearance of apoptotic cells [11, 12], with a similar response having been described in response to chemotherapy [13]. Although this inflammatory process is usually confined to the acute phase of the radiation response [14], long-term immune changes could also persist following irradiation, chemotherapy, or HSCT [15, 16]. As there is still limited evidence to support the existence of long-term chronic inflammation, the mechanisms responsible for long-term chronic immune disturbances in cancer survivors and their potential consequences on survivors' health still remain unknown.

We hypothesized that childhood cancer survivors, in particular when exposed to TBI/HSCT, present long-lasting immune alterations that could contribute to diseases later in life. Our results show that exposure to TBI/HSCT is associated with persistent chronic inflammation, a remodeling of immune cells epigenome and altered immune functions. We further establish that T cell from childhood cancer survivors presents an epigenetic signature consistent with accelerated aging. We propose that persistent alterations of the immune system in childhood cancer survivors contributes to higher risk of secondary diseases, including cardio-metabolic diseases.

Results

To study the long-term effect of cancer treatment on immune functions, we recruited childhood cancer survivors who had received chemotherapy alone or in combination with TBI/HSCT in the course of their treatment, with clinical characteristics and cancer history presented in Table 1. The majority of our population was composed of survivors of acute lymphoblastic or myeloid leukemia, as well as Hodgkin's and non-Hodgkin's lymphoma, and all survivors received chemotherapy. Our two groups were age-matched, with no difference in age at inclusion, at diagnosis, or in number of years on remission (Table 1). Survivors in the

TBI/HSCT group tended to be shorter and lighter ($p = 0.05$ and $p = 0.07$ respectively).

TBI/HSCT is associated with long-term epigenetic remodeling in T cell

Reports have suggested that inflammation could persist years after cancer treatments [17], potentially through a long-term "memory" of the treatment, implying epigenetic mechanisms. Thus, we assessed the DNA methylation profile of immune cells. CD4$^+$ ($p = 0.05$) and CD8$^+$ T cell ($p = 0.07$) tended to show lower global DNA methylation levels in CCS treated with TBI/HSCT, while monocytes tended to show higher methylation levels ($p = 0.06$), with no difference in other populations (Fig. 1a). We then tested if these changes in methylation were gene-specific and performed reduced representation bisulfite sequencing (RRBS) in CD4$^+$ T cell. We found differential methylation at cytosines which corresponded to 419 different neighboring genes in the TBI/HSCT group (Fig. 1b, Additional file 1: Table S1). Out of the 419 differentially methylated regions (DMRs), 9 were identified in enhancers and 47 in promoters (Additional file 1: Table S1). Differential methylation was also found at microRNA (miRNA) loci (Additional file 1: Table S1), including miR-942 and miR-378c, which have been implicated in acute response to irradiation, or miR-124 which is linked to T cell polarization and inflammation [18, 19]. Using GO analysis on our 419 coding genes containing differentially methylated cytosines, we identified enrichments for GO terms linked to oxidative stress (15/77 GO terms found in our data, Fig. 1c, Additional file 1: Table S2) and genes related to immune processes (21/77 terms) including *positive* and *negative regulation of cytokines production* (Fig. 1c, Additional file 1: Table S2). Transcriptomic analysis of CD4$^+$ T cell by RNA-seq returned a small subset of genes differentially expressed (29, Fig. 1d, Additional file 1: Table S3a). Although we did not detect differential methylation at the proximity of the differentially expressed genes, except for *adhesion G protein-coupled receptor G1* (also known as GPR56), we found enrichment for GO terms related to inflammation, similar to the DMR-associated genes (Fig. 1e, Additional file 1: Table S3B). Collectively, these results support that TBI/HSCT stably alters the epigenome of T cell.

Cancer survivors treated with TBI/HSCT show long-term altered immune function

To determine the consequences of the remodeling of the T cell epigenome, we analyzed T cell function (Fig. 2a). In mitogen-stimulated CD4$^+$ and CD8$^+$ T cell from the TBI/HSCT group, we found a greater frequency of interferon (IFN)-γ but not interleukin (IL)-4-producing cells (Fig. 2b, Additional file 1: Figure S1a). Intracellular signaling pathways, including mTOR (mammalian target of rapamycin) and MAPK (mitogen-activated protein

Table 1 Participants' characteristics

	Non-IRR	TBI/HSCT	p value (TBI/HSCT vs non-IRR)
Number of participants	30	14	
Sex (male/female)	15/15	9/5	0.25
Age (year, range)	22.1 (16–34)	25.1 (16–39)	0.48
Age at diagnosis (year, range)	7.2 (0.2–17.7)	7.7 (1.2–16.6)	0.78
Height (cm)	170 ± 9	163 ± 12	0.05
Weight (kg)	73.9 ± 18.8	62.0 ± 19.3	0.07
Body mass index (kg/m^2)	25.5 ± 5.7	23.2 ± 6.8	0.26
Waist-to-height ratio	50.8 ± 8.5	51.4 ± 11.1	0.84
Diagnosis (number of survivors, %)			
Acute lymphoblastic leukemia	12 (40%)	5 (36%)	
Relapse	0 (0%)	1 (7%)	
Acute myeloid leukemia	1 (3%)	6 (43%)	
Relapse	0 (0%)	1 (7%)	
Neuroblastoma	1 (3%)	2 (14%)	
Malignant histiocytosis	0 (0%)	1 (7%)	
Hodgkins lymphoma	2 (13%)	0 (0%)	
Non-Hogkins lymphoma	3 (10%)	0 (0%)	
Other type of cancer	11 (21%)	0 (0%)	
Treatments (number of survivors, %)			
Chemotherapy	30 (100%)	14 (100%)	
TBI	0 (0%)	14 (100%)	
Hematopoietic stem cell transplant	3 (10%)	14 (100%)	
Triglycerides (mmol/l)	1.03 ± 0.50	2.11 ± 2.08	0.01
Total cholesterol (mmol/l)	4.82 ± 0.79	5.14 ± 1.12	0.28
LDL-cholesterol (mmol/l)	2.86 ± 0.53	2.97 ± 1.13	0.67
HDL-cholesterol (mmol/l)	1.59 ± 0.71	1.17 ± 0.41	0.05
Glucose (mmol/l)	4.74 ± 0.47	6.04 ± 4.19	0.10
Insulin (mIU/l)	7.17 ± 5.76	11.3 ± 8.60	0.07
HOMA-IR	0.96 ± 0.73	1.84 ± 1.98	0.04

LDL low-density lipoprotein, HOMA-IR homeostatic model assessment insulin resistance index, Non-IRR non-irradiated, TBI total body irradiation, HSCT hematopoietic stem cell transplant

kinases), are critical regulators of T cell polarization and cytokines production (Fig. 2a). Quantification of p38, ribosomal protein S6 kinase1 (S6 k1), c-Jun N-terminal kinase (JNK) and Akt phosphorylation in CD4$^+$ and CD8$^+$ T cell showed a marked increase for all four proteins in both groups upon mitogen stimulation (Fig. 2c, Additional file 1: Figure S1b). However, the TBI/HSCT group showed over-activation of p38 and S6 k1 under resting conditions in CD4$^+$ (Fig. 2c) and CD8$^+$ cells (Additional file 1: Figure S1b), potentially linked to the increased frequency of type 1 cytokine-producing T cell. These functional changes in T cell from the TBI/HSCT group were associated with elevated systemic levels of IFN-γ and tumor necrosis factor (TNF)-α ($p < 0.05$,

Fig. 2d), suggesting a link between radiation, HSCT, and long-term inflammation.

Acute exposure to radiation triggers a transient stress response resulting in pro-inflammatory cytokines production [14]. Thus, we tested the contribution of direct irradiation to T cell polarization and MAPK/mTOR activation using an in vitro model (Fig. 3a). Direct irradiation did not affect p-p38 or pS6 k1 ($p > 0.05$, Fig. 3b), or pJNK, pAkt-Ser473, and the frequency of IL-4/IFN-γ-producing cells in Jurkat cells (Additional file 1: Figure S2a-b). We then investigated the indirect effect of irradiation by exposing mitogen-stimulated PBMCs collected from healthy donors to the conditioned media obtained from irradiated fibroblasts (Fig. 3c). We found

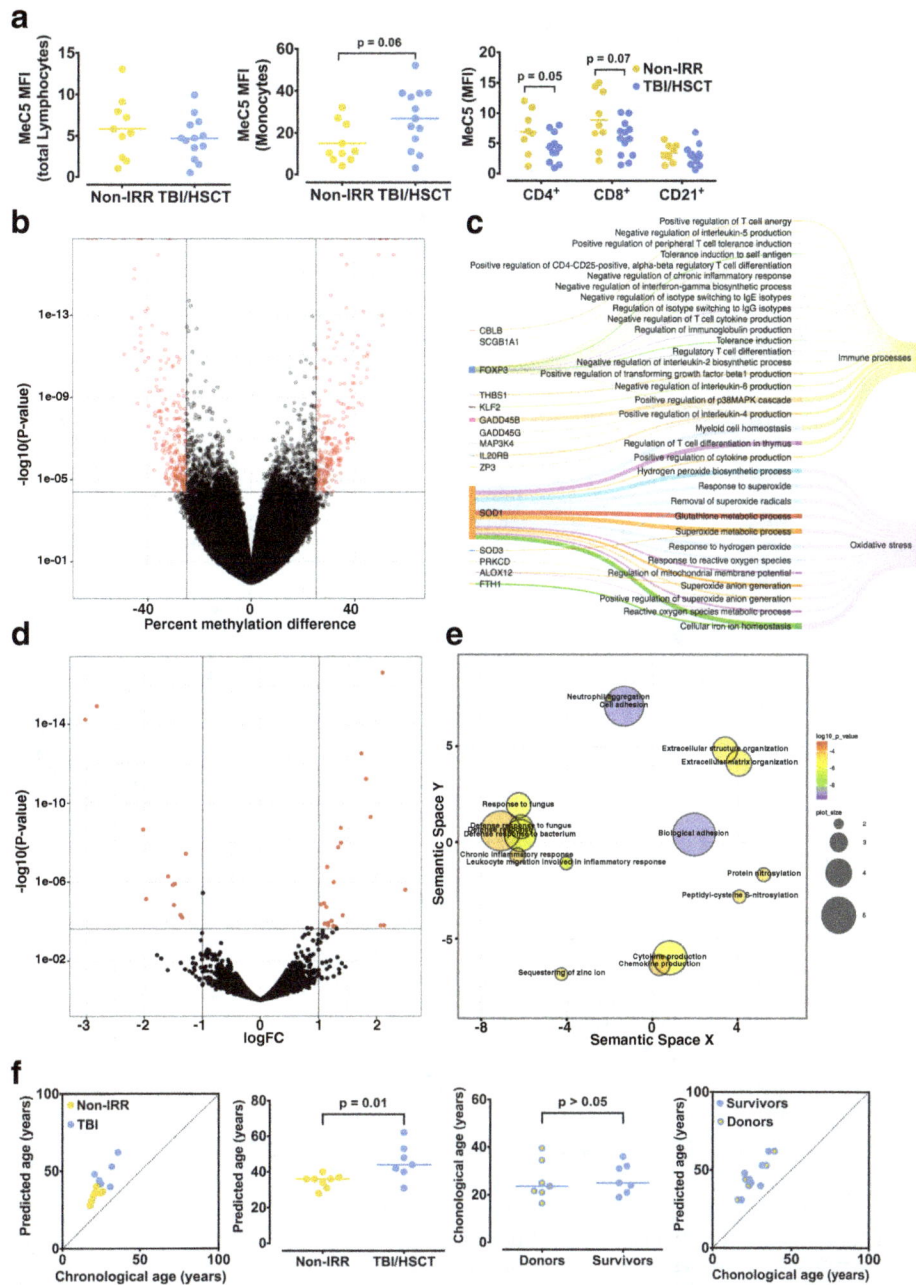

Fig. 1 Epigenetic and transcriptomic analysis of T cell in childhood cancer survivors (CCS). **a.** No difference in global DNA methylation was observed in total lymphocytes or B cells (CD3⁻CD21⁺) between CCS who received total body irradiation and hematopoietic stem cell transplant (TBI/HSCT) compared to those who received no irradiation (non-IRR, $p > 0.05$). CD4⁺ cells from CCS treated with TBI/HSCT showed global hypomethylation ($p = 0.05$), with a similar trend in CD8⁺ cells ($p = 0.07$), whereas monocytes tended to show hypermethylation ($p = 0.06$). **b.** Volcano plot representing the distribution of differentially methylated genes in the two groups of survivors, with more than 400 genes differentially methylated (represented in red, with a difference in methylation of more than 25%). **c.** Sankey diagram showing representative Gene Ontology (GO) terms clusters from differentially methylated genes, including all main GO terms related to immunological processes or oxidative stress. The width of the arrow is proportional to the contribution of the gene to the GO term and to the contribution of the GO term to immunological processes or oxidative stress **d.** Volcano plot reflecting the distribution of differentially expressed genes (in red) between the two groups of CCS. **e.** Representative GO terms clusters from differentially expressed genes showed a particular enrichment in GO terms related to immune processes and oxidative stress. **f.** Predicted biological age based on methylation levels on three specific CpG sites on *ASPA*, *ITGA2B*, and *PDE4C* was higher in CCS treated with TBI/HSCT. Both groups showed increased distance from the regression line, suggesting increased biological predicted age compared to chronological age. Chronological age was not different between the donors and the children who received hematopoietic stem cells transplant at the time of the experiment ($p > 0.05$)

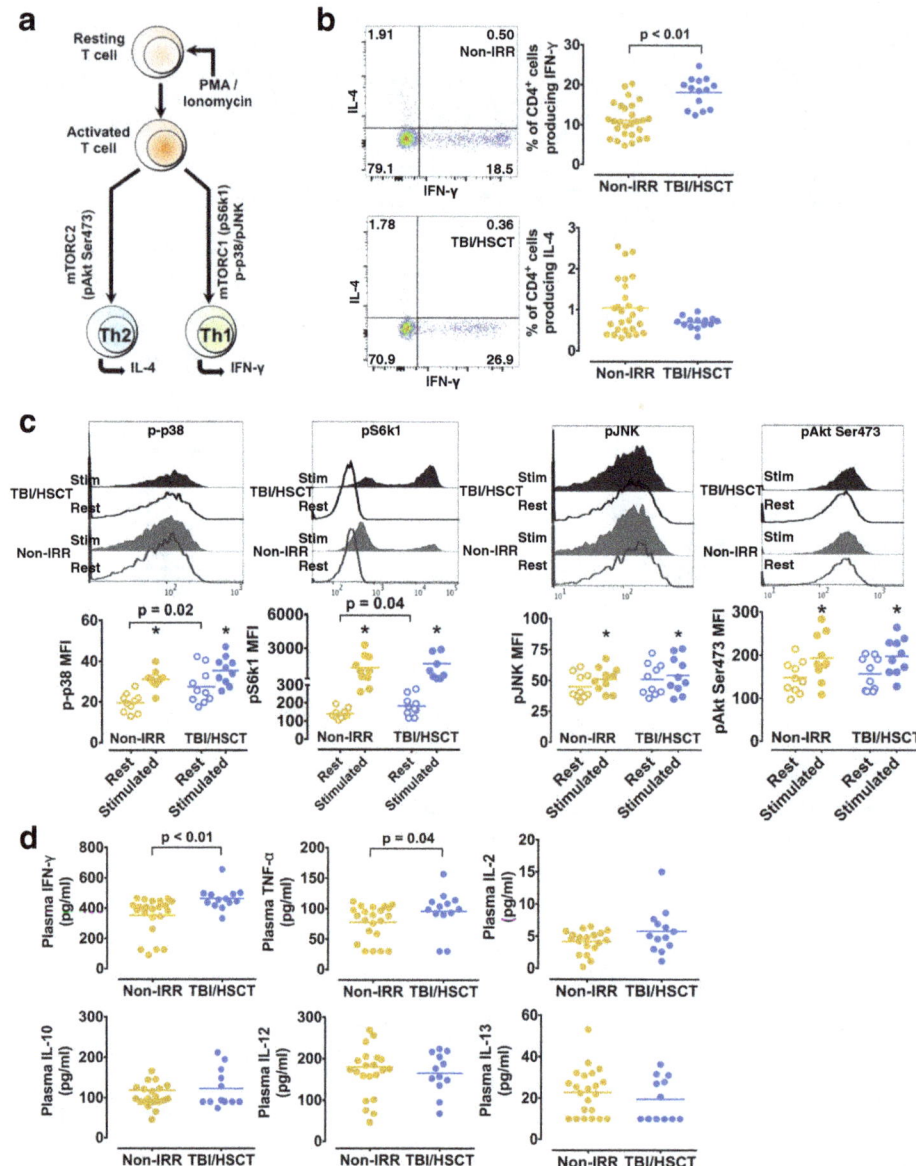

Fig. 2 CD4[+] T cell is altered in childhood cancer survivors (CCS) treated with TBI (total body irradiation)/HSCT (hematopoietic stem cell transplant). **a**. Schematic representation of intracellular signaling involved in polarized activation in T cells. **b**. Representative FACS dot plot of CD4[+] cells producing interferon (IFN)-γ (X-axis) or interleukin (IL)-4 (Y-axis) in CCS treated with TBI/HSCT (bottom) or no irradiation (non-IRR, top). The frequency of CD4[+] cells producing IFN-γ was higher in CCS treated with TBI/HSCT compared to non-IRR CCS ($p < 0.01$), with no difference in CD4[+] cells producing IL-4 ($p = 0.3$). **c**. Representative histograms for phosphorylated p38, phosphorylated ribosomal protein S6 kinase 1 (pS6 k1), phosphorylated c-Jun N-terminal kinase (pJNK), and phosphorylated Akt on Ser473 under resting condition (Rest) and upon mitogen stimulation (Stim). Upon mitogen stimulation, p-p38, pS6k1, pJNK, and pAkt Ser473 were all significantly increased (*$p < 0.05$, compared to resting condition) in CD4[+] cells in both groups ($n = 10$ in each group). Higher resting phosphorylation levels of p38 and S6 k1 were observed in CD4[+] cells from CCS treated with TBI ($p = 0.02$ and $p = 0.04$ respectively). **d**. Plasma levels of Th1 cytokines including interferon (IFN)-γ and tumor necrosis factor (TNF)-α were significantly elevated in CCS treated with TBI/HSCT ($p < 0.01$ and $p = 0.04$ respectively) whereas interleukin (IL)-10 and IL-13, or IL-2 and IL-12, did not differ between the two groups ($p > 0.05$)

that conditioned media from fibroblasts irradiated with a dose of 3Gy increased phosphorylation of p38 and S6 K1 in CD4[+] cells (Fig. 3d) but had no effect on pJNK or pAkt-Ser473 (Additional file 1: Figure S2c). Exposure to conditioned media from fibroblasts irradiated with a dose of 3Gy also had no effect on the frequency of CD4[+]

cells or CD8[+] cells producing IFN-γ ($p = 0.14$, Fig. 3d) or IL-4 ($p > 0.05$, Fig. 3d, Additional file 1: Figure S3a-b for CD8[+] cells). These results suggest that irradiation may exert its effect on T cell through secreted factors. To identify proteins secreted by irradiated cells, we analyzed cell culture supernatants from irradiated (1) fibroblasts

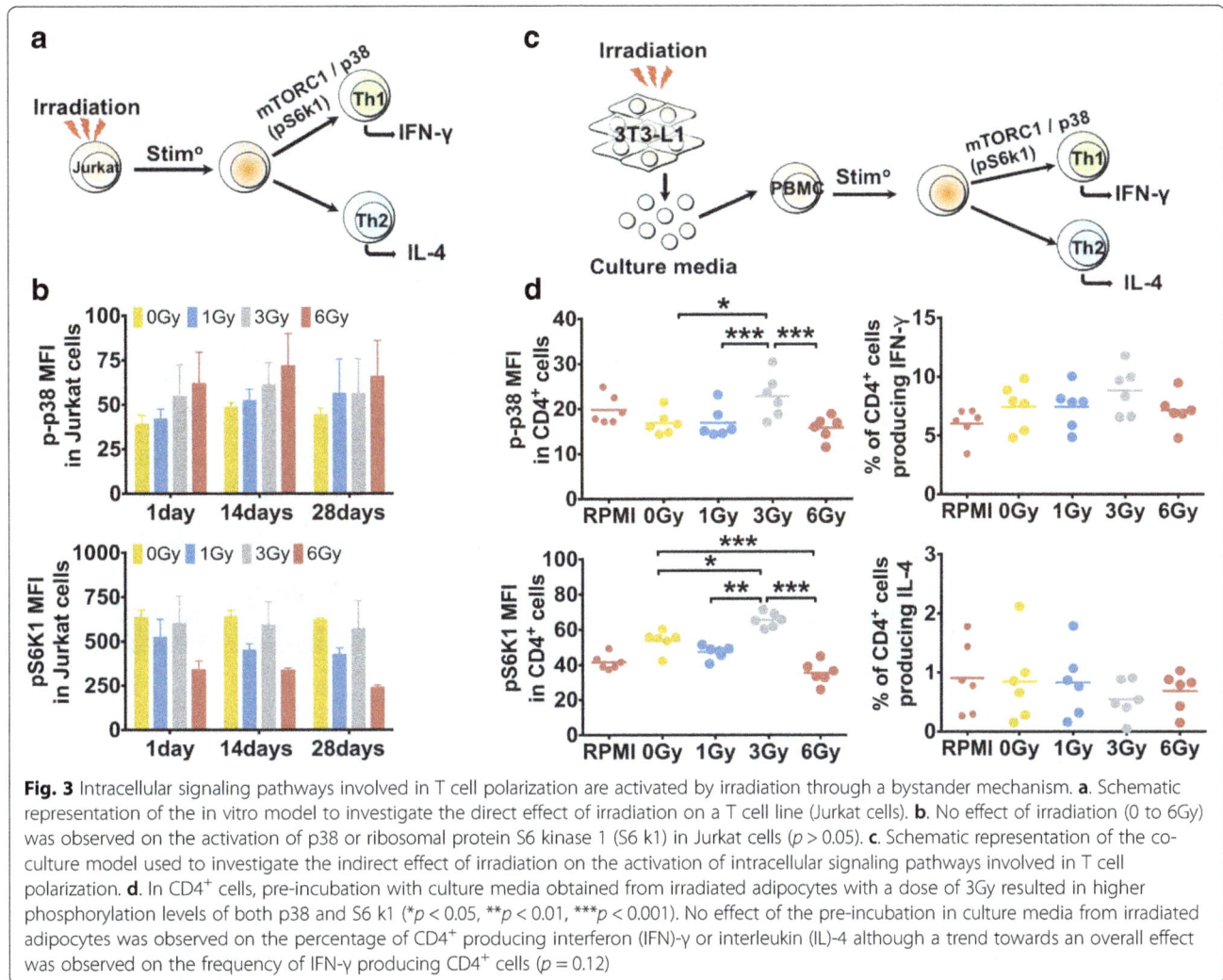

Fig. 3 Intracellular signaling pathways involved in T cell polarization are activated by irradiation through a bystander mechanism. **a.** Schematic representation of the in vitro model to investigate the direct effect of irradiation on a T cell line (Jurkat cells). **b.** No effect of irradiation (0 to 6Gy) was observed on the activation of p38 or ribosomal protein S6 kinase 1 (S6 k1) in Jurkat cells ($p > 0.05$). **c.** Schematic representation of the co-culture model used to investigate the indirect effect of irradiation on the activation of intracellular signaling pathways involved in T cell polarization. **d.** In CD4$^+$ cells, pre-incubation with culture media obtained from irradiated adipocytes with a dose of 3Gy resulted in higher phosphorylation levels of both p38 and S6 k1 (*$p < 0.05$, **$p < 0.01$, ***$p < 0.001$). No effect of the pre-incubation in culture media from irradiated adipocytes was observed on the percentage of CD4$^+$ producing interferon (IFN)-γ or interleukin (IL)-4 although a trend towards an overall effect was observed on the frequency of IFN-γ producing CD4$^+$ cells ($p = 0.12$)

or (2) fully differentiated adipocytes at 24 h and 7 days post-exposure using mass spectrometry (Fig. 4a). Most detected proteins were secreted in both irradiated or non-irradiated conditions (Fig. 4b), with some proteins uniquely detected in the irradiated or non-irradiated conditions, although this did not reach statistical significance (Additional file 1: Table S4). We next analyzed plasma samples from CCS and detected more than 50 proteins with a distinct expression pattern (Fig. 4c). GO analysis identified a specific enrichment for pathways related to *cell stress*, *immune processes* and *inflammation* (Fig. 4d). Of interest, the alpha-1-antitrypsin protein (encoded by the *SERPINA1* gene) was decreased in the TBI/HSCT group. Given the role of alpha-1 antitrypsin in the inhibition of pro-inflammatory cytokines secretion [20], decreased levels of this protein could participate in the immune changes in CCS treated with TBI/HSCT. Our cluster analysis suggested that the expression pattern of these proteins was group-specific. Collectively, our data suggest that secreted factors participate in a long-term alteration of the immune system in survivors exposed to irradiation and hematopoietic stem cell transplant.

Childhood cancer survivors are characterized by accelerated epigenetic aging

Given that T cell epigenetic remodeling specifically affected genes involved in inflammation and oxidative stress, two processes associated with aging, we investigated the contribution of epigenetic factors in cancer treatment-induced accelerated aging. Using the Epigenetic-Aging-Signature method [21], we found that both groups of survivors had increased predicted biological age (Fig. 1f), with CCS treated with TBI/HSCT showing a higher predicted biological age ($p = 0.01$, Fig. 1f). Moreover, the chronological age was correlated to the predicted age in non-irradiated CCS ($n = 8$, $r = 0.85$, $p < 0.01$, Fig. 1f) but not in the TBI/HSCT group ($n = 7$, $p > 0.05$, Fig. 1f). Since all survivors treated with TBI also received HSCT, our results could indicate that

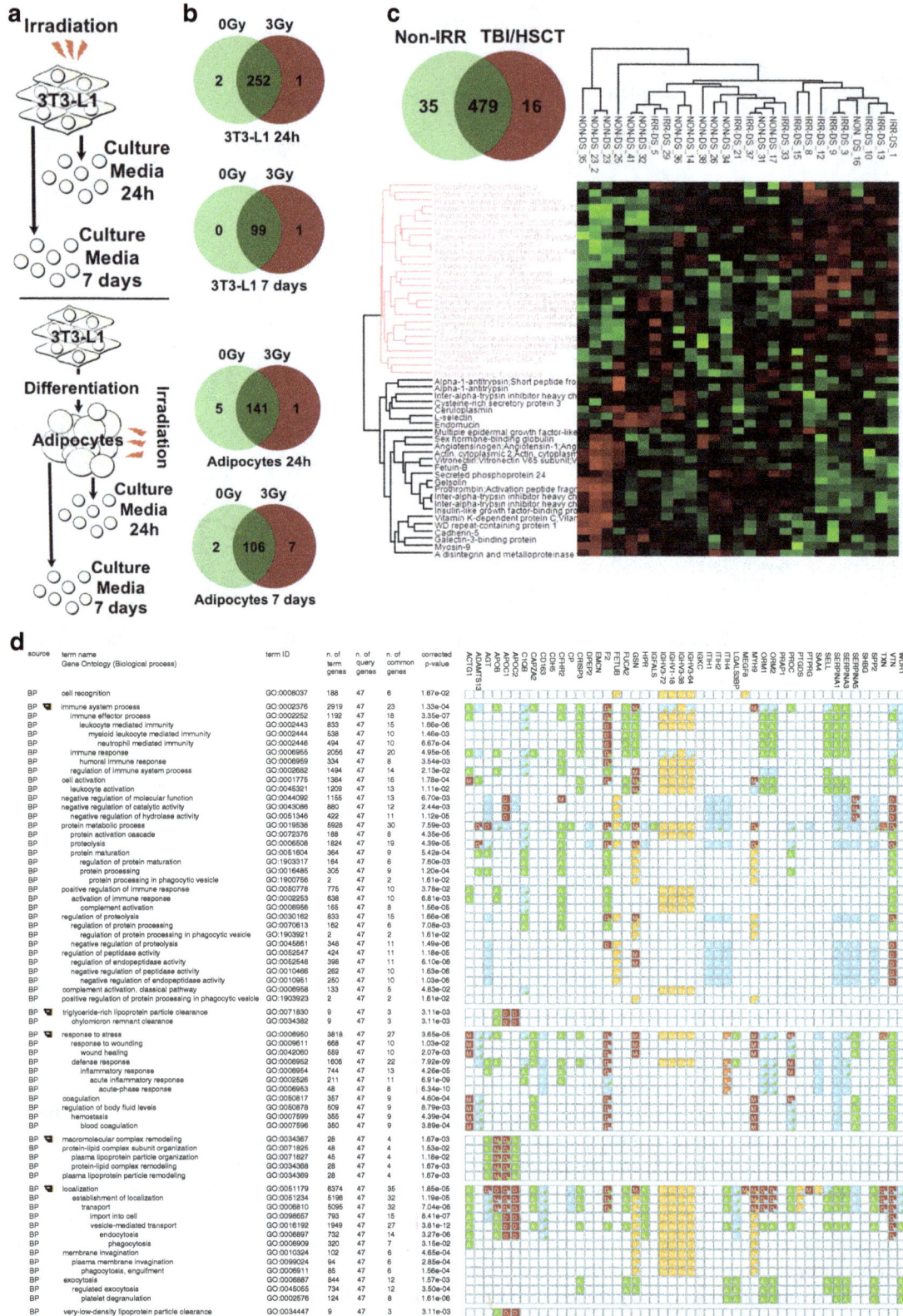

Fig. 4 (See legend on next page.)

(See figure on previous page.)
Fig. 4 Circulating factors involved on the indirect effect of irradiation on T cell function **a**. Schematic representation of the in vitro model to identify circulating factors responsible for the indirect effect of irradiation on T cell function. **b**. Venn diagram representing uniquely identified proteins in culture media from non-irradiated cells (0Gy, light green), from irradiated cells (3Gy, red), or in both conditions (dark green), in four different conditions (undifferentiated and differentiated fibroblasts at 24 h and seven days post-irradiation). **c**. Venn diagram representing uniquely identified proteins in plasma from non-irradiated (non-IRR, light green) or TBI/HSCT-treated survivors (TBI/HSCT, red), or found in both groups (dark green). Unsupervised hierarchical cluster analysis of protein abundance identifying specific patterns of proteins abundance profile in the two groups of survivors. **d**. Gene ontology analysis performed on proteins showing a different pattern of abundance between the two groups of survivors. S: Sequence or structural similarity [ISS]; Ba: biological aspect of ancestor [IBA]; A: traceable author [TAS]; e: electronic annotation [IEA]; D: direct assay [IDA]; M: mutant phenotype [IMP]; G: genetic interaction [IGI]; a: non-traceable author [NAS]; X: expression pattern [IEP]

the predicted biological age reflect the age of the donor as previously suggested [21]. However, we did not find any difference between the donors' and the recipients' chronological age (Fig. 1f). In addition, the inclusion of the donors' age in the model did not change the correlation between chronological and predicted age (Fig. 1f), suggesting that TBI/HSCT could be responsible for the accelerated epigenetic aging in T cell. When we compared the methylation levels on three specific CpG sites used to establish the Epigenetic-Aging-Signature, we found a hypermethylation only on *PDE4C* in the TBI/HSCT group ($p > 0.05$ for *ASPA* and *ITGA*, $p < 0.01$ for *PDE4C*, Additional file 1: Figure S1c). Consistent with the Epigenetic-Aging-Signature, transcriptomic analysis of T cells showed that more than 10% of differentially expressed genes belonged to the "innate and adaptive immunity, cytokine, and chemokine" cluster of genes, which constitutes genes previously reported to contribute to the aging signature of peripheral blood (Additional file 1: Table S3A) [22]. The present results support a role for cancer treatment in the accelerated aging of T cell in cancer survivors.

Multiple reports have suggested an increased prevalence of inflammatory diseases in cancer survivors. We thus investigated the presence of cardio-metabolic risk factors in our cohort. Consistent with previous studies [3, 7], CCS treated with TBI/HSCT had impaired metabolic profile, including increased triglycerides and reduced high-density lipoprotein cholesterol (HDL-C) levels ($p < 0.05$, Table 1). Importantly, these changes were not due to a difference in age, age at diagnosis, body mass index (BMI), or waist-to-hip ratio ($p > 0.05$, Table 1). The level of insulin resistance was also higher in the TBI/HSCT group ($p = 0.04$, Table 1), while fasting blood glucose and insulin levels also tended to be higher in that group ($p = 0.1$ and $p = 0.07$ respectively; Table 1). These results confirm that CCS, in particular those who received TBI/HSCT, are at increased cardio-metabolic risks with a potential link with chronic inflammation.

Discussion

Our results suggest that cancer treatment stably remodels the T cell epigenome at specific genes controlling

inflammation and oxidative stress in CCS. Using various markers of immune cell function and signaling pathways regulating pro-inflammatory cytokines production, we establish a link between T cell epigenetic remodeling and low-grade inflammation in survivors, in particular those who received TBI/HSCT. We identified that TBI/HSCT is associated with accelerated aging and propose a role for epigenetic changes in the elevated risk of age- and inflammation-related diseases long after treatment in CCS [23].

We found that CCS treated with TBI/HSCT are characterized by systemic inflammation. The secretion of cytokines by immune cells is regulated by epigenetic mechanisms [24]. Our global DNA methylation analysis of T cell from survivors supports a dramatic remodeling of the epigenome after TBI/HSCT. Radiation-induced long-term epigenetic changes have been reported in cultured human keratinocytes and rodents [25, 26] and could mediate the imprinting of a long-term "memory" of the radiation insult, potentially affecting immune cell function. HSCT has also been associated with an inflammatory response, although limited information regarding its long-term effect has been reported [16]. Nonetheless, it can be hypothesized that even sub-clinical levels of graft-versus-host disease could have contributed to the immune changes reported here. We have previously shown that the epigenome of lymphocytes is linked to environmental influences, notably nutritional [27, 28]. Epigenetic mechanisms including changes in DNA methylation, histone modifications, or even miRNAs are well-described as modulators of immune cell differentiation and function [29, 30]. For example, differentiation and polarized activation of T helper or cytotoxic cells are controlled by global DNA methylation at particular gene loci [31, 32]. Although we did not observe specific changes at previously reported gene loci, we identified several differentially methylated genes involved in critical pathways controlling T cell differentiation or cytokine production. It cannot be ruled out that by investigating epigenetic changes in global CD4$^+$ T cell, we might have missed DNA methylation changes specific to effector, memory, or regulatory T cell [31, 32]. In addition, these T cell subtypes present different epigenetic signature [31,

32]. Thus, our results could also suggest changes in the distribution of T cell subsets.

We found a greater frequency of type 1 cytokine-producing T cell in irradiated survivors, with these cells showing higher activation of p38 MAP kinase pathway and mTOR Complex 1 (mTORC1) signaling (S6 k1), potentially through a bystander effect. Direct and indirect exposure to ionizing radiation activate MAPKs (p38/JNK) and the PI3K (phosphoinositide 3-kinase)/Akt/mTOR pathways [12, 33], and both p38 and mTORC1 are critical for Th1 polarization and type 1 cytokines production [34, 35]. The over-activation of both p38 and mTORC1 is consistent with the greater frequency of Th1 cells and the higher levels of pro-inflammatory cytokines in survivors who received TBI/HSCT. The response to radiation involves the mobilization of immune cells and pro-inflammatory cytokine production, although these immune changes usually resolve within hours to days upon exposure [36]. Similarly, HSCT can be associated with an inflammatory response, though the long-term consequences remain unclear [16]. Delayed or chronic immune activation after radiation has been reported in atomic bomb survivors more than 50 years after exposure [37]. Impaired immune function has also been reported up to 10 years following radiation in long-term cancer survivors [15], although in both cases, the molecular mechanisms were not identified. Our results suggest that such immune changes could result from an indirect effect of irradiation, potentially due to circulating factors. This bystander effect has been previously suggested as playing a key role in the adaptations following irradiation [12]. Although we could not identify specific factors driving the epigenetic remodeling and altered immune function, it is likely that such factors might contribute to these phenomena [12]. We can speculate that the observed changes in the T cell methylome and T cell function could be involved in the perpetuation of the cancer treatment-induced pro-inflammatory programming. Limitations associated with our in vitro model to investigate the direct effect of irradiation, in particular the absence of the regulator of the Akt/mTOR pathway Phosphatase and TENsin homolog (PTEN) in Jurkat cells, forces us to caution when interpreting our results using this cell system. Further work is needed using other cell models to fully clarify the influence of irradiation on the epigenome.

Inflammation and oxidative stress are associated with several processes involved in aging [38]. Recently, changes in both the epigenome and the transcriptome of circulating leukocytes have been linked to the biological (rather than chronological) age of an individual [22, 39]. A marked remodeling of the epigenome encompassing global DNA hypomethylation and gene-specific hypermethylation at particular loci has been reported during aging [38], consistent with the hypomethylation we observed in T helper cells at the global DNA level. At the gene level, particular loci or even CpG sites have been identified as predictive markers of biological age [39] and allowed us to identify an increased predicted biological age in cancer survivors. Several components of the radiation response can contribute to accelerated aging or inflammatory diseases, including low-grade systemic inflammation, activation of MAPK/mTOR signaling, epigenetic remodeling, or oxidative stress [12, 33, 38, 40, 41]. In the present study, we identified the presence of such disturbances in cancer survivors more than 10 years post-treatment, which potentially explains the accelerated aging reported in this population [23]. We and others have previously shown that both reactive oxygen species and pro-inflammatory cytokines can affect DNA methylation [42, 43]. We can speculate that the initial inflammatory response and oxidative burst in response to treatment might have contributed to the epigenetic remodeling of immune cells, although the timing and nature of the events that might have led to this "long-term memory" are still to be unraveled. These changes in the T cell methylome might be involved in the perpetuation of the pro-inflammatory programming contributing to the early onset of cardio-metabolic complications in cancer survivors.

Conclusions

Improvements in childhood cancer survival are associated with higher prevalence of treatment-associated diseases later in life, notably of age-related conditions including cardiometabolic diseases. We identified low-grade inflammation and altered immune cell function in survivors treated with TBI/HSCT. This was associated with a dramatic remodeling of the T cell epigenetic signature and features of accelerated epigenetic aging. These immune changes could account for the increased risk of inflammatory and age-associated diseases later in life. A greater understanding of the mechanisms by which cancer treatments affect the epigenome of immune cells may help to decrease long-term complications in cancer survivors.

Methods
Participants
We recruited 44 childhood cancer survivors, diagnosed between 0 and 18 years, in full remission for more than 5 years and 16 years old and older at the time of enrolment. Survivors who had experienced graft-versus-host disease were not included in this study. This project was approved by the Human Research Ethics Committee (UNSW Sydney, HREC-10/017) and performed in accordance with Helsinki Declaration procedures. The nature of the project was explained and participants provided informed consent. Participants had received chemotherapy only (non-IRR) or a combination of chemotherapy with

TBI and HSCT (TBI/HSCT). Anthropometric data and medical history were recorded and BMI calculated.

Biological analyses

Fasting blood samples were collected and stored at − 80 °C. Serum insulin (Immulite 2000, Diagnostic Products Corporation, CA, USA), glucose levels, HDL-C, low-density lipoprotein cholesterol (LDL-C), and triglycerides were measured (LX20 analyzer, Beckman Coulter, CA, USA), and the insulin resistance index was calculated (Homeostasis Model Assessment, HOMA-IR) [44]. Systemic cytokine levels including IL-2, IL-4, IL-5, IL-10, IL-12, IL-13, IFN-γ, TNF-α, and granulocyte-monocyte colony stimulating factor were measured (Bio-Plex Pro Human Cytokine Th1/Th2 Assay, Bio-Rad Laboratories Inc., Australia, Intra-assay CV: 7–12% and Inter-assay CV: 6–10%). Results were reported only for cytokines that were detectable in more than 30% of the participants.

Flow cytometry

Peripheral blood mononuclear cells (PBMCs) were isolated from whole blood and cryopreserved [28]. PBMCs were thawed, left to recover overnight, and mitogen-stimulated for 6 h (2 µg/ml phorbol 12-myristate 13-acetate/ionomycin, Sigma-Aldrich, Australia), with the addition of monensin (BioLegend, CA, USA) after 2 h. PBMCs were then fixed (2% paraformaldehyde), stained for dead cells (ethidium monoazide bromide, Sigma-Aldrich), and permeabilized in ice-cold methanol. Cells were then stained using CD4-V500, CD-PE-Cy7, IL-4-PE, IFN-γ-Pacific blue (BD Biosciences, Australia), and phosphorylated pAkt-Ser473-AF647 (BD Biosciences), pS6k1-AF488, pJNK-AF488, and phosphorylated p38-AF647 (Cell Signaling Technology, MA, USA). PBMCs were analyzed on FACS CantoII (BD Biosciences), with data post-compensated and analyzed using FlowJo (Tree Star Inc., OR, USA). Results were expressed as percentage of IL-4⁺/IFN-γ⁺ cells or normalized median fluorescence intensity for pAkt, pS6k1, pJNK, and p-p38 in CD4⁺ and CD8⁺ cells.

In vitro and co-culture models

Jurkat cells (Clone E6–1, ATCC, VA, USA) were irradiated with doses of 0, 1, 3, or 6Gy (Xrad 320, Precision X-ray Inc., CT, USA) and left to recover for 24 h. At days 1, 14, and 28, post-irradiation cells were mitogen-stimulated and analyzed by flow cytometry as described above. Adipocytes (3 T3-L1, CL-173, ATCC) were irradiated with doses of 0, 1, 3, and 6Gy and left to recover for 24 h prior to the collection of culture media. PBMCs from six young healthy donors were mitogen-stimulated in conditioned media from irradiated adipocytes and analyzed by flow cytometry as described above.

Protein sample preparation and mass spectrometry

Plasma samples (14ul) from childhood cancer survivors were depleted from the 14 most abundant proteins (Sigma Seppro IgY14 Spin columns). Depleted plasma sample and conditioned media from cultured fibroblasts and fibroblasts differentiated into adipocytes (only 0/3Gy and at 24 h/7 days post-irradiation) were processed as previously described with slight modifications (see "Additional file 1") [45]. A survey scan m/z 350–1750 was acquired in the Orbitrap and lock mass enabled with data-dependent tandem MS analysis performed using a top-speed approach (cycle time of 2 s). MS² spectra were fragmented by HCD activation mode and the ion trap was selected as the mass analyzer. Peak lists were generated using Mascot Daemon and submitted to Mascot (version 2.5.1, Matrix Science). Label-free quantitation was carried out using MaxQuant (version 1.5.6.5) and Perseus (version 1.5.6.0) and pathway analysis using G-Profiler.

Epigenetic analyses

Global DNA methylation

Global DNA methylation was measured in PBMCs, using surface markers (CD3-PE, CD4, or CD21-APC, CD8, or CD14-PerCP, BD Biosciences) and anti-5-methylcytidine antibody (AbD Serotec, Bio-Rad) conjugated to AF488 (Zenon AF488 Mouse IgG1 labeling kit, Life Technologies, Australia) as previously described [28].

Gene-specific methylation

PBMCs were sorted on Influx Cell Sorter (BD Biosciences) using specific surface markers (CD4 and CD19/CD20-BV421, CD8-BV510, CD3-FITC, CD56-PE-CF594, CD45-PerCP-Cy5.5, and CD14-APC, BD Biosciences). Cells were then lysed before DNA/RNA extraction (AllPrep DNA/RNA/miRNA Universal kit on QIAcube, Qiagen, Australia). CD4⁺ T cell DNA was processed using reduced representation bisulfite sequencing with minor changes [46]. Genomic DNA was fragmented by overnight incubation with Msp1 restriction enzyme and adenylated with dATP and Klenow DNA polymerase (3′ to 5′ exo minus) before ligation to TruSeq adapters (Illumina, CA, USA). Twelve ligated samples were pooled and processed for bisulfite conversion using EZ DNA methylation kit (Zymo Research, CA, USA). Libraries were enriched by PCR, purified with AMPure beads, and sequenced on a HiSeq (50 bp single-end sequencing, Illumina, Danish National High-Throughput DNA Sequencing Centre, Denmark). Preprocessed reads were aligned to hg38 with Bismark [47], and differential methylation was analyzed with MethylKit [48]. All regions were annotated with the Bioconductor package ChIPseeker [49]. CpGs with more than 25% methylation change and q value < 0.01 were included for further analysis. Gene Ontology (GO) analysis was performed using a hypergeometric test on individual

CpGs and scatter plots generated with REVIGO [50]. T cell-specific enhancers were downloaded from SlideBase [51, 52] and lifted to hg38 using the UCSC liftOver tool [53], before counting overlaps with DMRs.

Epigenetic-Aging-Signature

DNA methylation was measured on sorted CD8$^+$ T cell at three specific CpG sites (*ASPA*, *ITGA2B*, and *PDE4C*) by bisulfite pyrosequencing. Beta values were then used in a multivariate model to estimate the predicted biological age as previously described [39].

Whole transcriptome sequencing

RNA from CD4$^+$ T cell was sequenced following standard protocol (Truseq Stranded total RNA protocol, Illumina). After depletion of ribosomal RNA and fragmentation, cDNA synthesis was performed on the first strand, followed by second strand synthesis. cDNA was cleaned using AMPure beads, adenylated and then ligated to adapters. Following an additional beads cleanup, DNA fragments were enriched by PCR and subjected to a final beads cleanup. Libraries were sequenced on a HiSeq (100 bp single-end sequencing, Illumina, Danish National High-Throughput DNA Sequencing Centre). Reads were aligned to hg38 using Rsubread aligner, and the number of reads aligning with Gencode (version 23) was counted with featureCounts [54]. Genes with less than 1 RPKM in half the samples were excluded. Differential expression was calculated with edgeR [55] using glmFit/glmLRT functions and tagwise dispersion, with correction for multiple testing using the Benjamini–Hochberg procedure. GO analysis was performed using GOrilla [56], and scatter plots were generated with REVIGO [50].

Statistical analysis

Data are expressed as mean +/− standard deviation and analyzed using SPSS Statistics (IBM, NY, USA). Normality of the distribution was tested using the Skewness and Kurtosis tests and anthropometric data, biological markers, cytokines levels, T cell polarization, and global DNA methylation or predicted age were compared using Student *t* test or Mann-Whitney *U* test. A chi-square test was used to compare the frequencies between the two groups. The effect of irradiation/mitogen stimulation on intracellular signaling was tested using two-way ANOVA for repeated measures or a combination of Friedman's ANOVA and Mann-Whitney *U* test. Correlation levels were tested using the Pearson or Spearman tests.

Acknowledgements

The authors are grateful to all the participants who contributed to the study. They also thank Dr. Barbara Cameron for her assistance with the Multiplex assay and Dr. Chris Brownly for his assistance with the flow cytometry and cell sorting experiments at the Biological Resources Imaging Laboratory (Flow Cytometry Facility, UNSW Australia, Australia). We would like to acknowledge The Danish National High-Throughput DNA Sequencing Centre for the sequencing.

Funding

This work was supported by a grant from the Cancer Institute New South Wales (09/RFG/2-21) to R.J. Cohn and D. Simar, an International Postgraduate Research Scholarship from UNSW Sydney to S. Daniel, and a research grant from the Danish Diabetes Academy supported by the Novo Nordisk Foundation to O. Fabre. The Novo Nordisk Foundation Center for Basic Metabolic Research is an independent Research Center at the University of Copenhagen partially funded by an unrestricted donation from the Novo Nordisk Foundation.

Authors' contributions

DS, RB, and RJC designed the study. SD, VN, LZ, OF, BC, KJ, RB, and DS collected and assembled the data. SD, VN, LRI, LZ, OF, BC, KJ, RJC, RB, and DS analyzed and interpreted the data. DS drafted the manuscript, and all authors contributed and approved the final manuscript.

Author details

[1]Mechanisms of Disease and Translational Research, School of Medical Sciences, UNSW Sydney, Wallace Wurth Building East Room 420, Sydney, NSW 2052, Australia. [2]The Novo Nordisk Foundation Center for Basic Metabolic Research, Faculty of Health and Medical Sciences, Panum, University of Copenhagen, 2200 Copenhagen N, Denmark. [3]Bioanalytical Mass Spectrometry Facility, Mark Wainwright Analytical Centre, UNSW Sydney, Sydney, Australia. [4]School of Women's and Children's Health, UNSW Sydney and Kids Cancer Centre, Sydney Children's Hospital Network, Randwick, Australia.

References

1. Coleman M, Forman D, Bryant H, Butler J, Rachet B, Maringe C, Nur U, Tracey E, Coory M, Hatcher J, et al. Cancer survival in Australia, Canada, Denmark, Norway, Sweden, and the UK, 1995–2007 (the International Cancer Benchmarking Partnership): an analysis of population-based cancer registry data. Lancet. 2011;377:127–38.
2. Hudson MM, Ness KK, Gurney JG, Mulrooney DA, Chemaitilly W, Krull KR, Green DM, Armstrong GT, Nottage KA, Jones KE, et al. Clinical ascertainment of health outcomes among adults treated for childhood cancer. JAMA. 2013;309:2371–81.
3. Diller L, Chow EJ, Gurney JG, Hudson MM, Kadin-Lottick NS, Kawashima TI, Leisenring WM, Meacham LR, Mertens AC, Mulrooney DA, et al. Chronic disease in the Childhood Cancer Survivor Study cohort: a review of published findings. J Clin Oncol. 2009;27:2339–55.
4. Ehrhardt MJ, Mulrooney DA. Metabolic syndrome in adult survivors of childhood cancer: the intersection of oncology, endocrinology, and cardiology. Lancet Diabetes Endocrinol. 2015;3:494–6.

5. Smith WA, Li C, Nottage KA, Mulrooney DA, Armstrong GT, Lanctot JQ, Chemaitilly W, Laver JH, Srivastava DK, Robison LL, et al. Lifestyle and metabolic syndrome in adult survivors of childhood cancer: a report from the St. Jude Lifetime Cohort Study. Cancer. 2014;120:2742–50.

6. Meacham LR, Sklar CA, Li S, Liu Q, Gimpel N, Yasui Y, Whitton JA, Stovall M, Robison LL, Oeffinger KC. Diabetes mellitus in long-term survivors of childhood cancer. Increased risk associated with radiation therapy: a report for the childhood cancer survivor study. Arch Intern Med. 2009;169:1381–8.

7. Neville KA, Cohn RJ, Steinbeck KS, Johnston K, Walker JL. Hyperinsulinemia, impaired glucose tolerance, and diabetes mellitus in survivors of childhood cancer: prevalence and risk factors. J Clin Endocrinol Metab. 2006;91:4401–7.

8. Nylander V, Ingerslev LR, Andersen E, Fabre O, Garde C, Rasmussen M, Citirikkaya K, Bæk J, Christensen GL, Aznar M, et al. Ionizing radiation potentiates high-fat diet-induced insulin resistance and reprograms skeletal muscle and adipose progenitor cells. Diabetes. 2016;65:3573–84.

9. Geng S, Chen K, Yuan R, Peng L, Maitra U, Diao N, Chen C, Zhang Y, Hu Y, Qi C-F, et al. The persistence of low-grade inflammatory monocytes contributes to aggravated atherosclerosis. Nat Commun. 2016;7:13436.

10. Winer DA, Winer S, Shen L, Wadia PP, Yantha J, Paltser G, Tsui H, Wu P, Davidson MG, Alonso MN, et al. B cells promote insulin resistance through modulation of T cells and production of pathogenic IgG antibodies. Nat Med. 2011;17:610–7.

11. Coates PJ, Lorimore SA, Wright EG. Damaging and protective cell signalling in the untargeted effects of ionizing radiation. Mutat Res. 2004;568:5–20.

12. Formenti SC, Demaria S. Systemic effects of local radiotherapy. Lancet Oncol. 2009;10:718–26.

13. Apetoh L, Ghiringhelli F, Tesniere A, Obeid M, Ortiz C, Criollo A, Mignot G, Maiuri MC, Ullrich E, Saulnier P, et al. Toll-like receptor 4–dependent contribution of the immune system to anticancer chemotherapy and radiotherapy. Nat Med. 2007;13:1050–9.

14. Stoecklein VM, Osuka A, Ishikawa S, Lederer MR, Wanke-Jellinek L, Lederer JA. Radiation exposure induces inflammasome pathway activation in immune cells. J Immunol. 2015;194:1178–89.

15. Fuks Z, Strober S, Bobrove A, Sasazuki T, McMichael A, Kaplan H. Long term effects of radiation of T and B lymphocytes in peripheral blood of patients with Hodgkin's disease. J Clin Invest. 1976;58:803.

16. Neven B, Leroy S, Decaluwe H, Le Deist F, Picard C, Moshous D, Mahlaoui N, Debre M, Casanova JL, Dal Cortivo L, et al. Long-term outcome after hematopoietic stem cell transplantation of a single-center cohort of 90 patients with severe combined immunodeficiency. Blood. 2009;113:4114–24.

17. Chow EJ, Simmons JH, Roth CL, Baker KS, Hoffmeister PA, Sanders JE, Friedman DL. Increased cardiometabolic traits in pediatric survivors of acute lymphoblastic leukemia treated with total body irradiation. Biol Blood Marrow Transplant. 2010;16:1674–81.

18. Chaudhry MA, Omaruddin RA, Brumbaugh CD, Tariq MA, Pourmand N. Identification of radiation-induced microRNA transcriptome by next-generation massively parallel sequencing. Jo Radiat Res. 2013;54:808–22.

19. Jiang S, Li C, McRae G, Lykken E, Sevilla J, Liu S-Q, Wan Y, Li Q-J. MeCP2 reinforces STAT3 signaling and the generation of effector CD4+ T cells by promoting miR-124-mediated suppression of SOCS5. Sci Signal. 2014;7:ra25.

20. Pott GB, Chan ED, Dinarello CA, Shapiro L. α-1-Antitrypsin is an endogenous inhibitor of proinflammatory cytokine production in whole blood. J Leukoc Biol. 2009;85:886–95.

21. Weidner CI, Ziegler P, Hahn M, Brummendorf TH, Ho AD, Dreger P, Wagner W. Epigenetic aging upon allogeneic transplantation: the hematopoietic niche does not affect age-associated DNA methylation. Leukemia. 2015;29:985–8.

22. Peters MJ, Joehanes R, Pilling LC, Schurmann C, Conneely KN, Powell J, Reinmaa E, Sutphin GL, Zhernakova A, Schramm K, et al. The transcriptional landscape of age in human peripheral blood. Nat Commun. 2015;6:8570.

23. Ness KK, Krull KR, Jones KE, Mulrooney DA, Armstrong GT, Green DM, Chemaitilly W, Smith WA, Wilson CL, Sklar CA, et al. Physiologic frailty as a sign of accelerated aging among adult survivors of childhood cancer: a report from the St Jude Lifetime Cohort Study. J Clin Oncol. 2013;31:4496–503.

24. Raghuraman S, Donkin I, Versteyhe S, Barrès R, Simar D. The emerging role of epigenetics in inflammation and immunometabolism. Trends Endocrinol Metab. 2016;27:782–95.

25. Koturbash I, Boyko A, Rodriguez-Juarez R, McDonald RJ, Tryndyak VP, Kovalchuk I, Pogribny IP, Kovalchuk O. Role of epigenetic effectors in maintenance of the long-term persistent bystander effect in spleen in vivo. Carcinogenesis. 2007;28:1831 8.

26. Kaup S, Kaup S, Grandjean V, Grandjean V, Mukherjee R, Mukherjee R, Kapoor A, Kapoor A, Keyes E, Keyes E, et al. Radiation-induced genomic instability is associated with DNA methylation changes in cultured human keratinocytes. Mutat Res. 2006;597:87–97.

27. Jacobsen MJ, Mentzel CMJ, Olesen AS, Huby T, Jorgensen CB, Barrès R, Fredholm M, Simar D. Altered methylation profile of lymphocytes is concordant with perturbation of lipids metabolism and inflammatory response in obesity. J Diabetes Res. 2016;2016:8539057.

28. Simar D, Versteyhe S, Donkin I, Liu J, Hesson L, Nylander V, Fossum A, Barrès R. DNA methylation is altered in B and NK lymphocytes in obese and type 2 diabetic human. Metabolism. 2014;63:1188–97.

29. Busslinger M, Tarakhovsky A. Epigenetic control of immunity. Cold Spring Harb Perspect Biol. 2014;6:a019307-a.

30. Kirchner H, Nylen C, Laber S, Barres R, Yan J, Krook A, Zierath JR, Naslund E. Altered promoter methylation of PDK4, IL1 B, IL6, and TNF after Roux-en Y gastric bypass. Surg Obes Relat Dis. 2014;10:671–8.

31. Mullen AC, Hutchins AS, High FA, Lee HW, Sykes KJ, Chodosh LA, Reiner SL. Hlx is induced by and genetically interacts with T-bet to promote heritable TH1 gene induction. Nat Immunol. 2002;3:652–8.

32. Lee DU, Agarwal S, Rao A. Th2 lineage commitment and efficient IL-4 production involves extended demethylation of the IL-4 gene. Immunity. 2002;16:649–60.

33. Multhoff G, Radons J. Radiation, inflammation, and immune responses in cancer. Front Oncol. 2012;2:58.

34. Waickman AT, Powell JD. mTOR, metabolism, and the regulation of T-cell differentiation and function. Immunol Rev. 2012;249:43–58.

35. Rincón M, Davis RJ. Regulation of the immune response by stress-activated protein kinases. Immunol Rev. 2009;228:212–24.

36. Shan Y-X, Jin S-Z, Liu X-D, Liu Y, Liu S-Z. Ionizing radiation stimulates secretion of pro-inflammatory cytokines: dose–response relationship, mechanisms and implications. Radiat Environ Biophys. 2006;46:21–9.

37. Kusunoki Y, Yamaoka M, Kubo Y, Hayashi T, Kasagi F, Douple EB, Nakachi K. T-cell immunosenescence and inflammatory response in atomic bomb survivors. Radiat Res. 2010;174:870–6.

38. López-Otín C, Blasco MA, Partridge L, Serrano M, Kroemer G. The hallmarks of aging. Cell. 2013;153:1194–217.

39. Weidner CI, Lin Q, Koch CM, Eisele L, Beier F, Ziegler P, Bauerschlag DO, ckel K-HJ, Erbel R, hleisen TWM, et al. Aging of blood can be tracked by DNA methylation changes at just three CpG sites. Genome Biol. 2014;15:R24.

40. Datta K, Suman S, Fornace J, Albert J. Radiation persistently promoted oxidative stress, activated mTOR via PI3K/Akt, and downregulated autophagy pathway in mouse intestine. Int J Biochem Cell Biol. 2014;57:167–76.

41. Kuzmina NS, Lapteva NS, Rubanovich AV. Hypermethylation of gene promoters in peripheral blood leukocytes in humans long term after radiation exposure. Environ Res. 2016;146:10–7.

42. Barrès R, Osler ME, Yan J, Rune A, Fritz T, Caidahl K, Krook A, Zierath JR. Non-CpG methylation of the PGC-1alpha promoter through DNMT3B controls mitochondrial density. Cell Metab. 2009;10:189–98.

43. Li Y, Gorelik G, Strickland FM, Richardson BC. Oxidative Stress, T cell DNA methylation, and lupus. Arthritis Rheumatol. 2014;66:1574–82.

44. Wallace TM, Levy JC, Matthews DR. Use and abuse of HOMA modeling. Diabetes Care. 2004;27:1487–95.

45. Unnikrishnan A, Guan YF, Huang Y, Beck D, Thoms JAI, Peirs S, Knezevic K, Ma S, de Walle IV, de Jong I, et al. A quantitative proteomics approach identifies ETV6 and IKZF1 as new regulators of an ERG-driven transcriptional network. Nucleic Acids Res. 2016;44:10644–61.

46. Gu H, Smith ZD, Bock C, Boyle P, Gnirke A, Meissner A. Preparation of reduced representation bisulfite sequencing libraries for genome-scale DNA methylation profiling. Nat Protoc. 2011;6:468–81.

47. Krueger F, Andrews SR. Bismark: a flexible aligner and methylation caller for Bisulfite-Seq applications. Bioinformatics. 2011;27:1571–2.

48. Akalin A, Kormaksson M, Li S, Garrett-Bakelman FE, Figueroa ME, Melnick A, Mason CE. methylKit: a comprehensive R package for the analysis of genome-wide DNA methylation profiles. Genome Biol. 2012;13:R87.

49. Yu G, Wang L-G, He Q-Y. ChIPseeker: an R/Bioconductor package for ChIP peak annotation, comparison and visualization. Bioinformatics. 2015;31:2382–3.

50. Supek F, Bošnjak M, Škunca N, Šmuc T. REVIGO summarizes and visualizes long lists of gene ontology terms. PLoS One. 2011;6:e21800.

51. Andersson R, Gebhard C, Miguel-Escalada I, Hoof I, Bornholdt J, Boyd M, Chen Y, Zhao X, Schmidl C, Suzuki T, et al. An atlas of active enhancers across human cell types and tissues. Nature. 2014;507:455–61.

52. Ienasescu H, Li K, Andersson R, Vitezic M, Rennie S, Chen Y, Vitting-Seerup K, Lagoni E, Boyd M, Bornholdt J, et al. On-the-fly selection of cell-specific enhancers, genes, miRNAs and proteins across the human body using SlideBase. Database. 2016;2016:baw144.

53. Hinrichs AS, Karolchik D, Baertsch R, Barber GP, Bejerano G, Clawson H, Diekhans M, Furey TS, Harte RA, Hsu F, et al. The UCSC Genome Browser Database: update 2006. Nucleic Acids Res. 2006;34:D590–D8.

54. Liao Y, Smyth GK, Shi W. The Subread aligner: fast, accurate and scalable read mapping by seed-and-vote. Nucleic Acids Res. 2013;41:e108-e.

55. Robinson MD, McCarthy DJ, Smyth GK. edgeR: a Bioconductor package for differential expression analysis of digital gene expression data. Bioinformatics. 2009;26:139–40.

56. Eden E, Navon R, Steinfeld I, Lipson D, Yakhini Z. GOrilla: a tool for discovery and visualization of enriched GO terms in ranked gene lists. BMC Bioinformatics. 2009;10:48.

18

A five-DNA methylation signature act as a novel prognostic biomarker in patients with ovarian serous cystadenocarcinoma

Wenna Guo[1†], Liucun Zhu[2†], Minghao Yu[1], Rui Zhu[2], Qihan Chen[1*] and Qiang Wang[1*]

Abstract

Background: Ovarian cancer is the most fatal tumor of the female reproductive system and the fifth leading cause of cancer death among women in the USA. The prognosis is poor due to the lack of biomarkers for treatment options.

Results: The methylation array data of 551 patients with ovarian serous cystadenocarcinoma (OSC) in The Cancer Genome Atlas (TCGA) database were assessed in this study to explore the methylation biomarkers associated with prognosis and improve the prognosis of patients. These patients were divided into training (first two thirds) and validation datasets (remaining one third). A five-DNA methylation signature was found to be significantly associated with the overall survival of patients with OSC using the Cox regression analysis in the training dataset. The Kaplan–Meier analysis showed that the five-DNA methylation signature could significantly distinguish the high- and low-risk patients in both training and validation sets. The receiver operating characteristic (ROC) analysis further confirmed that the five-DNA methylation signature exhibited high sensitivity and specificity to predict the prognostic survival of patients. Also, the five-DNA methylation signature was not only applicable in patients of different ages, stages, histologic grade, and size of residual tumor after surgery but also more accurate in predicting OSC prognosis compared with known biomarkers.

Conclusions: This five-DNA methylation signature demonstrated the potential of being a novel independent prognostic indicator and served as an important tool for guiding the clinical treatment of OSC to improve outcome prediction and management for patients. Hence, the findings of this study might have potential clinical significance.

Keywords: Biomarker, DNA methylation, OSC, Prognosis, Risk stratification

Background

Ovarian cancer is the most lethal cancer of the female reproductive system and the fifth leading cause of cancer death among women in the USA with an estimated 22,240 new cases and 14,070 deaths expected to occur in 2018 [1, 2]. Ovarian serous cystadenocarcinoma (OSC), a common type of ovarian cancer, accounts for about 90% of all ovarian cancers [2]. The standard treatment consists of cytoreductive surgery followed by a combination of platinum- and taxane-based chemotherapy [3]. Although

advances in treatment technology in the last few decades have substantially improved the average survival time, the cure rates remain relatively unchanged [4]. The overall 5-year survival probability of women diagnosed with ovarian cancer is still less than 50% (47%) [1]. Assessment of patients prior to therapy might enable a risk-adapted approach and hence offer an opportunity to provide improved personalized treatment. Physicians can direct low-risk patients to conventional treatments, while high-risk patients can be channeled to trials of novel therapies. This selection may enhance the ability of clinical trials to demonstrate clinical benefits. Therefore, determining high-risk patients with OSC and improving the clinical outcome are urgently needed for current clinical management. The identification of highly specific,

* Correspondence: lyonchenqihan@hotmail.com; wangq@nju.edu.cn
†Wenna Guo and Liucun Zhu contributed equally to this work.
[1]State Key Laboratory of Pharmaceutical Biotechnology, School of Life Sciences, Nanjing University, Nanjing, China
Full list of author information is available at the end of the article

sensitive, and independent predictive prognostic biomarkers that will allow the stratification of care is essential.

DNA methylation is well known to be associated with ovarian cancer and has great potential to serve as a biomarker in screening the disease, monitoring response to therapy, and predicting the prognosis [5, 6]. The methylation of particular subsets of CpG islands may have consequences for specific processes of tumorigenesis [7]. Aberrant DNA methylation occurs commonly in tumors and is recognized as one of the earliest distinguishing molecular characteristic in carcinogenesis [8, 9]. A number of genes have been identified as being hypermethylated or silenced in ovarian cancer [10]. Thus, cancer methylation studies hold great promise in revealing potential biomarkers for improving the survival rate. Using DNA methylation as a biomarker has several advantages over other molecular markers, including the relative stability of DNA methylation both in vivo and ex vivo [11]; need for a smaller amount of tissues to obtain adequate DNA for methylation analysis [12]; and relative accuracy thanks to quantitative assay because DNA methylation measurements can be compared with absolute reference points [13]. An increasing number of reports are available about the potential of DNA methylation as a prognostic biomarker [14]. For instance, patients with higher methylation levels of *ABCA1* have shorter overall survival [10]; hypomethylation of CpG sites within the *MSX1* gene is associated with resistant high-grade serous ovarian cancer [15]; and *OPCML* gene promoter methylation can serve as a useful biomarker for predicting the prognosis of patients with ovarian cancer [5]. However, the use of genome-wide methylation analysis in clinical practice is limited by the large sets of DNA methylation identified and the difficulties in complex statistical analyses. Moreover, the reproducibility of prognostic methylation signature identified is limited by different specimens and the lack of adjustment for major confounding factors [16].

Consequently, the whole-genome methylation profiles of tumor tissues from patients with OSC in The Cancer Genome Atlas (TCGA) database were analyzed in this study to identify DNA methylation biomarkers so as to explore the utility of DNA methylation analysis for cancer prognosis. The potential clinical significance of methylation biomarkers serving as molecular prognostic markers was examined using Kaplan–Meier method and receiver operating characteristic (ROC) analysis. Furthermore, the independence and reproducibility of identified methylation biomarkers in different groups were also investigated.

Results

Clinical characteristics of the patients
All 551 patients in this study were clinically and pathologically diagnosed with OSC. The median age and

median survival of these patients were 60 years (range, 30–89 years) and 1227 days, respectively. The 3-year overall survival (OS) rate of all patients was 51.60%. The clinical stage was defined according to the Federation Internationale des Gynaecologistes et Obstetristes (FIGO) staging system. The tumor histologic grade was assigned according to the World Health Organization criteria. OSC was divided into stages I, II, III, and IV, and the neoplasm histologic grade included G2, G3, and G4. Anatomic neoplasm subdivisions were obtained from different positions, including left, right, and bilateral. Tumor residual diseases were dichotomized into no macroscopic disease, 1–10 mm, 11–20 mm, and > 20 mm. The clinicopathological characteristics of patients are summarized in Table 1.

Identification of DNA methylation markers associated with the OS of patients in the training dataset
The univariate Cox proportional hazard regression analysis (see the "Materials and methods" section) was performed using the methylation levels as variables in the training dataset to identify DNA methylation markers associated with the OS of patients with OSC. As a result, a total of 1630 DNA methylation sites were found to be significantly associated with the OS of patients ($P < 0.05$). Subsequently, multivariate Cox regression, stepwise regression, and screening were performed for these 1282 DNA methylation sites, and a hazard ratio model consisting of 5 methylation sites (cg05254747, cg13652336, cg25123470, cg06038133, and cg04907664) was identified as the optimum prognostic model for predicting the OS of patients. In this model, these 5 methylation sites were all significantly ($P < 0.05$) associated with the OS of patients. The risk scoring formula of these 5 methylation sites was obtained: Risk score = $- 1.034 \times \beta$ value of cg05254747 + $2.433 \times \beta$ value of cg13652336 + $1.552 \times \beta$ value of cg25123470 + $2.284 \times \beta$ value of cg06038133 − $1.030 \times \beta$ value of cg04907664. Obviously, the hypermethylation levels of cg13652336, cg25123470, and cg06038133 were associated with a higher risk, whereas the hypomethylation levels of cg05254747 and cg04907664 were associated with a higher risk. The corresponding gene symbol of these 5 sites was *SLC39A14*, *PREX2*, *KCNIP2*, *CORO6*, and *EFNB1*, respectively. The chromosomal locations of these 5 methylation sites and related log-rank test *P* values are shown in Additional file 1: Table S1.

Association between five-DNA methylation signature and patient OS in the training and validation datasets
Hazard ratios (HRs) from the Cox regression analysis indicated that the five-DNA methylation signature was significantly associated with the OS of patients ($P < 0.001$, HR 2.72, 95% CI 2.03–3.65). The Kaplan–Meier analysis was performed in the training and validation datasets to determine the potential predictive value of this five-DNA

Table 1 Clinicopathological characteristics of OSC patients from TCGA

Characteristics	Groups	Patients					
		Total ($N = 551$)		Training dataset ($N = 368$)		Validation dataset ($N = 183$)	
		No.	%	No.	%	No.	%
Age at diagnosis	Median	59		60		59	
	Range	26–89		34–87		30–89	
	< 60	286	50.44	187	50.95	104	63.41
	≥ 60	265	46.74	182	49.59	79	48.17
FIGO stage	I	15	2.65	5	1.36	10	6.10
	II	27	4.76	12	3.27	15	9.15
	III	423	74.60	287	78.20	136	82.93
	IV	82	14.46	62	16.89	20	12.20
	Unknown	4	0.71	2	0.54	2	1.22
Histologic grade*	G2	69	12.17	25	6.81	44	26.83
	G3	478	84.30	341	92.92	137	83.54
	G4	1	0.18	1	0.27	0	0.00
	Others	3	0.53	1	0.27	2	1.22
Tumor residual (mm)	No macroscopic disease	116	20.46	67	18.26	49	29.88
	1–10	244	43.03	191	52.04	53	32.32
	11–20	33	5.82	16	4.36	17	10.37
	> 20	105	18.52	64	17.44	41	25.00
	Unknown	53	9.35	33	8.99	25	15.24
Anatomic subdivision	Bilateral	383	67.55	253	68.94	130	79.27
	Left	78	13.76	55	14.99	23	14.02
	Right	62	10.93	40	10.90	22	13.41
	Unknown	28	4.94	20	5.45	8	4.88

*G1 and GB/GX were excluded in this study as these tumors may have a different biological behavior

methylation signature in the prognosis. The five-DNA methylation signature was assigned to each patient in the high-risk ($N = 174$) or the low-risk ($N = 174$) group in the training dataset using the median of prognostic risk scores as the cutoff point. The mean OS in the high-risk and low-risk groups was 1080 days and 1499 days, respectively. The patients in the high-risk group had a significantly ($P < 0.001$) worse prognosis (Fig. 1a). A similar result was observed in the validation dataset (Fig. 1b). These results showed that the novel five-DNA methylation signature could distinguish high-risk patients from low-risk patients, implying its significance in the prognostic prediction of OSC. Meanwhile, the individual methylation levels of these five methylation sites in patients in the high- and low-risk groups were analyzed. As a result, high-risk patients exhibited significantly lower methylation levels for cg05254747 and cg04907664 and significantly higher methylation levels for the other three methylation sites in both training (Fig. 1c) and validation datasets (Additional file 1: Figure S1) ($P < 0.01$, Mann–Whitney U test), which were consistent with the previous results.

Evaluation of the predictive performance of the five-DNA methylation signature using ROC analysis

The sensitivity and specificity of the five-DNA methylation signature in predicting survival were evaluated using the ROC analysis to further assess the predictive accuracy of the five-DNA methylation signature in the validation dataset. The AUC of the five-DNA methylation signature was 0.715 ($P < 0.001$, 95% CI 0.62–0.81) (Fig. 2), indicating that the five-DNA methylation signature had high sensitivity and specificity. Therefore, it could be used to predict the prognostic survival of patients with OSC with high accuracy, and it might have potentially great significance in clinical application.

Predictive performance of the five-DNA methylation signature based on different regrouping methods

Furthermore, several factors were associated with prognostic survival, including age [1, 17], stage [18], histologic grade [19], and size of residual tumor after cytoreductive surgery [20], and the reproducibility was poor in the prognostic markers identified by different groups [5]. Regrouping was carried out based on different clinicopathological

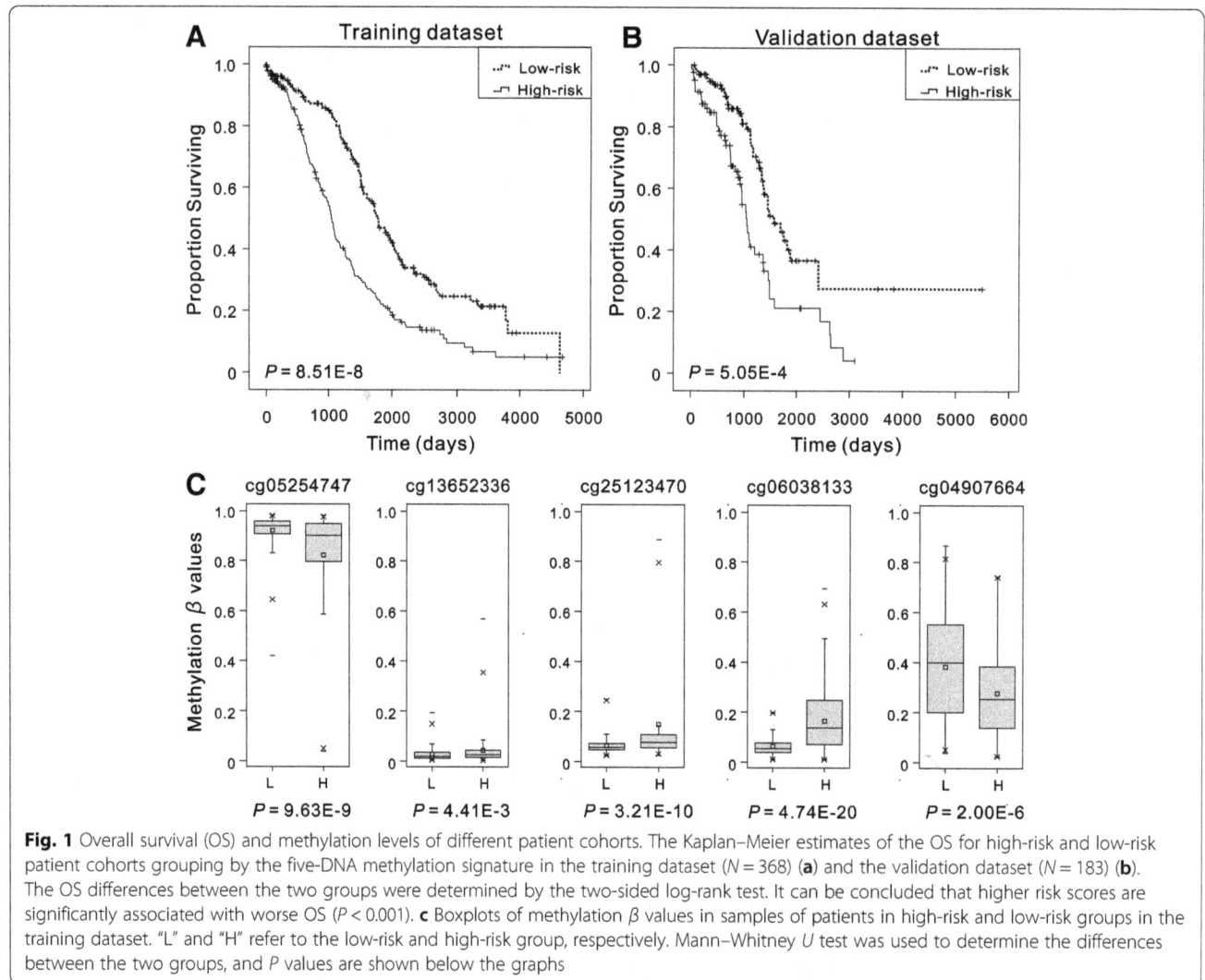

Fig. 1 Overall survival (OS) and methylation levels of different patient cohorts. The Kaplan–Meier estimates of the OS for high-risk and low-risk patient cohorts grouping by the five-DNA methylation signature in the training dataset ($N = 368$) (**a**) and the validation dataset ($N = 183$) (**b**). The OS differences between the two groups were determined by the two-sided log-rank test. It can be concluded that higher risk scores are significantly associated with worse OS ($P < 0.001$). **c** Boxplots of methylation β values in samples of patients in high-risk and low-risk groups in the training dataset. "L" and "H" refer to the low-risk and high-risk group, respectively. Mann–Whitney U test was used to determine the differences between the two groups, and P values are shown below the graphs

characteristics so as to confirm that this five-DNA methylation signature was of high applicability and could precisely predict the OS of patients. Gillen et al. found that increasing age was correlated with shorter survival [17], and Chi et al. found that patient age might serve as a significant prognostic factor for ovarian carcinoma [21]. Patients were divided into three cohorts based on their ages at initial diagnosis: ≤ 50 ($N = 127$, 23.05%), 51–60 ($N = 178$, 32.30%), and > 60 ($N = 246$, 44.65%), to analyze the clinical effect of the five-DNA methylation signature in patients with different ages. Kaplan–Meier curves showed that patients in the low-risk group had significantly ($P < 0.01$) longer OS, and the AUC value was 0.680, 0.774, and 0.720 respectively for the three age cohorts (Fig. 3), suggesting that the five-DNA methylation signature was independent of age. Patients in stages III and IV had significantly shorter OS compared with patients in stages I and II [22], and the 5-year survival of women diagnosed with distant-stage disease was only 29% [1]. Despite the

markedly different outcomes by the extent of disease, the OS was obviously different in high- and low-risk groups, and the AUC in stages I and II and stages III and IV cohorts was 0.778 and 0.735, respectively (Additional file 1: Figure S2). As for the histologic grade, considering the number of samples, we verified the predictive performance of the five-DNA methylation signature in G2 ($N = 69$) and G3 ($N = 478$). Irrespective of grades, the patients in the high-risk group had significantly ($P < 0.05$) shorter OS, and the AUC values were 0.696 and 0.740 (Additional file 1: Figure S3). The anatomic subdivisions from left alone and right alone were combined as unilateral cohorts for these analyses due to small numbers. The differences ($P < 0.001$) in the OS between the two groups were also observed, and the AUC values in all the subgroups were more than 0.72, in both unilateral ($N = 140$) and bilateral cohorts ($N = 383$) (Additional file 1: Figure S4). Recent investigations highlighted that the distribution of residual disease was an important predictor and a

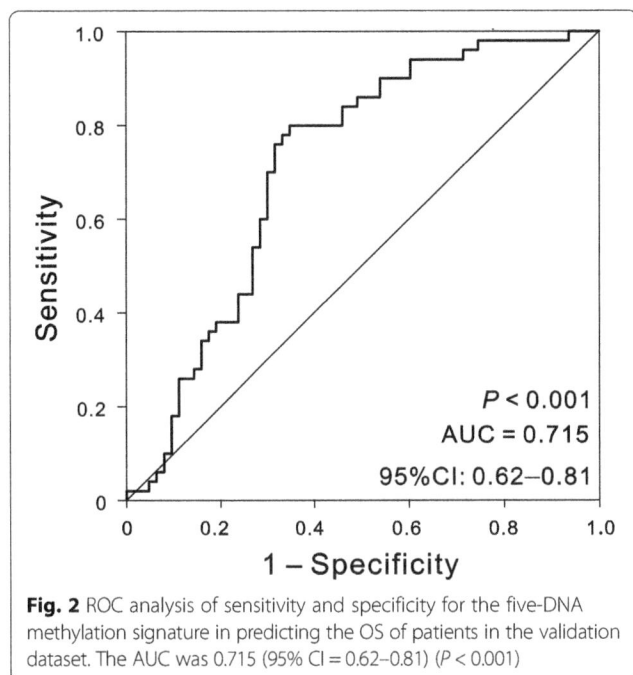

Fig. 2 ROC analysis of sensitivity and specificity for the five-DNA methylation signature in predicting the OS of patients in the validation dataset. The AUC was 0.715 (95% CI = 0.62–0.81) (*P* < 0.001)

determinant of OS of patients [23]. The present data showed that the five-DNA methylation signature could provide a fairly better reference for different residual disease cohorts owing to the effectiveness of risk stratification (Additional file 1: Figure S5). All these results indicated that the signature showed satisfactory applicability when patients were regrouped by different clinicopathological characteristics, suggesting that the signature was an independent applicable prognostic predictor of patient survival. The results are summarized in Table 2.

Comparison of the five-DNA methylation signature with other known prognostic biomarkers

In addition, several prognostic biomarkers were identified in previous studies. For instance, Luo et al. demonstrated that the expression of *HER2* was a predictor of poor prognosis for ovarian cancer [24]. The expression model of *MANF* combined with *DOCK11* was associated with the prognostic outcomes of patients with OSC, and the model could potentially serve as a novel prognostic indicator [25]. The methylation of the *BRCA1* promoter was associated with a poor patient outcome [26]. Expression of *HOTAIR* was an independent prognostic factor of OS, and its surrogate DNA methylation signature indicated carboplatin resistance in ovarian cancer [27, 28]. The sensitivity and specificity of known biomarkers from other studies were chosen to be evaluated in the validation dataset so as to verify whether the five-DNA methylation signature had the advantage of stable and reliable performance. The ROC analyses for other known biomarker is just as the analysis for our five-DNA methylation signature, and the results showed that the five-DNA methylation signature

outperformed other known prognostic biomarkers, including the types of mRNA, lncRNA, and DNA methylation. And statistical comparison using *Z* test revealed that our signature had significantly higher (*P* < 0.05) predictive performance than most of the other known biomarker. The AUCs of these biomarkers are shown in Fig. 4 and Additional file 1: Table S2. All these results inspiringly revealed that the five-DNA methylation signature provided better stability and reliability in predicting the OS of patients with OSC and was a superior predictor. Additionally, the expression of the genes corresponding to the five DNA methylation sites and genes in the five-mRNA signature [29] whose accuracy is second only to the five-DNA methylation signature were also analyzed. And the results demonstrated that the latter genes had higher fold changes in the comparison of high- and low-risk patients, and no difference was noted in the expression of almost all the former five genes in this study (Additional file 1: Figure S6).

Discussion

Molecular signatures have been proven to predict the clinical prognosis in different kinds of tumors [6, 10, 30, 31]. For instance, the methylation of *PCDH19* predicted a poor prognosis of hepatocellular carcinoma [31]; the methylation of *DFNA5* showed strong potential as a prognostic biomarker for breast cancer; and the signature of *CXCL11* combined with *HMGA2* could precisely predict the OS of patients with high-grade serous ovarian cancer [30]. However, many of these studies were limited by either small sample size or lack of validation of the biomarker as an independent prognostic biomarker. Some studies showed that combinations of DNA methylation as biomarkers achieved higher sensitivity and specificity compared with individual DNA methylation [12]. In the present study, a five-DNA methylation signature significantly associated with the OS of patients with OSC was predicted based on genome-wide DNA methylation analysis using the Cox regression and ROC analyses. The five-DNA methylation signature also performed well in differentiating low- and high-risk groups and in associated log-rank tests with significant *P* values, demonstrating that it was an independent predictor of patient survival when adjusted by age, FIGO stages, histologic grade, and residual disease after cytoreductive surgery. Furthermore, the results of the univariate Cox regression and Kaplan–Meier analyses for the five individual methylation sites were not as good as for the combination of these five-DNA methylation sites in both training and validation datasets, indicating that a combination of methylation sites might offer a better potential to fulfill much more sensitive and specific prognostic tests for patients with OSC.

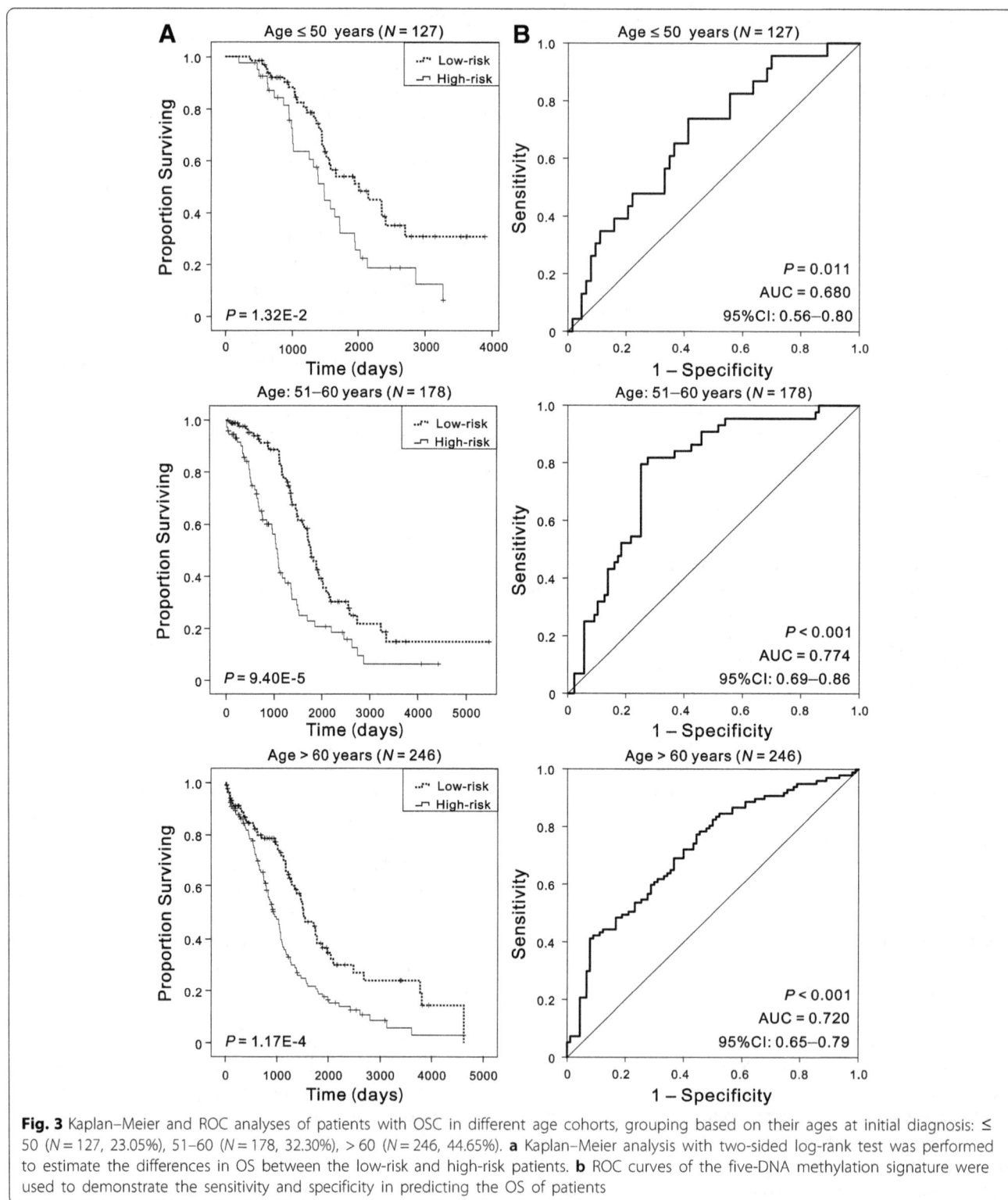

Fig. 3 Kaplan–Meier and ROC analyses of patients with OSC in different age cohorts, grouping based on their ages at initial diagnosis: ≤ 50 ($N = 127$, 23.05%), 51–60 ($N = 178$, 32.30%), > 60 ($N = 246$, 44.65%). **a** Kaplan–Meier analysis with two-sided log-rank test was performed to estimate the differences in OS between the low-risk and high-risk patients. **b** ROC curves of the five-DNA methylation signature were used to demonstrate the sensitivity and specificity in predicting the OS of patients

Researchers have revealed that the aforementioned five methylation sites may be crucial in cancer development. *SLC39A14* has been identified as an independent factor for predicting the biochemical recurrence-free survival of patients with prostate cancer, and the decreased expression of *SLC39A14* is associated with the tumor aggressiveness of human prostate cancer [32]. *PREX2* (also known as *P-Rex2*) was highly expressed in the brain, heart, skeletal muscle, placenta, and lymph node and promoted cancer cell migration and/or invasion [33–35].

Table 2 Results of Kaplan–Meier and ROC analysis based on different regrouping methods

Regrouping factors	Group	Sample size	Kaplan–Meier, P value	AUC	95% CI of AUC
Age at diagnosis	≤ 50	127	1.32E–02	0.680	0.56–0.80
	51–60	178	9.40E–05	0.774	0.69–0.86
	> 60	246	1.17E–04	0.720	0.65–0.79
FIGO stage	I and II	42	6.76E–02	0.778	0.59–0.96
	III and IV	505	1.03E–09	0.735	0.69–0.79
Histologic grade	G2	69	2.91E–02	0.696	0.53–0.86
	G3	478	3.26E–09	0.740	0.69–0.79
Anatomic subdivision	Unilateral	140	4.27E–04	0.753	0.66–0.85
	Bilateral	383	4.73E–07	0.727	0.67–0.79
Tumor residual disease (mm)	No macroscopic disease	116	1.17E–03	0.795	0.67–0.92
	1–10	255	1.16E–03	0.665	0.59–0.76
	> 10	138	5.18E–05	0.770	0.68–0.86

The *CORO6* promoter was frequently methylated in renal cell cancer [36]. The expression of *EFNB1* was related to the metastasis of breast cancer, and its enhanced expression conferred a poor prognosis [37]. The elevated co-expression of *NGFR*, *EFNB1*, and *APP* was associated with longer overall and metastasis-free survival of patients with breast cancer [38]. In addition, SLC39A14 participates in manganese ion transmembrane transporter activity; KCNIP2 regulates calcium ion binding; PREX2 and EFNB1 are involved in the G-protein coupled receptor signaling pathway and ephrin receptor signaling pathway, respectively. Although the functional mechanism of these five genes still needs further study, their methylation has significant correlations with the

prognosis of patients with OSC and may serve as a potential therapeutic target for OSC.

Meanwhile, a comparison of the five-DNA methylation signature with other known prognostic biomarkers showed that it had distinctly higher sensitivity and specificity in the outcome prediction of OSC. The five-mRNA signature identified in a previous study [29] also had high accuracy surpassed only by the five-DNA methylation signature. However, these five mRNAs were completely different from the genes that corresponded to the five DNA methylation sites in this study. The expression analysis of these ten genes between high- and low-risk patients indicated that one possible reason was that mRNAs acting as biomarkers had larger fold changes in the expression level to be captured by our statistical methods. Further, it is generally believed that DNA methylation has an effect on the gene regulation with several exceptions [6, 39]. The potential association between the methylation level and the gene expression levels of these five genes demonstrated that only the expression of *SLC39A14* and *CORO6* was significantly ($P < 0.05$) correlated with the methylation levels at cg05254747 and cg06038133 sites, respectively, and no statistically significant association was observed between the methylation level and the expression of the other three genes. Further studies should be performed to establish a better prognostic biomarker for the combination of mRNAs and DNA methylation signature.

Conclusion

In conclusion, using genome-wide analysis of DNA methylation data of 551 patients with OSC, this study showed that a five-DNA methylation signature was significantly associated with the OS of patients, and its practical value in patients with different ages, FIGO stages, histologic grades, and some other clinical features was confirmed. Therefore, the five-DNA methylation

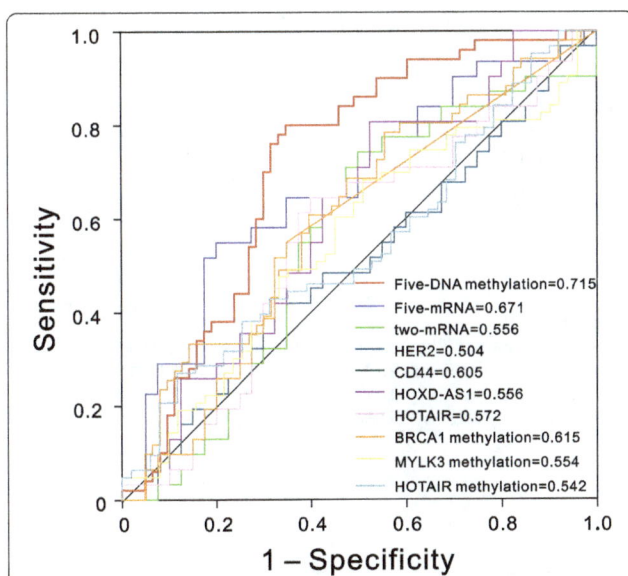

Fig. 4 ROC curves show the sensitivity and specificity of the five-DNA methylation signature and other known biomarkers in predicting the OS of patients

Legend for Fig. 4:
- Five-DNA methylation=0.715
- Five-mRNA=0.671
- two-mRNA=0.556
- HER2=0.504
- CD44=0.605
- HOXD-AS1=0.556
- HOTAIR=0.572
- BRCA1 methylation=0.615
- MYLK3 methylation=0.554
- HOTAIR methylation=0.542

signature may potentially be used as a novel independent prognostic biomarker to predict the OS of patients with OSC. Further clinical studies on the functional mechanism of the five-DNA methylation signature should be examined for the possibility of its participation in the carcinogenesis.

Materials and methods

DNA methylation data in OSC tissues from TCGA dataset

The DNA methylation data of patients with OSC were downloaded from TCGA database [40]. TCGA level 3 methylation data and related clinical information for patients were obtained. TCGA DNA methylation data (level 3) were obtained using Infinium HumanMethylation27 BeadChip (Illumina Inc., CA, USA), and the genomic coordinates of the CpGs were based on GRCh38. All DNA methylation levels were expressed as β values, calculated as $M/(M + U)$, where M is the signal from methylated beads, and U is the signal from unmethylated beads at the targeted CpG site. Only the data including patients with their clinical survival information were selected to analyze the correlation between DNA methylation levels and the corresponding survival in OSC. Considering that tumors in G1, GB, and GX may have a different biological behavior, they were excluded in this study. Ultimately, 551 samples containing information on 27,578 DNA methylation sites were included in this study, and the corresponding clinical information for each sample was also obtained from TCGA database. These 551 samples were separated into training dataset (first two thirds) and validation dataset (remaining one third) according to TCGA series number. The training dataset was applied for identifying and constructing prognostic biomarkers, and the validation dataset was used for verifying the accuracy of the biomarkers in predicting survival, thus determining the potential clinical predictive value.

Statistical analyses

All statistical analyses were conducted using the R statistical package (R version 3.4.4) unless otherwise stated. OS was defined as the interval from the date of patient's first diagnosis to the date of last known contact or death. The univariate Cox proportional hazard analysis was first performed in the training dataset to identify methylation markers significantly (P value cutoff < 0.05) correlated with patient survival as candidate markers. Then, the multivariate Cox regression analysis was carried out to further screen the factors associated with patient survival. In brief, two, three, four, five, and six genes were selected from the candidate markers exhaustively as covariates to construct models. Subsequently, AUC was used to measure and compare the model performance; the model with a higher predictive performance was

eventually selected out. The model could be used to construct a risk score formula that would be helpful to predict survival. The prognostic risk scores for each patient were calculated based on this formula. According to their prognostic risk scores, these patients were ranked and further separated into "low-risk" and "high-risk" groups using the median risk score as the cutoff point. Patients with risk score higher than the median risk score were assigned to the high-risk group, whereas patients with lower risk were assigned to the low-risk group. After that, the Kaplan–Meier estimator, a non-parametric statistic, with log-rank test (Mantel–Cox) was used to calculate the cumulative survival time and compare the differences in OS between the two groups. Kaplan–Meier curves were drawn using the "survival" package. Finally, the ROC analysis was conducted with the "pROC" package using a categorical variable for OS ≤ 3 years compared with methylation biomarkers. AUC was calculated along with 95% confidence interval (CI). The larger the AUC is, the better the model is for the risk prediction [41]. And Z test was used to further compare the AUC of different biomarkers [42]. Additionally, the potential association between methylation and gene expression level was evaluated using the Spearman's rank correlation test.

Abbreviations

AUC: Area under the ROC curve; CI: Confidence interval; OS: Overall survival; OSC: Ovarian serous cystadenocarcinoma; ROC: Receiver operating characteristic; TCGA: The Cancer Genome Atlas; FIGO: Federation Internationale des Gynaecologistes et Obstetristes

Acknowledgements

The results shown in this manuscript are based upon the data generated by TCGA Research Network: http://cancergenome.nih.gov/.

Funding

This work was supported by grants from the National Natural Science Foundation of China (Grant No. 31501045, 31471200 and 31741073). This work was also supported by the Graduate Research and Innovation Fund of Nanjing University (No. 2017CL06).

Authors' contributions

QW and QHC conceived and designed the study. WNG and LCZ carried out the data analysis, interpreted the entire results, and drafted the manuscript. MHY and RZ helped to carry out the data analysis. All authors read and approved the final manuscript.

Author details
[1]State Key Laboratory of Pharmaceutical Biotechnology, School of Life Sciences, Nanjing University, Nanjing, China. [2]School of Life Sciences, Shanghai University, Shanghai, China.

References

1. Siegel RL, Miller KD, Jemal A. Cancer statistics, 2018. CA Cancer J Clin. 2018; 68:7–30.
2. Cancer Genome Atlas Research N. Integrated genomic analyses of ovarian carcinoma. Nature. 2011;474:609–15.
3. Coccolini F, Campanati L, Catena F, Ceni V, Ceresoli M, Jimenez Cruz J, Lotti M, Magnone S, Napoli J, Rossetti D, De Iaco P, Frigerio L, Pinna A, Runnebaum I, Ansaloni L. Hyperthermic intraperitoneal chemotherapy with cisplatin and paclitaxel in advanced ovarian cancer: a multicenter prospective observational study. J Gynecol Oncol. 2015;26:54–61.
4. Coleman RL, Monk BJ, Sood AK, Herzog TJ. Latest research and treatment of advanced-stage epithelial ovarian cancer. Nat Rev Clin Oncol. 2013;10:211–24.
5. Zhou F, Tao G, Chen X, Xie W, Liu M, Cao X. Methylation of OPCML promoter in ovarian cancer tissues predicts poor patient survival. Clin Chem Lab Med. 2014;52:735–42.
6. Croes L, Beyens M, Fransen E, Ibrahim J, Vanden Berghe W, Suls A, Peeters M, Pauwels P, Van Camp G, Op de Beeck K. Large-scale analysis of DFNA5 methylation reveals its potential as biomarker for breast cancer. Clin Epigenetics. 2018;10:51.
7. Costello JF, Fruhwald MC, Smiraglia DJ, Rush LJ, Robertson GP, Gao X, Wright FA, Feramisco JD, Peltomaki P, Lang JC, Schuller DE, Yu L, Bloomfield CD, Caligiuri MA, Yates A, Nishikawa R, Su Huang H, Petrelli NJ, Zhang X, O'Dorisio MS, Held WA, Cavenee WK, Plass C. Aberrant CpG-island methylation has non-random and tumour-type-specific patterns. Nat Genet. 2000;24:132–8.
8. Ahluwalia A, Yan P, Hurteau JA, Bigsby RM, Jung SH, Huang TH, Nephew KP. DNA methylation and ovarian cancer. I. Analysis of CpG island hypermethylation in human ovarian cancer using differential methylation hybridization. Gynecol Oncol. 2001;82:261–8.
9. Wei SH, Balch C, Paik HH, Kim YS, Baldwin RL, Liyanarachchi S, Li L, Wang Z, Wan JC, Davuluri RV, Karlan BY, Gifford G, Brown R, Kim S, Huang TH, Nephew KP. Prognostic DNA methylation biomarkers in ovarian cancer. Clinical cancer research : an official journal of the American Association for Cancer Research. 2006;12:2788–94.
10. Chou JL, Huang RL, Shay J, Chen LY, Lin SJ, Yan PS, Chao WT, Lai YH, Lai YL, Chao TK, Lee CI, Tai CK, Wu SF, Nephew KP, Huang TH, Lai HC, Chan MW. Hypermethylation of the TGF-beta target, ABCA1 is associated with poor prognosis in ovarian cancer patients. Clin Epigenetics. 2015;7:1.
11. Keeley B, Stark A, Pisanic TR 2nd, Kwak R, Zhang Y, Wrangle J, Baylin S, Herman J, Ahuja N, Brock MV, Wang TH. Extraction and processing of circulating DNA from large sample volumes using methylation on beads for the detection of rare epigenetic events. Clinica Chimica Acta; International Journal of Clinical Chemistry. 2013;425:169–75.
12. Dai W, Teodoridis JM, Zeller C, Graham J, Hersey J, Flanagan JM, Stronach E, Millan DW, Siddiqui N, Paul J, Brown R. Systematic CpG islands methylation profiling of genes in the wnt pathway in epithelial ovarian cancer identifies biomarkers of progression-free survival. Clinical cancer research: an official journal of the American Association for Cancer Research. 2011;17:4052–62.
13. How Kit A, Nielsen HM, Tost J. DNA methylation based biomarkers: practical considerations and applications. Biochimie. 2012;94:2314–37.
14. Brown R, Curry E, Magnani L, Wilhelm-Benartzi CS, Borley J. Poised epigenetic states and acquired drug resistance in cancer. Nat Rev Cancer. 2014;14:747–53.
15. Bonito NA, Borley J, Wilhelm-Benartzi CS, Ghaem-Maghami S, Brown R. Epigenetic regulation of the Homeobox gene MSX1 associates with platinum-resistant disease in high-grade serous epithelial ovarian Cancer. Clinical cancer research: an official journal of the American Association for Cancer Research. 2016;22:3097–104.
16. Borley J, Wilhelm-Benartzi C, Brown R, Ghaem-Maghami S. Does tumour biology determine surgical success in the treatment of epithelial ovarian cancer? A systematic literature review British journal of cancer. 2012;107: 1069–74.
17. Gillen J, Gunderson C, Greenwade M, Rowland M, Ruskin R, Ding K, Crim A, Walter A, White E, Moore K. Contribution of age to clinical trial enrollment and tolerance with ovarian cancer. Gynecol Oncol. 2017;145:32–6.
18. Engel J, Eckel R, Schubert-Fritschle G, Kerr J, Kuhn W, Diebold J, Kimmig R, Rehbock J, Holzel D. Moderate progress for ovarian cancer in the last 20 years: prolongation of survival, but no improvement in the cure rate. Eur J Cancer. 2002;38:2435–45.
19. Peres LC, Cushing-Haugen KL, Kobel M, Harris HR, Berchuck A, Rossing MA, Schildkraut JM, Doherty JA. Invasive epithelial ovarian cancer survival by histotype and disease stage. J Natl Cancer Inst. 2018.
20. Chi DS, Eisenhauer EL, Zivanovic O, Sonoda Y, Abu-Rustum NR, Levine DA, Guile MW, Bristow RE, Aghajanian C, Barakat RR. Improved progression-free and overall survival in advanced ovarian cancer as a result of a change in surgical paradigm. Gynecol Oncol. 2009;114:26–31.
21. Chi DS, Liao JB, Leon LF, Venkatraman ES, Hensley ML, Bhaskaran D, Hoskins WJ. Identification of prognostic factors in advanced epithelial ovarian carcinoma. Gynecol Oncol. 2001;82:532–7.
22. Montavon C, Gloss BS, Warton K, Barton CA, Statham AL, Scurry JP, Tabor B, Nguyen TV, Qu W, Samimi G, Hacker NF, Sutherland RL, Clark SJ, O'Brien PM. Prognostic and diagnostic significance of DNA methylation patterns in high grade serous ovarian cancer. Gynecol Oncol. 2012;124:582–8.
23. Hamilton CA, Miller A, Miller C, Krivak TC, Farley JH, Chernofsky MR, Stany MP, Rose GS, Markman M, Ozols RF, Armstrong DK, Maxwell GL. The impact of disease distribution on survival in patients with stage III epithelial ovarian cancer cytoreduced to microscopic residual: a gynecologic oncology group study. Gynecol Oncol. 2011;122:521–6.
24. Luo H, Xu X, Ye M, Sheng B, Zhu X. The prognostic value of HER2 in ovarian cancer: a meta-analysis of observational studies. PLoS One. 2018;13: e0191972.
25. Zhang J, Xu M, Gao H, Guo JC, Guo YL, Zou M, Wu XF. Two protein-coding genes act as a novel clinical signature to predict prognosis in patients with ovarian serous cystadenocarcinoma. Oncol Lett. 2018;15:3669–75.
26. Chiang JW, Karlan BY, Cass L, Baldwin RL. BRCA1 promoter methylation predicts adverse ovarian cancer prognosis. Gynecol Oncol. 2006;101:403–10.
27. Qiu JJ, Lin YY, Ye LC, Ding JX, Feng WW, Jin HY, Zhang Y, Li Q, Hua KQ. Overexpression of long non-coding RNA HOTAIR predicts poor patient prognosis and promotes tumor metastasis in epithelial ovarian cancer. Gynecol Oncol. 2014;134:121–8.
28. Teschendorff AE, Lee SH, Jones A, Fiegl H, Kalwa M, Wagner W, Chindera K, Evans I, Dubeau L, Orjalo A, Horlings HM, Niederreiter L, Kaser A, Yang W, Goode EL, Fridley BL, Jenner RG, Berns EM, Wik E, Salvesen HB, Wisman GB, van der Zee AG, Davidson B, Trope CG, Lambrechts S, Vergote I, Calvert H, Jacobs IJ, Widschwendter M. HOTAIR and its surrogate DNA methylation signature indicate carboplatin resistance in ovarian cancer. Genome medicine. 2015;7:108.
29. Liu LW, Zhang Q, Guo W, Qian K, Wang Q, Five-Gene Expression A. Signature predicts clinical outcome of ovarian serous cystadenocarcinoma. Biomed Res Int. 2016;2016:6945304.
30. Jin C, Xue Y, Li Y, Bu H, Yu H, Zhang T, Zhang Z, Yan S, Lu N, Kong B. A 2-protein signature predicting clinical outcome in high-grade serous ovarian cancer. International journal of gynecological cancer: official Journal of the International Gynecological Cancer Society. 2018;28:51–8.
31. Zhang T, Guan G, Chen T, Jin J, Zhang L, Yao M, Qi X, Zou J, Chen J, Lu F, Chen X. Methylation of PCDH19 predicts poor prognosis of hepatocellular carcinoma. Asia-Pacific journal of clinical oncology. 2018.
32. Xu XM, Wang CG, Zhu YD, Chen WH, Shao SL, Jiang FN, Liao QD. Decreased expression of SLC 39A14 is associated with tumor aggressiveness and biochemical recurrence of human prostate cancer. OncoTargets and therapy. 2016;9:4197–205.
33. Fine B, Hodakoski C, Koujak S, Su T, Saal LH, Maurer M, Hopkins B, Keniry M, Sulis ML, Mense S, Hibshoosh H, Parsons R. Activation of the PI3K pathway in cancer through inhibition of PTEN by exchange factor P-REX2a. Science. 2009;325:1261–5.
34. Mense SM, Barrows D, Hodakoski C, Steinbach N, Schoenfeld D, Su W, Hopkins BD, Su T, Fine B, Hibshoosh H, Parsons R, PTEN inhibits PREX2-catalyzed activation of RAC1 to restrain tumor cell invasion. Sci Signal 2015; 8: ra32.

35. Srijakotre N, Man J, Ooms LM, Lucato CM, Ellisdon AM, Mitchell CA. P-Rex1 and P-Rex2 RacGEFs and cancer. Biochem Soc Trans. 2017;45:963–77.

36. Morris MR, Ricketts CJ, Gentle D, McRonald F, Carli N, Khalili H, Brown M, Kishida T, Yao M, Banks RE, Clarke N, Latif F, Maher ER. Genome-wide methylation analysis identifies epigenetically inactivated candidate tumour suppressor genes in renal cell carcinoma. Oncogene. 2011;30:1390–401.

37. Yin H, Lu C, Tang Y, Wang H, Wang H, Wang J. Enhanced expression of EphrinB1 is associated with lymph node metastasis and poor prognosis in breast cancer. Cancer biomarkers: section A of Disease markers. 2013;13: 261–7.

38. Fernandez-Nogueira P, Bragado P, Almendro V, Ametller E, Rios J, Choudhury S, Mancino M, Gascon P. Differential expression of neurogenes among breast cancer subtypes identifies high risk patients. Oncotarget. 2016;7:5313–26.

39. Phelps DL, Borley JV, Flower KJ, Dina R, Darb-Esfahani S, Braicu I, Sehouli J, Fotopoulou C, Wilhelm-Benartzi CS, Gabra H, Yazbek J, Chatterjee J, Ip J, Khan H, Likos-Corbett MT, Brown R, Ghaem-Maghami S. Methylation of MYLK3 gene promoter region: a biomarker to stratify surgical care in ovarian cancer in a multicentre study. Br J Cancer. 2017;116:1287–93.

40. International Cancer Genome C, Hudson TJ, Anderson W, Artez A, Barker AD, Bell C, et al. International network of cancer genome projects. Nature. 2010;464:993–8.

41. Mehdi T, Bashardoost N, Ahmadi M. Kernel smoothing for ROC curve and estimation for thyroid stimulating hormone. Inter J Env Res Pub Heal. 2011: 239–42.

42. Pandis N. Comparison of 2 means (independent z test or independent t test). American journal of orthodontics and dentofacial orthopedics, Official publication of the American Association of Orthodontists, its constituent societies, and the American Board of Orthodontics. 2015;148:350–1.

19

DNA methylation levels are associated with CRF$_1$ receptor antagonist treatment outcome in women with post-traumatic stress disorder

Julius C. Pape[1] (iD), Tania Carrillo-Roa[1], Barbara O. Rothbaum[2], Charles B. Nemeroff[3], Darina Czamara[1], Anthony S. Zannas[1,8], Dan Iosifescu[4,9,10], Sanjay J. Mathew[5], Thomas C. Neylan[6,7], Helen S. Mayberg[2], Boadie W. Dunlop[2] and Elisabeth B. Binder[1,2*]

Abstract

Background: We have previously evaluated the efficacy of the CRF$_1$ receptor antagonist GSK561679 in female PTSD patients. While GSK561679 was not superior to placebo overall, it was associated with a significantly stronger symptom reduction in a subset of patients with probable CRF system hyperactivity, i.e., patients with child abuse and *CRHR1* SNP rs110402 GG carriers. Here, we test whether blood-based DNA methylation levels within *CRHR1* and other PTSD-relevant genes would be associated with treatment outcome, either overall or in the high CRF activity subgroup.

Results: Therefore, we measured *CRHR1* genotypes as well as baseline and post-treatment DNA methylation from the peripheral blood in the same cohort of PTSD-diagnosed women treated with GSK561679 ($N = 43$) or placebo ($N = 45$). In the same patients, we assessed DNA methylation at the PTSD-relevant genes *NR3C1* and *FKBP5*, shown to predict or associate with PTSD treatment outcome after psychotherapy. We observed significant differences in *CRHR1* methylation after GSK561679 treatment in the subgroup of patients with high CRF activity. Furthermore, *NR3C1* baseline methylation significantly interacted with child abuse to predict PTSD symptom change following GSK561679 treatment.

Conclusions: Our results support a possible role of *CRHR1* methylation levels as an epigenetic marker to track response to CRF$_1$ antagonist treatment in biologically relevant subgroups. Moreover, pre-treatment *NR3C1* methylation levels may serve as a potential marker to predict PTSD treatment outcome, independent of the type of therapy. However, to establish clinical relevance of these markers, our findings require replication and validation in larger studies.

Keywords: CRF$_1$ receptor antagonist, DNA methylation, Epigenetics, PTSD, CRHR1, NR3C1, FKBP5

* Correspondence: binder@psych.mpg.de; ebinder@emory.edu
[1]Department of Translational Research in Psychiatry, Max Planck Institute of Psychiatry, Munich, Germany
[2]Department of Psychiatry and Behavioral Sciences, Emory University School of Medicine, Atlanta, GA, USA
Full list of author information is available at the end of the article

Background

Post-traumatic stress disorder (PTSD) is a common psychiatric disorder with a prevalence of about 5% in the general population and an overall lifetime prevalence of 7–12%. Key symptoms of the disorder include intrusive memories, avoidance, and numbing as well as hyperarousal. Typically, these symptoms are long lasting and occur after exposure to traumatic life events. Women are twice as likely to develop the disease than men. PTSD therapies include both evidence-based psychotherapies and pharmacology, but only few patients attain remission. Currently, only two medications, paroxetine and sertraline, are approved by the US Food and Drug Administration (FDA). These SSRIs are capable of significantly reducing PTSD symptoms, but with only 20–30% remission rates to these agents, there is a need for additional pharmacologic treatment options [1].

Among pathophysiologic mechanisms that have been investigated for PTSD, disruptions of regulation of the hypothalamic-pituitary-adrenal (HPA) axis are among the most frequently cited hypotheses [2]. A key regulator of the HPA axis is the corticotropin-releasing factor (CRF) and its type 1 receptor (CRF_1 receptor), and many studies have reported alterations in this system in PTSD [3]. Therefore, it represents a promising novel drug target for this disorder. In response to stress, CRF is secreted by nerve terminals of the paraventricular nucleus of the hypothalamus and binds to the CRF_1 receptor in the adenohypophysis to release adrenocorticotropic hormone (ACTH). This process acts as the initial step of HPA axis activation and leads to the release of a number of hormones from the adrenal cortex including cortisol. Numerous studies in laboratory animals as well as in humans indicate that abnormalities of these HPA axis regulators play a crucial role in stress-related disorders such as PTSD [4].

In humans, for example, a number of independent studies report increased cerebrospinal fluid concentrations of corticotropin-releasing factor in PTSD patients [5–7], suggesting hyperactivity of the hypothalamus and extra-hypothalamus CRF system. Moreover, previous investigations have found that genetic variants in the CRF receptor 1 gene (*CRHR1*) are associated with differences in CRF signaling and may also impact individual responses to environmental stressors [3]. The most studied are variants within a haplotype tagged by the intronic SNP rs110402 that also comprises rs242924 and rs7209436. Interactions with exposure to child abuse and this haplotype were shown to alter risk for major depression, with individuals homozygous for the G-allele of rs110402 and exposed to child abuse being at higher risk in several but not all studies (see [8] for review). This haplotype has also been associated with differences in the neural activation profile with emotional stimulus processing [9], as well as

neuroendocrine responses in psychological and pharmacological challenge tests [10–14], in which individuals who experienced childhood abuse and carry the G-allele display stronger HPA axis disturbances.

These preclinical and clinical results, taken together, support the role of CRF/CRF_1 receptor as a potential drug target in PTSD. However, antagonism of the CRF_1 receptor may only benefit those patients with initial increases in CRF signaling, which according to the above cited endocrine studies are likely to be those with exposure to child abuse and carrying the G-allele of rs110402.

We recently published a study evaluating the efficacy of a novel CRF_1 receptor antagonist (GSK561679) in a cohort of female PTSD patients in a double-blind, placebo-controlled trial. Although the drug was not superior to placebo overall, it was associated with a significantly stronger symptom reduction in a subset of patients with probable CRF_1 receptor hyperactivity, i.e., patients with childhood abuse and carriers of the GG genotype of the *CRHR1* SNP rs110402 [15, 16]. These patients may represent a biologically distinct subtype of PTSD and show distinct biomarker profiles. Markers that predict or monitor treatment outcome would represent an important tool to offer targeted treatment for individual patients. Despite great progress in identifying the underpinnings of the pathophysiology of PTSD and some very promising results in the biomarker field [17, 18], there is still no clinically applicable marker in PTSD, neither for diagnosis nor, perhaps even more significantly, to guide treatment selection. This is likely due to the complex pathophysiology of the disease that may include an interplay of genetics, environment, and epigenetic changes. It is therefore likely that not a single but rather a combination of different biological and clinical markers will need to be identified [18].

In addition to gene variants that predispose to PTSD development, epigenetic changes have been implicated in the pathophysiology of PTSD (for review, see [19]). These modifications may also serve as diagnostic marks as well as predicting and monitoring treatment outcome. Several studies highlight the possible use of epigenetic marks in peripheral tissues such as the blood and saliva as diagnostic markers in PTSD [18, 20, 21]. So far, epigenetic marks of only two genes, also within the HPA axis, *NR3C1*—encoding the glucocorticoid receptor (GR) and *FKBP5*—a co-chaperone of the GR, have been shown to associate with treatment response. More specifically, *NR3C1* baseline promoter methylation in peripheral blood predicted treatment outcome in PTSD, and in the same study, promoter methylation of *FKBP5* decreased in association with symptom improvement [22]. These findings were observed after 12 weeks of psychotherapy and have not yet been investigated in the context of pharmacological treatment.

Extending our previous study showing potential effects of a novel CRF_1 receptor antagonist (GSK561679) in a specific subset of women with PTSD (GG homozygous for rs110402 and with a history of childhood abuse) [16], we here use the same cohort to test whether blood-based epigenetic changes of PTSD relevant genes could serve as potential markers for treatment selection and outcome monitoring in biologically defined subgroups of patients. Given that the drug targets the CRF_1 receptor, we focused our analysis on the methylation of the *CRHR1* gene using the previous subgrouping of patients based on genetic and environmental risk factors. In addition, we explored whether methylation levels of two other genes within the stress hormone system (*NR3C1* and *FKBP5*), previously shown to predict and correlate with PTSD symptom improvement after psychotherapy [22], would also be associated with pharmacological treatment response in our study, again with specific focus on patients with probable CRF system hyperactivity (rs110402 GG-carriers and exposure to child abuse).

Results

Subgroup differences in *CRHR1* baseline methylation and change in *CRHR1* methylation from baseline to post-treatment

First, we tested a model with the main effects and interaction effect of child abuse and rs110402 carrier status on mean *CRHR1* baseline methylation. Seventy-nine subjects were included in this analysis due to missing genotype data in three samples. Neither the main effects nor the interaction effect showed significance ($n = 79$; $p > 0.05$). Next, we tested a model including main effects of treatment as well as interaction effects of treatment by child abuse, treatment by rs110402, child abuse by rs110402, and the three-way interaction of treatment by child abuse by rs110402 on changes in mean methylation levels of *CRHR1* from baseline to post-treatment. Due to missing methylation data in two baseline samples and one post-treatment sample, 57 subjects with baseline and post-treatment methylation data remained for this analysis. There was a significant interaction effect of child abuse by rs110402 carrier status ($n = 57$; $F (1, 41) = 9.05$; $p = 0.004$; $\beta = -0.449$; Cohen's $f = 0.47$; $R^2 = 0.38$; adj. $R^2 = 0.153$; post-hoc power = 0.94) on change in methylation. Further, the three-way interaction of treatment by child abuse by rs110402 showed a significant effect on *CRHR1* methylation levels from pre- to post-treatment ($n = 57$; $F (1, 41) = 4.86$; $p = 0.033$; $\beta = -0.297$; Cohen's $f = 0.344$; $R^2 = 0.38$; adj. $R^2 = 0.153$; post-hoc power = 0.72) (Fig. 1a, b).

Genotype by childhood abuse interaction on methylation change stratified by treatment

To further explore the significant three-way interaction on *CRHR1* methylation, we investigated the interaction

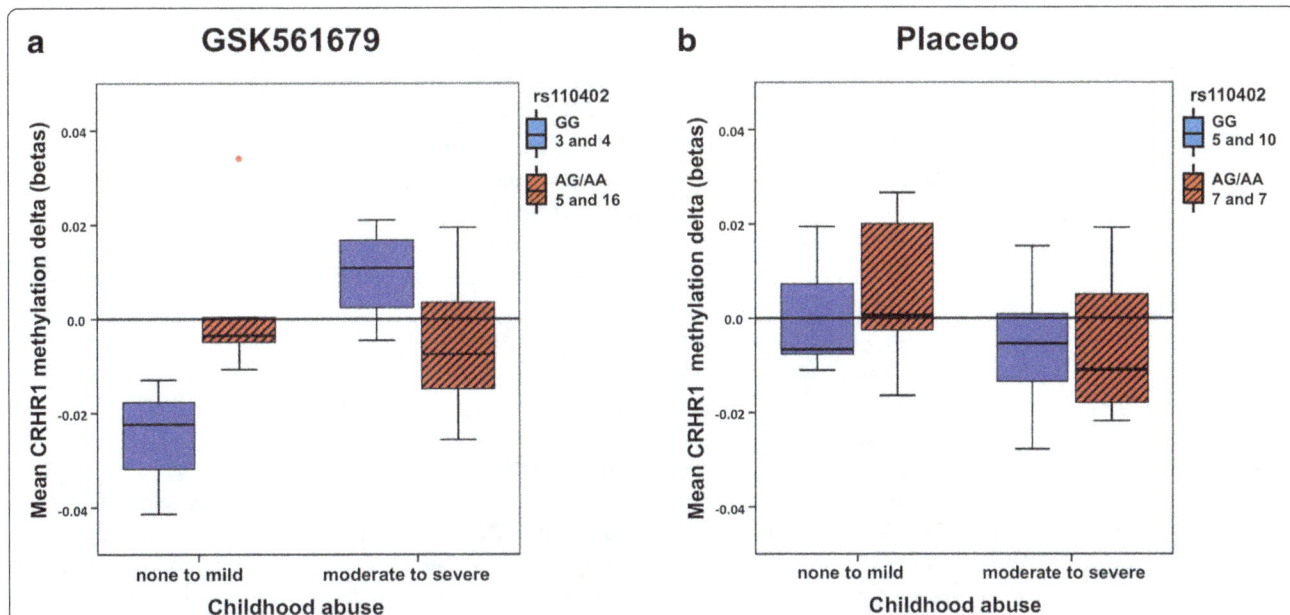

Fig. 1 The boxplots describe the mean change of CRHR1 methylation (top tertile of the most variable CpGs from pre- to post-treatment) in abused and non-abused patients treated with GSK561679 or placebo. GG carriers are shown in blue (plain boxes) and AA/AG in red (striped boxes). Positive values correspond to an increase, whereas negative values correspond to a decrease in methylation from baseline to endpoint. Dots indicate outliers. Three-way interaction of treatment × rs110402 A carrier status × child abuse was significantly associated with mean methylation change ($n = 57$; $p = 0.033$) (**a**, **b**). After treatment stratification, there was a significant interaction effect of rs110402 A carrier status and child abuse on mean methylation change in subjects treated with GSK561679 ($n = 28$; $p = 0.00005$) (**a**) but not with placebo ($n = 29$; $p > 0.05$) (**b**)

of rs110402 carrier status by child abuse on the change in methylation levels stratified by treatment. The interaction showed a significant effect on pre- to post-treatment CRHR1 methylation change only in patients treated with the CRF_1 receptor antagonist ($n = 28$; F (1, 16) $= 29.81$; $p = 0.00005$; withstands Bonferroni correction for multiple testing; $\beta = -0.913$; Cohen's $f = 1.366$; $R^2 = 0.73$; adj. $R^2 = 0.55$; post-hoc power $= 0.99$) (Fig. 1a).

Interestingly, the subset of patients with child abuse and who are also carriers of the GG genotype of rs110402 showed an increase in CRHR1 methylation with GSK561679 treatment. This subgroup was previously described to benefit most from the drug ([16] and Additional file 1: Figure S1). The other three subsets of patients (no abuse and rs110402 GG; no abuse and rs110402 AG/AA; abuse and rs110402 AG/AA) showed no change or decreased methylation after GSK561679 treatment. There was no significant effect in the placebo group ($n = 29$; $p > 0.05$) (Fig. 1b).

Baseline methylation by treatment interaction effects on PTSD symptom change

We next tested whether baseline methylation predicted %-change of PTSD symptoms from pre- to post-treatment. Seventy-nine (CAPS)/78 (PSS) subjects were included in the analysis due to missing genotype data in three samples and missing phenotype data (PSS %-change) in one sample. Neither NR3C1 ($n = 79/78$; $p > 0.05$) nor FKBP5 ($n = 79/78$; $p > 0.05$) showed a significant interaction effect of treatment by baseline methylation on symptom change.

Three-way interaction effects on PTSD symptom change with treatment, baseline methylation, and SNP/child abuse

Next, we included either rs110402 or child abuse in our analysis and tested for two three-way interaction effects (rs110402 × treatment × mean baseline methylation or child abuse × treatment × mean baseline methylation) on symptom reduction measured by change in Clinician-Administered PTSD Scale (CAPS) and PTSD Symptom Scale-Self-Report (PSS-SR) scores. Treatment by baseline methylation by rs110402 carrier status was not significantly associated with differences in PTSD symptom change for neither of the genes (NR3C1: $n = 79/78$, $p > 0.05$; FKBP5: $n = 79/78$, $p > 0.05$).

The three-way interaction that included child abuse was significant for NR3C1 baseline methylation ($n = 78$; F (1, 56) $= 4.26$; $p = 0.044$; $\beta = 0.276$; Cohen's $f = 0.277$; $R^2 = 0.33$; adj. $R^2 = 0.087$; post-hoc power $= 0.67$) and showed a trend towards significance for FKBP5 baseline methylation ($n = 79$, F (1, 57) $= 2.81$; $p = 0.099$; $\beta = 0.215$; Cohen's $f = 0.222$; $R^2 = 0.28$; adj. $R^2 = 0.017$; post-hoc power $= 0.38$).

More specifically, CRF_1 receptor antagonist-treated, abused patients with high baseline NR3C1 methylation levels showed the strongest PSS percent change and therefore the best treatment outcome overall (Fig. 2a, b). A post-hoc analysis revealed that the interaction of baseline NR3C1 methylation and child abuse was significantly associated with PSS percent change after CRF_1 receptor antagonist treatment ($n = 38$; F (1, 20) $= 4.58$; $p = 0.045$; $\beta = 0.331$; Cohen's $f = 0.478$; $R^2 = 0.67$; adj. $R^2 = 0.39$; post-hoc power $= 0.81$) (Fig. 2a) but not placebo ($n = 40$; $p > 0.05$) (Fig. 2b). Results from the same analysis using CAPS score %-change as treatment outcome showed the same direction of effects but did not reach significance (three-way interaction: $n = 79$; $p > 0.05$) (Fig. 2c, d).

For FKBP5, abused patients with high baseline methylation and treated with the CRF_1 receptor antagonist experienced the strongest CAPS percent change ($n = 79$, F (1, 57) $= 2.81$; $p = 0.099$). The post-hoc analysis, stratifying patients by treatment and testing the interaction effect of baseline methylation by child abuse on PTSD symptom change, did not reach significance in neither one of the treatment groups ($p > 0.05$ for all) (Fig. 3a–d).

Pre- to post-treatment methylation change by treatment interaction effects and three-way interaction effects including SNP or child abuse on PTSD symptom change

To examine the association between FKBP5/NR3C1 methylation change from baseline to post-treatment and symptom improvement, we tested for interaction effects of treatment by pre- to post-methylation change on %-change of PTSD symptoms from pre- to post-treatment. For NR3C1 and FKBP5, 57 subjects were included in the analysis due to missing methylation data in two baseline samples and one post-treatment sample. None of the tested interactions reached significance (FKBP5: $n = 57$, $p > 0.5$; NR3C1: $n = 57$, $p > 0.5$). Further, including either rs110402 or child abuse in our analysis to test for two three-way interactions (rs110402 × treatment × pre- to post-methylation change or child abuse × treatment × pre- to post-methylation change) on symptom reduction also did not show significant effects (FKBP5: $n = 57$, $p > 0.5$; NR3C1: $n = 57$, $p > 0.5$).

Discussion

The objective of this study was to investigate epigenetic marks of PTSD-related genes in association with PTSD symptom changes after CRF_1 receptor antagonist (GSK561679) treatment in female PTSD patients. In a first analysis, we observed significant differences in CRHR1 methylation levels after treatment among patients with probable CRF hyperactivity who previously demonstrated the greatest clinical benefit from the CRF_1 receptor antagonist [16]; this effect was not present among those who received placebo. This subgroup of patients who had experienced child abuse and were

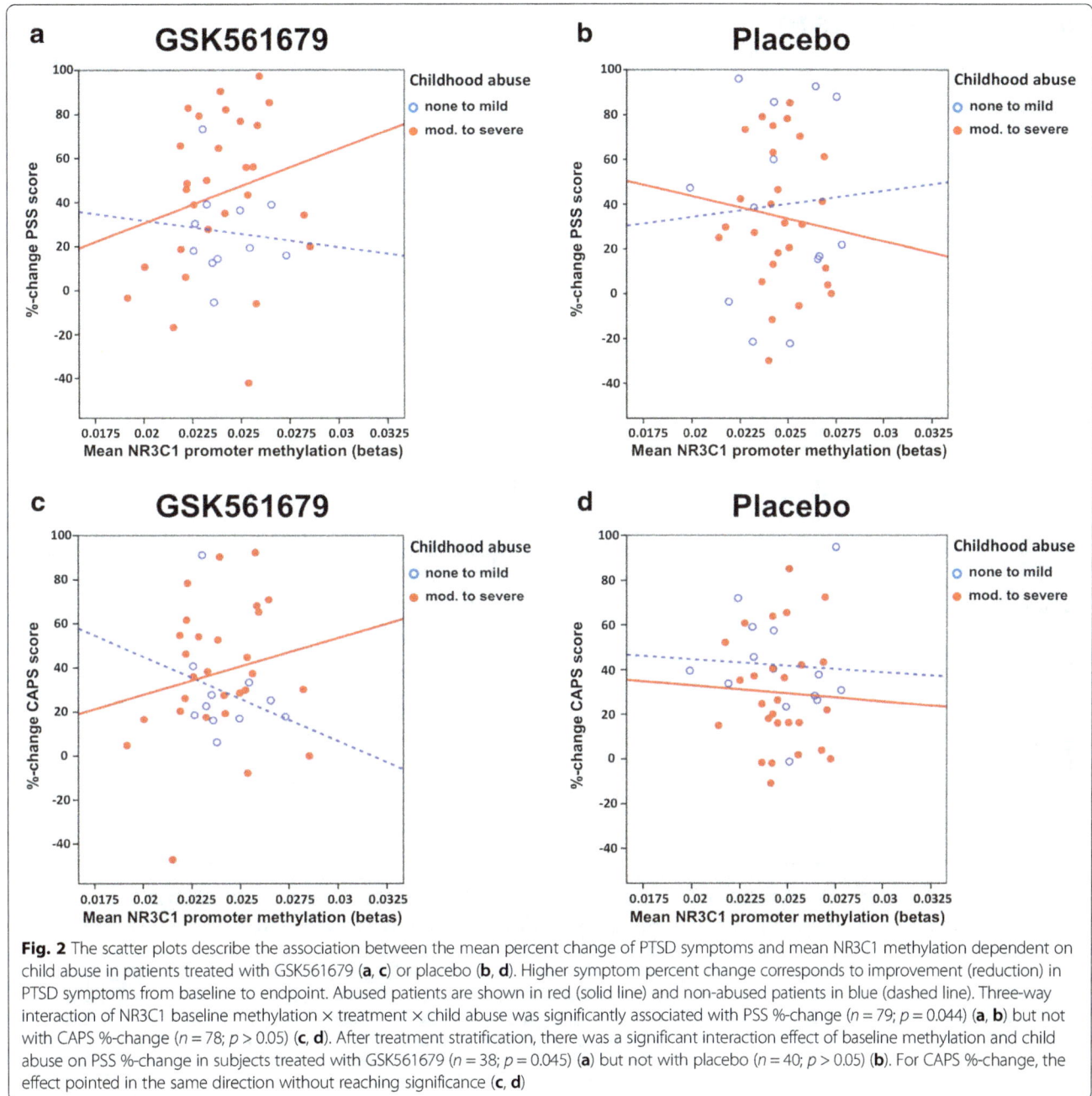

Fig. 2 The scatter plots describe the association between the mean percent change of PTSD symptoms and mean NR3C1 methylation dependent on child abuse in patients treated with GSK561679 (**a, c**) or placebo (**b, d**). Higher symptom percent change corresponds to improvement (reduction) in PTSD symptoms from baseline to endpoint. Abused patients are shown in red (solid line) and non-abused patients in blue (dashed line). Three-way interaction of NR3C1 baseline methylation × treatment × child abuse was significantly associated with PSS %-change ($n = 79$; $p = 0.044$) (**a, b**) but not with CAPS %-change ($n = 78$; $p > 0.05$) (**c, d**). After treatment stratification, there was a significant interaction effect of baseline methylation and child abuse on PSS %-change in subjects treated with GSK561679 ($n = 38$; $p = 0.045$) (**a**) but not with placebo ($n = 40$; $p > 0.05$) (**b**). For CAPS %-change, the effect pointed in the same direction without reaching significance (**c, d**)

homozygous for the rs110402 GG allele were the only individuals showing a significant increase in *CRHR1* methylation from baseline to the post-GSK561679 treatment time point. All other subjects either showed no change or a reduction in methylation over the time of treatment. On the other hand, baseline *CRHR1* methylation did not predict treatment outcome, suggesting that this epigenetic change may only serve as a potential tracker of symptom changes. The maximum difference in mean *CRHR1* methylation between the subgroups was more than 3%, a change comparable to or even larger than other studies examining

peripheral blood DNA methylation and psychiatric disorders or psychiatric treatment response. In fact, when examining the 11 CpGs composing the *CRHR1* variable methylation score, the maximal effects were observed in CpGs cg27410679 and cg04194664. In the subgroup of patients with child abuse and homozygous for the rs110402 GG allele, these CpGs showed an increase in methylation of up to 3.9% and a maximum methylation difference between the four subgroups of 9.9% (cg04194664) and 7.7% (cg27410679). Future studies should evaluate these optimized markers in larger samples.

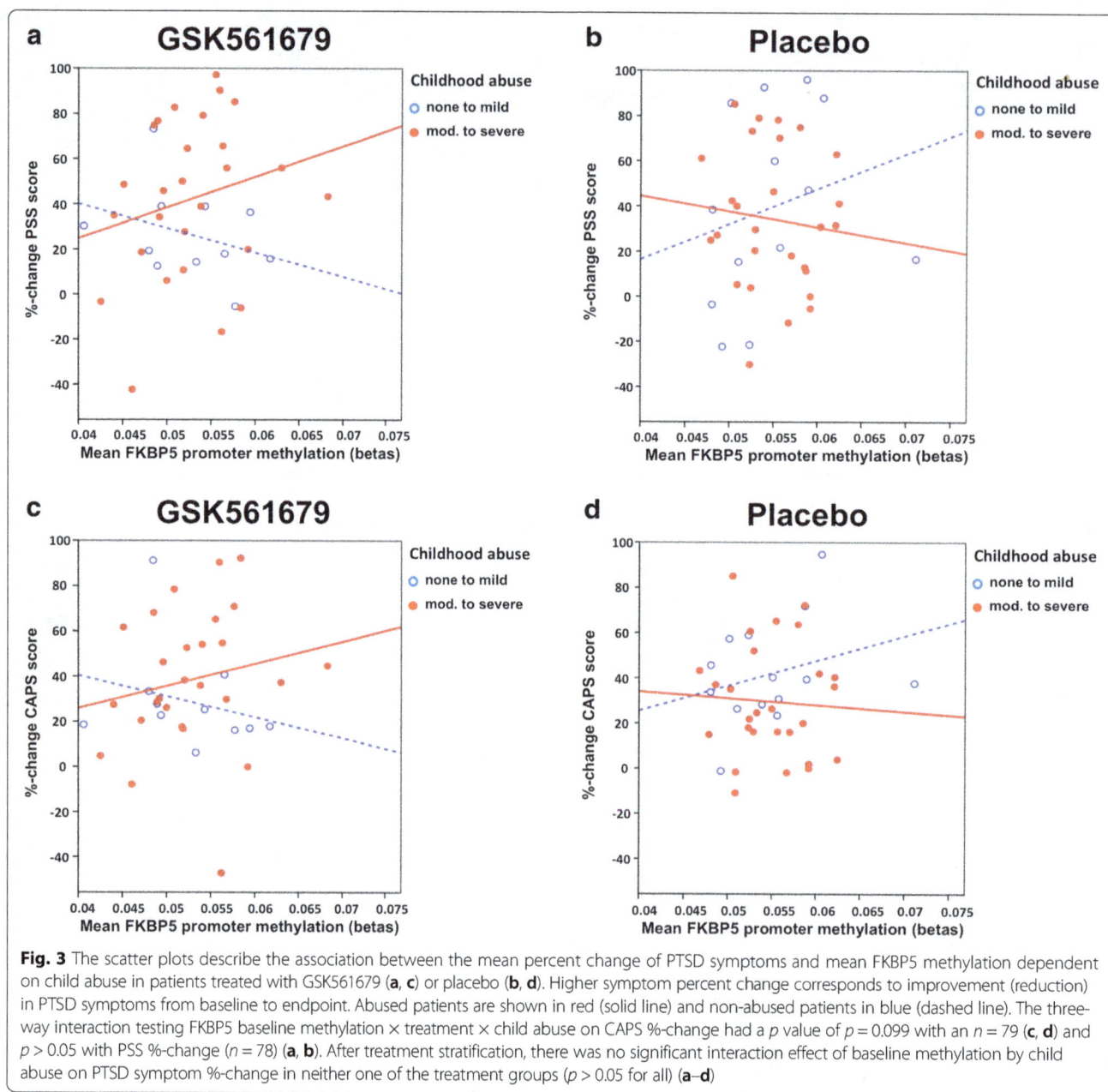

Fig. 3 The scatter plots describe the association between the mean percent change of PTSD symptoms and mean FKBP5 methylation dependent on child abuse in patients treated with GSK561679 (**a**, **c**) or placebo (**b**, **d**). Higher symptom percent change corresponds to improvement (reduction) in PTSD symptoms from baseline to endpoint. Abused patients are shown in red (solid line) and non-abused patients in blue (dashed line). The three-way interaction testing FKBP5 baseline methylation × treatment × child abuse on CAPS %-change had a p value of $p = 0.099$ with an $n = 79$ (**c**, **d**) and $p > 0.05$ with PSS %-change ($n = 78$) (**a**, **b**). After treatment stratification, there was no significant interaction effect of baseline methylation by child abuse on PTSD symptom %-change in neither one of the treatment groups ($p > 0.05$ for all) (**a–d**)

A number of factors can contribute to changes in DNA methylation. In a mixed tissue such as peripheral blood, the most likely contributor is the changes in immune cell subtype composition. Changes in immune responses have been reported in PTSD (reviewed by [23]), and symptom normalization may be associated with a change in immune function and cell type proportion [24–26]. We attempted to account for this using a bioinformatics deconvolution method for blood cell types from genome-wide methylation data [27] and adding the estimated cell type proportions as covariates. In addition, there has been increasing evidence suggesting that dynamic methylation changes, as observed in our study, may

be mediated by certain transcription factors [28–30]. Several studies have reported on the potential role of the glucocorticoid receptor as one of these transcription factors mediating glucocorticoid-induced DNA demethylation [31, 32]. CRF_1 receptor antagonists influence the regulation of the HPA axis and by that, ultimately, modulate GR activity. Our previously identified subgroup of patients with rs110402 GG genotype and a history of child abuse displayed a significant increase in *CRHR1* methylation after GSK561679 treatment. Previous studies have shown that this combination of environmental and genetic risk is associated with specific disruptions of HPA axis regulation, including an enhanced cortisol response to the

Trier Social Stress Test and the combined dexamethasone suppression/CRF stimulation test [11–14]. A combination of increased CRF activity and GR activation may exist in this subgroup and normalize with specific CRF$_1$ receptor antagonist treatment. In fact, a number of studies have also reported GR supersensitivity with PTSD [33, 34] and its normalization with effective treatment [35, 36]. Such a reversal of GR supersensitivity in the subset of patients with response to the antagonist may also lead to changes in GR-mediated DNA methylation. In fact, active GR response elements are shown in the ENCODE project for the *CRHR1* locus [37]. Finally, GSK561679 itself could directly impact *CRHR1* methylation. However, the *CRHR1* expression is low in peripheral blood cells (https://gtex portal.org/), suggesting that the epigenetic regulation of the locus indirectly via receptor blockade and adaptive transcriptional regulation is an unlikely mechanism for inducing this effect.

In our second analysis, we investigated peripheral blood DNA methylation of two genes, for which a previous study had found an association with improvement of PTSD symptoms after prolonged exposure therapy [22]. In a small cohort of combat veterans diagnosed with PTSD, the authors reported that pre-treatment *NR3C1* methylation significantly predicted treatment outcome, with higher *NR3C1* methylation at baseline associated with better response to psychotherapy. The authors also observed a decrease in *FKBP5* promoter methylation over treatment in patients showing clinical improvement [22].

Similar to Yehuda et al. [22], we also find that higher baseline methylation of *NR3C1* is associated with better treatment outcome with the antagonist. However, in our analysis, this is only seen in patients who had also experienced child abuse. No association was found for *FKBP5*, neither for baseline levels predicting treatment outcome nor for change in *FKBP5* methylation being associated with symptom improvement, as reported in Yehuda et al. [22]. While exploratory, our results support the conclusion that peripheral blood DNA methylation of *NR3C1* is associated with PTSD treatment response.

The major limitation of this study is the small sample size, particularly after biological subgrouping. Power calculation for our main hypothesis (change of CRHR1 methylation over treatment and prediction of treatment outcome), however, revealed that power would be sufficient to detect medium to large effect sizes, whereas smaller effect sizes would have been missed. A post-hoc power analysis for the specific effect sizes detected in our study showed that power ranged between 0.673 and 0.999. Further, due to the exploratory nature of our study, we did not apply a systematic correction for multiple testing, increasing the risk for false-positive associations. To identify smaller effects, confirm our results, and reduce the risk of a type I and type II error, much larger sample sizes will be required for future studies.

An additional limitation to this study, which represents a general issue in DNA methylation analyses of mixed tissues, is to rule out cell type composition variation as a potential confounding factor contributing to the observed epigenetic changes. As described, we applied a commonly used bioinformatics cell-type deconvolution method [27] to address this issue. However, this method only accounts for six different cell types in the blood, so that changes in subtypes not covered by this algorithm may still contribute to the observed changes in DNA methylation.

Conclusion

Overall, our results indicate that markers for PTSD likely will need to be an index, comprised of several combination markers. Here, we describe the association of *CRHR1* DNA methylation with treatment response, but only in a specific subset of patients defined by genetic and environmental risk factors. While our association of baseline *NR3C1* methylation with PTSD treatment outcome is supportive of previous findings, both studies are small. Given the exploratory nature of the study and the small sample size, larger studies that stratify patients by potential biomarker status will be needed to fully establish the clinical value of these measures.

Methods
Study overview

Detailed descriptions of the trial design and the study results were published previously [15, 16] and are summarized in the following.

Cohort

Patients were recruited at four academic sites (Emory University, Icahn School of Medicine at Mount Sinai, Baylor College of Medicine, University of California San Francisco/San Francisco Veterans Affairs Medical Center) in the USA. The institutional review boards at each study site approved the study. The cohort used for this study consisted of 88 female patients between 18 and 65 years of age. Males were excluded due to potential reproductive organ toxicity of the investigational medication. All subjects were free of psychotropic medication (except non-benzodiazepine hypnotics) for at least 2 weeks prior to randomization. Subjects had to fulfill criteria for a primary psychiatric diagnosis of DSM-IV-defined PTSD of at least 3 month's duration since the index trauma. PTSD status at the baseline (randomization) visit had to be of at least moderate severity, defined as Clinician-Administered PTSD Scale (CAPS) for DSM-IV [38] past-month and past-week total scores ≥ 50. Important exclusion criteria included current or past diagnosis of a psychotic disorder, bipolar disorder, or obsessive-compulsive disorder. Subjects with a positive test for drugs of abuse at the screening visit, or who met criteria for substance abuse or dependence within 3 months of the randomization visit, or who presented with significant current suicidal ideation were excluded. Pregnant or lactating women and subjects with an unstable medical condition were also excluded.

Study design

Subjects participated in a parallel-group, double-blind, placebo-controlled randomized clinical trial of a novel CRF_1 receptor antagonist (GSK561679). After randomization, patients were either treated with a nightly dose of 350 mg GSK561679 or placebo over 6 weeks. At the baseline visit (prior to treatment phase), numerous data including demographics, vital signs, and several psychiatric measures were assessed, e.g., level of childhood maltreatment was tested using the Childhood Trauma Questionnaire (CTQ). CAPS score and PTSD Symptom Scale-Self-Report (PSS-SR) [39] were assessed at weeks 1, 2, 4, and 6 after randomization to assess PTSD symptom severity, and the percent change of these scores from pre- to post-treatment were used to determine the degree of improvement in PTSD symptoms. For biological assessments (e.g., methylation levels, genotyping), whole blood was collected at baseline ($n = 88$) as well as after 5 weeks of treatment ($n = 60$ with both baseline and post-treatment) and DNA extraction was performed.

DNA extraction

DNA isolation from whole blood was performed with a *magnetic bead*-based technology on the chemagic 360 extraction robot using the chemagic DNA Blood Kit special (PerkinElmer Inc., Waltham, MA, USA). Quality and quantity of the extracted DNA were assessed using the Epoch Microplate Spectrophotometer (BioTek, Winooski, VT, USA).

Genotyping

Genome-wide SNP genotyping was performed for all subjects using Illumina HumanOmniExpress-24 BeadChips according to the manufacturer's protocol. We excluded the relatives of individual subjects from the whole sample ($n = 3$, Pihat ≥ 0.0625) based on mean identity by descent (IBD) in PLINK [40]. Eighty-five subjects remained for further QC. For the genome-wide analyses that were used to correct for population stratification, we only included individuals with a sample-wise call rate ≥ 0.98 and SNPs with call rate ≥ 0.98, Hardy Weinberg equilibrium test (HWE) p value $\geq 1 \times 10^{-5}$ and MAF ≥ 0.05, allowing for a total of 575,455 markers in 85 individuals. To correct for population stratification in an ethnically mixed sample, principal components (PC) for the genetic background were calculated from all

genotypes for each of the individuals using genome-wide complex trait analysis (GCTA) [41].

Methylation analysis

DNA methylation levels were assessed using the Illumina 450k array. After bisulfite conversion with the Zymo EZ-96 DNA Methylation Kit (Zymo Research, Irvine, CA. USA), genome-wide DNA methylation levels were assessed for 84 baseline samples and 60 matching post-treatment samples using Illumina 450K DNA methylation arrays (Illumina, San Diego, CA, USA) as previously published [42].

Quality control of DNA methylation

Minfi Bioconductor R package (version 1.10.2) was used to perform quality control of methylation data including normalization, intensity readouts, cell type composition estimation, and beta and M value calculation. A detection p value larger than 0.01 in at least 75% of the samples led to an exclusion of the probe. Probes that were located close (10 bp from query site) to a SNP which had a minor allele frequency of ≥ 0.05 in any of the populations represented in the sample were removed as well as X chromosome, Y chromosome, and non-specific binding probes. The data were then normalized using functional normalization, which is an extension of quantile normalization included in the minfi R package. The Bioconductor R package shinyMethyl version 0.99.3 was used to identify batch effects by inspecting the association of the first principal component of the methylation levels with plate, sentrix array, and position using linear regression and visual inspection of PCA plots. A linear regression model was fitted in R with the M values for each probe as the dependent variable and plate, sentrix array, and row as the independent variables as factors to remove batch effects. Two baseline samples and one post-treatment sample did not pass quality control, which resulted in 82 baseline samples and 57 matching pairs with 450K methylation data.

Statistical analyses

Statistical analysis was carried out using SPSS v.18.0 (IBM Corp., Armonk, NY, USA) and R software v 3.2 (https://www.r-project.org/). Genotype analysis (SNP rs110402): the intronic SNP rs110402 has been shown to be associated with HPA axis hyperactivity [11, 14, 43]. This may result in a different response to antagonizing the CRF system, depending on a patient's rs110402 genotype. We therefore focused on rs110402 genotype stratification in our analysis. Direct genotypes were taken from the HumanOmniExpress-24 array (rs110402 MAF = 0.401, HWE test p value = 0.52). According to our previous study [16], patients were categorized by rs110402 A-allele carrier status (GG = 33 carriers and 53

A-allele carriers, of which 38 patients had the AG genotype and 15 were homozygous for the A-allele). Grouping individuals carrying one or two copies of the minor A-allele of rs110402 has been used in previous studies [9, 11, 44] and helps to preserve power. Additive effects of that SNP have previously been reported [45]. Methylation analysis: *CRHR1*: From the *CRHR1* gene locus covered by 33 CpGs on the 450k array, the top tertile (11 CpGs) of the CpGs with the most variable methylation change from pre to post-treatment was selected (Additional file 1: Table S1). The mean methylation of these 11 CpGs was calculated and used for further analysis. *NR3C1*: Mean methylation of 5 CpG sites within the 1F promoter and exon present on the Illumina 450K array was used for the analysis (Additional file 1: Table S2). DNA methylation in the 1F promoter and exon had been shown to predict PTSD treatment outcome [22]. *FKBP5*: Mean methylation level of 3 CpG sites within the exon 1 promoter present on the Illumina 450K array was used for the analysis (Additional file 1: Table S3). DNA methylation of this locus was shown to track with symptom improvement [22]. Childhood trauma status was defined as previously described by categorizing individuals as having experienced either no or only mild abuse versus those having experienced at least one type of moderate to severe abuse (emotional abuse ≥ 13, physical abuse ≥ 10, sexual abuse ≥ 8) (57 = abused, 31 = non-abused) using the CTQ [45]. We performed linear regression models adjusted for age, smoking, ancestry PC, and estimated blood cell count to test for main/two-way and three-way interaction effects on methylation changes as well as main/two-way and three-way interactions effects on PTSD symptom %-change. For each of the analysis, only individuals with complete phenotype, methylation data, genotypes, and any additional covariates were included in the model. We calculated power post-hoc using G Power 3.1 [46]. Alpha was set to 0.05, and the number of groups, degrees of freedom, and eta squares were set according to the test-specific calculations performed in SPSS. Statistical significance was considered at $p < 0.05$. Due to the exploratory nature of the study, no correction for multiple testing was applied. As a measure of effect size, Cohen's f was calculated and interpreted as follows: $f < 0.25$ = small effect size; $0.25 < f < 0.4$ = medium effect size; $f > 0.4$ = large effect size [47].

Abbreviations

ACTH: Adrenocorticotropic hormone; CAPS: Clinician-Administered PTSD Scale; CpG: Cytosine-phosphate-guanine; CRF1: Corticotropin-releasing hormone receptor 1; *CRHR1*: Corticotropin-releasing hormone receptor 1 (gene); CTQ: Childhood Trauma Questionnaire; *FKBP5*: FK506-binding protein 51 kDa gene; GR: Glucocorticoid receptor; HPA: Hypothalamic-pituitary-adrenal; *NR3C1*: Nuclear receptor subfamily 3 group C member 1; PSS: PTSD symptom scale; PTSD: Post-traumatic stress disorder; QC: Quality control; *SKA2*: Spindle and kinetochore-associated complex subunit 2; SNP: Single nucleotide polymorphism

Acknowledgements

We thank Susann Sauer, Anne Löschner, and Maik Ködel for the excellent technical assistance with DNA extraction, genotyping, and DNA methylation assessment.

Funding

Funding for the study was provided from a grant from the National Institute of Mental Health, U19 MH069056 (BWD, HM). Additional support was received from K23 MH086690 (BWD) and VA CSRD Project ID 09S-NIMH-002 (TCN) and the Max Planck Society. The GSK561679 compound was currently licensed by Neurocrine Biosciences. GlaxoSmithKline contributed the study medication and matching placebo, as well as funds to support subject recruitment and laboratory testing, and Neurocrine Biosciences conducted the pharmacokinetic analyses. GlaxoSmithKline and Neurocrine Biosciences were not involved in the data collection, data analysis, or interpretation of findings.

Authors' contributions

EB and JP designed the research and coordinated the experimental work. BD, HM, CN, BR, DI, SM, and TN were responsible for the clinical trial and the different recruitment sites. JP performed the experimental work. JP, TC, and DC performed the statistical analysis. JP and EB prepared the initial manuscript. BR, CN, DC, AZ, DI, SM, TN, HM, and BD revised and edited the manuscript. All authors read and approved the final manuscript.

Competing interests

Dr. Mayberg reports grants from NIMH, grants, and other from GSK, during the conduct of the study; personal fees from Abbott Labs (previously St Jude Medical Inc), outside the submitted work.
Dr. Dunlop reports grants from the National Institute of Mental Health during the conduct of the study; grants from Takeda, grants from Janssen, grants from Acadia, grants from Axsome, outside the submitted work.
Dr. Mathew has served as a consultant to Allergan, Alkermes, and Fortress Biotech. He has received research support from NeuroRx.
Dr. Iosifescu reports grants from the National Institute of Mental Health, during the conduct of the study; personal fees from Axsome, personal fees from Alkermes, grants from Brainsway, grants from LiteCure, personal fees from Lundbeck, grants from Neosync, personal fees from Otsuka, personal fees from Sunovion, outside the submitted work.
Dr. Nemeroff has received research support from the National Institutes of Health (NIH) and Stanley Medical Research Institute. For the last 3 years, he was a consultant for Xhale, Takeda, Taisho Pharmaceutical Inc., Prismic Pharmaceuticals, Bracket (Clintara), Fortress Biotech, Sunovion Pharmaceuticals Inc., Sumitomo Dainippon Pharma, Janssen Research & Development LLC, Magstim, Inc., Navitor Pharmaceuticals, Inc., TC MSO, Inc., Intra-Cellular Therapies, Inc. He is a Stockholder of Xhale, Celgene, Seattle Genetics, Abbvie, OPKO Health, Antares, BI Gen Holdings, Inc., and Corcept Therapeutics Pharmaceuticals Company. Dr. Nemeroff is a member of the scientific advisory boards of the American Foundation for Suicide Prevention (AFSP), Brain and Behavior Research Foundation (BBRF) (formerly named National Alliance for Research on Schizophrenia and Depression [NARSAD]), Xhale, Anxiety Disorder Association of America (ADAA), Skyland Trail, Bracket (Clintara), Laureate Institute for Brain Research, Inc. and on the board of directors of AFSP, Gratitude America and ADAA. Dr. Nemeroff has income sources or equity of 10.000 USD or more from American Psychiatric Publishing, Xhale, Bracket (Clintara), CME Outfitters, Takeda, Intra-Cellular Therapies, Inc., and Magstim. Dr. Nemeroff holds the following patents: Method and devices for transdermal delivery of lithium (US 6,375,990B1) and Method of assessing antidepressant drug therapy via transport inhibition of monoamine neurotransmitter by ex vivo assay (US 7,148,027B2).
Dr. Binder, Dr. Rothbaum, Dr. Neylan, Dr. Pape, Dr. Carrillo-Roa, Dr. Czamara and Dr. Zannas have nothing to disclose.

Author details
[1]Department of Translational Research in Psychiatry, Max Planck Institute of Psychiatry, Munich, Germany. [2]Department of Psychiatry and Behavioral Sciences, Emory University School of Medicine, Atlanta, GA, USA. [3]Department of Psychiatry and Behavioral Sciences, University of Miami Miller School of Medicine, Miami, FL, USA. [4]Department of Psychiatry, Icahn School of Medicine at Mount Sinai, New York, NY, USA. [5]Menninger Department of Psychiatry & Behavioral Sciences, Baylor College of Medicine & Michael E. Debakey VA Medical Center, Houston, TX, USA. [6]Department of Psychiatry, University of California, San Francisco, San Francisco, CA, USA. [7]The San Francisco Veterans Affairs Medical Center, San Francisco, CA, USA. [8]Department of Psychiatry and Behavioral Sciences, Duke University Medical Center, Durham, NC, USA. [9]New York University School of Medicine, New York, NY, USA. [10]Nathan Kline Institute for Psychiatric Research, Orangeburg, NY, USA.

References

1. Krystal JH, Davis LL, Neylan TC, Raskind MA, Schnurr PP, Stein MB, et al. It is time to address the crisis in the pharmacotherapy of posttraumatic stress disorder: a consensus statement of the PTSD psychopharmacology working group. Biol Psychiatry. 2017. https://doi.org/10.1016/j.biopsych.2017.03.007.
2. Mehta D, Binder EB. Gene × environment vulnerability factors for PTSD: the HPA-axis. Neuropharmacology. 2012;62:654–62.
3. Binder EB, Nemeroff CB. The CRF system, stress, depression and anxiety-insights from human genetic studies. Mol Psychiatry. 2010;15:574–88.
4. Laryea G, Arnett MG, Muglia LJ. Behavioral studies and genetic alterations in corticotropin-releasing hormone (CRH) neurocircuitry: insights into human psychiatric disorders. Behav Sci (Basel, Switzerland). 2012;2:135–71.
5. Baker DG, West SA, Nicholson WE, Ekhator NN, Kasckow JW, Hill KK, et al. Serial CSF corticotropin-releasing hormone levels and adrenocortical activity in combat veterans with posttraumatic stress disorder. Am J Psychiatry. 1999;156:585–8.
6. Bremner JD, Licinio J, Darnell A, Krystal JH, Owens MJ, Southwick SM, et al. Elevated CSF corticotropin-releasing factor concentrations in posttraumatic stress disorder. Am J Psychiatry. 1997;154:624–9.
7. Sautter FJ, Bissette G, Wiley J, Manguno-Mire G, Schoenbachler B, Myers L, et al. Corticotropin-releasing factor in posttraumatic stress disorder (PTSD) with secondary psychotic symptoms, nonpsychotic PTSD, and healthy control subjects. Biol Psychiatry. 2003;54:1382–8.
8. Halldorsdottir T, Binder EB. Gene × environment interactions: from molecular mechanisms to behavior. Annu Rev Psychol. 2017;68:215–41.
9. Glaser YG, Zubieta J-K, Hsu DT, Villafuerte S, Mickey BJ, Trucco EM, et al. Indirect effect of corticotropin-releasing hormone receptor 1 gene variation on negative emotionality and alcohol use via right ventrolateral prefrontal cortex. J Neurosci. 2014;34:4099–107.
10. Cicchetti D, Rogosch FA, Oshri A. Interactive effects of corticotropin releasing hormone receptor 1, serotonin transporter linked polymorphic region, and child maltreatment on diurnal cortisol regulation and internalizing symptomatology. Dev Psychopathol. 2011;23:1125–38.
11. Heim C, Bradley B, Mletzko TC, Deveau TC, Musselman DL, Nemeroff CB, et al. Effect of childhood trauma on adult depression and neuroendocrine function: sex-specific moderation by CRH receptor 1 gene. Front Behav Neurosci. 2009;3:41.
12. Mahon PB, Zandi PP, Potash JB, Nestadt G, Wand GS. Genetic association of FKBP5 and CRHR1 with cortisol response to acute psychosocial stress in healthy adults. Psychopharmacology. 2013;227:231–41.
13. Sumner JA, McLaughlin KA, Walsh K, Sheridan MA, Koenen KC. CRHR1 genotype and history of maltreatment predict cortisol reactivity to stress in adolescents. Psychoneuroendocrinology. 2014;43:71–80.
14. Tyrka AR, Price LH, Gelernter J, Schepker C, Anderson GM, Carpenter LL. Interaction of childhood maltreatment with the corticotropin-releasing hormone receptor gene: effects on hypothalamic-pituitary-adrenal axis reactivity. Biol Psychiatry. 2009;66:681–5.
15. Dunlop BW, Rothbaum BO, Binder EB, Duncan E, Harvey PD, Jovanovic T, et al. Evaluation of a corticotropin releasing hormone type 1 receptor antagonist in women with posttraumatic stress disorder: study protocol for a randomized controlled trial. Trials. 2014;15:240.
16. Dunlop BW, Binder EB, Iosifescu D, Mathew SJ, Neylan TC, Pape JC, et al. Corticotropin-releasing factor type 1 receptor antagonism is ineffective for women with posttraumatic stress disorder. Biol Psychiatry. 2017;23: 5295–301.
17. Colvonen PJ, Glassman LH, Crocker LD, Buttner MM, Orff H, Schiehser DM, et al. Pretreatment biomarkers predicting PTSD psychotherapy outcomes: a systematic review. Neurosci Biobehav Rev. 2017;75:140–56.
18. Lehrner A, Yehuda R. Biomarkers of PTSD: military applications and considerations. Eur J Psychotraumatol. 2014;5. https://doi.org/10.3402/ejpt. v5.23797.
19. Klengel T, Pape J, Binder EB, Mehta D. The role of DNA methylation in stress-related psychiatric disorders. Neuropharmacology. 2014;80:115–32.
20. Labonté B, Azoulay N, Yerko V, Turecki G, Brunet A. Epigenetic modulation of glucocorticoid receptors in posttraumatic stress disorder. Transl Psychiatry. 2014;4:e368.
21. Yehuda R, Flory JD, Bierer LM, Henn-Haase C, Lehrner A, Desarnaud F, et al. Lower methylation of glucocorticoid receptor gene promoter 1F in peripheral blood of veterans with posttraumatic stress disorder. Biol Psychiatry. 2015;77: 356–64.
22. Yehuda R, Daskalakis NP, Desarnaud F, Makotkine I, Lehrner AL, Koch E, et al. Epigenetic biomarkers as predictors and correlates of symptom improvement following psychotherapy in combat veterans with PTSD. Front Psychiatry. 2013; 4:118.
23. Wang Z, Young MRI. PTSD, a disorder with an immunological component. Front Immunol. 2016;7:219.
24. Gill JM, Saligan L, Lee H, Rotolo S, Szanton S. Women in recovery from PTSD have similar inflammation and quality of life as non-traumatized controls. J Psychosom Res. 2013;74:301–6.
25. Gocan AG, Bachg D, Schindler AE, Rohr UD. Balancing steroidal hormone cascade in treatment-resistant veteran soldiers with PTSD using a fermented soy product (FSWW08): a pilot study. Horm Mol Biol Clin Invest. 2012;10: 301–14.
26. Morath J, Gola H, Sommershof A, Hamuni G, Kolassa S, Catani C, et al. The effect of trauma-focused therapy on the altered T cell distribution in individuals with PTSD: evidence from a randomized controlled trial. J Psychiatr Res. 2014;54: 1–10.
27. Houseman E, Accomando WP, Koestler DC, Christensen BC, Marsit CJ, Nelson HH, et al. DNA methylation arrays as surrogate measures of cell mixture distribution. BMC Bioinformatics. 2012;13:86.
28. Kirillov A, Kistler B, Mostoslavsky R, Cedar H, Wirth T, Bergman Y. A role for nuclear NF-kappaB in B-cell-specific demethylation of the Igkappa locus. Nat Genet. 1996;13:435–41.
29. Feldmann A, Ivanek R, Murr R, Gaidatzis D, Burger L, Schübeler D. Transcription factor occupancy can mediate active turnover of DNA methylation at regulatory regions. PLoS Genet. 2013;9:e1003994.
30. Weaver ICG, D'Alessio AC, Brown SE, Hellstrom IC, Dymov S, Sharma S, et al. The transcription factor nerve growth factor-inducible protein a mediates epigenetic programming: altering epigenetic marks by immediate-early genes. J Neurosci. 2007;27:1756–68.
31. Thomassin H, Flavin M, Espinás ML, Grange T. Glucocorticoid-induced DNA demethylation and gene memory during development. EMBO J. 2001;20: 1974–83.
32. Wiench M, John S, Baek S, Johnson TA, Sung M-H, Escobar T, et al. DNA methylation status predicts cell type-specific enhancer activity. EMBO J. 2011;30:3028–39.

DNA methylation levels are associated with CRF1 receptor antagonist treatment outcome in women...

233

33. de Kloet CS, Vermetten E, Heijnen CJ, Geuze E, Lentjes EGWM, Westenberg HGM. Enhanced cortisol suppression in response to dexamethasone administration in traumatized veterans with and without posttraumatic stress disorder. Psychoneuroendocrinology. 2007;32:215–26.

34. Yehuda R. Status of glucocorticoid alterations in post-traumatic stress disorder. Ann N Y Acad Sci. 2009;1179:56–69.

35. Olff M, de Vries G-J, Güzelcan Y, Assies J, Gersons BPR. Changes in cortisol and DHEA plasma levels after psychotherapy for PTSD. Psychoneuroendocrinology. 2007;32:619–26.

36. Yehuda R, Pratchett LC, Elmes MW, Lehrner A, Daskalakis NP, Koch E, et al. Glucocorticoid-related predictors and correlates of post-traumatic stress disorder treatment response in combat veterans. Interface Focus. 2014;4: 20140048.

37. ENCODE Project Consortium TEP. An integrated encyclopedia of DNA elements in the human genome. Nature. 2012;489:57–74.

38. Blake DD, Weathers FW, Nagy LM, Kaloupek DG, Gusman FD, Charney DS, et al. The development of a clinician-administered PTSD scale. J Trauma Stress. 1995;8:75–90.

39. Foa EB, Riggs DS, Dancu CV, Rothbaum BO. Reliability and validity of a brief instrument for assessing post-traumatic stress disorder. J Trauma Stress. 1993;6:459–73.

40. Purcell S, Neale B, Todd-Brown K, Thomas L, Ferreira MAR, Bender D, et al. PLINK: a tool set for whole-genome association and population-based linkage analyses. Am J Hum Genet. 2007;81:559–75.

41. Yang J, Lee SH, Goddard ME, Visscher PM. GCTA: a tool for genome-wide complex trait analysis. Am J Hum Genet. 2011;88:76–82.

42. Mehta D, Klengel T, Conneely KN, Smith AK, Altmann A, Pace TW, et al. Childhood maltreatment is associated with distinct genomic and epigenetic profiles in posttraumatic stress disorder. Proc Natl Acad Sci. 2013;110:8302–7.

43. Griebel G, Holsboer F. Neuropeptide receptor ligands as drugs for psychiatric diseases: the end of the beginning? Nat Rev Drug Discov. 2012; 11:462–78.

44. Hsu DT, Mickey BJ, Langenecker SA, Heitzeg MM, Love TM, Wang H, et al. Variation in the corticotropin-releasing hormone receptor 1 (CRHR1) gene influences fMRI signal responses during emotional stimulus processing. J Neurosci. 2012;32:3253–60.

45. Bradley RG, Binder EB, Epstein MP, Tang Y, Nair HP, Liu W, et al. Influence of child abuse on adult depression. Arch Gen Psychiatry. 2008;65:190.

46. Faul F, Erdfelder E, Lang A-G, Buchner A. G*power 3: a flexible statistical power analysis program for the social, behavioral, and biomedical sciences. Behav Res Methods. 2007;39:175–91.

47. Cohen J. Statistical power analysis for the behavioral sciences. 2nd ed. Hillsdale: Lawrence Erlbaum Associates, Publishers; 1988.

Permissions

All chapters in this book were first published in CE, by BioMed Central; hereby published with permission under the Creative Commons Attribution License or equivalent. Every chapter published in this book has been scrutinized by our experts. Their significance has been extensively debated. The topics covered herein carry significant findings which will fuel the growth of the discipline. They may even be implemented as practical applications or may be referred to as a beginning point for another development.

The contributors of this book come from diverse backgrounds, making this book a truly international effort. This book will bring forth new frontiers with its revolutionizing research information and detailed analysis of the nascent developments around the world.

We would like to thank all the contributing authors for lending their expertise to make the book truly unique. They have played a crucial role in the development of this book. Without their invaluable contributions this book wouldn't have been possible. They have made vital efforts to compile up to date information on the varied aspects of this subject to make this book a valuable addition to the collection of many professionals and students.

This book was conceptualized with the vision of imparting up-to-date information and advanced data in this field. To ensure the same, a matchless editorial board was set up. Every individual on the board went through rigorous rounds of assessment to prove their worth. After which they invested a large part of their time researching and compiling the most relevant data for our readers.

The editorial board has been involved in producing this book since its inception. They have spent rigorous hours researching and exploring the diverse topics which have resulted in the successful publishing of this book. They have passed on their knowledge of decades through this book. To expedite this challenging task, the publisher supported the team at every step. A small team of assistant editors was also appointed to further simplify the editing procedure and attain best results for the readers.

Apart from the editorial board, the designing team has also invested a significant amount of their time in understanding the subject and creating the most relevant covers. They scrutinized every image to scout for the most suitable representation of the subject and create an appropriate cover for the book.

The publishing team has been an ardent support to the editorial, designing and production team. Their endless efforts to recruit the best for this project, has resulted in the accomplishment of this book. They are a veteran in the field of academics and their pool of knowledge is as vast as their experience in printing. Their expertise and guidance has proved useful at every step. Their uncompromising quality standards have made this book an exceptional effort. Their encouragement from time to time has been an inspiration for everyone.

The publisher and the editorial board hope that this book will prove to be a valuable piece of knowledge for researchers, students, practitioners and scholars across the globe.

List of Contributors

Antoine G. van der Heijden, Cindy C. M. van Rijt-van de Westerlo, Jack A. Schalken, Lambertus A. L. M. Kiemeney and J. Alfred Witjes
Department of Urology Radboud University Medical Center, Nijmegen, The Netherlands

Lourdes Mengual, Mercedes Ingelmo-Torres, Montserrat Baixauli, Maria J. Ribal and Antonio Alcaraz
Laboratory and Department of Urology, Hospital Clinic of Barcelona, IDIBAPS, University of Barcelona, Barcelona, Spain

Juan J. Lozano
CIBERehd,Plataforma de Bioinformática, Centro de Investigación Biomédica en red de Enfermedades Hepáticas y Digestivas, Barcelona, Spain

Bogdan Geavlete, Cristian Moldoveanud and Cosmin Ene
Saint John Emergency Clinical Hospital, Bucharest, Romania

Colin P. Dinney and Bogdan Czerniaks
MD Anderson Cancer Center, Houston, Texas, USA

Antoine G. van der Heijden and Lourdes Mengual
Hospital Clínic de Barcelona, Centre de Recerca Biomèdica CELLEX, office B22, C/Casanova, 143, 08036 Barcelona, Spain

Janina Graule, Kristin Uth, Elia Fischer, Irene Centeno, José A. Galván, Micha Eichmann, Tilman T. Rau, Rupert Langer, Heather Dawson, Alessandro Lugli, Mario P. Tschan and Inti Zlobec
Institute of Pathology, University of Bern, Murtenstrasse 31, Room L310, 3008 Bern, Switzerland

Kristin Uth and Mario P. Tschan
Graduate School for Cellular and Biomedical Sciences, University of Bern, Freiestrasse 1, 3012 Bern, Switzerland

Ulrich Nitsche
Department of Surgery, Klinikum rechts der Isar, Technische Universität München, Ismaninger Strasse 22, Munich 81675, Germany

Peter Traeger
Careanesth AG, Nelkenstrasse 15, Zürich 8006, Switzerland

Martin D. Berger
Department of Medical Oncology, University Hospital of Bern, 3010 Bern, Switzerland Division of Medical Oncology, Norris Comprehensive Cancer Center, Keck School of Medicine, University of Southern California, Los Angeles 90033, CA, USA

Beat Schnüriger, Marion Hädrich and Peter Studer
Department of Visceral and Internal Medicine, University Hospital of Bern, 3008 Bern, Switzerland

Daniel Inderbitzin
University of Bern and Bürgerspital Solothurn, Schöngrünstrasse 42, 4500 Solothurn, Switzerland

Qihua Tan, Marianne Nygaard, Mette Soerensen, Kaare Christensen and Lene Christiansen
Epidemiology and Biostatistics, Department of Public Health, Faculty of Health Science, University of Southern Denmark, J. B. Winsløws Vej 9B, DK-5000 Odense, Denmark

Qihua Tan, Shuxia Li, Martin Larsen and Kaare Christensen
Unit of Human Genetics, Department of Clinical Research, University of Southern Denmark, Odense, Denmark

Morten Frost
Department of Endocrinology, Odense University Hospital, Odense, Denmark

Martin Larsen
Department of Clinical Genetics, Odense University Hospital, Odense, Denmark

Ding Peng, Yanqing Gong, Yonghao Zhan, Shiming He, Bao Guan, Yifan Li, Han Hao, Zhisong He, Gengyan Xiong, Cuijian Zhang, Xuesong Li and Liqun Zhou
Department of Urology, Peking University First Hospital, Beijing 100034, China

Ding Peng, Guangzhe Ge, Ziying Xu, Yue Shi, Yuanyuan Zhou and Weimin
Key Laboratory of Genomic and Precision Medicine, Beijing Institute of Genomics, Chinese Academy of Sciences, Beijing 100101, China

Ding Peng, Yanqing Gong, Yonghao Zhan, Shiming He, Bao Guan, Yifan Li, Han Hao, Zhisong He, Gengyan Xiong, Cuijian Zhang, Xuesong Li and Liqun Zhou
Institute of Urology, Peking University, Beijing 100034, China
National Urological Cancer Center, Beijing 100034, China
Urogenital Diseases (Male) Molecular Diagnosis and Treatment Center, Peking University, Beijing 100034, China

Guangzhe Ge and Weimin Ci
University of Chinese Academy of Sciences, Beijing 100049, China

Daniela Nasif, Richard Branham, Guillermo Urrutia and María T. Branham
IHEM, National University of Cuyo, CONICET, Mendoza, Argentina

Sergio Laurito and María Roqué
IHEM, Faculty of Exact and Natural Sciences, National University of Cuyo, CONICET, Mendoza, Argentina

Emanuel Campoy
IHEM, CONICET, Facultad de Ciencias Médicas, National University of Cuyo, Mendoza, Argentina

Richard Branham
IANIGLA, CONICET, Mendoza, Argentina

Wenji Yan, Xiuduan Xu, Yunsheng Yang and Mingzhou Guo
Department of Gastroenterology and Hepatology, Chinese PLA General Hospital, #28 Fuxing Road, Beijing 100853, China

Wenji Yan and Guanghai Dai
Department of Oncology, Chinese PLA General Hospital, #28 Fuxing Road, Beijing 100853, China

Kongming Wu
Department of Oncology, Tongji Hospital of Tongji Medical College, Huazhong University of Science and Technology, Wuhan 430030, China

James G. Herman
The Hillman Cancer Center, University of Pittsburgh Cancer Institute, 5117 Centre Ave, Pittsburgh, Pennsylvania 15213, USA

Alboukadel Kassambara, Stéphanie Boireau, Nicolas Robert, Guilhem Requirand, Jerome Moreaux, Giacomo Cavalli and Jerome Moreaux
Department of Biological Hematology, CHU Montpellier, Montpellier, France

Laurie Herviou, Alboukadel Kassambara, Stéphanie Boireau, Nicolas Robert, Guilhem Requirand, Giacomo Cavalli and Jerome Moreaux
IGH, CNRS, Univ Montpellier, Montpellier, France

Guillaume Cartron and Jerome Moreaux
UFR de Médecine, Univ Montpellier, Montpellier, France

Carsten Müller-Tidow, Anja Seckinger, Hartmut Goldschmidt and Dirk Hose
Medizinische Klinik und Poliklinik V, Universitätsklinikum Heidelberg, Heidelberg, Germany

Anja Seckinger, Hartmut Goldschmidt and Dirk Hose
Nationales Centrum für Tumorerkrankungen, Heidelberg, Germany

Laure Vincent and Guillaume Cartron
Department of Clinical Hematology, CHU Montpellier, Montpellier, France

Guillaume Cartron
UMR CNRS 5235, Univ Montpellier, Montpellier, France

Jerome Moreaux
Laboratory for Monitoring Innovative Therapies, Department of Biological Hematology, Hôpital Saint-Eloi-CHRU de Montpellier, 80, av. Augustin Fliche, 34295 Montpellier, Cedex 5, France

Emma Ahlén Bergman, Ciputra Adijaya Hartana, Ludvig B. Linton, Sofia Berglund, Christian Lundgren, Malin E. Winerdal, David Krantz, A. Ali Zirakzadeh, Per Marits and Ola Winqvist
Unit of Immunology and Allergy, Department of Medicine Solna, Karolinska Institutet, Karolinska University Hospital, Stockholm, Sweden

Markus Johansson
Department of Urology, Sundsvall Hospital, Sundsvall, Sweden

Markus Johansson, Karin Palmqvist, A. Ali Zirakzadeh and Amir Sherif
Department of surgical and perioperative Sciences, Urology and Andrology, Umeå University, Umeå, Sweden

Martin Hyllienmark
TLA Targeted Immunotherapies AB, Stockholm, Sweden

Benny Holmström
Department of Urology, Akademiska University Hospital, Uppsala, Sweden

Karin Palmqvist
Department of Surgery, Urology Section, Östersund County Hospital, Östersund, Sweden

Johan Hansson
Centre for Research and Development, Faculty of Medicine, Uppsala University, County Council of Gävleborg, Uppsala, Sweden

Farhood Alamdari
Department of Urology, Västmanland Hospital, Västerås, Sweden.

Ylva Huge and Firas Aljabery
Department of Clinical and Experimental Medicine, Division of Urology, Linköping University, Linköping, Sweden

Katrine Riklund and Amir Sherif
Department of Radiation Sciences, Diagnostic Radiology, Umeå University, Umeå, Sweden

Louise K. Sjöholm
Center for Molecular Medicine, Department of Clinical Neuroscience, Karolinska Institutet, Stockholm, Sweden

Lien-Hung Huang and Sung-Chou Li
Genomics and Proteomics Core Laboratory, Department of Medical Research, Kaohsiung Chang Gung Memorial Hospital, 12th Floor, Children's Hospital, No.123, Dapi Rd, Niaosong District, Kaohsiung 83301, Taiwan

Ho-Chang Kuo and Ying-Hsien Huang
Department of Pediatrics, Kaohsiung Chang Gung Memorial Hospital and Chang Gung University College of Medicine, Kaohsiung, Taiwan
Kawasaki Disease Center, Kaohsiung Chang Gung Memorial Hospital, Kaohsiung, Taiwan

Cheng-Tsung Pan and Yeong-Shin Lin
Institute of Bioinformatics and Systems Biology, National Chiao Tung University, Hsinchu, Taiwan

Yeong-Shin Lin
Department of Biological Science and Technology, National Chiao Tung University, Hsinchu, Taiwan

Sarah Gonzalez-Nahm and Sara E. Benjamin-Neelon
Department of Health, Behavior and Society, Johns Hopkins Bloomberg School of Public Health, 624 N Broadway, Baltimore, MD 21205, USA

Michelle A. Mendez
Department of Nutrition, Gillings School of Global Public Health, University of North Carolina at Chapel Hill, Chapel Hill, NC, USA

Susan K. Murphy
Department of Obstetrics and Gynecology, Duke University Medical Center, Durham, NC, USA

Vijaya K. Hogan
W.K. Kellogg Foundation, Battle Creek, MI, USA

Diane L. Rowley
Department of Maternal and Child Health, Gillings School of Global Public Health, University of North Carolina at Chapel Hill, Chapel Hill, NC, USA

Cathrine Hoyo
Department of Biological Sciences, North Carolina State University, Raleigh, NC, USA

Sang-Won Um, Kyung-Jong Lee and Hojoong Kim
Department of Internal Medicine, Samsung Medical Center, Sungkyunkwan University School of Medicine, Seoul 135-710, South Korea

Yujin Kim, Bo Bin Lee, Dongho Kim and Duk-Hwan Kim
Department of Molecular Cell Biology, Samsung Biomedical Research Institute, Sungkyunkwan University School of Medicine, Suwon 440-746, South Korea

Hong Kwan Kim and Young Mog Shim
Department of Thoracic and Cardiovascular Surgery, Samsung Medical Center, Sungkyunkwan University School of Medicine, Seoul 135-710, South Korea

Joungho Han
Department of Pathology, Samsung Medical Center, Sungkyunkwan University School of Medicine, Seoul 135-710, South Korea

Duk-Hwan Kim
Samsung Medical Center, Research Institute for Future Medicine, #50 Ilwon-dong, Kangnam-gu, Professor Rm #5, Seoul 135-710, South Korea

Pei-Chien Tsai and Craig A. Glastonbury, Alice Vickers, Massimo Mangino, Kirsten Ward, Kerrin S. Small and Jordana T. Bell
Department of Twin Research and Genetic Epidemiology, King's College London, London SE1 7EH, UK

Pei-Chien Tsai
Department of Biomedical Sciences, Chang Gung University, Taoyuan, Taiwan

Division of Allergy, Asthma, and Rheumatology, Department of Pediatrics, Chang Gung Memorial Hospital,Linkou, Taiwan

Craig A. Glastonbury
Big Data Institute at the Li Ka Shing Centre for Health Information and Discovery, University of Oxford, Oxford OX3 7LF, UK

Melissa N. Eliot
Department of Epidemiology, Brown University School of Public Health, Providence, RI 02912, USA

Alice Vickers
Centre for Stem Cells and Regenerative Medicine, King's College London, Floor 28, Tower Wing, Guy's Hospital, Great Maze Pond, London SE1 9RT, UK

Massimo Mangino
NIHR Biomedical Research Centre at Guy's and St Thomas' Foundation Trust, London SE1 9RT, UK

Eric B. Loucks and Karl T. Kelsey
Department of Epidemiology, Brown University School of Public Health, Providence, RI 02912, USA

Miina Ollikainen
Institute for Molecular Medicine Finland (FIMM) and Department of Public Health, University of Helsinki, Helsinki, Finland

Karl T. Kelsey
Department of Laboratory Medicine & Pathology, Brown University, Providence, RI 02912, USA

Katharina Bomans, Judith Schenz, Sandra Tamulyte, Dominik Schaack, Markus Alexander Weigand and Florian Uhle
Department of Anesthesiology, Heidelberg University Hospital, Im Neuenheimer Feld 110, 69120 Heidelberg, Germany

Heidi Marjonen and Pauliina Auvinen
Department of Medical and Clinical Genetics, Medicum, University of Helsinki, Helsinki, Finland

Hanna Kahila, Timo Tuuri, Viveca Söderström-Anttila, Andres Salumets and Aila Tiitinen
Department of Obstetrics and Gynecology, University of Helsinki and Helsinki University Hospital, Helsinki, Finland

Olga Tšuiko, Triin Viltrop and Andres Salumets
Department of Biomedicine, Institute of Biomedicine and Translational Medicine, University of Tartu, Tartu, Estonia

Olga Tšuiko and Andres Salumets
Competence Centre on Health Technologies, Tartu, Estonia

Sulev Kõks
Department of Pathophysiology, Institute of Biomedicine and Translational Medicine, University of Tartu, Tartu, Estonia
Department of Reproductive Biology, Estonian University of Life Sciences, Tartu, Estonia

Airi Tiirats and Andres Salumets
Department of Obstetrics and Gynaecology, Institute of Clinical Medicine, University of Tartu, Tartu, Estonia

Airi Tiirats
Department of Paediatric ICU, Tartu University Hospital, Tartu, Estonia

Viveca Söderström-Anttila and Anne-Maria Suikkari
The Family Federation of Finland, Fertility Clinic, Helsinki, Finland

Idoia Blanco-Luquin, Miren Altuna, Javier Sánchez-Ruiz de Gordoa, Amaya Urdánoz-Casado, Miren Roldán, María Elena Erro, Carmen Echavarri and Maite Mendioroz
Neuroepigenetics Laboratory-Navarrabiomed, Complejo Hospitalario de Navarra, Universidad Pública de Navarra (UPNA), IdiSNA (Navarra Institute for Health Research), C/ Irunlarrea, 3, 31008 Pamplona, Navarra, Spain

Miren Altuna, Javier Sánchez-Ruiz de Gordoa, María Cámara, María Elena Erro and Maite Mendioroz
Department of Neurology, Complejo Hospitalario de Navarra- IdiSNA (Navarra Institute for Health Research), C/ Irunlarrea, 3, 31008 Pamplona, Navarra, Spain

Victoria Zelaya
Department of Pathology, Complejo Hospitalario de Navarra- IdiSNA (Navarra Institute for Health Research), 31008 Pamplona, Navarra, Spain

Carmen Echavarri
Hospital Psicogeriátrico Josefina Arregui, 31800 Alsasua, Navarra, Spain

Robin Ortiz
Departments of Internal Medicine & Pediatrics, Johns Hopkins University School of Medicine, 600 North Wolfe Street, Harvey Bldg. Rm 805, Baltimore, MD 21287, USA

Joshua J. Joseph
Division of Endocrinology, Diabetes, and Metabolism, Department of Medicine, The Ohio State University Wexner Medical Center, 566 McCampbell Hall, 1581 Dodd Drive, Columbus, OH 43210, USA

Richard Lee
Department of Psychiatry and Behavioral Sciences, Johns Hopkins University School of Medicine, 720 Rutland Ave. Ross Bldg. 1068, Baltimore, MD 21205,USA

Gary S. Wand and Sherita Hill Golden
Division of Endocrinology, Diabetes and Metabolism, Department of Medicine, Johns Hopkins University School of Medicine, 1830 E. Monument Street Suite 333, Baltimore, MD 21287, USA

Sara Daniel, Briana Clifford, Romain Barres and David Simar
Mechanisms of Disease and Translational Research, School of Medical Sciences, UNSW Sydney, Wallace Wurth Building East Room 420, Sydney, NSW 2052, Australia

Vibe Nylander, Lars R. Ingerslev, Odile Fabre, Romain Barres and David Simar
The Novo Nordisk Foundation Center for Basic Metabolic Research, Faculty of Health and Medical Sciences, Panum, University of Copenhagen, 2200 Copenhagen N, Denmark

Ling Zhong
Bioanalytical Mass Spectrometry Facility, Mark Wainwright Analytical Centre, UNSW Sydney, Sydney, Australia

Karen Johnston and Richard J. Cohn
School of Women's and Children's Health, UNSW Sydney and Kids Cancer Centre, Sydney Children's Hospital Network, Randwick, Australia

Wenna Guo, Minghao Yu, Qihan Chen and Qiang Wang
State Key Laboratory of Pharmaceutical Biotechnology, School of Life Sciences, Nanjing University, Nanjing, China

Liucun Zhu and Rui Zhu
School of Life Sciences, Shanghai University, Shanghai, China

Julius C. Pape, Tania Carrillo-Roa, Anthony S. Zannas, Darina Czamara and Elisabeth B. Binder
Department of Translational Research in Psychiatry, Max Planck Institute of Psychiatry, Munich, Germany

Barbara O. Rothbaum and Elisabeth B. Binder
Department of Psychiatry and Behavioral Sciences, Emory University School of Medicine, Atlanta, GA, USA

Charles B. Nemeroff
Department of Psychiatry and Behavioral Sciences, University of Miami Miller School of Medicine, Miami, FL, USA

Sanjay J. Mathew
Menninger Department of Psychiatry & Behavioral Sciences, Baylor College of Medicine & Michael E. Debakey VA Medical Center, Houston, TX, USA

Thomas C. Neylan
Department of Psychiatry, University of California, San Francisco, San Francisco, CA, USA
The San Francisco Veterans Affairs Medical Center, San Francisco, CA, USA

Anthony S. Zannas
Department of Psychiatry and Behavioral Sciences, Duke University Medical Center, Durham, NC, USA

Dan Iosifescu
New York University School of Medicine, New York, NY, USA
Nathan Kline Institute for Psychiatric Research, Orangeburg, NY, USA
Department of Psychiatry, Icahn School of Medicine at Mount Sinai, New York, NY, USA

Index

www.ingramcontent.com/pod-product-compliance
Lightning Source LLC
Chambersburg PA
CBHW080512200326
41458CB00012B/4177